THE MEDICAL WORD BOOK

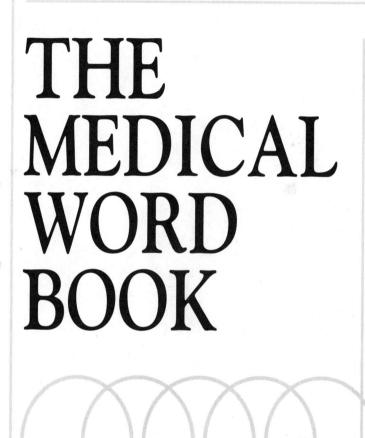

SHEILA B. SLOANE
Formerly, President, Medi-Phone, Inc.

THE
A spelling and
vocabulary guide
to medical transcription

MEDICAL
WORD
BOOK

1991
W.B. SAUNDERS COMPANY
Harcourt Brace Jovanovich, Inc.
Philadelphia London Toronto Montreal Sydney Tokyo

third edition

W. B. SAUNDERS COMPANY
Harcourt Brace Jovanovich Inc.

The Curtis Center
Independence Square West
Philadelphia, PA 19106

Library of Congress Cataloging-in-Publication Data
Sloane, Sheila B.
    The medical word book : a spelling and vocabulary guide to medical
transcription / Sheila B. Sloane. — 3rd ed.
        p.   cm.
    ISBN 0-7216-3243-2
    1. Medicine — Terminology.   I. Title.
    [DNLM: 1. Nomenclature.   W 15 S634m]
R123.S57   1991
610'.14 — dc20
DNLM/DLC   90-8903

Editor: Margaret M. Biblis
Designer: Karen O'Keefe
Production Manager: Carolyn Naylor
Manuscript Editor: Martha Tanner
Illustration Coordinator: Cecelia Kunkle
Cover Designer: Ellen Bodner

The Medical Word Book, 3/E   ISBN 0-7216-3243-2

Printed in the United States of America

Last digit is the print number: 9   8   7   6   5   4   3   2   1

To
Evan, Lindsay, Alex, and Nicole
For the Joy They Give

Preface

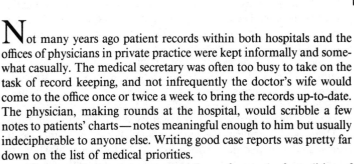

Not many years ago patient records within both hospitals and the offices of physicians in private practice were kept informally and somewhat casually. The medical secretary was often too busy to take on the task of record keeping, and not infrequently the doctor's wife would come to the office once or twice a week to bring the records up-to-date. The physician, making rounds at the hospital, would scribble a few notes to patients' charts—notes meaningful enough to him but usually indecipherable to anyone else. Writing good case reports was pretty far down on the list of medical priorities.

The preceding paragraph opened the preface to the first edition of *The Medical Word Book.* Since its publication in 1973 there have been many important advances in the effectiveness of medical transcription, many of which have been brought about by the excellent teaching programs of the American Association for Medical Transcription. Today, the understanding and acceptance of professional competence of the transcriptionist are a far cry from the early days of the first *Medical Word Book.*

All of the new material in this third edition has been carefully researched. There are approximately 18,000 new entries in the various sections, and a new section entitled Immunology—With Special Reference to AIDS has been introduced. The immune system is an extremely complex network of specialized organs and cells that defends the body against foreign invaders. Not only is the system itself complex but the vocabulary describing its numerous functions is equally complex. The circumstance of AIDS further complicates both the responses of the immune system and its terminology.

The basic purposes of the book remain unchanged: to introduce the newcomer and the seasoned transcriptionist to the available information and to provide, collected in one place, the essentials necessary to make their task of transcribing medical reports an easier one. The transcriptionist new to the profession is relieved of the responsibility of guessing whether a disease entity, an instrument, or the like is listed in one particular specialty rather than another. If a word applies to several specialties, it is listed in each of the appropriate sections. In this respect, repetition of terms has not been avoided; rather, it has been sought out. For example, "sarcoidosis" appears in Cardiovascular System, Internal Medicine, Orthopedics, and Respiratory System, thus making it unnecessary to flip pages back and forth between sections to find a proper spelling.

As in the past, no attempt has been made to make this a complete listing of medical terms. Such an undertaking would be overwhelming and cumbersome. The attempt here is to give the reader a listing of commonly used uncommon medical terms to ease the burden of searching through many books.

The book is divided into three major parts. The first comprises Anatomy, Illustrated, a series of color plates showing human structure; General Medical Terms, consisting of words common to all specialties; and General Surgical Terms, dealing with such topics as incisions, dressings, sutures, positions, and anesthetics. The alphabetical listing in Drugs and Chemistry includes radionuclides, chemotherapeutic agents, and the experimental drugs used in the treatment of AIDS and other immune-related diseases. Specific tests and pathogenic organisms are listed in Laboratory Terminology, concluding with Normal Laboratory Values.

The second part is divided into 15 specialties or organ systems. These are arranged alphabetically so that the desired subject can be readily located by flipping through the pages and noting the section title at the top of the page. Within each section, words are listed so that the familiar term will lead to the unfamiliar; that is, unfamiliar terms are given as subentries under familiar main entries. If, for example, the term "Mönckeberg's degeneration" is used in a cardiovascular report, one need only turn to the section on the cardiovascular system to find the proper spelling under "degeneration."

The third section includes abbreviations and symbols, combining forms, and rules for forming plurals. The appendix provides a table of elements and tables of weights, measures, and conversions.

Selected entries and combining forms are given in two ways: the correct spelling and, at its own alphabetical place, a phonetic spelling. The latter is given in italics, with a cross-reference to the proper spelling. If, for example, the term "pterygium" is used in an ophthalmology report, the transcriptionist may turn to the ophthalmology section and look for what sounds like "terijeum." At that place, there appears the entry "terijeum. See pterygium."

I should like to express my sincere appreciation to Margaret Biblis and the staff of the W. B. Saunders Company for their skillful help and guidance. For his patience, support, and constant encouragement, I offer my deepest gratitude to my husband, John Dusseau. Many reference books, too, have been of significant help. Among the many consulted, the following have been, in their authority and wide-ranging scope, the most useful:

AIDS, A Basic Guide for Clinicians, Ebbesen, Biggar & Melbye, W. B. Saunders Company, 1984

Cecil's Textbook of Medicine, Volumes I and II, 18th Edition, Wyngaarden & Smith, W. B. Saunders Company, 1988

Dermatology, Volumes I and II, 2nd Edition, Moschella & Hurley, W. B. Saunders Company, 1985

Dictionary of Immunology, Rosen, Steiner & Unanue, Elsevier Science Publishing Company, Inc., 1989

Dorland's Illustrated Medical Dictionary, 27th Edition, W. B. Saunders Company, 1988

Fundamentals of Otolaryngology, A Textbook of Ear, Nose & Throat Diseases, 6th Edition, Adams, Boies & Hilger, W. B. Saunders Company, 1989

Gastrointestinal Disease, 4th Edition, Sleisenger & Fordtran, W. B. Saunders Company, 1989

Heart Disease, A Textbook of Cardiovascular Medicine, 3rd Edition, Braunwauld, W. B. Saunders Company, 1988

Immunology III, Bellanti, W. B. Saunders Company, 1985

Nelson's Textbook of Pediatrics, 13th Edition, Behrman & Vaughan, W. B. Saunders Company, 1989

Respiratory Function in Disease, 3rd Edition, Bates, W. B. Saunders Company, 1989

Rheumatology and Immunology, 2nd Edition, Cohen & Bennett, Grune & Stratton, 1986

To the thousands of users of the first two editions of *The Medical Word Book*, my thanks. It is my hope that this third edition will continue to answer the needs of transcriptionists and health-care personnel in all areas of medicine in their challenging quest for the correct spelling of the often puzzling, sometimes elusive medical term.

SHEILA B. SLOANE

Contents

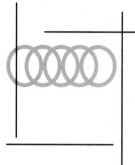

THE
MEDICAL
WORD
BOOK

Anatomy, Illustrated

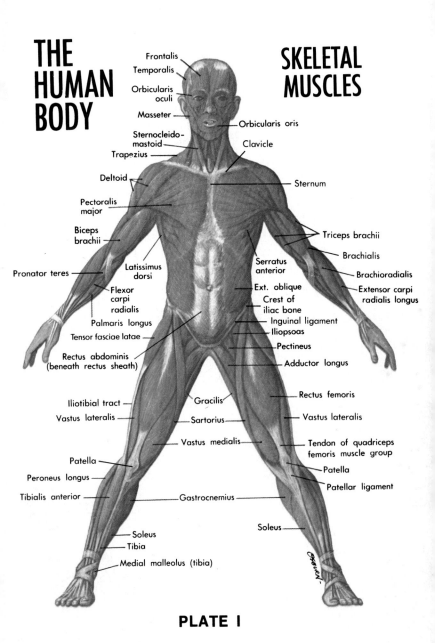

THE HUMAN BODY

SKELETAL MUSCLES

Frontalis
Temporalis
Orbicularis oculi
Masseter
Orbicularis oris
Sternocleido-mastoid
Clavicle
Trapezius
Deltoid
Sternum
Pectoralis major
Biceps brachii
Triceps brachii
Brachialis
Pronator teres
Latissimus dorsi
Serratus anterior
Brachioradialis
Flexor carpi radialis
Ext. oblique
Extensor carpi radialis longus
Crest of iliac bone
Palmaris longus
Inguinal ligament
Tensor fasciae latae
Iliopsoas
Rectus abdominis (beneath rectus sheath)
Pectineus
Adductor longus
Gracilis
Rectus femoris
Iliotibial tract
Vastus lateralis
Sartorius
Vastus lateralis
Vastus medialis
Tendon of quadriceps femoris muscle group
Patella
Patella
Peroneus longus
Patellar ligament
Tibialis anterior
Gastrocnemius
Soleus
Soleus
Tibia
Medial malleolus (tibia)

PLATE I

BONES

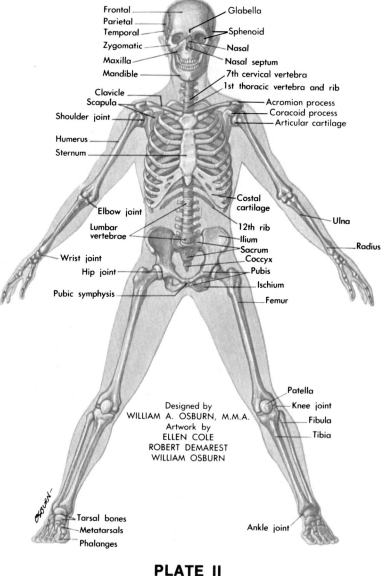

Frontal — Glabella
Parietal — Sphenoid
Temporal
Zygomatic — Nasal
Maxilla — Nasal septum
Mandible — 7th cervical vertebra
— 1st thoracic vertebra and rib
Clavicle — Acromion process
Scapula — Coracoid process
Shoulder joint — Articular cartilage
Humerus
Sternum
Costal cartilage
Elbow joint — Ulna
Lumbar vertebrae — 12th rib
— Ilium
Wrist joint — Sacrum
— Coccyx — Radius
Hip joint — Pubis
Pubic symphysis — Ischium
— Femur

Patella
Knee joint
Fibula
Tibia

Designed by
WILLIAM A. OSBURN, M.M.A.
Artwork by
ELLEN COLE
ROBERT DEMAREST
WILLIAM OSBURN

Tarsal bones
Metatarsals — Ankle joint
Phalanges

PLATE II

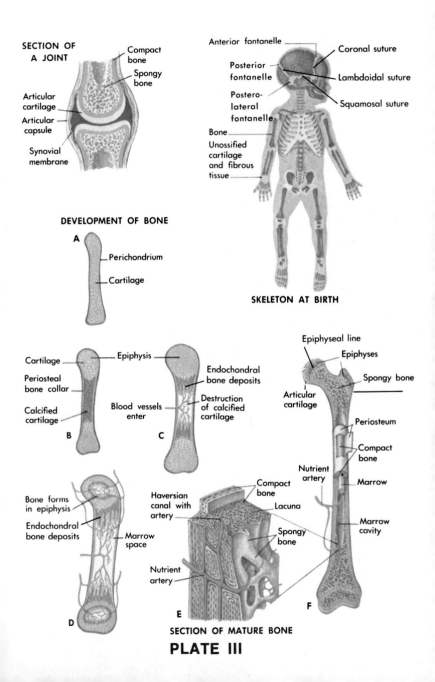

SECTION OF A JOINT

Compact bone
Spongy bone
Articular cartilage
Articular capsule
Synovial membrane

Anterior fontanelle
Coronal suture
Posterior fontanelle
Lambdoidal suture
Postero-lateral fontanelle
Squamosal suture
Bone
Unossified cartilage and fibrous tissue

SKELETON AT BIRTH

DEVELOPMENT OF BONE

A
Perichondrium
Cartilage

Cartilage
Epiphysis
Endochondral bone deposits
Periosteal bone collar
Blood vessels enter
Destruction of calcified cartilage
Calcified cartilage

B

C

Epiphyseal line
Epiphyses
Spongy bone
Articular cartilage
Periosteum
Compact bone
Nutrient artery
Marrow
Marrow cavity

Bone forms in epiphysis
Endochondral bone deposits
Marrow space

Haversian canal with artery
Compact bone
Lacuna
Spongy bone
Nutrient artery

D

E

F

SECTION OF MATURE BONE

PLATE III

THE ORGANS OF DIGESTION

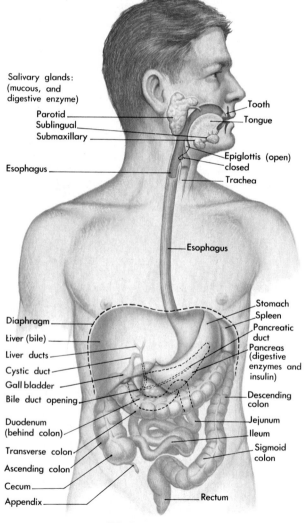

Salivary glands:
(mucous, and
digestive enzyme)

Parotid

Sublingual

Submaxillary

Esophagus

Tooth

Tongue

Epiglottis (open)
closed

Trachea

Esophagus

Diaphragm

Liver (bile)

Liver ducts

Cystic duct

Gall bladder

Bile duct opening

Duodenum
(behind colon)

Transverse colon

Ascending colon

Cecum

Appendix

Stomach

Spleen

Pancreatic
duct

Pancreas
(digestive
enzymes and
insulin)

Descending
colon

Jejunum

Ileum

Sigmoid
colon

Rectum

PLATE IV

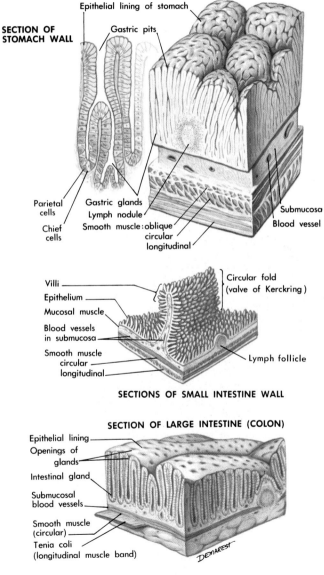

SECTION OF STOMACH WALL

Epithelial lining of stomach

Gastric pits

Parietal cells

Chief cells

Gastric glands

Lymph nodule

Smooth muscle: oblique
circular
longitudinal

Submucosa

Blood vessel

Villi

Epithelium

Mucosal muscle

Blood vessels in submucosa

Smooth muscle
circular
longitudinal

Circular fold (valve of Kerckring)

Lymph follicle

SECTIONS OF SMALL INTESTINE WALL

SECTION OF LARGE INTESTINE (COLON)

Epithelial lining

Openings of glands

Intestinal gland

Submucosal blood vessels

Smooth muscle (circular)

Tenia coli (longitudinal muscle band)

DEMAREST

PLATE V

THE ORGANS OF RESPIRATION AND THE HEART

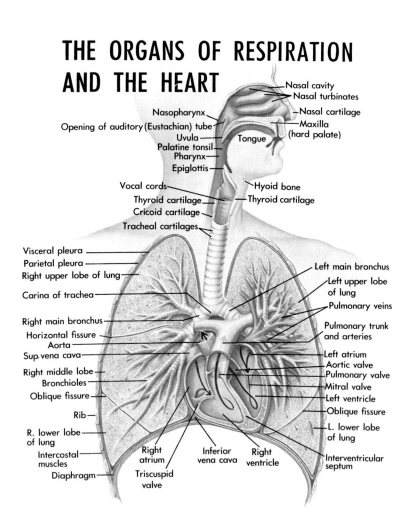

Nasal cavity
Nasal turbinates
Nasal cartilage
Nasopharynx
Opening of auditory (Eustachian) tube
Maxilla (hard palate)
Uvula
Tongue
Palatine tonsil
Pharynx
Epiglottis
Vocal cords
Hyoid bone
Thyroid cartilage
Thyroid cartilage
Cricoid cartilage
Tracheal cartilages
Visceral pleura
Parietal pleura
Left main bronchus
Right upper lobe of lung
Left upper lobe of lung
Carina of trachea
Pulmonary veins
Right main bronchus
Pulmonary trunk and arteries
Horizontal fissure
Aorta
Sup. vena cava
Left atrium
Aortic valve
Right middle lobe
Pulmonary valve
Bronchioles
Mitral valve
Oblique fissure
Left ventricle
Oblique fissure
Rib
L. lower lobe of lung
R. lower lobe of lung
Interventricular septum
Intercostal muscles
Right atrium
Inferior vena cava
Right ventricle
Diaphragm
Triscuspid valve

PLATE VI

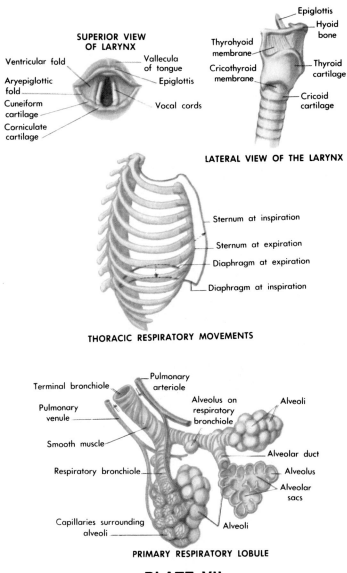

SUPERIOR VIEW OF LARYNX

Ventricular fold
Aryepiglottic fold
Cuneiform cartilage
Corniculate cartilage
Vallecula of tongue
Epiglottis
Vocal cords

Epiglottis
Hyoid bone
Thyrohyoid membrane
Cricothyroid membrane
Thyroid cartilage
Cricoid cartilage

LATERAL VIEW OF THE LARYNX

Sternum at inspiration
Sternum at expiration
Diaphragm at expiration
Diaphragm at inspiration

THORACIC RESPIRATORY MOVEMENTS

Terminal bronchiole
Pulmonary arteriole
Alveolus on respiratory bronchiole
Alveoli
Pulmonary venule
Smooth muscle
Respiratory bronchiole
Capillaries surrounding alveoli
Alveolar duct
Alveolus
Alveolar sacs
Alveoli

PRIMARY RESPIRATORY LOBULE

PLATE VII

THE MAJOR BLOOD VESSELS

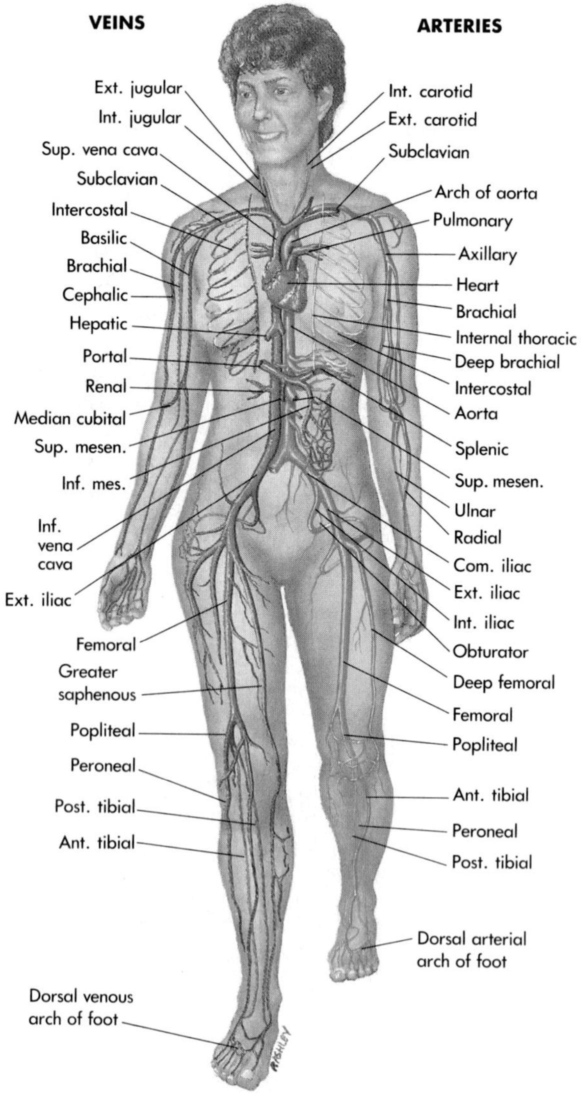

VEINS

ARTERIES

Ext. jugular
Int. jugular
Sup. vena cava
Subclavian
Intercostal
Basilic
Brachial
Cephalic
Hepatic
Portal
Renal
Median cubital
Sup. mesen.
Inf. mes.
Inf. vena cava
Ext. iliac
Femoral
Greater saphenous
Popliteal
Peroneal
Post. tibial
Ant. tibial
Dorsal venous arch of foot

Int. carotid
Ext. carotid
Subclavian
Arch of aorta
Pulmonary
Axillary
Heart
Brachial
Internal thoracic
Deep brachial
Intercostal
Aorta
Splenic
Sup. mesen.
Ulnar
Radial
Com. iliac
Ext. iliac
Int. iliac
Obturator
Deep femoral
Femoral
Popliteal
Ant. tibial
Peroneal
Post. tibial
Dorsal arterial arch of foot

PLATE VIII

DETAILS OF CIRCULATORY STRUCTURES

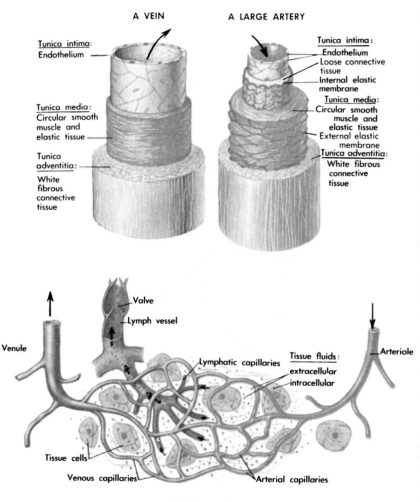

A VEIN

Tunica intima:
Endothelium

Tunica media:
Circular smooth
muscle and
elastic tissue

Tunica
adventitia:
White
fibrous
connective
tissue

A LARGE ARTERY

Tunica intima:
Endothelium
Loose connective
tissue
Internal elastic
membrane
Tunica media:
Circular smooth
muscle and
elastic tissue
External elastic
membrane
Tunica adventitia:
White fibrous
connective
tissue

Valve
Lymph vessel

Venule

Lymphatic capillaries
Tissue fluids:
extracellular
intracellular

Arteriole

Tissue cells

Venous capillaries

Arterial capillaries

A CAPILLARY BED

PLATE IX

THE BRAIN AND SPINAL NERVES

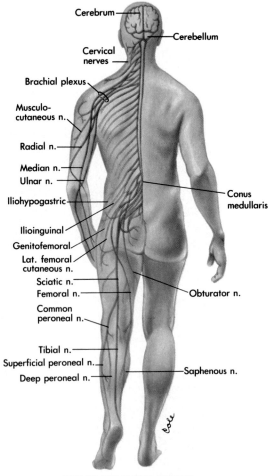

Cerebrum

Cerebellum

Cervical nerves

Brachial plexus

Musculo-cutaneous n.

Radial n.

Median n.

Ulnar n.

Iliohypogastric

Ilioinguinal

Genitofemoral

Lat. femoral cutaneous n.

Sciatic n.

Femoral n.

Common peroneal n.

Tibial n.

Superficial peroneal n.

Deep peroneal n.

Conus medullaris

Obturator n.

Saphenous n.

THE MAJOR SPINAL NERVES

PLATE X

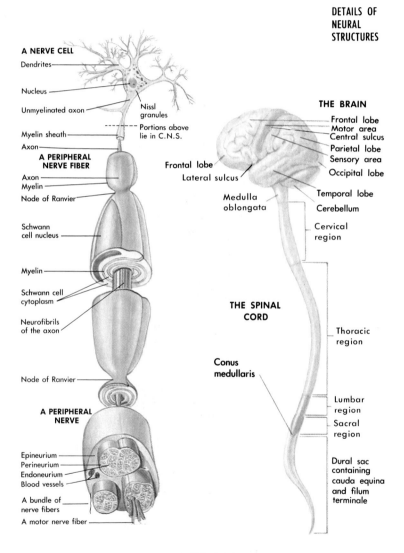

DETAILS OF
NEURAL
STRUCTURES

A NERVE CELL

Dendrites

Nucleus

Unmyelinated axon

Nissl granules

Portions above lie in C.N.S.

Myelin sheath

Axon

A PERIPHERAL NERVE FIBER

Axon
Myelin
Node of Ranvier

Schwann cell nucleus

Myelin

Schwann cell cytoplasm

Neurofibrils of the axon

Node of Ranvier

A PERIPHERAL NERVE

Epineurium
Perineurium
Endoneurium
Blood vessels

A bundle of nerve fibers

A motor nerve fiber

THE BRAIN

Frontal lobe
Motor area
Central sulcus
Parietal lobe
Sensory area
Occipital lobe

Frontal lobe
Lateral sulcus

Temporal lobe
Cerebellum

Medulla oblongata

Cervical region

THE SPINAL CORD

Thoracic region

Conus medullaris

Lumbar region

Sacral region

Dural sac containing cauda equina and filum terminale

PLATE XI

ORGANS OF SPECIAL SENSE THE EAR

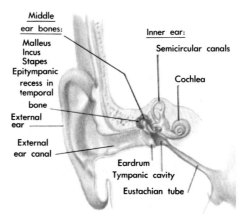

Middle
ear bones:

Malleus
Incus
Stapes
Epitympanic
recess in
temporal
bone

External
ear

External
ear canal

Inner ear:

Semicircular canals

Cochlea

Eardrum
Tympanic cavity
Eustachian tube

THE ORGAN OF HEARING

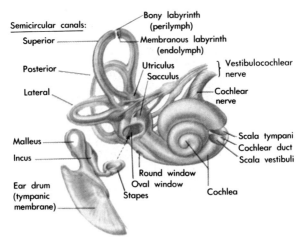

Semicircular canals:

Superior

Posterior

Lateral

Malleus

Incus

Ear drum
(tympanic
membrane)

Bony labyrinth
(perilymph)
Membranous labyrinth
(endolymph)
Utriculus
Sacculus

Vestibulocochlear
nerve

Cochlear
nerve

Scala tympani
Cochlear duct
Scala vestibuli

Round window
Oval window
Stapes

Cochlea

THE MIDDLE EAR AND INNER EAR

PLATE XII

THE LACRIMAL APPARATUS AND THE EYE

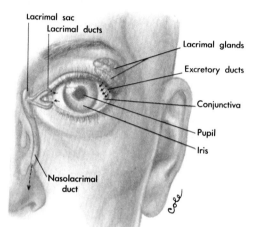

Lacrimal sac
Lacrimal ducts
Lacrimal glands
Excretory ducts
Conjunctiva
Pupil
Iris
Nasolacrimal duct

Cole

THE LACRIMAL APPARATUS

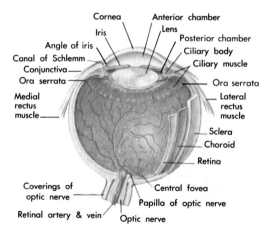

Cornea
Iris
Angle of iris
Canal of Schlemm
Conjunctiva
Ora serrata
Medial rectus muscle
Anterior chamber
Lens
Posterior chamber
Ciliary body
Ciliary muscle
Ora serrata
Lateral rectus muscle
Sclera
Choroid
Retina
Coverings of optic nerve
Central fovea
Papilla of optic nerve
Retinal artery & vein
Optic nerve

HORIZONTAL SECTION OF THE EYE

PLATE XIII

STRUCTURAL DETAILS

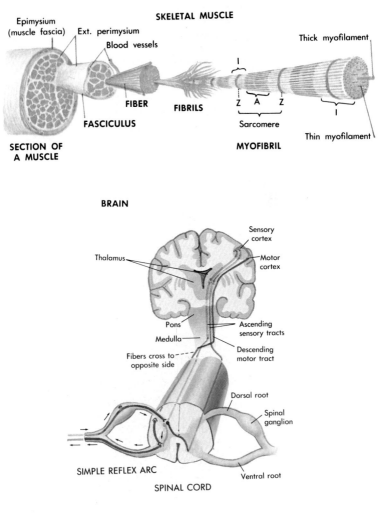

SKELETAL MUSCLE

Epimysium (muscle fascia)
Ext. perimysium
Blood vessels
FIBER
FIBRILS
FASCICULUS
SECTION OF A MUSCLE
I
Z   A   Z
Sarcomere
MYOFIBRIL
Thick myofilament
Thin myofilament
I

BRAIN

Sensory cortex
Motor cortex
Thalamus
Pons
Medulla
Ascending sensory tracts
Descending motor tract
Fibers cross to opposite side
Dorsal root
Spinal ganglion
SIMPLE REFLEX ARC
Ventral root
SPINAL CORD

PLATE XIV

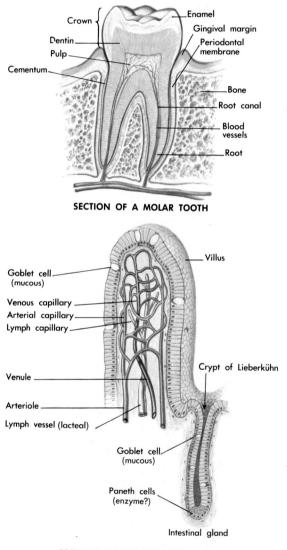

SECTION OF A MOLAR TOOTH

Crown
Enamel
Gingival margin
Dentin
Periodontal membrane
Pulp
Cementum
Bone
Root canal
Blood vessels
Root

Villus
Goblet cell (mucous)
Venous capillary
Arterial capillary
Lymph capillary
Crypt of Lieberkühn
Venule
Arteriole
Lymph vessel (lacteal)
Goblet cell (mucous)
Paneth cells (enzyme?)
Intestinal gland

SECTIONS OF SMALL INTESTINE WALL

PLATE XV

THE PARANASAL SINUSES

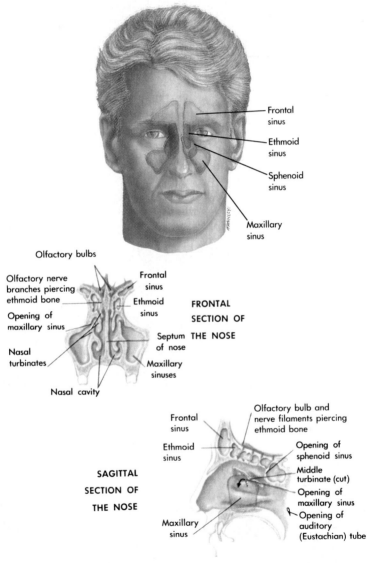

Frontal sinus

Ethmoid sinus

Sphenoid sinus

Maxillary sinus

Olfactory bulbs

Olfactory nerve branches piercing ethmoid bone

Frontal sinus

Ethmoid sinus

FRONTAL SECTION OF THE NOSE

Opening of maxillary sinus

Septum of nose

Nasal turbinates

Maxillary sinuses

Nasal cavity

Olfactory bulb and nerve filaments piercing ethmoid bone

Frontal sinus

Ethmoid sinus

Opening of sphenoid sinus

SAGITTAL SECTION OF THE NOSE

Middle turbinate (cut)

Opening of maxillary sinus

Opening of auditory (Eustachian) tube

Maxillary sinus

PLATE XVI

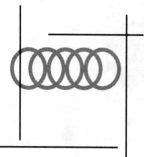

Part One

General Terms

General Medical Terms

abacterial
abaissement
abasia
abate
abatement
abdomen
abdominal
abducens
abducent
abduct
abduction
aberrant
aberration
abeyance
abirritant
ablate
ablation
abluent
abnormal
abnormality
abradant
abrasion
abrasive
abscess
absorbent
absorption
a capite ad calcem
acatastasia
acathectic
acathexia
accentuation
accessory
accommodation
accretion
achalasia
ache
acinus
acne

acosmia
acoustic
acquired
acrid
aculosure
acuminate
acute
adaptation
adduct
adduction
adenitis
adenocarcinoma
adenoma
adenomatous
adenopathy
adhere
adherent
adhesion
adhesive
adhesiveness
adipose
adiposis
aditus
adjunct
adjunctive
adjuvant
ad nauseam
adnerval
adnexa
adolescence
adolescent
adrenal
adsorb
adventitia
adventitious
adynamia
adynamic
aerate

aerophagia
afebrile
afferent
afunction
agenesis
agitated
agonal
agonist
ailment
akinesia
akinetic
ala
alae
alar
alba
albinism
algogenesia
alignment
alimentary
alimentation
allergic
allergy
allotype
alopecia
altricious
alveolus
ambidexterity
ambidextrous
ambient
ambiguous
ambulant
ambulatory
ambustion
amebiasis
amelioration
amnesia
amorphous
ampule
ampulla
ampullae
anabolism
anacatharsis
analgesia
analgesic
analogous
analogue
analysis

anaphylactic
anaphylactoid
anaphylaxis
anasarca
anastomosis
anatomical
anatomy
anemia
anemic
anergy
anesthesia
aneurysm
angulus
anhidrosis
anicteric
annectent
annular
annulus
anomalous
anomaly
anorectic
anorexia
anoxemia
anoxia
ansa
antacid
antagonist
antecedent
ante cibum – before meals
anteflexion
antegrade
anterior
anteroexternal
anterograde
anteroinferior
anterointernal
anterolateral
anteromedian
anteroposterior
anterosuperior
anteroventral
anteversion
anteverted
antexed
anthorisma
antibiotic
antibody

anticholinergic
anticoagulant
antidepressant
antidote
antigen
antihistamine
antipyretic
antisepsis
antiseptic
antitoxin
antitussive
antral
antrum
anus
anxiety
apertura
aperture
apex
aphagia
    a. algera
aphasia
aphasic
apical
apices
aplasia
apnea
apocrine
apogee
aponeurosis
apposition
approximal
approximate
apyretic
apyrexia
apyrexial
apyrogenetic
apyrogenic
aqueduct
aqueductus
aqueous
arcate
archetype
arciform
arctation
arcual
arcuate
arcuation

arcus
areola
areolar
arrhythmia
arrhythmic
arterial
arteriola
arteriole
arteriosclerosis
artery
arthritis
articulate
articulation
articulo
    a. mortis
artifact
artificial
ascending
ascertainment
ascites
asepsis
aseptic
aspect
    dorsal a.
    ventral a.
asphyxia
asphyxiation
aspirate
aspiration
aspirator
asterixis
asteroid
asthenia
asthenic
asthma
asymmetrical
asymmetry
asymptomatic
asynchronism
ataractic
ataraxia
ataxia
atelectasis
atonic
atonicity
atony
atopic

atopy
atraumatic
atresia
atretic
atrial
atrophy
attenuant
attenuate
attenuation
attrition
atypia
atypical
aura
auscultation
autogenesis
autogenous
autopsy
autosomal
autosome
auxiliary
avascular
avulsion
axilla
axillae
axillary
axis
azotemia
azygos
bacteria
ballotable
basal
base line
basilar
belching
benign
bifid
bifurcate
bifurcation
bigeminal
bigeminy
bilateral
bilious
biliousness
bimanual
biochemistry
biochemorphology
biology

biomicroscopy
biophysics
biophysiology
biopsy
bleb
blennogenic
blister
bolus
borborygmus
boss
bosselated
bout
BP–blood pressure
bradycardia
bradykinesia
breadth
brisement
bronchitis
bruise
bruit
bruxism
brwe. See bruit.
buccal
bulbar
bulboid
bulbous
bulla
bursa
buttock
cachectic
cachexia
cacoethic
cadaver
caduceus
calcification
calix
calor
calorie
canaliculus
canalis
cannula
capillary
capsule
caput
carcinogenesis
carcinoma
cardiomegaly

cardiomyopathy
cardiovascular
carphology
cartilage
cartilaginous
caruncle
catabolism
catamnesis
catharsis
catheter
Caucasian
cauda
caudad
caudae
caudal
caudalis
caudalward
causalgia
cauterization
cautery
cavum
CC–chief complaint
    clinical course
cecal
cellula
cellular
cellulitis
centrad
cephalad
cephalalgia
cephalic
cervical
channel
chemotherapy
chorda
chorea
chromosome
chronic
cicatricial
cicatrix
circadian
circinate
circulation
circulus
circumferential
circumflex

circumscribed
cirrhosis
claudication
cleft
clinical
clonus
closure
clubbing
clysis
coagulate
coagulation
coalesce
coalescence
coapt
coarctate
coccygeal
coccyx
coherent
coitus
colic
colicky
collagen
colostomy
coma
comatose
commissura
compatible
compensation
competence
complaint
compress
compression
computerized
concavity
concentric
concha
concomitant
concrescence
configuration
confluent
congenital
congested
conical
conjugate
consanguinity
conscious
consciousness

conservative
constipated
constipation
constitutional
constriction
consultant
consultation
contagious
contamination
contiguity
contiguous
contour
contractility
contraction
contraindication
contralateral
contusion
convalescence
convalescent
convexity
convoluted
convolution
convulsion
coroner
corpse
corpus
corpuscle
cortex
cortical
corticosteroid
coryza
cranial
crepitant
crepitation
crepitus
crescent
cribriform
crisis
criterion
critical
croupette
crus
cryoprecipitability
cryoprecipitate
cryotherapy
crypt
cryptogenetic

cul-de-sac
curet
curettage
cutaneous
cyanosis
cyanotic
cyst
cytoid
debilitate
debility
débouchement
debride
debridement
debris
deceleration
deciduous
decompression
decontamination
decortication
decrement
decrepitate
decrepitation
decrudescence
decrustation
decubation
decubitus
defecation
defervescence
defervescent
deformity
degeneration
degenerative
deglutition
dehiscence
dehydration
deleterious
delineate
delirious
delirium
delitescence
deltoid
demarcation
demise
demulcent
dendritic
denervation
density

denudation
depression
deprivation
dermatitis
dermis
descending
desiccate
deterioration
detumescence
deviation
dextroposition
diadochokinesia
diadochokinesis
diagnose
diagnosis
    biological d.
    clinical d.
    cytohistologic d.
    cytologic d.
    differential d.
    d. ex juvantibus
    niveau d.
    pathologic d.
    provocative d.
    roentgen d.
    serum d.
diagnostic
diagnostician
dialysis
dialyzed
diameter
diaphoresis
diaphoretic
diaphragm
diarrhea
diastasis
diathermy
diathesis
dichotomy
dietitian
differentiate
differentiation
diffuse
digestion
digestive
digit
digital

dilatation
dilation
dilator
dilution
diminution
dimpling
diplopia
disciform
discoid
discrete
discus
disease
disesthesia
disinfect
disintegration
dislocated
disorganization
disorientation
disparate
displacement
disposition
disseminated
dissociation
dissolution
dissonance
distad
distal
distalis
distally
distention
distortion
diuresis
diuretic
diurnal
divergent
diverticulum
divulsion
dizziness
donor
dorsal
dorsum
dressing
droplet
duct
ductulus
dysarthria
dysbarism

dyschezia
dyscrasia
dysentery
dysesthesia
dysfunction
dyspepsia
dysphagia
dysphasia
dysplasia
dyspnea
dyspneic
dysponderal
dyspragia
dysrhythmia
dyssymmetry
dystonia
dystonic
dysuria
ebrietas
ebriety
eccentric
ecchymoses
ecchymosis
ecchymotic
eclampsia
écouvillon
écouvillonage
ectad
ectal
ectoentad
ectopic
eczema
edema
edematous
edentulous
efferent
efficacy
efflux
effraction
effusion
egophony
elastica
elasticity
elective
electrocautery
electrophoresis
electropyrexia

electrotherapy
elicited
elongation
elucidate
emaciated
emanate
embedding
embolism
embryo
embryonic
emesis
emetic
emetocathartic
empiric
en bloc
encapsulated
endemic
endocardium
endocrine
endogenous
endoplasm
endoscopy
engorged
engorgement
enigmatic
entad
ental
enucleate
enucleation
environment
eparsalgia
epidemic
epigastric
epigastrium
epiphenomenon
epistaxis
epithelial
epithelium
equilibrium
equivocal
erosion
erosive
eructation
eruption
erythema
esophagitis
esophagus

ethanol
etiological
etiology
eucrasia
euphoria
eupnea
euthanasia
euthyroid
evacuation
evanescent
eversion
evert
evisceration
exacerbation
excavation
excise
excoriation
excrescence
excretion
excretory
exenteration
exhaustion
exogenous
exophytic
expiration
expire
exsanguinate
exsanguination
exstrophy
extraocular
extravasation
extremity
extrinsic
extrude
extubate
extubation
exudate
facial
facies
facilitation
Fahrenheit thermometer
fahrma. See words beginning
    pharma-.
falces
falciform
falx
familial

fascia
fascial
fascicle
fasciculation
fasciculus
fatigability
fatigue
FB – foreign body
        fingerbreadth
febrile
fecal
feces
fenestra
fenestrated
fenomenon. See *phenomenon.*
fervescence
fetal
fetid
fetor
fever
FH – family history
fiber
fibra
fibrillation
fibroma
fimbria
fimbriated
fingerbreadth
fissure
fistula
flaccid
flank
flatulence
flatus
flexibility
flexion
flexure
florid
fluctuant
fluctuation
fluoroscope
folium
follicle
follicular
folliculus
fontanel, fontanelle
fonticulus

foramen
foramina
forme
    f. fruste
    f. tardive
fornix
fossa
fovea
foveola
fragility
fremitus
frenulum
friable
frontal
fulgurate
fulguration
fulminant
fulminate
fumigation
function
functional
fundus
funduscopy
funiculus
FUO–fever of undetermined
      origin
    fever of unknown origin
furuncle
fusiform
fusion
gait
ganglion
gangrene
gangrenous
gaseous
gauze
genetic
geniculum
genitalia
genu
glomerulus
glomus
gonorrhea
gracile
gracilis
gradient

gram
granulation
grumous
guaiac
halitosis
haustrum
helminthic
hemangioma
hematemesis
hematochezia
hematocrit
hematogenous
hematoma
hematopoiesis
hematopoietic
hemiparesis
hemiplegia
hemoglobin
hemolysis
hemoptysis
hemorrhage
hemostasis
hepatic
hepatitis
hepatomegaly
hepatorenal
hereditary
heredity
heterogenic
heterotopia
heterotopic
hiatus
hiccup
hidradenoma
hidrorrhea
hilum
hilus
hirsute
hirsutism
histamine
histology
homogeneous
homogenous
homologous
homonymous
horizontal

hormone
hospital
H & P – history and physical
HPE – history and physical
          examination
HIP – history of present illness
hyaline
hyalinization
hydration
hydrotherapy
hygiene
hygienic
hygroma
hypalgesia
hypasthenia
hyperemia
hyperesthesia
hyperglycemia
hyperhidrosis
hyperplasia
hyperthermia
hypertonic
hypertonicity
hypertrophy
hyperventilation
hypervolemia
hypochondriac
hypodermic
hypodermoclysis
hypogastric
hypoglycemia
hypoplasia
hypothermal
hypothermia
hypothesis
hypotonia
hypotonic
hypoxia
iatrogenic
icteric
icterus
ictus
idiopathic
idiopathy
idiosyncrasy
illumination

IM – intramuscularly
imbed
imbricated
imbrication
immature
immediate
immobility
immobilization
immune
immunity
immunization
impalpable
impatency
impatent
imperforate
impermeable
impingement
implant
implantation
impressio
in articulo mortis
incarcerated
incidence
incipient
incisura
incompatibility
incompetence
incontinence
incubation
incurable
indigenous
indigestion
indisposition
indolent
induced
indurated
induration
inebriation
inebriety
inert
inertia
in extremis
infantile
infarct
infarction
infection

infectious
inferior
inferolateral
inferomedian
inferoposterior
infestation
infiltrate
infiltration
infirm
infirmity
inflammation
inflammatory
inflation
inflexion
infundibulum
infusion
ingestion
ingravescent
inguinal
inhalation
inherent
inhomogeneous
initial
injection
injury
innominate
inoculate
inoculation
insalubrious
insenescence
insidious
in situ
insomnia
inspiration
inspissated
instillation
insufficiency
insufflation
integration
integument
integumentary
intensity
intensive
intention
intercostal
intermittent
interstitial

intestine
intima
intolerance
in toto
intoxication
intractable
intramuscular
intrathecal
intravenous
intra vitam
intrinsic
introflexion
introversion
intubate
intubation
intumescence
intumescent
invaginate
inversion
in vivo
involuntary
ipsilateral
irradiation
irreducible
irregular
irregularity
irreversible
irrigation
irritability
irritant
ischemia
isolate
isolateral
isolation
Isolette
isotonia
isotonic
isotope
    radioactive i.
isthmus
IV – intravenous
jactitation
jaundice
joule
jugular
jugulation
junction

junctura
juvenile
juxtaposition
kahkekseah. See *cachexia.*
kahkektik. See *cachectic.*
kakoethik. See *cacoethic.*
keloid
keratosis
kilogram
kinetic
kyphosis
labile
labium
labyrinth
labyrinthus
lacerated
laceration
lacuna
lamina
laminated
lancinating
laparotomy
laser
lassitude
laterad
lateral
lateralis
latissimus
lavage
lesion
lethal
lethargy
limbus
limen
linear
lipoma
liquefaction
lobe
lobule
lobulus
lobus
longitudinal
lumbar
lumen
lymph
lymphadenopathy
lymphangiogram

lymphatic
lyse
lysis
ma – milliampere
maceration
macula
maim
malabsorption
malacia
malady
malaise
malar
malformation
malfunction
malignancy
malignant
malingerer
malleable
malnutrition
malposition
malpractice
malum
mandible
mandibula
maneuver
manipulation
manual
marasmus
marcid
margin
marginal
margo
marital
marsupialization
masculine
maser
massa
massage
mastication
masticatory
matrix
maxillary
maximum
meatus
medial
medialis
median

medianus
mediastinum
medicable
medicate
medication
medications. See *Drugs and
    Chemistry* section.
medicinal
medicochirurgic
mediolateral
medius
medulla
medusa
melanemesis
melanoma
melena
melu. See *milieu.*
membrana
membrane
membranous
membrum
meniscus
mentoanterior
mentoposterior
mentotransverse
mEq – milliequivalent
meridian
meridianus
meridional
meromelia
mesad
mesal
mesentery
mesiad
mesial
metabolic
metabolism
metamorphosis
metastases
metastasis
metastasize
metastatic
MFB – metallic foreign body
mg – milligram
MH – marital history
        medical history
mication

microbiology
microgram
milieu
milliampere
millicurie
milliequivalent
milligram
milliliter
millimeter
millimicrocurie
millimicrogram
millisecond
milliunit
millivolt
mittelschmerz
ml – milliliter
mm – millimeter
μmm – micromillimeter
modality
mongolism
mongoloid
monitor
morbid
morbidity
morcellated
morcellation
moribund
morphology
mortality
motile
motility
ms – millisecond
mucopurulent
mucosa
mucosal
mucosanguineous
mucus
multifactorial
mummification
mummying
mural
murmur
muscle
mutilation
myalgia
myelitis
myelogram

myeloma
myelopathy
myoma
myositis
myxedema
myxoma
nausea
nauseous
nebulization
necropsy
necrosis
neoplasm
neoplastic
nerve
neural
neurasthenia
nexus
niche
nidus
nocturia
nocturnal
node
nodular
nodule
nodulus
nodus
nonspecific
normoactive
normocephalic
normotensive
normothermia
normotonia
normotopia
normotrophic
nosocomial
noxious
NPO – nothing by mouth (nil
        per os)
NTP – normal temperature and
        pressure
nucha
nucleic
nucleoplasm
nucleus
nutrition
N & V – nausea and vomiting
obese

obesity
    exogenous o.
obfuscation
oblique
obliteration
obsolescence
obsolete
obstipation
obstruction
obtund
obturation
obtuse
occipital
occiput
occlusion
occult
oncology
opacity
opaque
OPD – outpatient department
optimum
orbicular
organic
organism
organomegaly
orifice
orthopnea
orthostatic
orthotopic
os
oscillation
oscitation
osculum
osteoarthritis
osteoid
osteolysis
ostium
P & A – percussion and
        auscultation
pain
    lancinating p.
palliate
palliative
pallor
palpable
palpate
palpation

palpitation
pancreas
panhidrosis
panhyperemia
panniculus
papilla
papilloma
papule
paracenesthesia
paracentesis
paracentral
paradoxical
paralyses
paralysis
paralytic
parasite
parasympathetic
parenchyma
parenchymal
parenteral
paresis
paresthesia
paries
parietal
pari passu
paroxysm
paroxysmal
pars
patent
pathogen
pathogenesis
pathognomonic
pathologic
pathological
pathology
pathosis
patulous
paucity
PC – after meals (post cibum)
PE – physical examination
peau
    p. d'orange
pectinate
pedal
pedicle
peduncle

peduncular
pedunculated
pelvic
pendulous
percussible
percussion
percutaneous
perfusion
pericardium
periosteum
peripheral
periphery
peritoneal
peritoneum
permeability
permeation
pernicious
per os – by mouth
per primam intentionem
per rectum
perspiration
per tubam
pestilence
petechia
petekeah. See *petechia.*
petrous
PH – past history
pharmaceutical
pharmacist
phenomenon
phlebitis
phthisis
physician
physiologic
physiological
physique
pica
piggy backing
pillion
placebo
plantar
plaque
platelet
plethora
plethoric
pleural

pleurisy
plexiform
plexus
plica
plication
PO – period of onset
po dorahnj. See *peau d'orange.*
polydipsia
polyleptic
polyuria
posterior
posteroinferior
posterolateral
posteromedial
postictal
postmortem
postnatal
postprandial
poudrage
poultice
prandial
preagonal
precursor
premonitory
preponderance
prescription
preventive
primary
procedure
process
prodromal
prodrome
prodromic
profundus
progeny
progeria
prognosis
proliferation
promontorium
promontory
pronation
prone
prophylactic
prophylaxis
proprioceptive
prostate

prosthesis
prosthetics
prostration
protuberance
provisional
provocative
proximal
proximalis
pruritus
psychic
psychogenic
psychosomatic
ptosis
puberty
pulsatile
pulsion
punctate
punctum
purulent
pustular
pustule
putative
putrescence
putrid
pyelogram
pyemesis
pyemia
pyknic
pyogenesis
pyogenic
pyramid
pyramidal
pyretic
pyrexia
pyrosis
quadrant
qualitative
quantitative
quarantine
quiescent
radial
radialis
radiant
radiate
radiathermy
radiatio

radiation
radical
radioactivity
radioisotope
radiology
radiolucent
radiotherapy
radix
rakoma. See *rhacoma.*
rale
ramification
ramus
raphe
rarefaction
rebound
recapitulation
recidivation
recrudescence
recrudescent
rectus
recumbent
recuperation
recurrence
reducible
redundant
refractory
regimen
regio
regional
regma. See *rhegma.*
regurgitant
regurgitation
rehabilitation
rehydration
reksis. See *rhexis.*
relapse
remedy
remission
remittent
renal
rentgen. See *roentgen.*
resection
reservoir
residual
residue
resilience
resolution

resorption
respiration
respiratory
restitutio
    r. integrum
restitution
restoration
resuscitation
retching
rete
retention
retrograde
retroperitoneal
retroversion
reversion
rhacoma
rhegma
rheumatic
rheumatism
rheumatoid
rhexis
rhonchal
rhonchial
rhonchus
rhythm
rictus
rigidity
    nuchal r.
rigor
    r. mortis
rigors
rima
roentgen
rong. See words beginning *rhonc-.*
rongeur
rostrum
rotation
rotexion
rubedo
rubefacient
rubella
rubor
ructus
rudiment
rudimentary
ruga
rugae

rugosity
rumination
rupture
sac
saccular
sacculus
saccus
sacral
sacroiliac
sacrum
sagittal
saliva
salivary
salivation
salubrious
salutary
sanative
sanatorium
sanguine
sanguineous
sarcoma
satellite
satiety
scalpel
scanning
      radioisotope s.
scanography
scaphoid
sciatica
scirrhous
scirrhus
sclerosing
sclerosis
sclerotic
scyphoid
scythropasmus
sebaceous
seborrhea
secretion
secretory
sedation
sedative
sedentary
seizure
semicomatose
semilunar
senescence

senile
senility
sensitivity
sensitization
sensorium
sensory
sepsis
septic
septicemia
septulum
sequela
sequelae
serial
serially
seriatim
seroma
seropurulent
seropus
serosa
serosanguineous
serous
serpiginous
serrated
sersinat. See *circinate.*
serum
sessile
sexual
sexuality
shivering
shock
        anaphylactic s.
SI – seriously ill
sibling
sign
      vital s's
Silastic
sinister
sinistrad
sinus
siphon
sithropazmus. See
   scythropasmus.
skeleton
skeletonized
skew
slough
sloughing

sluf. See *slough.*
soluble
somatic
somnolence
spasm
spasmodic
species
specific
specimen
spes
      s. phthisica
sphenoid
spheroid
sphincter
splenomegaly
spontaneous
sporadic
spurious
squamous
stability
stamina
stasis
stat–statim (immediately)
status
steatorrhea
steatosis
stellate
stenosis
stenotic
stereoscopic
sterile
sterilely
stigma
stigmata
stimulant
stimulation
stimulus
stoma
strangulation
stratum
stria
striae
striated
stricture
stridor
stroma
stupor

stuporous
subacute
subcostal
subcutaneous
subcuticular
subluxation
sulcus
superficial
superficialis
supernumerary
supination
supine
suppuration
suppurative
susceptible
symbiosis
symmetrical
symphysis
symptom
symptomatic
symptomatology
syncopal
syncope
syndrome
synechia
synergetic
synkinesis
synthesis
systemic
tabes
tabescent
tabez. See *tabes.*
tachycardia
tachypnea
tactile
takipneah. See *tachypnea.*
tampon
technique
tegmen
tela
telangiectasis
temperature
tenacious
tenaculum
ter in die
terminal
terminus

tertiary
tessellated
tetralogy
texture
therapeutic
therapist
therapy
thermometer
    centigrade t.
    Fahrenheit t.
thoracic
thoracocentesis
thorax
threshold
throbbing
thyroid
thyromegaly
tigroid
tinnitus
tisis. See *phthisis.*
tissue
titration
tolerance
tomogram
tomography
tonicity
tonus
topical
topography
torpid
torpidity
torpor
torsion
tortuous
torus
tosis. See *ptosis.*
tourniquet
toxemia
toxic
toxicity
trabecula
trachea
tract
tractus
trajector
tranquilizer
transfusion

transient
transillumination
translucent
transmigration
transmissible
transmission
transplantation
transudate
transverse
trauma
traumatic
treatment
tremor
tremulous
trigeminy
trigone
trigonum
trocar
troche
trochlea
trochlear
truncus
tuba
tubal
tubercle
tuberculum
tuberosity
tubule
tubulus
tumefacient
tumefaction
tumescence
tumid
tumor
tunic
tunica
tunnel
turbid
turbidity
turgescence
turgescent
turgid
turgor
tussive
twinge
twitch
tympanic

tympanitic
uforeah. See *euphoria.*
ukraseah. See *eucrasia.*
ulcerate
ulceration
ultrasonic
ultrasonography
ultrasound
ultraviolet
umbilical
umbilicus
umbo
unciform
unconscious
unction
undernutrition
undifferentiated
undulation
unicentral
unilateral
upnea. See *eupnea.*
uremia
ureter
ureteral
URI – upper respiratory
        infection
urinalysis
urogenital
urticaria
uthahnazeah. See *euthanasia.*
uthiroid. See *euthyroid.*
uvula
vaccinate
vaccine
vacillate
vallecula
valve
variability
variable
variant
varix
vas
vascular
velamen
velamentum
velum

venter
ventral
ventralis
venule
verge
vertebra
vertebrae
vertebral
vertex
vertical
vertigo
vesicle
vesicula
vestibule
vestibulum
vestigial
viable
villus
vincula
vinculum
viral
virile
virulent
virus
viscera
visceral
viscid
viscus
vital
vitality
vitamin
vitium
vitreous
volar
volvulate
vomica
vomit
vomiting
vomitus
        v. cruentus
vortex
vulsella
vulsellum
wakefulness
wart
well-developed

well-nourished
wheal
wheeze
whelk
whorl
wound

xiphoid
zifoid. See *xiphoid.*
zona
zonula
zoster

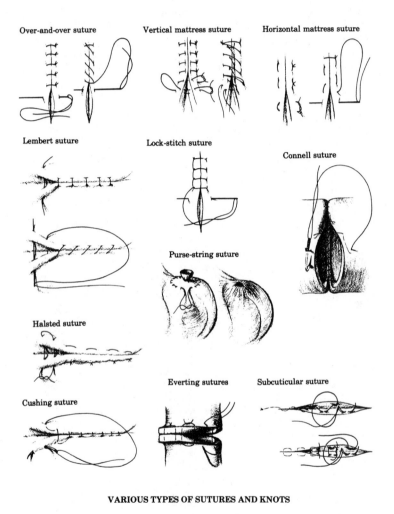

Over-and-over suture

Vertical mattress suture

Horizontal mattress suture

Lembert suture

Lock-stitch suture

Connell suture

Purse-string suture

Halsted suture

Cushing suture

Everting sutures

Subcuticular suture

VARIOUS TYPES OF SUTURES AND KNOTS

(Courtesy of Dorland's Illustrated Medical Dictionary, 27th ed. Plate 44. Philadelphia, W. B. Saunders Company, 1988.)

General Surgical Terms

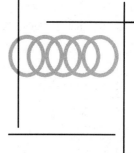

Aaron's sign
Abbe's
    operation
    rings
Abbott-Rawson tube
abdomen
abdominal
abdominocentesis
abdominoperineal
abdominoscopy
Abernethy's operation
aberrant
ablate
ablation
abrader
abrasion
abscess
    amebic a.
    appendiceal a.
    ischiorectal a.
    mammary a.
    perianal a.
    perirectal a.
    pyogenic a.
    subphrenic a.
absorbable
absorbent
abutment
accessory
Ace bandage
achalasia
    pelvirectal a.
    sphincteral a.
ACMI
    forceps
    gastroscope
    laparoscope
    proctoscope

ACMI (continued)
    telescope
    valve
Acrel's ganglion
ACTH – adrenocorticotropic
    hormone
actinomycosis
acupuncture
acusection
acusector
Acutrol sutures
Adair's forceps
Adams'
    operation
    position
Adaptic gauze dressing
adenectomy
adenitis
    mesenteric a.
adenocarcinoma
adenofibroma
adenoma
adenomammectomy
adenomatosis
adenomatous
adenomyosis
adenopathy
    axillary a.
adhesion
    attic a's.
adhesiotomy
adhesive
adipectomy
adipocele
adipose
adiposis
adjacent
adnexa

adnexopexy
adrenal
adrenalectomize
adrenalectomy
adrenalorrhaphy
adrenalotomy
Adson's forceps
advancement
adventitia
adventitious
aerate
aeration
aerogram
aerography
Aeroplast dressing
afferent
agenesis
agglutination
Agnew-Verhoeff incision
agraffe
akahlazea. See *achalasia.*
Åkerlund deformity
akinesia
akinesis
alar
Albert's
    position
    suture
albuginea
Alcon's suture
Alexander's incision
alignment
alimentary
alimentation
Allarton's operation
Allen's
    clamp
    trocar
Allingham's
    operation
    speculum
    ulcer
Allis' forceps
Allis-Ochsner forceps
Allison's suture
allograft
Alm's retractor

alveolar
Americaine anesthetic agent
ampulla
    a. of Vater
amputation
Amussat's operation
Amytal anesthetic agent
anal
anastomosis
    antiperistaltic a.
    Braun's a.
    Clado's a.
    end-to-end a.
    end-to-side a.
    Furniss' a.
    intestinal a.
    isoperistaltic a.
    side-to-end a.
    side-to-side a.
anastomotic
anatomical
anchorage
Andrews' operation
Anectine anesthetic agent
Anestacon anesthetic agent
anesthesia
    absorption a.
    angiospastic a.
    axillary a.
    basal a.
    Bier's local a.
    block a.
    brachial a.
    caudal a.
    chloroform a.
    closed a.
    colonic a.
    compression a.
    conduction a.
    Corning's a.
    electric a.
    endobronchial a.
    endotracheal a.
    epidural a.
    extradural a.
    field block a.
    fractional a.

anesthesia (continued)
    general a.
    Gwathmey's oil-ether a.
    high pressure a.
    hyperbaric a.
    hypnosis a.
    hypobaric a.
    hypotensive a.
    hypothermic a.
    infiltration a.
    inhalation a.
    insufflation a.
    intercostal a.
    intramedullary a.
    intranasal a.
    intraoral a.
    intraosseous a.
    intrapulpal a.
    intraspinal a.
    intratracheal a.
    intravenous a.
    intubation a.
    isobaric a.
    Kulenkampff's a.
    local a.
    lumbar epidural a.
    Meltzer's a.
    mixed a.
    nasoendotracheal a.
    nasotracheal intubation a.
    nerve blocking a.
    open a.
    paracervical block a.
    paraneural a.
    parasacral a.
    paravertebral a.
    partial a.
    peridural a.
    perineural a.
    periodontal a.
    permeation a.
    plexus a.
    presacral a.
    pressure a.
    pudendal block a.
    rectal a.
    refrigeration a.

anesthesia (continued)
    regional a.
    retrobulbar a.
    sacral a.
    saddle block a.
    semiclosed a.
    semiopen a.
    spinal a.
    splanchnic a.
    stellate block a.
    subarachnoid a.
    surface a.
    surgical a.
    sympathetic block a.
    topical a.
    transsacral a.
    transtracheal a.
    twilight a.
anesthesiologist
anesthesiology
anesthetic
anesthetic agents
    alcohol
    alphaprodine
    Americaine
    amethocaine
    amobarbital
    Amytal
    Anectine
    Anestacon
    anticholinesterase
    Avertin
    benoxinate hydrochloride
    benzocaine
    benzoquinonium chloride
    Blockain
    Brevital
    bupivacaine hydrochloride
    butacaine sulfate
    butethamine
      hydrochloride
    Butyn
    Carbocaine hydrochloride
    carbon dioxide
    Cetacaine
    chloramine-T
    chloroform

anesthetic agents (continued)
  chloroprocaine
    hydrochloride
  cinchocaine
  Citanest
  cocaine
  cocaine hydrochloride
  curare
  Cyclaine
  cyclomethycaine sulfate
  cyclopentane
  cyclopropane
  decamethonium bromide
  decamethonium iodide
  Demerol
  dibucaine hydrochloride
  diethyl oxide
  Dilaudid
  divinyl ether
  Duranest
  Dyclone
  dyclonine hydrochloride
  edrophonium chloride
  ether
  ether in oil
  ethocaine
  Ethrane
  ethyl chloride
  ethyl ether
  ethyl oxide
  ethyl vinyl ether
  ethylene
  etidocaine hydrochloride
  Evipal
  Fluoromar
  Fluothane
  Forane
  gallamine
  halothane
  helium
  hexobarbital
  hexylcaine hydrochloride
  Holocaine
  Innovar
  ketamine hydrochloride
  lidocaine hydrochloride

anesthetic agents (continued)
  lignocaine
  Lorfan
  Marcaine hydrochloride
  meperidine hydrochloride
  mepivacaine
    hydrochloride
  methohexital sodium
  methoxyflurane
  Metycaine hydrochloride
  morphine
  narcotic agents
  narcotic antagonists
  Nembutal
  Nesacaine-CE
  Nisentil
  nitrous oxide
  Novocain
  Nupercaine hydrochloride
  Ophthaine
  Oxaine
  oxethazaine
  Penthrane
  pentobarbital
  Pentothal
  Percaine
  piperocaine hydrochloride
  Pontocaine
  pramoxine hydrochloride
  prilocaine hydrochloride
  procaine hydrochloride
  proparacaine
    hydrochloride
  propoxycaine
    hydrochloride
  secobarbital
  Seconal
  sodium pentothal
  succinylcholine chloride
  Surfacaine
  Tensilon
  tetracaine hydrochloride
  thialbarbitone
  thiamylal sodium
  thiopental sodium

anesthetic agents (continued)
    topical cocaine
    trichloroethylene
    Trilene
    Trimar
    Tronothane hydrochloride
    vinyl ether
    vinyl ethyl ether
    Xylocaine with
      epinephrine
anesthetist
anesthetize
aneurysm
aneurysmal
aneurysmectomy
aneurysmoplasty
aneurysmorrhaphy
aneurysmotomy
Angelchik prosthesis
angiitis
angiopancreatitis
angulation
ankyloproctia
annular
annulorrhaphy
annulus
anoperineal
anoplasty
anorectal
anorectocolonic
anorectum
anoscope
    Bacon's a.
    Bodenheimer's a.
    Boehm's a.
    Brinkerhoff's a.
    Buie-Hirschman a.
    Fansler's a.
    Goldbacher's a.
    Hirschman's a.
    Ives' a.
    Muer's a.
    Otis' a.
    Pratt's a.
    Pruitt's a.
    rotating a.

anoscope (continued)
    Sims' a.
    speculum a.
    Welch-Allyn a.
anoscopy
anosigmoidoscopic
anosigmoidoscopy
anospinal
Anson-McVay operation
antecolic
antecubital
anteflexion
anterolateral
anteromedial
anteversion
antimesenteric
antiperistalsis
antiperistaltic
antral
antrectomy
antrum
    pyloric a.
    a. pyloricum
    a. of Willis
anus
apepsia
    achlorhydria a.
aperture
apex
apical
aplooshahzh. See *épluchage.*
aponeurosis
aponeurotic
aponeurotomy
appendalgia
appendectomy
appendekthlipsia
appendical
appendiceal
appendicealgia
appendicectasis
appendicectomy
appendices
appendicism
appendicitis
    acute a.

appendicitis (continued)
 chronic a.
 a. by contiguity
 fulminating a.
 gangrenous a.
 a. granulosa
 helminthic a.
 a. larvata
 myxoglobulosis a.
 necro-purulent a.
 a. obliterans
 perforating a.
 perforative a.
 stercoral a.
 subperitoneal a.
 suppurative a.
 syncongestive a.
 verminous a.
appendiclausis
appendicocecostomy
appendicocele
appendicoenterostomy
appendicolithiasis
appendicolysis
appendicopathia
appendicopathy
appendicosis
appendicostomy
appendicular
appendiculoradiography
appendix
 auricular a.
 cecal a.
 a. cerebri
 ensiform a.
 vermiform a.
 a. vermiformis
appendolithiasis
appendoroentgenography
appendotome
Appolito's
 operation
 suture
apposition
approximate
approximation
aqueduct

areola
areolae
areolar
areolitis
Argyll-Robertson pupil, suture
Aries-Pitanguy mammaplasty
Arlt's suture
Armsby's operation
arrhythmia
artery
 appendicular a.
 brachial a.
 calcareous a.
 epigastric a.
 femoral a.
 hepatic a.
 intramural a.
 sternocleidomastoid a.
 suprascapular a.
 temporal a.
 thoracoacromial a.
Asch's forceps
ascites
asepsis
aseptic
Ashford's mamilliplasty
Ashley's breast prosthesis
aspirate
aspiration
aspirator
 Thorek's a.
assimilation
asymmetry
asymptomatic
atheromatosis
 a. cutis
athyreosis
atonicity
atony
atraumatic
atresia
atretic
atrial
Atroloc suture
atrophy
augmentation
auricle

auricular
auscultation
Austin's knife
autogenous
autograft
autologous
autotransfusion
autotransplantation
    pancreatic a.
Auvray's incision
avascular
avascularization
Avertin anesthetic agent
avulsion
aw bissahk. See *en bissac.*
awl
    curved a.
Axenfeld's suture
axilla
axillae
axillary
axis
Babcock's
    clamp
    forceps
    operation
    suture
Backhaus' forceps
Bacon's anoscope
Bainbridge's forceps
Baker's
    cyst
    tube
Bakes' dilator
Balfour's
    gastroenterostomy
    retractor
balloon
    Grüntzig-type b.
ballooning
ballottement
    abdominal b.
Ball's operation
bandage. See also *dressing.*
    Ace b.
    adhesive b.
    Barton's b.

bandage (continued)
    capeline b.
    circular b.
    compression b.
    cotton elastic b.
    cotton-wool b.
    cravat b.
    crepe b.
    crucial b.
    Curad plastic b.
    demigauntlet b.
    elastic b.
    Elasticon b.
    Elastoplast b.
    Esmarch's b.
    figure-of-eight b.
    fixation b.
    four-tailed b.
    gauntlet b.
    gauze b.
    Gibney's b.
    hammock b.
    immobilizing b.
    Kerlix b.
    Kling b.
    many-tailed b.
    Marlex b.
    Martin's b.
    oblique b.
    plaster b.
    pressure b.
    recurrent b.
    reversed b.
    roller b.
    Scultetus' b.
    spica b.
    spiral b.
    stockinette b.
    Surgiflex b.
    suspensory b.
    T bandage
    Thillaye's b.
    triangular b.
    Velpeau's b.
    Y bandage
Band-aid dressing
Bardenheuer's incision

Bard-Parker blade
Barnes'
    dilator
    trocar
Barraquer's suture
Barrett's
    esophagus
    forceps
Barr's
    hook
    probe
    speculum
Barth's hernia
Barton's bandage
basal
Bassini's operation
"basting stitch"
    Parker-Kerr b.s.
bath
    sitz b.
Battle-Jalaguier-Kammerer
    incision
Battle's
    incision
    operation
Baynton's operation
Beardsley's clamp
Beatson's operation
Beaver's blades
Beck-Jianu gastrostomy
Beckman's retractor
Beck's gastrostomy scoop
Béclard's
    hernia
    suture
bedsore
Beebe's forceps
Bell's suture
Belmas' operation
Benedict's gastroscope
benign
Berbridge's scissors
Berens'
    retractor
    scoop
Bergman-Israel incision

Bergmann's incision
Berna's retractor
Bernstein's gastroscope
Best's
    clamp
    operation
Bevan's
    forceps
    incision
    operation
Beyea's operation
bezoar
Bier's local anesthesia
Biesenberger's operation
bifrontal
bifurcation
bilateral
biliary
Billroth's
    forceps
    gastroenterostomy I and II
    operation
bilobate
bimanual
binder
    Velcro b.
biopsy
    aspiration b.
    excisional b.
    fractional b.
    needle b.
    punch b.
    sponge b.
    surface b.
Bircher's operation
Birkett's hernia
bisection
bistoury
    b. blade
blade
    Bard-Parker b's.
    Beaver's b's.
    bistoury b.
Blair's knife
Blake's forceps
Blalock-Hanlon operation
Blalock-Taussig operation

Blanchard's
    cryptotome
    forceps
bleeders
Blockain anesthetic agent
Bloodgood's operation
bloodless
blotchy
Blumer's shelf
Boari's button
Bobb's operation
Bochdalek's foramen
Bodenheimer's anoscope
body
    malpighian b's.
Boehm's
    anoscope
    proctoscope
    sigmoidoscope
boggy
Bogue's operation
bolus
Bonner's position
Bonta's knife
borborygmus
Bose's operation
bosselated
bougie
    acorn-tipped b.
    common duct b.
    olive-tipped b.
    polyvinyl b.
    soluble b.
    tunneled b.
    wax-tipped b.
    whistle b.
Bovie unit
bowel
Boyce's position
Boys-Allis forceps
Bozeman's
    position
    suture
Brackin's incision
Bradford's forceps
Braun and Jaboulay
    gastroenterostomy

Braun's anastomosis
Brenner's operation
Brevital anesthetic agent
Bricker's operation
Brinkerhoff's anoscope
Brinton's disease
Brock's incision
Brooks' scissors
Brophy's forceps
Brown-Adson forceps
Brown's forceps
bruit
    b. de clapotement (*brwe duh klahpotmaw*)
Brunner's
    dissector
    forceps
Brunschwig's operation
brwe. See *bruit.*
Bryant's operation
bubo
Buckstein's insufflator
Buerger's disease
Buie-Hirschman
    anoscope
    clamp
Buie's
    clamp
    forceps
    irrigator
    position
    probe
    procedure
    scissors
    sigmoidoscope
    technique
    tube
Buie-Smith
    retractor
    speculum
bunion
bunionectomy
Bunnell's suture
Burnham's scissors
bursa
bursectomy
bursocentesis

bursotomy
Butcher's saw
buttock
button
    Boari's b.
    Chlumsky's b.
    Jaboulay's b.
    Lardennois's b.
    Murphy's b.
    peritoneal b.
    polyethylene collar b.
    Villard's b.
Butyn anesthetic agent
Byford's retractor
cadaver
calcifectomy
calcific
calcificectomy
calculus
Caldwell's position
caliper
Callisen's operation
Calot's triangle
Camper's fascia
canal
    crural c.
    c. of Nuck
canaliculus
canalization
cannula
    Ingals' c.
    perfusion c.
cannulation
canthus
Cantor's tube
capitonnage
capsule
Carbocaine hydrochloride
  anesthetic agent
carbuncle
carcinoma
    basal cell c.
    ductal c.
    infiltrating ductal cell c.
    lobular c.
    metastatic c.
    squamous cell c.

Cargile's membrane
Carmalt's forceps
Carman's tube
Carmody's forceps
carrier
    Deschamps' c.
    Lahey's c.
    Mayo's c.
    Wangensteen's c.
Carter's
    clamp
    splenectomy
cartilage
cartilaginous
caruncle
caruncula
Casselberry's position
Cassidy-Brophy forceps
catheter
    Foley c.
    Groshong's c.
    Hickman's c.
    indwelling c.
    Lane's c.
    mushroom c.
    retention c.
    self-retaining c.
    Virden's c.
    Weber's c.
    whistle-tip c.
catheterization
catheterize
cathode
Cattell's
    operation
    tube
cauterization
cautery
cavernous
cavity
    peritoneal c.
cecal
cecectomy
cecocele
cecocolic
cecocolon
cecocoloplicopexy

cecocolostomy
cecofixation
cecoileostomy
cecopexy
cecoplication
cecoptosis
cecorectal
cecorrhaphy
cecosigmoidostomy
cecostomy
cecotomy
cecum
      hepatic c.
      c. mobile
celiac
celiectomy
celiocentesis
celioenterotomy
celiogastrotomy
celioparacentesis
celiopyosis
celiorrhaphy
celioscopy
celiotomy
      ventral c.
Cellolite
cellophane dressing
cellulitus
cellulocutaneous
celluloid
centesis
cephalad
cephalic
Cetacaine anesthetic agent
Chaffin-Pratt tube
Chaput's operation
Chelsea-Eaton speculum
chemosurgery
Cherney's incision
Chernez' incision
Chevalier-Jackson gastroscope
Cheyne's operation
Chiazzi's operation
Chiba needle
Chiene's incision
Child's operation
Childs-Phillips needle

Chlumsky's button
cholangiectasis
cholangioadenoma
cholangiocarcinoma
cholangiocholecysto-
    choledochectomy
cholangioenterostomy
cholangiogastrostomy
cholangiogram
cholangiography
      operative c.
cholangiohepatitis
cholangiohepatoma
cholangiojejunostomy
      intrahepatic c.
cholangioma
cholangiostomy
cholangiotomy
cholangitis
      c. lenta
cholecyst
cholecystalgia
cholecystatony
cholecystectasia
cholecystectomy
cholecystelectrocoagulectomy
cholecystendysis
cholecystenteric
cholecystenteroanastomosis
cholecystenterorrhaphy
cholecystenterostomy
cholecystgastrostomy
cholecystic
cholecystis
cholecystitis
      c. emphysematosa
      follicular c.
      gaseous c.
      c. glandularis proliferans
cholecystnephrostomy
cholecystocholangiogram
cholecystocolonic
cholecystocolostomy
cholecystocolotomy
cholecystoduodenostomy
cholecystoenterostomy
cholecystogastric

cholecystogastrostomy
cholecystogram
cholecystography
cholecystoileostomy
cholecystojejunostomy
cholecystokinetic
cholecystolithiasis
cholecystolithotripsy
cholecystopathy
cholecystopexy
cholecystoptosis
cholecystopyelostomy
cholecystorrhaphy
cholecystosis
cholecystostomy
cholecystotomy
choledochal
choledochectomy
choledochitis
choledochocele
choledochocholedochorrhaphy
choledochocholedochostomy
choledochoduodenostomy
choledochoenterostomy
choledochogastrostomy
choledochogram
choledochography
choledochohepatostomy
choledochoileostomy
choledochojejunostomy
choledocholith
choledocholithiasis
choledocholithotomy
choledocholithotripsy
choledochoplasty
choledochorrhaphy
choledochoscope
choledochosphincterotomy
choledochostomy
choledochotomy
choledochus
cholelith
cholelithiasis
cholelithotomy
cholelithotripsy
cholelithotrity
cholemesis

cholemia
cholepathia
choleperitoneum
cholescintography
chordee
chyle
cicatrectomy
cicatricial
cicatricotomy
cicatrix
cicatrization
circumcision
circumflex
cirsectomy
cirsenchysis
cirsodesis
cirsotome
cirsotomy
cisterna
Citanest anesthetic agent
Clado's anastomosis
Clagett's operation
clamp
      Allen's c.
      Babcock's c.
      Beardsley's c.
      Best's c.
      Buie-Hirschman c.
      Buie's c.
      C. clamp
      Carter's c.
      Cope's c.
      Crile's c.
      Daniel's c.
      DeMartel-Wolfson c.
      Dennis' c.
      Dixon-Thomas-Smith c.
      Doyen's c.
      Eastman's c.
      Fehland's c.
      Foss' c.
      Friedrich-Petz c.
      Furniss' c.
      Furniss-Clute c.
      Furniss-McClure-Hinton
        c.
      Gant's c.

clamp (continued)
  Glassman's c.
  Hayes' c.
  Heaney c.
  Herff's c.
  Hunt's c.
  Hurwitz's c.
  Jarvis' c.
  Kapp-Beck c.
  Kelly's c.
  Kocher's c.
  Lahey's c.
  Lane's c.
  Linton's c.
  Lockwood's c.
  MacDonald's c.
  Martel's c.
  Mastin's c.
  Mikulicz's c.
  Moreno's c.
  mosquito c.
  Moynihan's c.
  Nussbaum's c.
  Ochsner's c.
  Parker's c.
  Payr's c.
  Pean's c.
  Pemberton's c.
  Pennington's c.
  Phillips' c.
  Pott's c.
  Rankin's c.
  Ranzewski's c.
  Roosevelt's c.
  Schoemaker's c.
  Scudder's c.
  Stevenson's c.
  Stone-Holcombe c.
  Stone's c.
  von Petz's c.
  Wangensteen's c.
  Watts' c.
  W. Dean McDonald c.
  Wolfson's c.
  Yellen c.
  Zachary Cope–DeMartel
    c.

claudication
clavicle
clavicular
cleavage
cleft
clitoral
clitoridectomy
clitoridotomy
clitoritomy
cloaca
Cloquet's
    fascia
    hernia
    node
    septum
closure
    Smead-Jones c.
clove-hitch
Cloward's retractor
Clute's incision
clysis
coagulate
coagulation
Coakley's suture
coalescence
coapt
coaptation
coarctation
coarctotomy
cobalt
coccyx
Codman's incision
Coffey's incision
colectomy
Cole's retractor
colic
colicky
colitis
Collin's forceps
collodion
colloid
collum
    c. vesicae felleae
colocentesis
coloclysis
colocolostomy
colocutaneous

colofixation
colohepatopexy
coloileal
cololysis
colon
    c. ascendens
    ascending c.
    c. descendens
    descending c.
    irritable c.
    lead-pipe c.
    pelvic c. of Waldeyer
    sigmoid c.
    c. sigmoideum
    thrifty c.
    transverse c.
    c. transversum
colonorrhagia
colonorrhea
colonoscope
colonoscopy
colopexostomy
colopexotomy
colopexy
coloplication
coloproctectomy
coloproctostomy
coloptosis
colorectostomy
colorrhaphy
colosigmoidostomy
colostomy
    ileotransverse c.
    Wangensteen's c.
colotomy
comedocarcinoma
comedomastitis
comminuted
comminution
concretion
condyloma
    c. acuminatum
confluent
Connell's suture
constriction
    duodenopyloric c.

contracture
    Dupuytren's c.
    Volkmann's c.
convolution
Cook's speculum
Cooper's
    hernia
    ligament
    operation
Cope's clamp
cord
    spermatic c.
Corning's anesthesia
Cornish wool dressing
corpora
corpus
cortex
Cotting's operation
cottonoid patty
Courvoisier's
    gallbladder
    incision
Craig's needle
cremaster
cremasteric
cribriform
Crile's
    clamp
    forceps
    retractor
Cripps'
    obturator
    operation
crural
crus
Cruveilhier's ulcer
cryocautery
cryosurgery
cryotherapy
crypt
    c's of Lieberkühn
    Luschka's c's
cryptitis
cryptotome
    Blanchard's c.
cul-de-sac

Curad plastic bandage
curettage
curetted
Curtis' forceps
curvature
    lesser c.
Curvoisier's gastroenterostomy
Cushing's
    forceps
    suture
    ulcer
cutaneous
cuticle
Cyclaine anesthetic agent
cyst
    Baker's c.
    blue dome c.
    branchial c.
    echinococcus c.
    inclusion c.
    involution c.
    pilonidal c.
    retention c.
    sacrococcygeal c.
    thyroglossal c.
cystauchenotomy
cystduodenostomy
cystectomy
cystic
cysticolithectomy
cysticolithotripsy
cysticorrhaphy
cysticotomy
cystidolaparotomy
cystis
    c. fellea
cystjejunostomy
cystocele
cystocolostomy
cystodiaphanoscopy
cystoduodenostomy
cystogastrostomy
cystojejunostomy
    Roux-en-Y c.
cystosarcoma
    c. phylloides

Czerny-Lembert suture
Czerny's
    operation
    suture
dabreedmaw. See *débridement.*
Dacron graft
Dallas' operation
Daniel's clamp
David's speculum
Deaver's
    incision
    retractor
    scissors
DeBakey's scissors
Debove's tube
débride
débridement
decompression
decubitus
defecation
deformity
    Åkerlund d.
dehiscence
    wound d.
dehisens. See *dehiscence.*
DeLee's forceps
Delphian node
DeMartel-Wolfson clamp
Demerol anesthetic
    agent
Denans' operation
Dennis'
    clamp
    forceps
denudation
DePage-Janeway
    gastrostomy
Depage's position
dermabraded
dermabrasion
Dermalene suture
Dermalon suture
descensus
    d. ventriculi
Deschamps' carrier
desiccate

desiccation
Desjardin's
 forceps
 probe
Dexon suture
diaphragm
diaphragmatic
diastalsis
diastasis
 d. recti abdominis
Dieffenbach's operation
dieresis
Dieulafoy's
 erosion
 ulcer
digital
dilation
 digital d.
dilator
 Bakes' d.
 Barnes' d.
 Ferris' d.
 Kron's d.
 Mantz's d.
 Murphy's d.
 Ottenheimer's d.
 pneumatic balloon d.
 Ramstedt's d.
 Savary-Gilliard d.
 Wales' d.
 Young's d.
Dilaudid anesthetic agent
dimpling
director
 Larry's d.
 Pratt's d.
discission
discrete
disease. See *Medical Specialty*
 sections.
dissection
 blunt d.
 radical neck d.
 sharp d.
 supraomohyoid neck d.
dissector
 Brunner's d.

dissector (continued)
 Kocher's d.
 Wangensteen's d.
disseminated
distention
diverticula
diverticulectomy
diverticulitis
diverticulogram
diverticulopexy
diverticulosis
diverticulum
 Meckel's d.
Dixon-Thomas-Smith clamp
Dowell's operation
Doyen's
 clamp
 forceps
 scissors
drain
 accordion d.
 cigarette d.
 Hemovac d.
 latex d.
 Penrose d.
 polyethylene d.
 polyvinyl d.
 rubber-dam d.
 stab wound d.
 suction d.
 sump d.
 whistle-tip d.
dressing. See also *bandage.*
 absorbable d.
 Adaptic gauze d.
 adhesive d.
 Aeroplast d.
 Band-aid d.
 barrel d.
 bolus d.
 brassiere-type d.
 bulky d.
 butterfly d.
 cellophane d.
 cocoon d.
 collar d.
 collodion d.

dressing (continued)
>   compound d.
>   compression d.
>   Cornish wool d.
>   dry pressure d.
>   felt d.
>   fine mesh d.
>   fluff d.
>   fluffy compression d.
>   foam rubber d.
>   four-tailed d.
>   Gelfilm d.
>   Gelfoam d.
>   Gelocast d.
>   impregnated d.
>   Lister's d.
>   Lubafax d.
>   many-tailed d.
>   Mersilene d.
>   mustache d.
>   Nu-gauze d.
>   occlusive d.
>   paraffin d.
>   patch d.
>   petrolatum gauze d.
>   plastic d.
>   pressure d.
>   propylene d.
>   Raytec d.
>   sheepskin d.
>   stent d.
>   stockinette d.
>   Styrofoam d.
>   Surgicel gauze d.
>   Telfa d.
>   tulle gras d.
>   Vaseline gauze d.
>   Velrco d.
>   Vioform d.
>   Wangensteen's d.
>   Xeroform d.

drugs. See *Drugs and Chemistry* section.

Drummond-Morison operation

duct
>   alveolar d.

duct (continued)
>   biliary d.
>   common bile d.
>   common hepatic d.
>   cystic d.
>   efferent d.
>   excretory d.
>   lacrimal d.
>   lactiferous d.
>   mammary d.
>   nasolacrimal d.
>   pancreatic d.
>   papillary d.
>   parotid d.
>   prostatic d.
>   salivary d.
>   d. of Santorini
>   semicircular d.
>   Stensen's d.
>   Wharton's d.
>   d. of Wirsung

Dudley's hook
Dudley-Smith speculum
Dührssen's incision
Duke's trocar
Duncan's position
Dunhill's hemostat
duodenal
duodenectomy
duodenitis
duodenocholangeitis
duodenocholecystostomy
duodenocholedochotomy
duodenocolic
duodenocystostomy
duodenoduodenostomy
duodenoenterostomy
duodenogram
duodenohepatic
duodenoileostomy
duodenojejunostomy
duodenolysis
duodenorrhaphy
duodenoscopy
duodenostomy
duodenotomy
duodenum

Dupuytren's
    contracture
    enterotome
    suture
Duranest anesthetic agent
DuVal's procedure
Duvergier's suture
Dyclone anesthetic agent
dye laser
dysfunction
dyskinesia
    biliary d.
dysplasia
Earle's probe
Eastman's clamp
ecchymosis
echinococcosis
echinococcotomy
ectocolostomy
ectokelostomy
ectopic
ectropion
Edebohl's
    incision
    position
edema
edematous
Eder-Chamberlin gastroscope
Eder-Hufford gastroscope
Eder-Palmer gastroscope
Eder's
    gastroscope
    laparoscope
Edwards' hook
Ekehorn's operation
Elasticon bandage
Elastoplast bandage
electrocautery
electrocholecystectomy
electrocholecystocausis
electrocoagulation
electrodesiccation
electrogastroenterostomy
electrosurgery
Elliot's position
Elliott's forceps
Ellsner's gastroscope

Elsberg's incision
embolectomy
embolism
embolus
Emerson's stripper
Emmet's suture
en bissac
en bloc
encapsulated
endocholedochal
endoscopy
endothyropexy
engorgement
en masse
enterauxe
enterectasis
enterectomy
enterelcosis
enteritis
enteroanastomosis
enteroapokleisis
enterocele
enterocentesis
enterochirurgia
enterocholecystostomy
enterocholecystotomy
enterocleisis
enteroclysis
enterocolectomy
enterocolitis
enterocolostomy
enteroenterostomy
    Parker-Kerr e.
enteroepiplocele
enterogastritis
enterohepatopexy
enterolith
enterolithiasis
enteropexy
enteroplasty
enteroptosis
enterorrhaphy
enterostomy
    Witzel's e.
enterotome
    Dupuytren's e.
enterotomy

enucleation
epauxesiectomy
epidermoid
epigastric
epigastrium
epigastrocele
epigastrorrhaphy
epiglottis
epiplocele
epiploectomy
epiploenterocele
epiploic
epiploitis
epiplomerocele
epiplomphalocele
epiploon
epiplopexy
epiploplasty
epiplorrhaphy
epiplosarcomphalocele
epiploscheocele
epithelialization
epithelialize
epithelium
épluchage
eponychium
Equisetene suture
erosion
    Dieulafoy's e.
erythema
erythematous
eschar
Esmarch's
    bandage
    scissors
esofa-. See words beginning
    esopha-.
esogastritis
esophagectomy
esophagocardiomyotomy
esophagocologastrostomy
esophagoduodenostomy
esophagoenterostomy
esophagofundopexy
esophagogastrectomy
esophagogastroanastomosis
esophagogastroplasty

esophagogastroscopy
esophagogastrostomy
esophagojejunogastrostomosis
esophagojejunostomy
esophagus
    Barrett's e.
Ethibond suture
Ethicon suture
Ethiflex suture
Ethilon suture
Ethrane anesthetic agent
euthyroid
evagination
eventration
Evipal anesthetic agent
evisceration
excavation
excision
    wound e.
excoriation
excrement
exenteration
exenteritis
exploratory
exsanguination
exsanguinotransfusion
exteriorize
extirpation
extravasation
extrusion
extubate
exudate
falciform
fanenstel. See *Pfannenstiel.*
Fansler's
    anoscope
    proctoscope
    speculum
Farris' forceps
fascia
    Camper's f.
    Cloquet's f.
    cremasteric f.
    cribriform f.
    external oblique f.
    infundibuliform f.
    f. lata femoris

fascia (continued)
    pectineal f.
    prepubic f.
    Scarpa's f.
    f. transversalis
    transverse f.
fascial
fasciaplasty
fascioplasty
fasciorrhaphy
fasciotomy
FB – fingerbreadth
    foreign body
fecal
fecalith
fecopurulent
Federoff's splenectomy
Fehland's clamp
Feilchenfeld's forceps
felon
femoral
femorocele
fenestra
Fenger's probe
feokromositoma. See
    pheochromocytoma.
Ferguson-Coley operation
Ferguson-Moon retractor
Ferguson's
    forceps
    operation
    scissors
    scoop
Fergusson's incision
Ferris'
    dilator
    scoop
Ferris-Smith forceps
fibercolonoscope
fibergastroscope
fiberoptic
fiberscope
    Hirschowitz's f.
fibrin
fibrinopurulent
fibroadenoma
fibroadenosis

fibrocystic
fibroma
fibromatoid
fibromectomy
fibromyoma
fibromyomectomy
fibromyotomy
fibrosis
fimbria
fimbriated
fingerbreadth
Finney's
    operation
    pyloroplasty
fissure
fistula
fistulectomy
fistulization
fistuloenterostomy
fistulotomy
fistulous
fitobezor. See phytobezoar.
flap
    cellulocutaneous f.
    island f.
    musculocutaneous f.
    skin f.
    sliding f.
    surgical f.
Flaxedil suture
flebektomee. See phlebectomy.
flebitis. See phlebitis.
flebo-. See words beginning
    phlebo-.
flegmon. See phlegmon.
Flexiton suture
Flexon suture
flexure
    duodenojejunal f.
    hepatic f.
    iliac f.
    sigmoid f.
    splenic f.
fluctuant
fluctuation
Fluoromar anesthetic agent
Fluothane anesthetic agent

Foerster's forceps
Foley catheter
follicle
    Lieberkühn's f's
follicular
folliculi
    f. lymphatici aggregati
    f. lymphatici aggregati
      appendicis vermiformis
    f. lymphatici gastrici
    f. lymphatici lienales
    f. lymphatici recti
    f. lymphatici solitarii
      intestini crassi
    f. lymphatici solitarii
      intestini tenuis
folliculus
foramen
    f. of Bochdalek
    Morgagni's f.
    f. of Winslow
Forane anesthetic agent
forceps
    ACMI f.
    Adair's f.
    Adson's f.
    Allis' f.
    Allis-Ochsner f.
    Asch's f.
    Babcock's f.
    Backhaus' f.
    Bainbridge's f.
    Barrett's f.
    Beebe's f.
    Bevan's f.
    Billroth's f.
    Blake's f.
    Blanchard's f.
    Boys-Allis f.
    Bradford's f.
    Brophy's f.
    Brown-Adson f.
    Brown's f.
    Brunner's f.
    Buie's f.
    Carmalt's f.
    Carmody's f.

forceps (continued)
    Cassidy-Brophy f.
    Collin's f.
    Crile's f.
    Curtis' f.
    Cushing's f.
    DeLee's f.
    Dennis' f.
    Desjardin's f.
    Doyen's f.
    Elliott's f.
    Farris' f.
    Feilchenfeld's f.
    Ferguson's f.
    Ferris-Smith f.
    Foerster's f.
    Foss' f.
    Frankfeldt's f.
    Fulpit's f.
    Glassman-Allis f.
    Glassman's f.
    Gray's f.
    Halsted's f.
    Harrington's f.
    Healy's f.
    Heaney's f.
    Hirschman's f.
    Hoxworth's f.
    Hudson's f.
    Jackson's f.
    Jones' f.
    Judd-Allis f.
    Judd-DeMartel f.
    Kelly's f.
    Kerrison's f.
    Kocher's f.
    Lahey-Pean f.
    Lahey's f.
    Leksell's f.
    Lillie's f.
    Lockwood's f.
    Lovelace's f.
    Lower's f.
    Maier's f.
    Martin's f.
    Mayo-Blake f.
    Mayo-Ochsner f.

forceps (continued)
    Mayo-Robson f.
    Mayo's f.
    McNealy-Glassman-
      Babcock f.
    McNealy-Glassman-
      Mixter f.
    Mixter's f.
    Moynihan's f.
    New's f.
    Ochsner-Dixon f.
    Ochsner's f.
    Parker-Kerr f.
    Péan's f.
    Pennington's f.
    Percy's f.
    Porter's f.
    Potts-Smith f.
    Pratt-Smith f.
    Providence f.
    Rankin's f.
    Ratliff-Blake f.
    Rochester-Ewald f.
    Rochester-Mixter f.
    Rochester-Rankin f.
    Rochester's f.
    Roeder's f.
    Russian f.
    Schoenberg's f.
    Schutz's f.
    Scudder's f.
    Semken's f.
    Shallcross' f.
    Singley's f.
    Spencer Wells f.
    Steinmann's f.
    Stille's f.
    Stone's f.
    Strassmann's f.
    sucker iris f.
    Thoms' f.
    Thorek-Mixter f.
    Virtus' f.
    Walter's f.
    Walther's f.
    Wangensteen's f.
    Watze's f.

forceps (continued)
    Weisenbach's f.
    Welch-Allyn f.
    Williams' f.
    Yeomans' f.
    Young's f.
    Zenker's f.
    Zollinger's f.
Foss'
    clamp
    forceps
    retractor
fossa
    duodenal f.
    epigastric f.
    Hartmann's f.
    ischiorectal f.
    Landzert's f.
    Mohrenheim's f.
    subsigmoid f.
Fowler's
    incision
    position
Fowler-Weir incision
fragmentation
Frankfeldt's
    forceps
    needle
    sigmoidoscope
    snare
Frank's operation
Franz's retractor
Fredet-Ramstedt
    operation
    pyloromyotomy
fren-. See words beginning *phren-.*
frenulum
frenum
Freund's operation
friable
Friedrich-Petz clamp
Frost's suture
FSH – follicle-stimulating
    hormone
Fuchs' position
fulguration
fulminant

fulminate
Fulpit's forceps
fundoplication
    Nissen f.
fundus
fundusectomy
funiculopexy
funiculus
Furniss'
    anastomosis
    clamp
    incision
Furniss-Clute clamp
Furniss-McClure-Hinton clamp
furuncle
furunculosis
Gabriel's proctoscope
Gaillard-Arlt suture
galactocele
gallbladder
    Courvoisier's g.
Gallie's
    operation
    transplant
gallstone
Gambee's suture
Gamgee tissue
Gamna nodules
Gandy-Gamna nodules
ganglion
    Acrel's g.
ganglionectomy
ganglionostomy
gangliosympathectomy
gangrene
gangrenous
Gant's clamp
gasserectomy
gastrectomy
    von Haberer-Aguirre g.
gastritis
    cirrhotic g.
    hypertrophic g.
gastrocele
gastrocolic
gastrocolitis
gastrocolostomy

gastrocolotomy
gastrodiaphany
gastroduodenal
gastroduodenoscopy
gastroduodenostomy
gastroenteritis
gastroenteroanastomosis
gastroenterocolostomy
gastroenteroplasty
gastroenterostomy
    Balfour's g.
    Billroth's g. I and II
    Braun and Jaboulay g.
    Curvoisier's g.
    Heineke-Mikulicz g.
    Hofmeister's g.
    Polya's g.
    Roux's g.
    Schoemaker's g.
    von Haberer-Finney g.
    Wölfler's g.
gastroenterotomy
gastroepiploic
gastroesophagostomy
gastrogalvanization
gastrogastrostomy
gastrogavage
gastrohepatic
gastroileitis
gastroileostomy
gastrointestinal
gastrojejunocolic
gastrojejunostomy
gastrolysis
gastromegaly
gastromyotomy
gastronesteostomy
gastropexy
gastroplasty
gastroplication
gastroptosis
gastropylorectomy
gastropyloric
gastrorrhaphy
gastrorrhexis
gastroscope
    ACMI g.

gastroscope (continued)
    Benedict's g.
    Bernstein's g.
    Chevalier-Jackson g.
    Eder's g.
    Eder-Chamberlin g.
    Eder-Hufford g.
    Eder-Palmer g.
    Ellsner's g.
    fiberoptic g.
    flexible g.
    Herman-Taylor g.
    Housset-Debray g.
    Janeway's g.
    Kelling's g.
    Schindler's g.
    Wolf-Schindler g.
gastroscopy
gastrosplenic
gastrostomy
    Beck-Jianu g.
    Beck's g.
    DePage-Janeway g.
    Janeway's g.
    Kader's g.
    Marwedel's g.
    Spivack's g.
    Ssabanejew-Frank g.
    Stamm's g.
    Witzel's g.
gastrotome
gastrotomy
Gatellier's incision
gauze
Gelfilm dressing
Gelfoam dressing
Gelocast dressing
Gély's suture
Gersuny's operation
GI – gastrointestinal
Gibbon's hernia
Gibney's bandage
Gibson-Balfour retractor
Gibson's
    incision
    suture
Gill's operation

Gimbernat's ligament
gland
    adrenal g's
    Lieberkühn's g.
    parotid g.
    pineal g.
    pituitary g.
    salivary g.
    sublingual g.
    submaxillary g.
    thyroid g.
Glassman-Allis forceps
Glassman's
    clamp
    forceps
glioma
glossectomy
glossitis
glossoplasty
glossorrhaphy
glossotomy
Goelet's retractor
goiter
    adenomatous g.
    colloid g.
    cystic g.
    exophthalmic g.
    fibrous g.
    nodular g.
    papillomatous g.
    parenchymatous g.
    substernal g.
    toxic g.
Goldbacher's
    anoscope
    needle
    proctoscope
    speculum
Gosset's retractor
Gould's suture
Goyrand's hernia
graft
    autogenous g.
    bifurcation g.
    cutis g.
    Dacron g.
    fascial g.

graft (continued)
    fiber glass g.
    full-thickness skin g.
    Marlex g.
    split-thickness skin g.
    tantalum mesh g.
    Teflon g.
Graham-Roscie operation
granulation
granuloma
granulomatous
Gray's forceps
Greenhow's incision
Green's retractor
Greiling's tube
gridiron incision
Grieshaber's retractor
Grondahl-Finney operation
Gronshong's catheter
Gruber's hernia
Grüntzig-type balloon
Grynfelt's hernia
guarding
Gudebrod's suture
Guild-Pratt speculum
Gussenbauer's
    operation
    suture
Guyton-Friedenwald
    suture
Gwathmey's oil-ether
    anesthesia
gynecomastia
Hagedorn's needle
Hahn's operation
hallux
    h. malleus
    h. valgus
    h. varus
Halsted's
    forceps
    hemostat
    incision
    operation
    suture
hamartoma

Handley's
    incision
    operation
Harmon's incision
Harrington-Pemberton
    retractor
Harrington's
    forceps
    retractor
Harris' suture
Hartmann's
    fossa
    point
    pouch
haustra coli
haustration
haustrum
Hayes' clamp
healing
    h. by first intention
    h. by granulation
    h. by second intention
    h. by third intention
Healy's forceps
Heaney's
    clamp
    forceps
Heaton's operation
Heerman's incision
Heineke-Mikulicz
    gastroenterostomy
    operation
    pyloroplasty
Heineke's operation
Heller's operation
hemangioma
hemangiosarcoma
hematemesis
hematoma
hemicolectomy
hemicorporectomy
hemigastrectomy
hemihepatectomy
hemipylorectomy
hemisection
hemithyroidectomy
hemoptysis

hemorrhage
hemorrhagic
hemorrhoid
    combined h.
    external h.
    internal h.
    lingual h.
    mixed h.
    mucocutaneous h.
    prolapsed h.
    strangulated h.
    thrombosed h.
hemorrhoidal
hemorrhoidectomy
hemostasis
hemostat
    Dunhill's h.
    Halsted's h.
    Maingot's h.
Hemovac drain
Henke's triangle
Henry's
    incision
    operation
    splenectomy
hepatectomize
hepatectomy
hepatic
hepaticocholangiochole-
   cystenterostomy
hepaticocholangiojejunostomy
hepaticodochotomy
hepaticoduodenostomy
hepaticoenterostomy
hepaticogastrostomy
hepaticojejunostomy
hepaticolithotomy
hepaticolithotripsy
hepaticostomy
hepaticotomy
hepatitis
hepatobiliary
hepatocele
hepatocholangio-
   cystoduodenostomy
hepatocholangioduodenostomy
hepatocholangioenterostomy

hepatocholangiogastrostomy
hepatocholangiostomy
hepatocirrhosis
hepatoduodenostomy
hepatoenterostomy
hepatogastric
hepatolithectomy
hepatomegaly
hepatopexy
hepatorrhaphy
hepatosplenomegaly
hepatostomy
hepatotomy
Herff's clamp
Herman-Taylor gastroscope
hernia
    abdominal h.
    acquired h.
    h. adiposa
    amniotic h.
    Barth's h.
    Béclard's h.
    Birkett's h.
    cecal h.
    Cloquet's h.
    congenital h.
    Cooper's h.
    crural h.
    diaphragmatic h.
    diverticular h.
    duodenojejunal h.
    encysted h.
    epigastric h.
    extrasaccular h.
    femoral h.
    foraminal h.
    funicular h.
    gastroesophageal h.
    Gibbon's h.
    gluteal h.
    Goyrand's h.
    Gruber's h.
    Grynfelt's h.
    Hesselbach's h.
    Hey's h.
    hiatal h.
    hiatus h.

hernia (continued)
 Holthouse's h.
 incarcerated h.
 incisional h.
 indirect h.
 infantile h.
 inguinal h.
 inguinocrural h.
 inguinofemoral h.
 inguinoproperitoneal h.
 inguinosuperficial h.
 h. in recto
 intermuscular h.
 interparietal h.
 intersigmoid h.
 interstitial h.
 irreducible h.
 ischiatic h.
 ischiorectal h.
 Krönlein's h.
 Küster's h.
 labial h.
 Laugier's h.
 levator h.
 linea alba h.
 Littré-Richter h.
 Littré's h.
 lumbar h.
 Maydl's h.
 mesenteric h.
 mesocolic h.
 mucosal h.
 oblique h.
 obturator h.
 omental h.
 ovarian h.
 pantaloon h.
 paraduodenal h.
 paraesophageal h.
 paraperitoneal h.
 parasaccular h.
 h. par glissement
 parietal h.
 paraumbilical h.
 pectineal h.
 perineal h.
 Petit's h.

hernia (continued)
 properitoneal h.
 pudendal h.
 pulsion h.
 rectal h.
 reducible h.
 retrocecal h.
 retrograde h.
 retroperitoneal h.
 Richter's h.
 Rieux's h.
 Rokitansky's h.
 sciatic h.
 scrotal h.
 sliding h.
 spigelian h.
 strangulated h.
 subpubic h.
 synovial h.
 thyroidal h.
 tonsillar h.
 Treitz's h.
 tunicary h.
 umbilical h.
 uterine h.
 vaginal h.
 vaginolabial h.
 Velpeau's h.
 ventral h.
 vesical h.
 voluminous h.
 Von Bergmann's h.
 W h.
hernial
herniary
herniated
herniation
hernioappendectomy
hernioenterotomy
hernioid
herniolaparotomy
hernioplasty
herniopuncture
herniorrhaphy
herniotome
herniotomy

Hesselbach's
   hernia
   ligament
   triangle
heteroautoplasty
Heyer-Schulte prosthesis
Hey-Grooves' operation
Hey's hernia
hiatal
hiatopexy
hiatus
Hickman's catheter
hidradenitis
   h. suppurativa
Higgins' incision
Hill-Ferguson retractor
hilum
hilus
Hinckle-James speculum
Hirschman-Martin proctoscope
Hirschman's
   anoscope
   forceps
   proctoscope
Hirschowitz's fiberscope
Hochenegg's operation
Hofmeister's gastroenterostomy
Hoguet's
   maneuver
   operation
Holocaine anesthetic agent
Holthouse's hernia
homograft
homoplastic
homoplasty
Hood and Kirklin incision
hook
   Barr's h.
   Dudley's h.
   Edwards' h.
   Linton's h.
   Pratt's h.
   Rosser's h.
   Stewart's h.
   Welch-Allyn h.
Hopkins' operation
Horsley's pyloroplasty

Hotchkiss' operation
Housset-Debray gastroscope
Houston's valve
Hoxworth's forceps
Hudson's forceps
Hunt's
   clamp
   operation
Hurwitz's clamp
hydrocele
hydrocelectomy
hydroperitoneum
hydrops
   h. abdominis
hygroma
hyperemic
hyperinsulinism
hyperparathyroidism
hyperpituitarism
hyperplasia
hyperthyroidism
hypertonic
hypertrophic
hypertrophy
hypochondrium
hypocystotomy
hypodermatomy
hypogastric
hypoparathyroidism
hypophysectomy
hypopituitarism
hypoplasia
hypothermia
hypothyroidism
hypotonic
Hyrtl's sphincter
^{131}I – radioactive iodine
I & D – incision and drainage
ileac
ileal
ileectomy
ileitis
   distal i.
   regional i.
   terminal i.
ileocecal
ileocecostomy

ileocecum
ileocolic
ileocolitis
ileocolostomy
ileocolotomy
ileocystoplasty
ileoileostomy
ileoproctostomy
ileorectal
ileorectostomy
ileorrhaphy
ileosigmoid
ileosigmoidostomy
ileostomy
    Koch i.
ileotomy
ileotransversostomy
ileum
    terminal i.
ileus
iliocolotomy
iliohypogastric
ilioinguinal
iliolumbocostoabdominal
iliopectineal
iliopubic
imbricated
imbrication
impaction
implant
    Silastic i.
incarcerated
incarceration
incised
incision
    abdominal i.
    abdominothoracic i.
    ab externo i.
    Agnew-Verhoeff i.
    alar i.
    Alexander's i.
    angular i.
    aortotomy i.
    arcuate i.
    areolar i.
    arteriotomy i.
    Auvray's i.

incision (continued)
    backcut i.
    Bardenheuer's i.
    Bar's i.
    Battle-Jalaguier-
      Kammerer i.
    Battle's i.
    bayonet i.
    Bergman-Israel i.
    Bergmann's i.
    Bevan's i.
    bivalved i.
    Brackin's i.
    Brock's i.
    bur-hole i.
    buttonhole i.
    celiotomy i.
    cervical i.
    Cherney's i.
    Chernez' i.
    Chiene's i.
    circular i.
    circumareolar i.
    circumcisional i.
    circumferential i.
    circumlimbal i.
    circumscribing i.
    Clute's i.
    Codman's i.
    Coffey's i.
    collar i.
    confirmatory i.
    conjunctival i.
    corneoscleral i.
    cortical i.
    Courvoisier's i.
    crescent i.
    crosshatch i.
    crucial i.
    cruciate i.
    curved i.
    curvilinear i.
    Deaver's i.
    deltopectoral i.
    dorsolateral i.
    Dührssen's i.
    dural i.

incision (continued)

    Edebohls' i.
    elliptical i.
    Elsberg's i.
    endaural i.
    enterotomy i.
    exploratory i.
    Fergusson's i.
    fishmouth i.
    flank i.
    flexed i.
    Fowler's i.
    Fowler-Weir i.
    Furniss' i.
    Gatellier's i.
    Gibson's i.
    Greenhow's i.
    gridiron i.
    guillotine i.
    Halsted's i.
    Handley's i.
    Harmon's i.
    Heerman's i.
    hemitransfixion i.
    Henry's i.
    Higgins' i.
    hockey-stick i.
    Hood and Kirklin i.
    horizontal i.
    inframammary i.
    infraumbilical i.
    inguinal i.
    intercartilaginous i.
    intracapsular i.
    Jackson's i.
    J-shaped i.
    Kammerer's i.
    Kehr's i.
    Kocher's i.
    Küstner's i.
    lamellar i.
    Lamm's i.
    Langenbeck's i.
    lateral flank i.
    lateral rectus i.
    lazy-S i.
    Lempert's i.

incision (continued)

    Lilienthal's i.
    limbal i.
    linear i.
    Linton's i.
    longitudinal i.
    Lonquet's i.
    Mackenrodt's i.
    Mason's i.
    Maylard i.
    Mayo-Robson i.
    McArthur's i.
    McBurney's i.
    McLaughlin's i.
    McVay's i.
    meatal i.
    median i.
    Meyer's hockey stick i.
    midline i.
    Mikulicz' i.
    Morison's i.
    muscle splitting i.
    myringotomy i.
    Nagamatsu i.
    oblique i.
    Ollier's i.
    Orr's i.
    paracostal i.
    parainguinal i.
    paramedian i.
    paramuscular i.
    parapatellar i.
    pararectus i.
    parasagittal i.
    parascapular i.
    paraumbilical i.
    paravaginal i.
    Parker's i.
    Péan's i.
    perianal i.
    periareolar i.
    perilimbal i.
    periscapular i.
    peritoneal i.
    Perthes' i.
    Pfannenstiel's i.
    Phemister's i.

incision (continued)
    popliteal i.
    postauricular i.
    posterior i.
    posterolateral i.
    proximal i.
    pyelotomy i.
    racquet i.
    radial i.
    rectus muscle splitting i.
    recumbent i.
    relaxing i.
    relief i.
    retroauricular i.
    rim i.
    Risdon's extraoral i.
    Rocky-Davis i.
    Rodman's i.
    Rollet's i.
    Rosen's i.
    Roux-en-Y jejunal loop i.
    saber-cut i.
    salmon backcut i.
    Sanders' i.
    Schobinger's i.
    Schuchardt's i.
    scratch type i.
    semicircular i.
    semiflexed i.
    semilunar i.
    serpentine i.
    Shambaugh's i.
    shelving i.
    shoulder-strap i.
    Simon's i.
    Singleton's i.
    Sloan's i.
    Smith-Peterson i.
    spiral i.
    stab-wound i.
    stellate i.
    sternal splitting i.
    Stewart's i.
    Strombeck's i.
    subcostal i.
    subinguinal i.
    submammary i.

incision (continued)
    subtrochanteric i.
    subumbilical i.
    supracervical i.
    suprapubic i.
    supraumbilical i.
    temporal i.
    Thomas-Warren i.
    thoracoabdominal i.
    thoracotomy i.
    Timbrall-Fisher i.
    transection i.
    transmeatal i.
    transrectus i.
    transverse i.
    trap-door i.
    T-shaped i.
    U-shaped i.
    vertical i.
    Vischer's i.
    V-shaped i.
    Warren's i.
    Watson-Jones i.
    Weber-Fergusson i.
    wedge i.
    Whipple's i.
    Wilde's i.
    Willie-Meyer i.
    W-shaped i.
    Y-type i.
    Z-flap i.
    Z-plasty i.
    Z-shaped i.
incisional
incisive
incisura
    i. angularis ventriculi
    i. cardiaca ventriculi
inclusion
incontinence
indurated
induration
infarction
    intestinal i.
infiltration
inflammation
inframamillary

inframammary
infundibula
infundibuliform
infundibulopelvic
infundibulum
Ingals' cannula
inguinal
inguinoabdominal
inguinocrural
inguinolabial
inguinoscrotal
Innovar anesthetic agent
inoperable
in situ
instillation
insufflation
insufflator
    Buckstein's i.
    Weber's i.
intercostal
interfemoral
interstitial
intestinal
intestine
intima
intractable
intracystic
intraductal
intubation
intumescence
intussusception
intussusceptum
intussuscipiens
invagination
inversion
inverted
irradiation
irrigator
    Buie's i.
ischioanal
ischiococcygeal
ischiorectal
ischochymia
island
    i's of Langerhans
isograft

Israel's retractor
isthmectomy
isthmus
Ivalon's suture
Ives' anoscope
Jaboulay's
    button
    operation
    pyloroplasty
Jackson's
    forceps
    incision
    retractor
Jacobs-Palmer laparoscope
Jam-Shidi needle
Janeway's
    gastroscope
    gastrostomy
Jarvis' clamp
jaundice
jejunectomy
jejunitis
jejunocecostomy
jejunocolostomy
jejunoileitis
jejunoileostomy
jejunojejunostomy
jejunorrhaphy
jejunostomy
jejunotomy
jejunum
Jelk's operation
Jenckel method
Jobert's suture
Jobst stocking
Johnson's tube
Jones'
    forceps
    position
    scissors
Jonge's position
Jonnesco's operation
Jorgenson's scissors
J-shaped incision
Judd-Allis forceps
Judd-DeMartel forceps
Judd's pyloroplasty

juncture
    saphenofemoral j.
Jutte tube
Kader-Senn operation
Kader's gastrostomy
Kalt's suture
Kammerer's incision
Kapp-Beck clamp
Keeley's stripper
Keel's operation
Keen's operation
Kehr's incision
Keith's needle
Kelling's gastroscope
Kelly's
    clamp
    forceps
    proctoscope
    retractor
    sigmoidoscope
    suture
    tube
keloid
keloplasty
kelotomy
kemo-. See words beginning
    chemo-.
keratosis
Kerlix bandage
Kerrison's
    forceps
    punch
    retractor
    rongeur
kyl. See *chyle.*
Killian-King retractor
King's retractor
Kirby's suture
Kirschner's
    suture
    wire
Klatskin's needle
Kleenspec sigmoidoscope
Klemme's retractor
Kling bandage
knife
    Austin's k.

knife (continued)
    Blair's k.
    Bonta's k.
Knowles' scissors
Koch ileostomy
Kocher-Crotti retractor
kocherization
Kocher's
    clamp
    dissector
    forceps
    incision
    operation
    ulcer
koilonychia
kol-. See words beginning *chol-.*
kolangi-. See words beginning
    cholangi-.
kole-. See words beginning *chole-.*
kolo-. See words beginning *cholo-.*
Kondoleon operation
Kraske's
    operation
    position
    retractor
Krönlein's hernia
Kron's
    dilator
    probe
Kulenkampff's anesthesia
Kurten's stripper
Küster's hernia
Küstner's incision
laceration
lacuna
    l. musculorum
    l. vasorum
lacunar
Lahey-Péan forceps
Lahey's
    carrier
    clamp
    forceps
    operation
    retractor
    tenaculum
lamella

lamina
Lamm's incision
Landzert's fossa
Lane's
    catheter
    clamp
    operation
Langenbeck's incision
Langerhans' islands
laparectomy
laparocholecystotomy
laparocolostomy
laparocolotomy
laparocystectomy
laparocystidotomy
laparoenterostomy
laparoenterotomy
laparogastroscopy
laparogastrostomy
laparogastrotomy
laparohepatotomy
laparoileotomy
laparomyomectomy
laparorrhaphy
laparoscope
    ACMI l.
    Eder's l.
    Jacobs-Palmer l.
    Lent's l.
laparoscopic
laparoscopy
laparosplenectomy
laparosplenotomy
laparotomaphilia
laparotome
laparotomy
laparotrachelotomy
laparotyphlotomy
Lardennois's button
La Roque's technique
Larry's
    director
    probe
laser
Laugier's hernia
lavage
Law's position

Le Dran's suture
Le Fort's suture
leiomyoma
leiomyomata
Leksell's
    forceps
    rongeur
Lembert's suture
Lempert's incision
Lempka's stripper
Lent's laparoscope
lesion
leukonychia
Levin's tube
Lieberkühn's
    crypts
    follicles
    glands
Lieberman's
    proctoscope
    sigmoidoscope
lien
    l. accessorius
    l. mobilis
lienal
lienculus
lienopancreatic
lienorenal
ligament
    arcuate l.
    Cooper's l.
    gastrocolic l.
    gastrohepatic l.
    gastrolienal l.
    gastrophrenic l.
    Gimbernat's l.
    hepatogastric l.
    Hesselbach's l.
    inguinal l.
    lacunar l.
    lienorenal l.
    pancreaticosplenic l.
    pectineal l.
    phrenicocolic l.
    phrenicolienal l.
    phrenicosplenic l.
    Poupart's l.

ligament (continued)
    splenocolic l.
    splenorenal l.
    l. of Treitz
ligation
    high saphenous vein l.
ligature
    McGraw's elastic l.
Lilienthal's incision
Lillie's forceps
Lincoff's sponge
line
    iliopectineal l.
    median l.
    pectinate l.
    pectineal l.
    Spieghel's l.
linea
    l. alba
    l. semilunaris
linitis
    l. plastica
Linton's
    clamp
    hook
    incision
    operation
    retractor
    tube
lipectomy
lipoma
Lister's
    dressing
    scissors
lithotome
lithotomy
lithotony
lithotresis
Littauer's scissors
Little's retractor
Littré-Richter hernia
Littré's
    hernia
    suture
lobe
    Riedel's l.
lobectomy

lobular
lobule
lobulette
lobulus
Lockwood's
    clamp
    forceps
Löffler's suture
Lonquet's incision
Lord's operation
Loreta's operation
Lorfan anesthetic agent
Lotheissen-McVay technique
Lotheissen's operation
Lovelace's forceps
Lower's forceps
Lubafax dressing
Luer-Korte scoop
lumen
lunula
Luschka's crypts
lymphadenectomy
lymphadenitis
lymphadenopathy
    giant follicular l.
lymphosarcoma
Lynch's operation
lyse
lysis
MacDonald's clamp
Macewen's operation
Mackenrodt's incision
Mackid's operation
Madden technique
Maier's forceps
    operation
Maingot's hemostat
Mair's operation
malacotomy
malignant
malpighian bodies
mamilla
mammaplasty
    Aries-Pitanguy m.
    augmentation m.
mammary
mammectomy

mammiform
mamilliplasty
     Ashford's m.
mammogram
mammography
mammoplasia
mammoplasty
maneuver
     Hoguet's m.
Mann-Williamson ulcer
Manson's schistosomiasis
Mantz's dilator
Marcaine hydrochloride
   anesthetic agent
Marcy's operation
Marlex
     bandage
     graft
     mesh
     suture
marsupialization
Martel's clamp
Martin's
     bandage
     forceps
     needle
     retractor
     speculum
Marwedel's
     gastrostomy
     operation
Mason's incision
mastadenitis
mastadenoma
mastectomy
masthelcosis
Mastin's clamp
mastitis
mastocarcinoma
mastochondroma
mastodynia
mastogram
mastography
mastoncus
mastopathia
     m. cystica
mastopathy
     cystic m.

mastopexy
mastoplastia
mastoplasty
mastoptosis
mastorrhagia
mastoscirrhus
mastosis
mastostomy
mastotomy
Mathew's speculum
matrix
Maunsell's suture
maxilla
Maydl's
     hernia
     operation
Mayer's position
Maylard incision
Mayo-Blake forceps
Mayo-Collins retractor
Mayo-Harrington
     scissors
Mayo linen suture
Mayo-Lovelace retractor
Mayo-Noble scissors
Mayo-Ochsner forceps
Mayo-Robson
     forceps
     incision
     operation
     position
     scoop
Mayo-Sims scissors
Mayo's
     carrier
     forceps
     needle
     operation
     probe
     retractor
     scissors
     scoop
     stripper
McArthur's
     incision
     method
     operation

McBurney's
    incision
    operation
    point
McDonald, W. Dean
    clamp
McEvedy's operation
McGraw's elastic ligature
McLaughlin's incision
McNealy-Glassman-Babcock
    forceps
McNealy-Glassman-Mixter
    forceps
McVay's
    incision
    operation
Meckel's diverticulum
mediastinal
mediastinum
medications. See *Drugs and
    Chemistry* section.
Medrafil's wire suture
medulla
medusa
megacolon
megalogastria
Meigs' suture
Meltzer's anesthesia
membrane
    Cargile m.
membranous
Menghini's needle
Mercurio's position
Mermingas' operation
Mersilene
    gauze dressing
    suture
mesenteric
mesenteriopexy
mesenteriorrhaphy
mesenteriplication
mesentery
mesentorrhaphy
mesh
    Marlex m.
    tantalum m.
    Teflon m.
mesoappendicitis

mesoappendix
mesocecum
mesocolon
    ascending m.
    descending m.
    sigmoid m.
    transverse m.
mesocoloplication
mesogastrium
mesorectum
mesosigmoid
mesosigmoidopexy
metastases
metastasis
metastatic
metatarsal
method
    Jenckel m.
    McArthur's m.
    Morison's m.
Metycaine hydrochloride
    anesthetic agent
Metzenbaum's scissors
Meyerding's retractor
Meyer's
    hockey stick incision
    retractor
MFB – metallic foreign
    body
microcalcification
microcalcificectomy
microgastria
microsurgery
Mikulicz's
    clamp
    incision
    operation
Miles' operation
milium
    colloid m.
Miller-Abbott tube
Miller's scissors
Mixter's forceps
Mohrenheim's fossa
Montague's
    proctoscope
    sigmoidoscope
Moore's scoop

Moreno's clamp
Morgagni's foramen
Morison's
    incision
    method
    pouch
Morton's toe
Moschcowitz's operation
motility
Moynihan's
    clamp
    forceps
    operation
    position
    probe
    scoop
mucocutaneous
    m. hemorrhoid
mucopurulent
mucosa
Mueller-Frazier tube
Mueller-Pool tube
Mueller-Pynchon tube
Mueller-Yankauer tube
Muer's anoscope
multilocular
Murphy's
    button
    dilator
    needle
    retractor
    treatment
muscle
    cremaster m.
    deltoid m.
    external oblique m.
    internal oblique m.
    latissimus dorsi m.
    masseter m.
    pectineus m.
    pectoralis major m.
    pectoralis minor m.
    pyramidalis m.
    rectococcygeus m.
    rectus m.
    scalene m.
    serratus anterior m.

muscle (continued)
    serratus magnus m.
    sternohyoid m.
    sternothyroid m.
    subscapularis m.
    transversus m.
Myers' stripper
myoma
myomectomy
myotomy
Nabatoff's stripper
Nachlas' tube
Nagamatsu incision
Narath's operation
narcosis
    Nussbaum's n.
narcotic
navel
necropsy
necropurulent
necrosis
necrotic
needle
    Chiba n.
    Childs-Phillips n.
    Craig's n.
    Frankfeldt's n.
    Goldbacher's n.
    Hagedorn's n.
    Jam-Shidi n.
    Keith's n.
    Klatskin's n.
    Martin's n.
    Mayo's n.
    Menghini's n.
    Murphy's n.
    pop-off n.
    Reverdin's n.
    Rochester's n.
    Silverman's n.
    Vim-Silverman n.
Nembutal anesthetic agent
neoplasm
neoplastic
nerve
    hypogastric n.
    iliohypogastric n.

nerve (continued)
    ilioinguinal n.
    phrenic n.
Nesacaine-CE anesthetic agent
neurectomy
    gastric n.
Neurolon suture
nevus
    melanocytic n.
    pigmented n.
Newman's proctoscope
New's
    forceps
    scissors
nipple
    invaginated n.
Nisentil anesthetic agent
Nissen fundoplication
Noble's position
node
    axillary n's
    cervical lymph n's
    Cloquet's n.
    delphian n.
nodular
nodule
    Gamna n's
    Gandy-Gamna n's
nonfunctioning
nonperforating
Northbent's scissors
Norwood's snare
Novocain anesthetic agent
NPO – nothing by mouth (*nil per os*)
Nuck's canal
Nu-gauze dressing
Nupercaine hydrochloride anesthetic agent
Nussbaum's
    clamp
    narcosis
Nuttall's operation
O'Beirne's
    sphincter
    tube

Oberst's operation
oblique
    external o.
    internal o.
obliteration
obstruction
    intestinal o.
obturator
    Cripps' o.
occlusion
    enteromesenteric o.
occult
Ochsner-Dixon forceps
Ochsner's
    clamp
    forceps
    scissors
    tube
Oddi's sphincter
Ogilvie's operation
Ollier's incision
omentectomy
omentopexy
omentoplasty
omentorrhaphy
omentosplenopexy
omentotomy
omentum
    gastrocolic o.
    gastrohepatic o.
    gastrosplenic o.
    splenogastric o.
omphalectomy
omphalelcosis
omphalic
omphalitis
omphalocele
onychauxis
onychectomy
onychia
onychomycosis
onychorrhexis
onychotomy
operable
operation
    Abbe-Estlander o.
    Abbe's o.

operation (continued)

Abernethy's o.
Adams' o.
Alexander's o.
Allarton's o.
Allingham's o.
Amussat's o.
Andrews' o.
Anson-McVay o.
Appolito's o.
Armsby's o.
Babcock's o.
Ball's o.
Bassini's o.
Battle's o.
Baynton's o.
Beatson's o.
Belmas' o.
Best's o.
Bevans' o.
Beyea's o.
Biesenberger's o.
Billroth's o.
Bircher's o.
Blalock-Hanlon o.
Blalock-Taussig o.
Bloodgood's o.
Bobb's o.
Bogue's o.
Bose's o.
Brenner's o.
Bricker's o.
Brunschwig's o.
Bryant's o.
Callisen's o.
Cattell's o.
Chaput's o.
Cheyne's o.
Chiazzi's o.
Child's o.
Clagett's o.
Cooper's o.
Cotting's o.
Cripps' o.
Czerny's o.
Dallas' o.
Denans' o.

operation (continued)

Dieffenbach's o.
Dowell's o.
Drummond-Morison o.
Ekehorn's o.
Ferguson-Coley o.
Ferguson's o.
Finney's o.
Frank's o.
Fredet-Ramstedt o.
Freund's o.
Gallie's o.
Gersuny's o.
Gill's o.
Graham-Roscie o.
Grondahl-Finney o.
Gussenbauer's o.
Hahn's o.
Halsted's o.
Handley's o.
Heaton's o.
Heineke-Mikulicz o.
Heineke's o.
Heller's o.
Henry's o.
Hey-Grooves o.
Hochenegg's o.
Hoguet's o.
Hopkins' o.
Hotchkiss' o.
Hunt's o.
interval o.
Jaboulay's o.
Jelk's o.
Jonnesco's o.
Kader-Senn o.
Keel's o.
Keen's o.
Kocher's o.
Kondoleon o.
Kraske's o.
Lahey's o.
Lane's o.
Linton's o.
Lord's o.
Loreta's o.

operation (continued)
Lotheissen's o.
Lynch's o.
Macewen's o.
Mackid's o.
Mair's o.
Marcy's o.
Marwedel's o.
Maydl's o.
Mayo-Robson o.
Mayo's o.
McArthur's o.
McBurney's o.
McEvedy's o.
McVay's o.
Mermingas' o.
Mikulicz's o.
Miles' o.
Moschcowitz's o.
Moynihan's o.
Narath's o.
Nuttall's o.
Oberst's o.
Ogilvie's o.
Pirogoff's o.
Polya's o.
Poth's o.
radical o.
Ramstedt's o.
Rehn-Delorme o.
Rose's o.
Routier's o.
Roux-en-Y o.
Scarpa's o.
Schede's o.
Schlatter's o.
Senn's o.
Sotteau's o.
State o.
subcutaneous o.
Swenson's o.
Talma's o.
Tanner's o.
Tansini's o.
Textor's o.
Thiersch's o.
Torek's o.

operation (continued)
Travel's o.
Trendelenburg's o.
Treves' o.
Turner's o.
van Buren's o.
Vermale's o.
Verneuil's o.
Vidal's o.
Wangensteen's o.
Warren's o.
Watson's o.
Waugh's o.
Weir's o.
Whipple's o.
Whitehead's o.
Winiwarter's o.
Wise's o.
Witzel's o.
Wölfler's o.
Wützer's o.
Wyeth's o.
Wyllys-Andrews o.
Zieman's o.
Zimmerman's o.
Z-plasty
Ophthaine anesthetic agent
OR – operating room
organomegaly
Orr's incision
os pubis
O'Sullivan-O'Connor retractor
O'Sullivan's retractor
Otis' anoscope
Ottenheimer's dilator
Owen's position
Oxaine anesthetic agent
Oxycel pack
oxygen
    o. therapy
oxygenation
oxygenator
oxyuriasis
Oxyuris
    O. vermicularis
Pagenstecher's linen thread
Palfyn's suture

palliate
palliative
palma
p. manus
palmar
palpation
pampiniform
Pancoast's suture
pancolectomy
pancreas
aberrant p.
accessory p.
p. divisum
Willis' p.
Winslow's p.
pancreatectomy
pancreatic
pancreaticoduodenostomy
pancreaticoenterostomy
pancreaticogastrostomy
pancreaticojejunostomy
pancreaticosplenic
pancreatitis
pancreatoduodenectomy
pancreatoduodenostomy
pancreatoenterostomy
pancreatography
pancreatolithectomy
pancreatolithotomy
pancreatotomy
pancreolithotomy
panniculus
panproctocolectomy
Panzer's scissors
papilla
p. of Vater
papillae
papillary
papillate
papillectomy
papilloma
papillosphincterotomy
paracentesis
abdominal p.
p. abdominis
p. vesicae
parathyroid

parathyroidectomy
Paré's suture
parenchyma
paries
parietal
parietes
Parker-Kerr
"basting stitch"
enteroenterostomy
forceps
suture
Parker's
clamp
incision
retractor
Parkinson's position
paronychia
parotid
parotidectomy
parotitis
pars
p. pylorica
p. superior duodeni
paste
Unna's p.
patency
patent
patulous
Paul-Mixter tube
Payr's clamp
Péan's
clamp
forceps
incision
position
peau d'orange
pectenotomy
pectineal
pectoral
pectoralis
pedicle
peduncle
pedunculated
pelvis
Pemberton's clamp
pendulous

Pennington's
   clamp
   forceps
   speculum
Penrose drain
Penthrane anesthetic agent
Pentothal anesthetic agent
peptic
Percaine anesthetic agent
percutaneous
Percy's forceps
perforation
perianal
periappendicitis
perigastric
perineal
perineorrhaphy
perineum
periphery
perirectal
peristalsis
peristaltic
peritoneal
peritonealize
peritoneocentesis
peritoneoclysis
peritoneography
peritoneoplasty
peritoneoscope
      Wolf's p.
peritoneoscopy
peritoneotomy
peritoneum
    parietal p.
    visceral p.
peritonitis
peritonization
peritonize
perityphlitis
    p. actinomycotica
periumbilical
per primam intentionem
Perthes' incision
Petit's
   hernia
   suture
Pfannenstiel's incision

phalanx
Phemister's incision
pheochromocytoma
Phillips' clamp
phlebectomy
phlebitis
phlebolith
phlebolithiasis
phleboplasty
phlebosclerosis
phlebothrombosis
phlebotomy
phlegmon
phrenemphraxis
phrenic
phrenicectomized
phrenicectomy
phreniclasis
phrenicoexeresis
phreniconeurectomy
phrenicotomy
phrenicotripsy
phytobezoar
pillar
pilonidal
pinealectomy
pinealoma
Pirogoff's operation
pituitectomy
plantar
platysma
pledget
plexus
    brachial p.
    pampiniform p.
plica
    p. duodenalis
    p. duodenojejunalis
    p. duodenomesocolica
    p. epigastrica
    p. gastropancreatica
    p. ileocecalis
    p. paraduodenalis
    p. umbilicalis
plication
plombage

plug
    p. gastrostomy
po dorahnj. See *peau d'orange.*
point
    Hartmann's p.
    McBurney's p.
pollicization
Polya's
    gastroenterostomy
    operation
Polydek suture
polyethylene
polyp
polypectomy
polypoid
polyposis
    p. gastrica
    p. intestinalis
    p. ventriculi
polypotome
polyunguia
Ponka technique
pons
    p. hepatis
Pontocaine anesthetic agent
Pool's tube
porta
    p. hepatis
    p. lienis
portacaval
portal
    intestinal p.
Porter's forceps
position
    Adams' p.
    Albert's p.
    anatomical p.
    arm-extension p.
    Bonner's p.
    Boyce's p.
    Bozeman's p.
    Buie's p.
    Caldwell's p.
    Casselberry's p.
    coiled p.
    decortical p.
    decubitus p.
    Depage's p.

position (continued)
    dorsal p.
    dorsal elevated p.
    dorsal inertia p.
    dorsal lithotomy p.
    dorsal recumbent p.
    dorsal rigid p.
    dorsodecubitus p.
    dorsolithotomy p.
    dorsorecumbent p.
    dorsosacral p.
    dorsosupine p.
    Duncan's p.
    Edebohls' p.
    Elliot's p.
    emprosthotonos p.
    fetal p.
    Fowler's p.
    frog-legged p.
    Fuchs' p.
    genucubital p.
    genufacial p.
    genupectoral p.
    head dependent p.
    hinge p.
    horizontal p.
    hornpipe p.
    jackknife p.
    Jones' p.
    Jonge's p.
    kidney p.
    knee-chest p.
    knee-elbow p.
    kneeling-squatting p.
    Kraske's p.
    lateral decubitus p.
    lateral prone p.
    lateral recumbent p.
    Law's p.
    leapfrog p.
    lithotomy p.
    Mayer's p.
    Mayo-Robson p.
    Mercurio's .
    Moynihan's p.
    neck extension p.
    Noble's p.

position (continued)
    opisthotonos p.
    orthopnea p.
    orthotonos p.
    Owen's p.
    Parkinson's p.
    Péan's p.
    Proetz's p.
    prone p.
    Robson's p.
    Rose's p.
    Samuel's p.
    Schüller's p.
    Scultetus' p.
    semi-Fowler p.
    semiprone p.
    semireclining p.
    shoe-and-stocking p.
    Simon's p.
    Sims' p.
    Stenver's p.
    Stern's p.
    supine p.
    Trendelenburg's p.
    upright p.
    Valentine's p.
    Walcher's p.
    Waters-Waldron p.
    Wolfenden's p.
Poth's operation
Pott's
    clamp
Potts-Smith
    forceps
    scissors
pouch
    Hartmann's p.
    Morison's p.
Poupart's
    ligament
    shelving edge, of P's
      ligament
Pratt-Smith forceps
Pratt's
    anoscope
    director
    hook
    probe

Pratt's (continued)
    scissors
    speculum
prepped and draped
probe
    Barr's p.
    Buie's p.
    Desjardin's p.
    Earle's p.
    Fenger's p.
    Kron's p.
    Larry's p.
    Mayo's p.
    Moynihan's p.
    Pratt's p.
    Welch-Allyn p.
procedure
    Buie's p.
    DuVal's p.
    Puestow-Gillesby p.
procidentia
proctalgia
    p. fugax
proctectasia
proctectomy
procteurynter
procteurysis
proctitis
proctococcypexy
proctocolectomy
proctocolitis
proctocolpoplasty
proctocystoplasty
proctocystotomy
procto-elytroplasty
proctologic
proctology
proctoperineoplasty
proctopexy
proctoplasty
proctoptosis
proctorrhaphy
proctoscope
    ACMI
    Boehm's p.
    Fansler's p.
    Gabriel's p.
    Goldbacher's p.

proctoscope (continued)
  Hirschman-Martin p.
  Hirschman's p.
  Kelly's p.
  Lieberman's p.
  Montague's p.
  Newman's p.
  Pruitt's p.
  Strauss' p.
  Turell's p.
  Tuttle's p.
  Vernon-David p.
  Welch-Allyn p.
  Yeomans' p.
proctoscopy
proctosigmoidectomy
proctosigmoiditis
proctosigmoidoscopy
proctostenosis
proctostomy
proctotome
proctotomy
proctovalvotomy
Proetz's position
prolapse
  rectal p.
prolapsus
  p. ani
  p. recti
proliferation
properitoneal
prosthesis
  Angelchik p.
  Ashley's breast p.
  Heyer-Schulte p.
protrusion
Providence forceps
Pruitt's
  anoscope
  proctoscope
pruritus
  p. ani
pseudocyst
  pancreatic p.
psoas
pubic
pubioplasty

pubiotomy
pubis
pudendal
pudic
Puestow-Gillesby procedure
pulsatile
punch
  Kerrison's p.
punctate
puncture
  epigastric p.
pupil
  Argyll-Robertson p.
Purcell's retractor
purulent
pylon
pylorectomy
pyloric
pyloristenosis
pylorodilator
pylorodiosis
pyloroduodenitis
pylorogastrectomy
pyloromyotomy
  Fredet-Ramstedt p.
pyloroplasty
  Finney's p.
  Heineke-Mikulicz p.
  Horsley's
  Jaboulay's p.
  Judd's p.
  Ramstedt's p.
pyloroptosis
pyloroscopy
pylorospasm
pylorostomy
pylorotomy
pylorus
Pynchon's tube
pyocelia
pyramid
  p. of thyroid
pyramidalis
raclage
radioisotope
rafe. See raphe.
Ramdohr's suture

Ramstedt's
    dilator
    operation
    pyloroplasty
ramus
Rankin's
    clamp
    forceps
Ranzewski's clamp
ranula
    pancreatic r.
raphe
Ratliff-Blake forceps
Raytec gauze dressing
rectal
rectectomy
rectocele
rectorectostomy
rectoromanoscopy
rectoscopy
rectosigmoid
rectosigmoidectomy
rectostomy
rectovaginal
rectovesical
rectum
redundant
Rehn-Delorme operation
reperitonealize
resection
    gastric r.
retinaculum
retractor
    Alm's r.
    Balfour's r.
    Beckman's r.
    Berens' r.
    Berna's r.
    Buie-Smith r.
    Byford's r.
    Cloward's r.
    Cole's r.
    Crile's r.
    Deaver's r.
    Ferguson-Moon r.
    Foss' r.
    Franz's r.

retractor (continued)
    Gibson-Balfour r.
    Goelet's r.
    Gosset's r.
    Green's r.
    Grieshaber's r.
    Harrington-Pemberton r.
    Harrington's r.
    Hill-Ferguson r.
    Israel's r.
    Jackson's r.
    Kelly's r.
    Kerrison's r.
    Killian-King r.
    King's r.
    Klemme's r.
    Kocher-Crotti r.
    Krasky's r.
    Lahey's r.
    Linton's r.
    Little's r.
    Martin's r.
    Mayo-Collins r.
    Mayo-Lovelace r.
    Mayo's r.
    Meyerding's r.
    Meyer's r.
    Murphy's r.
    O'Sullivan's r.
    Parker's r.
    Purcell's r.
    Richardson-Eastman r.
    Richardson's r.
    Rigby's r.
    Rochester-Ferguson r.
    Roux's r.
    Senn's r.
    Sistrunk's r.
    Sloan's r.
    Smith-Buie r.
    Theis' r.
    Volkmann's r.
    Walker's r.
    Walter-Deaver r.
    Webster's r.
    Weinberg's r.
    Weitlaner's r.

retractor (continued)
   Wolfson's r.
retrocecal
retroflexion
retrograde
retromammary
retroperitoneal
retroversion
Reverdin's needle
Richardson-Eastman retractor
Richardson's
   retractor
   suture
Richter's
   hernia
   suture
Riedel's
   lobe
   struma
Rieux's hernia
Rigal's suture
Rigby's retractor
rima
ring
   Abbe's r's
   inguinal r.
Ringer's lactate solution
Risdon's extraoral incision
Ritisch's suture
Rives' splenectomy
Robson's position
Rochester-Ewald forceps
Rochester-Ferguson
   retractor
   scissors
Rochester-Mixter forceps
Rochester-Rankin forceps
Rochester's
   forceps
   needle
Rocky-Davis incision
Rodman's incision
Roeder's forceps
Rokitansky's hernia
Rollet's incision
rongeur
   Kerrison's r.

rongeur (continued)
   Leksell's r.
Roosevelt's clamp
Rosen's
   incision
   operation
Rose's position
rosette
Rosser's hook
Routier's operation
Roux-en-Y
   cystojejunostomy
   jejunal loop incision
   operation
Roux's
   gastroenterostomy
   retractor
   sign
Rovsing's sign
RR – Recovery Room
Rubin's tube
ruga
   r. gastrica
rugae
Rumel's tourniquet
rupture
Russian forceps
Ryle's tube
sac
   hernial s.
   serous s.
saccular
sacculation
sacculus
Saenger's suture
Samuel's position
Sanders' incision
sanguineous
Santorini's duct
saphenectomy
saphenofemoral
saphenous
sarcoid
sarcoma
saucerization
Savary-Gilliard dilator

saw
    Butcher's s.
scalene
scalenectomy
scalenotomy
scalenus
scalpel
Scarpa's
    fascia
    operation
    sheath
    triangle
Schede's operation
Schindler's gastroscope
schistosomiasis
    intestinal s.
    Manson's s.
Schlange's sign
Schlatter's operation
Schobinger's incision
Schoemaker's
    clamp
    gastroenterostomy
Schoenberg's forceps
Schuchardt's incision
Schüller's position
Schutz's forceps
scirrhous
scirrhus
scissors
    Berbridge's s.
    Brooks' s.
    Buie's s.
    Burnham's s.
    Deaver's s.
    DeBakey's s.
    Doyen's s.
    Esmarch's s.
    Ferguson's s.
    Jones' s.
    Jorgenson's s.
    Knowles' s.
    Lister's s.
    Littauer's s.
    Mayo-Harrington s.
    Mayo-Noble s.
    Mayo-Sims s.

scissors (continued)
    Mayo's s.
    Metzenbaum's s.
    Miller's s.
    New's s.
    Northbent's s.
    Ochsner's s.
    Panzer's s.
    Potts-Smith s.
    Pratt's s.
    Rochester-Ferguson s.
    Shortbent's s.
    Sistrunk's s.
    Thorek-Feldman s.
    Thorek's s.
    Vezien's s.
sclerotherapy
sclerosis
    gastric s.
scoop
    Beck's s.
    Berens' s.
    Desjardin's s.
    Ferguson's s.
    Ferris' s.
    Luer-Korte s.
    Mayo-Robson s.
    Mayo's s.
    Moore's s.
    Moynihan's s.
Scribner's shunt
scrotal
scrotectomy
scrotocele
scrotoplasty
scrotum
Scudder's
    clamp
    forceps
Scultetus' position
scybalous
scybalum
sebaceous
Seconal anesthetic agent
section
    frozen s.
semi-Fowler position

Semken's forceps
Senn's
    operation
    retractor
sentinel pile
sepsis
septum
    Cloquet's s.
    crural s.
    s. femorale
serosa
serosanguineous
serositis
serous
sessile
sfinkter-. See words beginning
    sphincter-.
Shallcross' forceps
Shambaugh's incision
sheath
    rectus s.
    s. of rectus abdominis
      muscle
    Scarpa's s.
shelf
    Blumer's s.
Shortbent's scissors
shotty nodes
shunt
    portacaval s.
    postcaval s.
    Scribner's s.
sibah-. See words beginning
    scyba-.
sigmoid
sigmoidectomy
sigmoiditis
sigmoidopexy
sigmoidoproctostomy
sigmoidorectostomy
sigmoidoscope
    Boehm's s.
    Buie's s.
    disposable s.
    fiberoptic s.
    Frankfeldt's s.
    Kelly's s.

sigmoidoscope (continued)
    Kleenspec s.
    Lieberman's s.
    Montague's s.
    Solow's s.
    Turell's s.
    Tuttle's s.
    Vernon-David s.
    Welch-Allyn s.
    Yeomans' s.
sigmoidoscopy
sigmoidosigmoidostomy
sigmoidostomy
sigmoidotomy
sigmoidovesical
sign
    Aaron's s.
    Roux's s.
    Rovsing's s.
    Schlange's s.
    Stokes' s.
    Tansini's s.
    Thomayer's s.
    Toma's s.
    Volkovitsch's s.
    Wachenheim-Reder s.
    Wahl's s.
    Wölfler's s.
    Wolkowitsch's s.
    Wreden's s.
Silastic implant
silicone
Silverman's needle
Simon's
    incision
    position
    suture
Sims'
    anoscope
    position
    speculum
    suture
Singleton's incision
Singley's forceps
sinus
    pilonidal s.
    sacrococcygeal s.

sinus (continued)
 thyroglossal s.
siphon
Sistrunk's
 retractor
 scissors
situs
 s. inversus viscerum
 s. perversus
 s. solitus
 s. transversus
skeletization
skeletonize
Sloan's
 incision
 retractor
sloughing
sluffing. See *sloughing.*
Smead-Jones closure
Smith-Buie retractor
Smith-Peterson incision
snare
 Frankfeldt's s.
 Norwood's s.
sois. See *psoas.*
Solow's sigmoidoscope
solution
 Ringer's lactate s.
Sotteau's operation
Southey's trocar
speculum
 Allingham's s.
 Barr's s.
 Buie-Smith s.
 Chelsea-Eaton s.
 Cook's s.
 David's s.
 Dudley-Smith s.
 Fansler's s.
 Goldbacher's s.
 Guild-Pratt s.
 Hinckle-James s.
 Martin's s.
 Mathew's s.
 Pennington's s.
 Pratt's s.
 proctoscopic s.

speculum (continued)
 Sims' s.
 Vernon-David s.
Spencer Wells forceps
sphincter
 Hyrtl's s.
 O'Beirne's s.
 Oddi's s.
 prepyloric s.
sphincteralgia
sphincterectomy
sphincterismus
sphincteritis
sphincteroplasty
sphincteroscope
sphincteroscopy
sphincterotome
sphincterotomy
 choledochal s.
spicular
spiculated
spicule
spiculum
Spieghel's line
Spivack's gastrostomy
splanchnicectomy
spleen
 accessory s.
splenectomize
splenectomy
 Carter's thoraco-
  abdominal s.
 Federoff's s.
 Henry's s.
 Rives' s.
 subcapsular s.
splenectopia
splenic
splenitis
splenocele
splenocleisis
splenomegaly
splenoncus
splenopexy
splenoportography
splenoptosis
splenorenal

splenorrhagia
splenorrhaphy
splenotomy
splenulus
sponge
    Lincoff's s.
Ssabanejew-Frank gastrostomy
Stamm's gastrostomy
stapler
    TA-30
    TA-55
stasis
State operation
steatorrhea
Steinmann's forceps
stenosis
    pyloric s.
stenotic
Stensen's duct
Stenvers' position
stent
stercoraceous
sterile
sterilely
sterility
sterilize
Steri-strip
Stern's position
sternal
sternum
Stevenson's clamp
Stewart's
    hook
    incision
Stille's forceps
stocking
    Jobst s.
Stokes' sign
stoma
stomach
    dumping s.
    leather bottle s.
Stone-Holcombe clamp
Stone's
    clamp
    forceps
strangulation

Strassmann's forceps
stratum
Strauss' proctoscope
stria
stricture
stripper
    Emerson's s.
    intraluminal s.
    Keeley's s.
    Kurten's s.
    Lempka's s.
    Mayo's s.
    Myers' s.
    Nabatoff's s.
    Webb's s.
    Wilson's s.
stroma
Strombeck's incision
struma
    Riedel's s.
strumectomy
stump
    invaginated s.
Sturmdorf's suture
subareolar
subcutaneous
submammary
subscapular
sudosist. See *pseudocyst.*
sulcus
    s. intermedius
superficial
superficialis
supernumerary
supination
supine
suppuration
suppurative
Supramid suture
Surfacaine anesthetic agent
surgical procedures. See
    operation.
Surgical gauze dressing
Surgiflex bandage
Surgilene suture
Surgilon suture
Surgilope suture

suspension
suture
    absorbable s.
    Acutrol s.
    Albert's s.
    Alcon's s.
    Allison's s.
    alternating s.
    anchoring s.
    angle s.
    Appolito's s.
    apposition s.
    Argyll-Robertson s.
    Arlt's s.
    atraumatic s.
    Atroloc s.
    Axenfeld's s.
    Babcock's s.
    back-and-forth s.
    Barraquer's s.
    baseball s.
    Béclard's s.
    Bell's s.
    biparietal s.
    black-braided s.
    black silk s.
    blanket s.
    bolster s.
    Bozeman's s.
    braided s.
    bregmatomastoid s.
    bridle s.
    bunching s.
    Bunnell's s.
    buried s.
    button s.
    cable wire s.
    capitonnage s.
    cardiovascular s.
    catgut s.
    celluloid s.
    chain s.
    chromic catgut s.
    circular s.
    circumcision s.
    clavate s.
    Coakley's s.

suture (continued)
    coaptation s.
    cobbler's s.
    collagen s.
    compound s.
    Connell's s.
    continuous s.
    corneoscleral s.
    coronal s.
    Cushing's s.
    cushioning s.
    cutaneous s.
    cuticular s.
    Czerny-Lembert s.
    Czerny's s.
    dacron s.
    dekalon s.
    deknatel s.
    delayed s.
    dentate s.
    dermal s.
    Dermalene s.
    Dermalon s.
    Dexon s.
    double-armed s.
    double-button s.
    dulox s.
    Dupuytren's s.
    Duvergier's s.
    edge-to-edge s.
    elastic s.
    Emmet's s.
    Equisetene s.
    Ethibond s.
    Ethicon s.
    Ethiflex s.
    Ethilon s.
    ethmoidomaxillary s.
    everting s.
    far-and-near s.
    figure-of-eight s.
    fixation s.
    Flaxedil s.
    Flexiton s.
    Flexon s.
    free ligature s.
    Frost's s.

suture (continued)

    furrier's s.
    Gaillard-Arlt s.
    Gambee's s.
    Gély's s.
    Gibson's s.
    glover's s.
    Gould's s.
    guy s.
    groove s.
    Gudebrod's s.
    Gussenbauer's s.
    gut chromic s.
    Guyton-Friedenwald s.
    Halsted's s.
    Harris' s.
    helical s.
    hemostatic s.
    horizontal mattress s.
    horsehair s.
    imbricated s.
    interlocking s.
    intermaxillary s.
    interrupted s.
    intradermal s.
    inverted s.
    Ivalon's s.
    Jobert's s.
    Kalt's s.
    kangaroo tendon s.
    Kelly's s.
    Kirby's s.
    Kirschner's s.
    lace s.
    lambdoid s.
    Le Dran's s.
    Le Fort's s.
    Lembert's s.
    ligation s.
    limbal s.
    Littré's s.
    living s.
    locking s.
    lock-stitch s.
    Löffler's s.
    loop s.

suture (continued)

    Marlex s.
    mattress s.
    Maunsell's s.
    Mayo-linen s.
    Medrafil's wire s.
    Meigs' s.
    Mersilene s.
    monofilament s.
    multifilament s.
    multistrand s.
    near-and-far s.
    Neurolon s.
    nonabsorbable s.
    noose s.
    nylon monofilament s.
    over-and-over s.
    overlapping s.
    Palfyn's s.
    Pancoast's s.
    Paré's s.
    Parker-Kerr s.
    pericostal s.
    Petit's s.
    pin s.
    plain catgut s.
    plastic s.
    plicating s.
    plication s.
    Polydek s.
    polyester s.
    polyethylene s.
    polyfilament s.
    polypropylene s.
    presection s.
    primary s.
    Prolene s.
    pulley s.
    pull-out wire s.
    pursestring s.
    quilled s.
    quilted s.
    Ramdohr's s.
    reinforcing s.
    relaxation s.
    retention s.

suture (continued)
  ribbon gut s.
  Richardson's s.
  Richter's s.
  Rigal's s.
  Ritisch's s.
  rubber s.
  running continuous s.
  Saenger's s.
  sagittal s.
  secondary s.
  seminal s.
  seromuscular s.
  seroserosal silk s.
  seroserous s.
  serrated s.
  shotted s.
  silk s.
  silk-braided s.
  silkworm gut s.
  silver wire s.
  Simon's s.
  simple s.
  Sims' s.
  single-armed s.
  sling s.
  spiral s.
  stainless steel s.
  staple s.
  stay s.
  steel mesh s.
  stick-tie s.
  Sturmdorf's s.
  subcuticular s.
  superficial s.
  support s.
  Supramid s.
  surgical s.
  Surgilene s.
  Surgilon s.
  Surgilope s.
  tantalum-wire s.
  Taylor's s.
  tendon s.
  tension s.
  Tevdek s.

suture (continued)
  Thermo-flex s.
  Thiersch's s.
  through-and-through s.
  tiger gut s.
  Tom-Jones s.
  tongue-and-groove s.
  traction s.
  transfixing s.
  transfixion s.
  twisted s.
  Tycron s.
  unabsorbable s.
  uninterrupted s.
  Verhoeff's s.
  vertical mattress s.
  Vicryl s.
  Viro-Tec s.
  visceroparietal s.
  whipstitch s.
  white braided s.
  white silk s.
  wire s.
  Wölfler's s.
  Wysler's s.
  Y-s.
  Z-s.
  Zytor's s.
Swenson's operation
sympathectomy
syndrome. See *Medical Specialty
  sections.*
syngraft
syringe
syringectomy
syringotome
syringotomy
Talma's operation
tamponade
Tanner's operation
Tansini's
  operation
  sign
tantalum mesh
Taylor's suture
T-bandage

technique
    Buie t.
    La Roque's t.
    Lotheissen-McVay t.
    Madden t.
    Ponka t.
    time diffusion t.
    vest-over-pants t.
Teflon
    graft
    mesh
Telfa dressing
tenaculum
    Lahey's t.
tendon
    conjoined t.
tenectomy
tenesmus
tenomyoplasty
tenotomy
Tensilon anesthetic agent
teratoma
testicle
Tevdek suture
Textor's operation
thalamectomy
thalamotomy
Theis' retractor
theleplasty
thelerethism
thelitis
thelorrhagia
thenar eminence
Thermo-flex suture
Thiersch's
    operation
    suture
Thillaye's bandage
Thomas-Warren incision
Thomayer's sign
Thoms' forceps
thoracotomy
Thorek-Feldman scissors
Thorek-Mixter forceps
Thorek's
    aspirator
    scissors

thread
    celluloid t.
    Pagenstecher's linen t.
thrombectomy
thrombophlebitis
thymectomize
thymectomy
thymus
thyroglossal
thyrohyal
thyroid
thyroidea
    t. accessoria
    t. ima
thyroidectomize
thyroidectomy
thyroiditis
thyroidotomy
thyromegaly
thyroparathyroidectomy
thyrotomy
thyrotoxicosis
Timbrall-Fisher incision
tissue
    Gamgee t.
toe
    Morton's t.
toilet
Toma's sign
Tom-Jones suture
Torek's operation
torsion
tortuous
tourniquet
    Rumel's t.
trabeculae
    t. lienis
    t. of spleen
trabecular
tracheostomy
tracheotomy
tract
    alimentary t.
    biliary t.
transduodenal
transection
transfixion

transfusion
transplant
    Gallie's t.
transplantation
transposition
transversalis
transversostomy
Travel's operation
treatment
    Murphy's t.
Treitz's
    hernia
    ligament of T.
Trendelenburg's
    operation
    position
Treves' operation
triangle
    Calot's t.
    Henke's t.
    Hesselbach's t.
    Scarpa's t.
trigone
trigonectomy
Trilene anesthetic agent
Trimar anesthetic agent
trocar
    Allen's t.
    Barnes' t.
    Duke's t.
    Ochsner's t.
    Southey's t.
Tronothane hydrochloride
  anesthetic agent
TSH – thyroid-stimulating
  hormone
T-shaped incision
T-tube
tube
    Abbott-Rawson t.
    Baker's t.
    Buie's t.
    Cantor t.
    Carman's t.
    Cattell's t.
    Chaffin-Pratt t.
    Debove's t.

tube (continued)
    Greiling's t.
    Johnson's t.
    Jutte's t.
    Kelly's t.
    Levin's t.
    Linton's t.
    Miller-Abbott t.
    Mueller-Frazier t.
    Mueller-Pool t.
    Mueller-Pynchon t.
    Mueller-Yankauer t.
    Nachlas' t.
    O'Beirne's t.
    Ochsner's t.
    Paul-Mixter t.
    Pool's t.
    Pynchon's t.
    Rubin's t.
    Ryle's t.
    Wangensteen t.
    Yankauer's t.
tuber
    t. omental
tubercle
    pubic t.
tumor
tumorectomy
tunica
    t. abdominalis
    t. adventitia
    t. albuginea
    t. dartos
    t. fibrosa hepatis
    t. fibrosa lienis
    t. mucosa ventriculi
    t. mucosa vesicae felleae
    t. muscularis coli
    t. muscularis intestini
      tenuis
    t. muscularis recti
    t. muscularis ventriculi
    t. serosa
    t. serosa coli
    t. serosa hepatis
    t. serosa intestini tenuis
    t. serosa lienis

tunica (continued)
    t. serosa peritonei
    t. serosa ventriculi
    t. serosa vesicae felleae
Turell's
    proctoscope
    sigmoidoscope
Turner's operation
Tuttle's
    proctoscope
    sigmoidoscope
Tycron suture
ulcer
    Allingham's u.
    Cruveilhier's u.
    Cushing's u.
    decubitus u.
    Dieulafoy's u.
    duodenal u.
    follicular u.
    gastric u.
    gastroduodenal u.
    gastrojejunal u.
    jejunal u.
    Kocher's u.
    Mann-Williamson u.
    marginal u.
    peptic u.
    perforating u.
    stomal u.
ulceration
ultrasonography
ultrasound
umbilectomy
umbilical
umbilicus
unguis
    u. incarnatus
Unna's paste
unit
    Bovie u.
urachus
U-shaped incision
uthiroid. See *euthyroid.*
vagal
vagotomy
vagus

Valentine's position
valve
    Houston's v.
valvula
    v. ileocolica
    v. pylori
van Buren's operation
varicocele
varicose
varicosity
varicotomy
varix
vas deferens
vasa
    v. brevia
vascular
vasectomy
Vaseline gauze dressing
Vater's
    ampulla
    papilla
vein
    azygos v.
    femoral v.
    portal v.
    saphenous v.
Velcro binder
Velpeau's
    bandage
    hernia
Velroc dressing
vena
    v. cava
venesection
venipuncture
venoperitoneostomy
ventral
ventrocystorrhaphy
verge
    anal v.
Verhoeff's suture
Vermale's operation
vermicular
vermiculation
vermiculous
vermiform
vermifugal

Verneuil's operation
Vernon-David
    proctoscope
    sigmoidoscope
    speculum
verruca
    v. acuminata
    v. digitata
    v. filiformis
    v. plana
    v. plantaris
    v. vulgaris
vesicointestinal
vessel
    circumflex v.
    external pudic v.
    hypogastric v.
    iliac v.
    pudendal v.
    pudic v.
vest-over-pants technique
Vezien's scissors
Vicryl suture
Vidal's operation
Vi-drape
Villard's button
villoma
villus
villusectomy
Vim-Silverman needle
Virden's catheter
Vioform dressing
Viro-Tec suture
Virtus' forceps
viscera
visceral
visceroparietal
visceroperitoneal
visceropleural
visceroptosis
viscerosensory
viscerotome
Vischer's incision
viscid
viscidity
viscus
Vitallium

Volkmann's
    contracture
    retractor
Volkovitsch's sign
volvulus
vomica
Von Bergmann's hernia
von Haberer-Aguirre gastrectomy
von Haberer-Finney
    gastroenterostomy
von Petz's clamp
V-shaped incision
Wachenheim-Reder sign
Wahl's sign
Walcher's position
Waldeyer's colon
Wales' dilator
Walker's retractor
Walter-Deaver retractor
Walter's forceps
Walther's forceps
Wangensteen's
    carrier
    clamp
    colostomy
    dissector
    dressing
    forceps
    operation
    tube
Warren's
    incision
    operation
wart
    plantar w.
Waters-Waldron position
Watson-Jones incision
Watson's operation
Watts' clamp
Watze's forceps
Waugh's operation
Webb's stripper
Weber-Fergusson incision
Weber's
    catheter
    insufflator
Webster's retractor

Weinberg's retractor
Weir's operation
Weisenbach's forceps
Weitlaner's retractor
Welch-Allyn
    anoscope
    forceps
    hook
    probe
    proctoscope
    sigmoidoscope
Wharton's duct
W hernia
Whipple's
    incision
    operation
Whitehead's operation
whitlow
    melanotic w.
    thecal w.
Wilde's incision
Williams' forceps
Willie-Meyer incision
Willis'
    antrum
    pancreas
Wilson's stripper
Winiwarter's operation
Winslow's
    foramen
    pancreas
wire
    Kirschner's w.
Wirsung's duct
Wise's operation
Witzel's
    enterostomy
    gastrostomy
    operation
Wolfenden's position
Wölfler's
    gastroenterostomy
    operation
    sign

Wölfler's (continued)
    suture
Wolf-Schindler gastroscope
Wolfson's
    clamp
    retractor
Wolf's peritoneoscope
Wolkowitsch's sign
Wreden's sign
W-shaped incision
Wützer's operation
Wyeth's operation
Wyllys-Andrews operation
Wysler's suture
Xeroform gauze dressing
xiphoid
Xylocaine with epinephrine
    anesthetic agent
xyster
Yankauer's tube
Y bandage
Yellen clamp
Yeomans'
    forceps
    proctoscope
    sigmoidoscope
Young's dilator
    forceps
Y-suture
Y-type incision
Zachary Cope-DeMartel clamp
Zenker's forceps
Z-flap incision
Zieman's operation
Zimmerman's operation
zister. See xyster.
Zollinger's forceps
Z-plasty
    incision
    operation
Z-shaped incision
Z-suture
Zytor's suture

Drugs and Chemistry

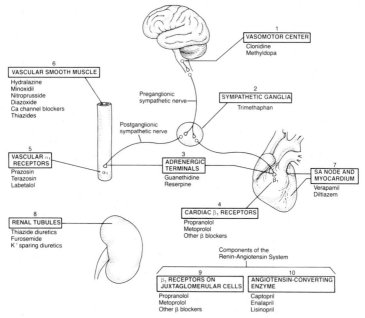

(Courtesy of Lehne, R. A., Crosby, L. J., Hamilton, D. B., and Moore, L. A.: Pharmacology for Nursing Care. Philadelphia, W. B. Saunders Company, 1990.)

Drugs and Chemistry

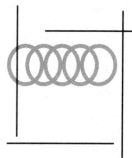

Abbocillin
Abbokinase
acarbose
Accelerase
Accurbron
Accutane
acebutol
acenocoumarin
acenocoumarol
acetaminophen
acetazolamide
acetic acid
acetohexamide
acetohydroxamic acid
acetone
acetosulfone sodium
Acetonide
acetophenazine
acetylcholine chloride
acetylcysteine
acetyldigitoxin
acetylsalicylic acid
Achromycin
    A. V
Achrostatin V
Acidophilus
Acidulin
Aci-Jel jelly
Acnaveen
Acne-Dome
acrisorcin
ACTH – adrenocorticotropic
   hormone
Acthar
Acticort
Actidil
Actifed
actinomycin

actinomycin (continued)
    a. D
Activase
Actrapid
acycloguanosine
acyclovir
Acylanid
Adapin
adenine
    a. arabinoside
adenosine
    a. deaminase
    a. diphosphate
    a. monophosphate
    a. triphosphate
Adipex-P
adrenalin chloride
Adriamycin
adriamycinone
Adroyd
Adrucil
Advil
Aerolone
Aeroseb-Dex
Aeroseb-HC
aerosolized pentamidine
Aerosporin
Afrin
Afrinol
aggregated albumin (human)
aggregated radioiodinated
    (I 131) albumin (human)
    (MAAI 131)
Agoral
A-hydroCort
Akineton
Akrinol
AL-721

alanine
Alba-3
Albamycin
Albatussin
albendazole
Albuminar-5
albumin microspheres (human)
Albumotope ^{125}I, ^{131}I
    A. L-S
albuterol
alcohol
Alconefrin
Aldactazide
Aldactone
Aldoclor
Aldomet
Aldoril
aldosterone
Alerin-TD
Alka-Seltzer
alkavervir
Alkeran
Alkets
allantoin
Allecur
allobarbital
allopurinol
Allpyral
Alpha Chymar
alpha-chymotrypsin
Alphaderm
alpha-difluoro-
    methylornithine
alpha-interferon
Alpha Keri
Alpha 1-thymosin
alphaprodine
alprazolam
alprenolol
alseroxylon
AlternaGEL
Aludrine
Aludrox
aluminum
    a. acetate
    a. hydroxide
    a. nicotinate

aluminum (continued)
    a. phosphate
    a. sulfate
Alupent
Alzinox
amantadine hydrochloride
Ambenyl
Ambilhar
Ambodryl
Amcill
Amen
Americaine-Otic
Amesec
A-MethaPred
amethocaine
Amicar
amikacin sulfate
Amikin
amiloride hydrochloride
aminacrine hydrochloride
amino acid
aminocaproic acid
Amino-Cerv
Aminodur
Aminophyllin
aminophylline
aminopterin
aminopyrine
aminosalicylate sodium
aminosalicylic acid
amiodarone
Amipaque
Amitid
amitriptyline hydrochloride
ammonia
ammonium biphosphate
    a. carbonate
    a. chloride
    a. ichthyosulfonate
    a. mandelate
    a. tartrate
Amnestrogen
amobarbital
amoxapine
amoxicillin
Amoxil
Amphedroxyn

amphetamine
    a. aspartate
    a. saccharate
    a. sulfate
Amphojel
amphotericin B
ampicillin
amrinone
amsacrine
Amsustain
amyl nitrite
Amytal
Anadrol
Ananase
Anaspaz
Ancef
Ancobon
Android
Anectine
    A. Flo-Pack
Anestacon
Anesthesin
Angio-CONRAY (contrast material)
angiotensin
Anhydron
anhydrous
    a. theophylline
anileridine
anisindione
anisotropine methylbromide
anistreplase
Ansaid
ansamycin
Ansolysen Bitartrate
Anspor
A-N stannous aggregated albumin
Antabuse
antazoline
Antepar
anthracycline
Anthra-Derm
anthralin
Antifoam A Compound
Antilirium
Antiminth

Antistine
Antivert
Antrenyl
    A. Bromide
Antrypol
Antuitrin "S"
Anturane
APC with codeine
A.P.L.
apomorphine hydrochloride
apothesine
A-Poxide
Apresazide
Apresoline
    A.-Esidrix
Aquacare
AquaMEPHYTON
Aquaphor
Aquaphyllin
Aquatag
Aquatensen
ara-C (cytosine arabinoside)
Aralen
Aramine
Arco-Lase
Arfonad
arginine glutamate
Argyrol
Aristocort
Aristoderm
Aristospan
Arlidin
Artane
Arthralgen
Asbron G Inlay-Tab
Ascodeen
ascorbic acid
Ascriptin
Asendin
asparaginase
L-asparaginase
aspartame
aspirin
astemizole
Atabrine
Atarax
atenolol

Athemol
Athrombin
Ativan
ATPase
Atromid-S
atropine
    a. methyl nitrate
    a. sulfate
attapulgite
Attenuvax
^{198}Au (gold)
Auralgan
Aureomycin
Aureotope
Auroloid-198
aurothioglucose
AVC cream
Aveeno bath
Aventyl HCl
Avertin
Avitene
azapetine phosphate
azaribine
azatadine maleate
azathioprine
Azene
azidothymidine
azlocillin
azodicarbonamide
Azo-Gantanol
Azo-Gantrisin
Azolid
Azo-Mandelamine
Azotrex
AZT-3′-azido-3′-deoxythymidine
aztemizole
aztreonam
Azulfidine
Azulfidine EN-tabs
Bacimycin
Bacitracin
baclofen
Bactrim
BAL in Oil
Balneol
Balnetar
Banthine

Barachlor
Basaljel
basis soap
BCNU–
    bischloroethylnitrosourea
beclomethasone dipropionate
Beclovent
Belganyl
Belladenal
belladonna
Bellergal
benactyzine hydrochloride
Benadryl
Bendectin
bendroflumethiazide
Benemid
Benisone
Benodaine
benoxaprofen
benoxinate
Bentyl
Benylin
Benzagel
benzalkonium chloride
benzathine
    penicillin G b.
Benzedrine
benzene hexachloride
benzestrol
benzocaine
benzodiazepine
benzoic acid
benzonatate
benzothiadiazine
benzoyl peroxide
benzphetamine
benzthiazide
benztropine mesylate
benzyl benzoate
benzylpenicilloyl-polylysine
Betadine
Betagan
betahistine
Betalin
betamethasone
    b. benzoate
    b. valerate

Betapen-VK
betaxolol
bethanechol chloride
bethanidine
Betoptic
Bicillin
BiCNU
Bilarcil
Bilopaque
Bio-Heprin
Biomydrin
Biozyme-C Ointment
biperiden
    b. hydrochloride
    b. lactate
bipyridine
bisacodyl
bischloroethylnitrosourea
bishydroxycoumarin
bismuth
    b. subcarbonate
    b. subsalicylate
bis-Tropamide
Blefcon
Blenoxane
bleomycin
    b. sulfate
Blephamide
Blocadren
Bonadoxin
Bonine
Bontril PDM
boracic acid
boric acid
Borofax
B & O suppositories
botulinum
Bradosol
Breokinase
Breonesin
Brethine
bretylium tosylate
Bretylol
Brevicon
Brevital
Bricanyl
Bristamycin

bromelain
bromide
bromocriptine
    b. mesylate
bromodiphenhydramine
bromophenol blue
brompheniramine
Brondecon
Bronkaid
Bronkephrine
Bronkodyl
Bronkosol
Bronkotabs
buclizine
Bufferin
bumetanide
Bumex
bupivacaine
Buprenex
buprenorphine
bupropion
Burow's solution
buserelin acetate
buspirone
busulfan
butabarbital sodium
butacaine
butadiene
butambem picrate
butaperazine
Butazolidin
    B. Alka
Butesin Picrate
butethamine
Buticaps
Butisol
butorphanol tartrate
butyl nitrite
Butyn
cade oil
Cafergot
caffeine
Caladryl cream
calamine
Calan
Calcidrine syrup
calcifediol

Calciferol
Calcimar
calcitonin-salmon
calcitriol
calcium carbonate
    c. chloride
    c. fluconate
    c. gluceptate
    c. glycerophosphate
    c. iodide
CaldeCort
Calderol
Caldesene
Calphosan
Cama Inlay-Tab
Camalox
Camoquin
Campho-phenique
camphorated parachlorophenol
Candeptin
Candex
candicidin
canrenoate
canrenone
cantharidin
Cantharone
Cantil
Capastat Sulfate
Capital
Capitrol
Capla
Capoten
capreomycin
capreomycin sulfate
Caprokol
captodiame
captopril
Carafate
carbachol
carbamazepine
carbarsone
carbenicillin disodium
    c. indanyl sodium
carbenoxolone
carbetapentane citrate
carbidopa
carbinoxamine

Carbocaine Hydrochloride
carbol-fuchsin
carbon 11
carbon dioxide
carboplatin
Carbo-Resin
Carboxin
Carbrital
carbromal
Carcholin
Cardilate
Cardiocreme
Cardioquin
Cardrase
carisoprodol
Carmol HC
carmustine
Carnitor
carotene
carphenazine
Cartrax
casanthranol
cascara sagrada
castor oil
Catapres
Cathomycin
Ceclor
Cedilanid-D
CeeNU
cefaclor
cefadroxil
    c. monohydrate
Cefadyl
cefamandole nafate
cefazolin sodium
cefixime
cefmenoxime
cefoperazone
cefotaxime
cefotetan
cefoxitin sodium
cefsulodin sodium
ceftazidime
ceftizoxime
ceftriaxone
Celestone
Cellothyl

celluvisc
Celontin
Cenadex
Cenalene
Centrax
cephalexin
cephaloridine
cephalosporin
cephalothin sodium
cephapirin sodium
cephradine
Cerebro-Nicin
Cerespan
Cerubidine
Cetacaine
Cetaphil
Cetapred
charcoal
Chardonna
chemotoxin
chenodiol
Chestamine
Chlo-Amine
chlophedianol hydrochloride
chloracne
chloral hydrate
Chloramate
chlorambucil
chloramine-T
chloramphenicol
Chloraseptic
chlorcyclizine
chlordane
chlordantoin
chlordiazepoxide hydrochloride
chlorhexidine
chlorhydroxyquinolin
chlormerodrin
    c. Hg 197
    c. Hg 203
chlormezanone
chloroform
Chloromycetin
Chloromyxin
chlorophenothane
chlorophyll
chloroprocaine hydrochloride

Chloroptic-P
chloroquine hydrochloride
chlorothen
chlorothiazide
chlorotrianisene
chlorpheniramine maleate
chlorphenoxamine
chlorpromazine
chlorpropamide
chlorprothixene
chlorquinaldol
chlortetracycline hydrochloride
chlorthalidone
Chlor-Trimeton
chlorzoxazone
Cho-Free
Choledyl
cholestyramine
choline magnesium trisalicylate
Choloxin
Cholybar
chondroitin sulfate
Chorex
chorionic gonadotropin
Chromalbin
chromic phosphate P 32
Chromitope Sodium
chromium Cr 51 serum albumin
chrysarobin
chrysazin
Chymar
chymopapain
Chymoral
chymotrypsin
cimetidine
cinnamedrine hydrochloride
cinoxacin
ciprofloxacin
Circanol
Circubid
cisapride
cisplatin
cis-platinum
cis-retinoic acid
Citanest
citrate of magnesia
citric acid

clemizole
Cleocin
clidinium bromide
clindamycin hydrochloride
Clinistix
Clinoril
Clistin
clofazimine
clofibrate
Clomid
clomiphene citrate
clonazepam
clonidine hydrochloride
Clonopin
clorazepate dipotassium
       c. monopotassium
Chlorpactin XCB
clonazepam
Clonopin
clortermine hydrochloride
clotrimazole
cloxacillin sodium
CMF (Cytoxan, methotrexate,
    5-fluorouracil)
C-MOPP (cyclophosphamide,
    vincristine, procarbazine,
    prednisone)
CoAdvil
cobalamin
^{57}Co, ^{58}Co, ^{60}Co (cobalt)
cobalt
cocaine
       c. hydrochloride
Codalan
codeine
       c. phosphate
Codimal
Cogentin
Colace
ColBENEMID
colchicine
colestipol
colistemethate sodium
colistin
collagenase
colloidal sulfur
Collo Kit

Coly-Mycin
Combid
Combipres
compactin
Compazine
Conestron
Congespirin
Conjutabs
COP (Cytoxan, Oncovin,
    prednisone)
Copavin
copper 62
copper oleate
       c. sulfate
Co-Pyronil
Coramine
Cordran
Corgard
Coricidin
Cor-Tar-Quin
Cort-Dome
Cortef
Corticaine
corticotropin
Cortifar
cortisol
cortisone
Cortisporin
Cortogen
Cortone
Cortril
Co-salt
Cosmegen
cosyntropin
Cotazym
co-trimoxazole
CoTylenol
Coumadin
coumarin
Co-Xan
C-Quins
cranberry juice
Cresatin
cromolyn sodium
crotamiton
Cruex
cryptenamine

crystalline warfarin sodium
crystal violet
Crysticillin
Crystodigin
Cuemid
cupric sulfate
Cuprimine
curare
CVP (Cytoxan, vincristine, prednisone)
cyanocobalamin Co 57, Co 58, Co 60
     radioactive c.
cyclacillin
Cyclaine
cyclamate
Cyclamycin
cyclandelate
Cyclapen-W
cyclizine lactate
cyclobenzaprine hydrochloride
Cyclogyl
Cyclohexane
cycloheximide
cyclomethycaine
Cyclomydril
Cyclopar
cyclopentane
cyclopentolate
cyclophosphamide
cyclopropane
cycloserine
Cyclospasmol
cyclosporin A
cyclosporine
cyclothiazide
cycrimine hydrochloride
Cylert
cyproheptadine hydrochloride
cyproterone acetate
Cystospaz
cytarabine
Cytellin
cytoketatin
Cytomel
Cytosar-U
cytosine arabinoside

Cytotec
Cytoxan
dacarbazine
Dacriose
Dactil
dactinomycin
Dalmane
danazol
Danex shampoo
Danilone
Danocrine
danthron
Dantrium
dantrolene sodium
dapsone
Daranide
Daraprim
Darbid
Daricon
Daro Tablets
Dartal
Darvocet
Darvon
Datril
Daunomycin
daunorubicin hydrochloride
Davoxin
Dayalets
dazoxiben
Deaner
deanol acetamidobenzoate
debrisoquin
Decadron
Deca-Durabolin
Decholin
Declomycin
Declostatin
Decubitex
dehydrocholate
dehydrocholic acid
dehydroemetine
dehydroepiandrosterone
Deladumone
Delalutin
Delatestryl
Delestrogen
Delfen

Delta-Cortef
Deltasone
Deltra
Delvex
demecarium
demeclocycline hydrochloride
Demerol
Demser
Demulen
Dendrid
Depakene
Depen
Depo-Medrol
Depo-Provera
Depo-Testosterone
Deprol
Dermacort
Dermatan
dermatomycin
Dermoplast
DES–diethylstilbestrol
Desenex
deserpidine
Desferal
desferrioxamine
desipramine hydrochloride
deslanoside
desmopressin
desonide
desoximetasone
desoxycorticosterone acetate
Desoxyn
desoxyribonuclease
Desquam-S
Desyrel
deuterium oxide
Devegan
dexamethasone
dexbrompheniramine
dexchlorpheniramine maleate
Dexedrine
dexpanthenol
dextran
dextroamphetamine
dextromethorphan
    hydrobromide
dextropantothenyl alcohol

dextropropoxyphene
dextrose
dextrothyroxine sodium
Diabeta
Diabinese
Diafen
Dialog
Dialose
diaminodiphenylsulfone
Diamox
diamthazole
Dianabol
Diazepam
diazoxide
Dibenzyline
dibucaine hydrochloride
dicarbazine
dichloracetate
dichloralphenazone
dichlorphenamide
dicloxacillin
    d. sodium
       monohydrate
Dicodid
Dicopac
Dicorvin
dicumarol
dicyclomine hydrochloride
dideoxycytidine
Didrex
Didronel
dienestrol
diethylcarbamazine
diethylstilbestrol
    d. diphosphate
diflorasone diacetate
diflunisal
Digitaline Nativelle
digitalis
digitoxin
digoxin
dihydrocodeinone bitartrate
dihydroergotamine
dihydrohydroxycodeinone
dihydromorphinone
dihydrotachysterol
dihydroxyacetone

dihydroxyaluminum aminoacetate
dihydroxystibamidine
diiodohydroxyquin
Diiodohydroxyquinoline
diisopropyl fluorophosphate
Dilantin
Dilatrate-SR
Dilaudid
Dilor
diloxanide
diltiazem
dimenhydrinate
dimercaprol
Dimetane
Dimetapp
dimethindene maleate
dimethisoquin hydrochloride
Dimethpyrindine
dimethyl sulfoxide
Dimocillin
dinitrochlorobenzene
dioctyl calcium sulfosuccinate
     d. sodium sulfosuccinate
Diodoquin
Diodrast
Dionosil
dioxyline phosphate
diphemanil methylsulfate
diphenhydramine hydrochloride
diphenidol
diphenoxylate hydrochloride
diphenylhydantoin
diphenylpyraline
dipivefrin
Diprosone
dipyridamole
Disalcid
Disomer
disopyramide phosphate
disulfiram
dithiazanine iodide
Ditropan
Diucardin
Diulo
Diupres

Diuretin
Diuril
Diutensen
DNCB – dinitrochlorobenzene
dobutamine hydrochloride
Dobutrex
docusate sodium
Dolene
Dolonil
Dolophine
Domeboro
domiphen bromide
domperidone
Donnagel
Donna-sed
Donnatal
Donnazyme
Dopamine
dopexamine
Dopram
Dorbane
Doriden
Dorsacaine
doxapram hydrochloride
doxazosin
doxepin hydrochloride
Doxinate
doxorubicin hydrochloride
doxycycline
doxylamine
Dramamine
Drinalfa
Drize
Drolban
dromostanolone propionate
droperidol
DTIC-Dome
Dulcolax
Duofilm
Duoprin
Duosterone
Duotrate
Duphaston
Durabolin
Duracillin
Duragesic
Duranest

Duraquin
Duricef
Duvoid
Dyazide
Dyclone
dyclonine
Dymelor
Dynacaine
Dynapen
dyphylline
Dyrenium
ecothiophate
econazole
Econopred
Edecrin
edetate
Edrisal
edrophonium chloride
E.E.S.
Efroxine
Efudex
Elase
Elavil
Elixicon
Elixophyllin
Elorine
Elspar
Elutek
emetine
Emetrol
Eminase
Emivan
Empirin
Empracet
Emprazil
Emulave
E-Mycin
enalapril
enanthate
Enarax
encainide
Endep
Endoxin
endralazine
Enduron
Enduronyl
enflurane

Enovid
enoximone
ephedrine hydrochloride
E-Pilo
epinephrine
        e. bitartrate
epinephryl borate
Epitrate
Eppy
Equagesic
Equanil
ergocalciferol
Ergomar
ergonovine maleate
Ergostat
ergotamine tartrate
Ergotrate
erythrityl tetranitrate
Erythrocin
        E. Lactobionate
        E. Stearate
erythrol tetranitrate
erythromycin
        e. estolate
        e. ethylsuccinate
        e. lactobionate
        e. propionate
        e. stearate
eserine
Esgic
Esidrix
Esimil
Eskalith
esmolol
Estar
Estinyl
Estivin
Estrace
estradiol
        e. valerate
Estradurin
estramustine
        e. phosphate
Estratest
estriol
estrogen
Estrone

Estrovarin
Estrovis
Estrugenone
Estrusol
Eta-Lent
Etamon
ethacrynic acid
ethambutol hydrochloride
ethamivan
ethanol
Ethaquin
Ethatab
ethaverine hydrochloride
ethchlorvynol
ether
ethinamate
ethinyl estradiol
ethionamide
ethmozine
ethosuximide
ethotoin
ethoxazene hydrochloride
Ethril
ethyl aminobenzoate
ethylene glycol
ethylenediamine
etidronate disodium
etoglucid
etoposide
Etrafon
etretinate
eucatropine
eugenol
Eumydrin
Eurax
Euresol
Euthroid
Eutonyl
Eutron
Evex
Excedrin
Exna
Extendryl
Exzit
^{18}F (fluorine)
Factorate
famotidine

Fansidar
F-Cortef
Fedrazil
Feldman buffer solution
Femogen
fenfluramine
fenoprofen calcium
fentanyl
Feosol
Fergon
Fer-In-Sol
Fero-Folic-500
Fero-Grad-500
Fero-Gradumet
ferrous
     f. citrate Fe 59
     f. gluconate
     f. sulfate
Festalan
fibrinolysin
Fiorinal
Flagyl
Flavin
flavoxate hydrochloride
flecainide
Fleet enema
Flexeril
florantyrone
Floraquin
Florinef
Floropryl
flucytosine
fludarabine
Fludrocortisone
fludrocortisone acetate
flumethasone pivalate
flunitrazepam
fluocinolone acetonide
Fluonid
fluorescein
fluoride
fluorine
     f. F 18
Fluoritab
5-fluorocytosin
2-Fluoro-2-deoxyglucose
fluorodeoxyuridine

fluorometholone
Fluoroplex
fluorouracil
   5-f.
fluoxetine
fluoxymesterone
fluphenazine hydrochloride
flurandrenolide
flurazepam hydrochloride
flurbiprofen
flurothyl
flutamide
folic acid
folinic acid
Folvite
Forhistal
formaldehyde
formalin
formocresol
Fortaz
foscarnet
fosfestrol
Fostex
Fostril
Fototar
Fourneau 309
frusemide
5-FU – 5-fluorouracil
FUDR – fluorodeoxyuridine
Fulvicin
fumagillin
Fungizone
Furacin
Furadantin
furamide
furazolidone
furocoumarin
furosemide
Furoxone
furtrethonium
gallamine
^{67}Ga (gallium)
gallium citrate Ga 67
gallium-68
Gallogen
Gamastan
Gammagee

gamma globulin
Gammar
Gamimune
Gamulin Rh
ganciclovir
Gantanol
Gantrisin
Garamycin
Gaviscon
Gaysal
Gelfoam
Gelusil
gemfibrozil
Gemonil
gentamicin
gentian violet
Geocillin
Geopen
Gerandrest
Germanin
Gexane
Gifford and Smith buffer solution
Gitaligin
gitalin
Glaucon
glibenclamide
glipizide
Glofil-125
glucagon
glucosamine hydrochloride
glutamic acid hydrochloride
Glutest
glutethimide
glyburide
glycerin
glyceryl guaiacolate
      α-g. guaiacol ether
      g. trinitrate
glycine
glycopyrrolate
Gly-Oxide
Glyrol
gold Au 198
      g. sodium thiomalate
gramicidin
Granulex
Grifulvin V

Grisactin
griseofulvin
Gris-PEG
G-strophanthin
Guaianesin
guaifenesin
guanabenz
guanadrel
guanethidine monosulfate
      g. sulfate
guanfacine
Gustase
Gyne-Lotrimin
Gynergen
Gynetone
Haemate P
Hague solution
Halcion
Haldane
Haldol
Haldrone
Halog
haloperidol
haloprogin
Halotestin
Halotex
halothane
Harmonyl
Hasacode
Hasamal
Hedspa
Hedulin
Hema-Combistix
Hemo-Vite
heparin
Hepathrom
Hep-B-Gammagee
heroin
Herplex
Hesper
hetacillin
Hetrazan
Hexa-Betalin
hexachlorophene
Hexadrol
Hexalet
hexamethonium

hexamethylene
      h. diisocyanate
hexamethylmelamine
Hexamine
hexocyclium methylsulfate
hexylresorcinol
Hippuran
Hipputope
Hiprex
Hismanal
Hispril
Histabid
Histachlor
Histadur
Histadyl
Histalog
histamine
      h. diphosphate
      h. phosphate
Histaspan
Histionex
Historal
Histrey
homatropine
Hormonin
Humorsol
Hycodan
Hycomine
Hycotuss
Hydeltrasol
Hydeltra-T.B.A.
Hydergine
hydralazine hydrochloride
Hydrillyn
hydriodic acid
hydrochloric acid
hydrochlorothiazide
hydrocodone bitartrate
hydrocortisone
      h. sodium succinate
      h. valerate
Hydrocortone
HydroDIURIL
hydroflumethiazide
Hydrolose
hydromorphone hydrochloride
Hydromox

Hydropres
hydroxocobalamin
hydroxyamphetamine
hydroxychloroquine sulfate
hydroxydaunomycin
14-Hydroxydihydrocodeinone
hydroxyethyl cellulose
hydroxymesterone
17α-hydroxyprogesterone
hydroxyurea
hydroxyzine hydrochloride
　　h. pamoate
Hygroton
Hykinone
Hylorel
hyoscine
hyoscyamine sulfate
Hyperab
Hyperstat
Hyper-Tet
hypoxanthine
Hytone
^{125}I, ^{131}I (iodine)
Iberet-Folic-500
Iberol Filmtab
ibopamine
Ibrin
ibuprofen
ichthammol
Ichthyol
idoxuridine
ifosfamide
^{131}I-HSA
Iletin
Ilidar
Ilopan
Ilosone
Ilotycin
　　I. Gluceptate
Ilozyme
^{131}I-MAA
Imferon
imidazole
imipenem
imipramine
　　i. hydrochloride
　　i. pamoate

Immu-G
Immuglobin
immune serum globulin
immunovar
Imodium
Imuran
^{131m}In(indium)
Inapsine
^{113m}In-colloid
indacrinone
indapamide
Inderal
Inderide
indigo carmine
indium
Indocin
indocyanine green
Indoklon
indomethacin
Indon
indoramin
^{111}In-DTPA
Inflamase
INH (isonicotine hydrazine)–
　　isoniazid
Innovar
inosine pranobex
inositol niacinate
insulin
Intal
interferon
interleukin-2
Intron A
Intropin
Inversine
iodinated glycerol
　　i. I 125 fibrinogen
　　i. I 131 aggregated
　　　albumin (human)
　　i. I 125 serum albumin
　　i. I 131 serum albumin
　　　(human)
iodine
　　radioactive i.
iodochlorhydroxyquin
iodohippurate sodium I 131
iodoquinol

Iodotope
iopanoic acid
[131]I-ortho-iodohippurate
ipecac
ipratropium bromide
Iprenol
iridium-191-M
[131]I-rose bengal
Ismelin
isoamyl nitrite
Iso-Bid
isobucaine
isobutylallylbarbituric acid
isocarboxazid
isoetharine hydrochloride
isoflurane
isoflurophate
Isohist
isoleucine
isometheptene
Isomil
isoniazid
isonicotinic acid hydrazide
isoprenaline
Isoprinosine
isopropamide iodide
isopropylarterenol
isoproterenol hydrochloride
        i. sulfate
Isoptin
Isopto Cetapred
Isordil
        I. Tembids
        I. Titradose
isosorbide dinitrate
isothipendyl
isotretinoin
isoxsuprine hydrochloride
isradipine
Isuprel
Ivadantin
ivermectin
Janimine
Jectofer
juniper tar
Kalpec
kanamycin sulfate

Kantrex
Kanulase
Kaochlor
kaolin
Kaon
Kaon-Cl
Kaopectate
Kay Ciel
Kayexalate
KEFF
Keflex
Keflin
Kefzol
Kemadrin
Kenalog
Kenacort
Keralyt
Ketaject
Ketalar
ketamine hydrochloride
ketoconazole
ketotifen
khellin
Klaron
Klor
Klorvess
Klotrix
K-Lyte
Koāte
Komed
Komex
Konakion
Kondremul
Konsyl
Konȳne
K-Phos
krypton Kr 81m
K-Tabs
Kudrox
Ku-Zyme
Kwell
labetalol hydrochloride
LāBID
Labstix
Lacril
LactAid

Lactobacillus acidophilus
lanatoside C
Lanoxicaps
Lanoxin
Largon
Larodopa
Larotid
Larylgan
Lasix
Lassar's zinc paste
lauryl sulfoacetate
lecithin
Ledercillin VK
Lentard
Lente Iletin
Lentopenil
Leritine
leucovorin calcium
Leukeran
levallorphan tartrate
levamisole
levarterenol bitartrate
levocarnitine
levodopa
Levo-Dromoran
Levoid
levonorgestrel
Levophed
Levoprome
levopropoxyphene napsylate
levorphanol tartrate
Levothroid
levothyroxine sodium
Levsin
Librax
Libritabs
Librium
Lidaform
lidamidine
Lidex
lidocaine
    l. hydrochloride
Lidone
Lidosporin
lignocaine
Limbitrol
lime solution

Lincocin
lincomycin hydrochloride
lindane
Lioresal
liothyronine sodium
liotrix
Lipancreatin
Lipo-Hepin
Lipo-Nicin
Liquaemin Sodium
Liquamar
Liquiprin
lisinopril
Lithane
lithium carbonate
Lithonate
LM 427
lobeline
Locorten
Loestrin
Lofenalac
lofexidine
Lomotil
lomustine
Loniten
Lo/Ovral
loperamide hydrochloride
Lopid
Lopressor
Lopurin
lorazepam
lorcainide hydrochloride
Lorelco
Lorfan
Loridine
Loroxide
Losec
Lotrimin
lovastatin
Lowila Cake
loxapine hydrochloride
    l. succinate
Loxitane
Lozol
Ludiomil
Lufyllin
Lugol's solution

Lullamin
Luminal
Lungaggregate Reagent
Lutrexin
lututrin
lypressin
lysergic acid diethylamide (LSD)
lysine
      l. hydrochloride
Lysodren
Lyteers
MAA Kit
Maalox
Macrodantin
Macroscan-131
Macrotec
mafenide acetate
magaldrate
Magan
Magnesia Magma
magnesium carbonate
      m. citrate
      m. gluconate
      m. oxide
      m. salicylate
      m. sulfate
      m. trisilicate
Mandacon
Mandalay
Mandelamine
mandelic acid
Mandol
manganese chloride
mannitol
Mantadil Cream
maprotiline
Marax
Marcaine
Marezine
Marplan
Matropinal
Matulane
Maxair
Maxidex
Maxiflor
Maxitrol
mazindol

Mebaral
mebendazole
mebutamate
mecamylamine
mechlorethamine hydrochloride
Mecholyl
meclizine hydrochloride
meclofenamate sodium
Meclomen
Mediatric
Medihaler-Iso
Medrol
medroxyprogesterone acetate
medrysone
mefenamic acid
mefloquine
Mefoxin
Megace
megestrol acetate
meglumine
Mektec 99
Mellaril
melphalan
menadiol sodium diphosphate
menadione
menaquinone
Menest
Menformon
Menic
Menrium
mepacrine
mepenzolate bromide
Mepergan
meperidine hydrochloride
mephenesin
mephentermine
mephenytoin
mephobarbital
mepivacaine hydrochloride
meprobamate
Meprospan
meprylcaine
meralluride
Meratran
merbromin
mercaptomerin sodium
6-mercaptopurine

Mercodinone
Mercuhydrin
Mercurochrome
mercury, ammoniated
Meromyosin
Merthiolate
Mesantoin
mescaline
Mesopin
mesoridazine besylate
Mestinon
mestranol
Mesulphen
metabutethamine
metabutoxycaine
metaclopramide
metacresol acetate
Metahydrin
Metamine
Metamucil
Metandren
metanephrine
Metaprel
metaproterenol sulfate
metaraminol bitartrate
Metatensin
methacholine
methacycline hydrochloride
methadone
methahydrin
methallenestril
methaminodiazepoxide
methamphetamine hydrochloride
methandrostenolone
methantheline bromide
methapyrilene
methaqualone
metharbital
methazolamide
methdilazine
Methedrine
methemalbumin
methenamine
    m. hippurate
    m. mandelate
Methergine
methicillin sodium

methimazole
methisazone
methixene hydrochloride
methocarbamol
methohexital sodium
Methorate
methotrexate
methotrimeprazine
methoxamine
methoxsalen
methoxyflurane
methscopolamine bromide
methsuximide
methyclothiazide
methyl
    m. isocyanate
methylcellulose
methylcobalamin
methyldopa
methyldopate hydrochloride
methylene blue
methylergonovine maleate
methylparaben
methylphenidate hydrochloride
methylphenylethylhydan-
    toin
methylphenylsuccinimide
methylprednisolone
    m. acetate
    m. sodium succinate
Methyl red – bromothymol blue
    reagent
methylrosaniline
methyltestosterone
methylthionine chloride
methyl violet
methylxanthine
methyprylon
methysergide maleate
Meticortelone
Meticorten
Metimyd
metoclopramide
metocurine iodide
metolazone
Metopirone
metoprolol tartrate

Metrazol
Metreton
metrifonate
metrizamide
metronidazole – misonidazole
metroxamine
Metubine
Metycaine
metyrapone
metyrosine
Mevacor
Mexate
mexiletine
mezlocillin
      m. sodium
MicaTin
miconazole
Micrainin
MICRhoGAM
microNEFRIN
Microsulfon
Midamor
midazolam
Midol
Midrin
Migral
Migralam
milk of magnesia
Milontin
Milpath
Milprem
milrinone
Miltown
Miltrate
Minipress
Minitec
Minizide
Minocin
minocycline hydrochloride
Minotal
minoxidil
Mintezol
Miochol
Miradon
misoprostol
Mithracin
mithramycin

mitomycin C
mitotane
mitoxantrone
Mixtard
Moban
Mobidin
Modane
Moderil
Modicon
molindone hydrochloride
Monistat
Monocaine
Monodral
monosodium glutamate
Monsel's solution
MOPP (nitrogen mustard,
      Oncovin, prednisone,
      procarbazine)
Moranyl
Moricizine
morphine
      m. hydrochloride
      m. sulfate
Motilium
Motrin
Moxalactam
6-MP – 6-mercaptopurine
MPI Iodine 123
MPI stannous diphosphonate
MTX – methotrexate
Mucilose
Mucomyst
Mudrane
Murine
Muro 128
Mustargen
Mutamycin
Myambutol
Mycelex
Mycifradin
Mycitracin
Mycolog
Mycostatin
Mydriacyl
Mylanta
Myleran
Mylicon

Myochrysine
Myodigin
Myophen
Myotonachol
Mysoline
Mysteclin
Mytrex

Nacton
nadolol
Nafcil
nafcillin sodium
Naganol
nalbuphine hydrochloride
Naldecon
Nalfon
Nal I 125
nalidixic acid
Nalline
nalorphine
naloxone hydrochloride
naltrexone
nandrolone decanoate
      n. phenpropionate
naphazoline
Naphuride
Naprosyn
naproxen
Naqua
Naquival
Narcan
narcotine
Nardil
Naturetin
Navane
Nebcin
Nectadon
NegGram
Nembutal
Neo-Antergan
NeoCalglucon
Neo-Cobefrin
Neo-Cortef
Neo-cultol
NeoDECADRON
Neo-Delta-Cortef
Neo-Deltef

Neohetramine
Neo-Hydeltrasol
Neolax
Neolin
Neo-Medrol
neomycin
Neo-Polycin
Neosone
Neosporin
neostigmine methylsulfate
Neo-Synephrine
Neothylline
Nephrox
Neptazane
Nesacaine
netilmicin sulfate
Neutrogena
niacin
niacinamide
nialamide
Niamid
nicardipine
niclosamide
Nico-400
Nicobid
Nicolar
Nico-Metrazol
Niconyl
Nico-Span
nicotinamide
nicotine
nicotinic acid
nicotinyl alcohol
nifedipine
Niferex
nifurtimox
nikethamide
Nilstat
Nipride
niridazole
Nisentil
Nitranitol
nitrazepam
Nitrazine
Nitretamin
nitrobenzene
Nitro-Bid

nitrofurantoin
      n. macrocrystals
      n. sodium
nitrofurazone
nitrogen mustard
nitroglycerin
Nitroglyn
nitroimidazole
Nitrol Ointment
Nitrong Ointment
Nitropress
nitroprusside
nitrosamide
Nitrospan
Nitrostat
nitrous oxide
Nizoral
Noctec
Nolamine
Noludar
Nolvadex
nomifensine
nonoxynol-9
nonvatrone
noradrenaline
Nordette
norepinephrine bitartrate
norethindrone
      n. acetate
Norflex
norfloxacin
Norgesic
norgestrel
Norinyl
Norisodrine
Norlestrin
Norlutate
Norlutin
normeperidine
Normodyne
Norodin
Noroxin
Norpace
Norpramin
Nor-Q.D.
Norquen
nortriptyline hydrochloride

noscapine
Novafed
Novahistine
Novatrin
novobiocin
Novocain
Novrad
Nubain
5-nucleotidase
Nucofed
Numorphan
Nupercainal
Nupercaine
Nutramigen
Nydrazid
nylidrin hydrochloride
Nystaform
nystatin
Obetrol
Ocufen
Ocusert
ofloxacin
Ogen
oleic acid I 125
omeprazole
Omnipen
Oncovin
Ophthaine
Ophthalgan
Ophthetic
Ophthochlor
Ophthocort
opium
Optef
Optilets-500
Oracaine
Orasone
Ora-Testryl
Oratrol
Orenzyme
Oretic
Oreticyl
Oreton
Organidin
Orimune
Orinase
Orlex Otic Solution

Ornade
Ornex
orphenadrine citrate
orthoboric acid
Ortho-mune
Ortho-Novum
Osmitrol
Osmoglyn
Osteolate
Osteoscan
Otrivin
ouabain
Ovcon
Ovral
Ovrette
Ovulen
oxacillin sodium
Oxaine
Oxalid
oxamniquine
oxandrolone
oxantel
oxatomide
oxazepam
ox bile extract
oxethazaine
oxprenolol
Oxsoralen
oxtriphylline
oxybutynin chloride
oxycodone
Oxydess
oxygen
oxymesterone
oxymetazoline hydrochloride
oxymetholone
oxymorphone hydrochloride
oxyphenbutazone
oxyphencyclimine hydrochloride
oxyphenisatin
oxyphenonium bromide
oxypurinol
oxytetracycline hydrochloride
oxytocin
^{32}P (potassium)
PABA – para-aminobenzoic acid
Pabalate

Pabirin
Pagitane
PAM (melphalan) –
    phenylalanine mustard
Pamelor
Pamine
Pamisyl
Panaquin
Pancrease
pancreatin
pancrelipase
pancuronium bromide
Panheprin
Panitol
Panmycin
PanOxyl
Panteric
panthenol
Pantopon
Pantothenylol
Panwarfin
papain
papaverine hydrochloride
para-aminobenzoic acid
para-aminosalicylic acid
paracetaldehyde
paracetamol
parachlormetaxylenol
Paradione
Paradol
Paraflex
Parafon Forte
paraldehyde
paramethadione
paramethasone acetate
Para-Pas
Parasal
Paredrine
paregoric
pargyline hydrochloride
Parlodel
Parnate
paromomycin
PAS – para-aminosalicylic acid
Pathibamate
Pathilon
Pathocil

Pavabid
Pavakey
Paveril
Pavulon
PBZ Lontabs
PBZ-SR
pectin
Pediacof
Pedialyte
Pediamycin
Pediazole
Peganone
pemoline
Penbritin
penicillamine
penicillin
        p. G benzathine
        p. G procaine
        p. V potassium
Pensyn
pentaerythritol tetranitrate
pentagastrin
Pentam 300
pentamidine
        p. isethionate
pentapiperide methylsulfate
pentapyrrolidinium bitartrate
pentazocine hydrochloride
        p. lactate
penthienate bromide
Pentids
pentobarbital sodium
pentolinium tartrate
pentostatin
pentoxifylline
Pentritol
pentylenetetrazol
Pen-Vee K
Pepcid
Pepto-Bismol
Perandren
Perazil
Perchloracap
Percocet-5
Percodan
Percogesic
Percorten

Pergonal
perhexiline
Periactin
Peri-Colace
Peritrate
Permapen
Permitil
Pernox
perphenazine
Persantine
Persistin
Pertofrane
Pertscan
peruvian balsam
PETN (pentaerythritol
    tetranitrate)
Petrogalar
peyote
Pfi-Lith
Phazyme
phenacemide
phenacetin
phenaglycodol
Phenaphen
phenaphthazine
phenazopyridine hydrochloride
phencyclidine
phendimetrazine tartrate
phenelzine sulfate
Phenergan
Phenetron
phenindamine
phenindione
pheniramine
phenmetrazine hydrochloride
phenobarbital
phenol
phenolphthalein
phenol red
phenolsulfonphthalein
phenothiazine
phenoxybenzamine
    hydrochloride
phenprocoumon
phensuximide
phentolamine

Phenurone
phenylalanine mustard
L-phenylalanine mustard
phenylbutazone
phenylephrine hydrochloride
phenylhydantoin
phenylhydrazine
phenylpropanolamine
    hydrochloride
phenyl salicylate
phenyltoloxamine citrate
phenytoin sodium
pHisoDerm
pHisoHex
pHos-pHaid
Phosphocol P 32
Phospholine Iodide
phosphonoformate
phosphorus
Phosphotec
Phosphotope
Phrenilin
Phyllocontin
phylloquinone
physostigmine salicylate
Physpan
phytonadione
picrotoxin
pilocarpine
Pilopine
Pima
pindolol
pipazethate hydrochloride
pipenzolate bromide
piperacetazine
piperacillin
piperazine
    p. citrate
    p. estrone sulfate
piperidolate hydrochloride
piperocaine
piperoxan
pipradrol
Piptal
pirbuterol
pirenzepine
piretanide

piroxicam
piroximone
Pitocin
Pitressin
Pituitrin
pix juniperi
Placidyl
Plaquenil
Platinol
Plegisol
Pnu-Imune
podophyllin
podophyllum resin
Polaramine
poldine methylsulfate
Polycillin
Polycitra
Polycycline
polyestradiol phosphate
polyethylene glycol
Poly-histine
Polymox
polymyxin B and E
Polysporin
Polytar
polythiazide
Poly-Vi-Flor
Poly-Vi-Sol
POMP (prednisone, Oncovin,
    methotrexate, 6-mercap-
    topurine)
Ponstel
Pontocaine
Potaba
potassium
    p. acetate
    p. *p*-aminobenzoate
    p. chloride
    p. gluconate
    p. hydroxide
    p. iodide
    p. perchlorate
    p. permanganate
    p. phosphate
Povan
practolol
Pragmatar

pralidoxime chloride
Pramosone
pramoxine
Prantal
prazepam
praziquantel
prazosin hydrochloride
Pred Forte
Prednefrin
prednimustine
prednisolone
      p. tebutate
prednisone
pregnanediol
pregnanetriol
pregnenolone succinate
Pregnyl
Prelu-2
Preludin
Premarin
Pre-Mens
prenalterol
pre-Pen
Pressonex
prilocaine
Primacaine
primaquine phosphate
primidone
Principen
Prinivil
Priscoline
Privine
prixoline
Pro-Banthine
probenecid
probucol
procainamide hydrochloride
procaine hydrochloride
Procan
procarbazine hydrochloride
Procardia
prochlorperazine
Procholon
procyclidine hydrochloride
Prodox
Profenil
Progestasert

progesterone
Progestin
Progestoral
Proglicem
Progynon
Proketazine
Proklar
proline
Prolixin
Prolixin Decanoate
Proloid
Proloprim
Proluton
promazine
promethazine hydrochloride
Pronestyl
propafenone
propantheline bromide
proparacaine hydrochloride
Propine
Propion Gel
propoxycaine
propoxyphene hydrochloride
      p. napsylate
propranolol hydrochloride
propylbutyldopamine
Propylparaben
propylthiouracil
Prostaphlin
Prostigmin
Protalba
protamine sulfate
Protopam Chloride
protoveratrine A
protriptyline hydrochloride
Provell
Provera
Provest
Prozac
pseudoephedrine
      p. hydrochloride
      p. sulfate
psilocybin
psyllium hydrophilic mucilloid
      p. seed
Pulmolite
Purinethol

Purodigin
Pyocidin-Otic
pyrantel pamoate
pyrazinamide
Pyribenzamine
Pyridium
pyridostigmine bromide
pyridoxal
pyridoxamine
pyridoxine hydrochloride
pyrilamine
pyrimethamine
pyrimidine
Pyrolite
Pyronil
pyrrobutamine
pyrrocaine
pyrvinium pamoate
Quaalude
Quadetts
Quadnite
Quadramin
Quadramoid
Quadrinal
Quadsul
Quan-III
Quarzan
Quelicin
Quelidrine
Queltuss
Questran
Quibron
Quide
Quilene
quinacrine
Quinaglute
Quinamm
quinazoline
Quine
quinestrol
quinethazone
Quinidex
quinidine
    q. gluconate
    q. polygalacturonate
    q. sulfate

quinine
    q. sulfate
Quinite
Quinora
Quintess
Quiphile
Quotane
racephedrine
Rachromate-51
Racobalamin[57]
Racobalamin[60]
radioiodinated I 125 serum
    albumin (human)
        r.s.a. (h.) (IHSA I 125,
        I 131)
radioiodine
radionuclide-labeled 125 I
    fibrinogen (human)
Rafampin
ranitidine
Raphetamine
Raudixin
Rau-Sed
Rautensin
Rautina
Rauwiloid
Rauwoldin
rauwolfia serpentina
Rauzide
Ravocaine
razoxane
Reactrol
Regitine
Regonol
Regroton
Remsed
Renacidin
Renelate
Renese
Renotec (Tc 99m-Iron-
    Ascorbate-DTPA)
Repan
Repoise
rescinnamine
reserpine
Reserpoid

resorcin
resorcinol
Respaire
Restophen
Restrol
retinoic acid
retinol
Retrovir
Rezamid
RhoGAM
ribavirin
riboflavin
rifabutine
Rifadin
Rifaldazine
Rifamate
rifampicin
rifampin
rifamycin
Rimactane
rimantadine
Rimifon
Rimso-50
Ringer's lactate
Riopan
RISA-125-H
RISA-131-H
ristocetin
Ritalin
ritodrine hydrochloride
Robalate
Robamox
Robaxin
Robaxisal
Robenogatope
Robicillin VK
Robimycin
Robinul
Robitussin
Rocaltrol
Roma-Nol
Romilar
Rondec-DM
Rondomycin
Roniacol
rose bengal sodium

rotoxamine
rovamycin
rubidium 81, 82
Rubratope[57]
Rubratope[60]
Rum-K
Ru-Tuss
Rythmol
salbutamol
salicylate
salicylazosulfapyridine
salicylic acid
Salpix
Salrin
salsalate
Saluron
Salutensin
Sandimmune
Sandril
Sanorex
Sansert
Sarapin
Scarlet Red Ointment
ScintiCheck
scopolamine
[75]Se (selenium)
Sebizon
Sebucare
Sebulex
Sebutone
secobarbital
Seconal
Sectral
selenium
    s. sulfide
selenomethionine Se 75
Selsun
Semikon
Semilente Iletin
Semitard
Semoxydrine
senna
Senokot
Septra
Ser-Ap-Es
Serax

Serc
Serenium
Serentil
Serfin
Seromycin
Serpasil
    S.-Apresoline
    S.-Esidrix
Sethotope
Setrol
Sidonna
Sigesic
Silain
Silvadene
silver nitrate
    s. sulfadiazine
Simeco
simethicone
Sine-Aid
Sinemet
Sinequan
Singlet
Singoserp
Sintrom
Sinulin
sitosterols
SK-Pramine
Slo-Phyllin
Slow-K
sodium acetate
    s. bicarbonate
    s. biphosphate
    s. butabarbital
    s. chloride
    s. chromate Cr 51
    s. cyanate
    s. ethylmercuri-
       thiosalicylate
    s. fluoride
    s. hyposulfite
    s. indigotin disulfonate
    s. iodide I 123, I 125, I 131
    s. iodohippurate I 131
    s. iothalamate I 125
    s. levothyroxine
    s. nitrite
    s. nitroprusside

sodium acetate (continued)
    s. oxychlorosene
    s. para-aminohippurate
    s. pentobarbital
    s. pertechnetate Tc 99 m
    s. phosphate P 32
    s. polystyrene sulfonate
    s. rose bengal I 131
    s. salicylate
    s. sulfathiazole
    s. thiosulfate
Softran
Solacen
Solganal
Solu-Cortef
Solu-Medrol
Soma
Somnafac
Somnos
Somophyllin
Sonilyn
sorbitol
Sorbitrate
sotalol
Sparine
sparteine
Spartocin
spectinomycin
Spectrocin
spiramycin
spironolactone
Sporostacin
^{85}Sr, ^{87m}Sr (strontium)
SSKI (supersaturated solution of
    potassium iodine)
Stadol
stanozolol
Staphcillin
Staticin
Statobex
Statrol
Steclin
Stelazine
Stemutrolin
Sterane
stilbestrol
Stilbetin

Stilphostrol
Stoxil
Streptase
streptokinase
streptomycin
streptozocin
Stronscan-85
strontium nitrate Sr 85
strontium Sr 87m
strophanthin
Strotope
strychnine
Suavitil
Sublimaze
succinate
succinylcholine chloride
Sucostrin
sucralfate
sucrose
Sudafed
Sudan IV
Suladrin
Sulamyd
sulfacetamide sodium
Sulfacet-R
sulfadiazine
sulfadoxine
Sulfadrin
sulfamethizole
sulfamethoxazole
Sulfamylon
sulfapyridine
sulfasalazine
sulfathiazole
sulfinpyrazone
sulfisoxazole
    s. diolamine
sulfobromophthalein
sulfonamide
sulfonylurea
sulfosalicylic acid
sulfur
sulindac
sulmazole
sulpiride
Sultrin
Sumycin

Supac
Superinone
Suprax
suramin
Surfacaine
Surfak
Surgicel
Surmontil
Sus-Phrine
Sustaire
Suvren
Symmetrel
Synalar
Synalgos
Synatan
Syncillin
Syncuma
Syndrox
Synemol
Synestrol
Synirin
Synkayvite
Synophylate
Synthroid
Syntocinon
Syntrogel
syrosingopine
Tabron
Tacaryl
TACE
Tagamet
Tagathen
Taka-diastase
Talwin
tamoxifen citrate
Tandearil
TAO – triacetyloleandomycin
    troleandomycin
Tapazole
Taractan
Tavist
Taxol
^{99m}Tc (technetium)
^{99m}Tc-albumin
^{99m}Tc-albumin microspheres
^{99m}Tc-dimercaptosuccinate
^{99m}Tc-DTPA

^{99m}Tc-glucoheptonate
^{99m}Tc-iron ascorbate
^{99m}Tc-MAA
^{99m}Tc-pertechnetate
^{99m}Tc-phosphate
^{99m}Tc-pyrophosphate
^{99m}Tc-sulfur colloid
Tc 99m sulfur colloid
TechneColl
TechneScan MAA
TechneScan PYP
technetated albumin (human)
    lung aggregate
technetium Tc 99 m
        t. Tc 99m aggregated
            albumin
        t. Tc 99m diphosphonate
        t. 99m DTPA
        t. Tc 99m etidronate
            sodium
        t. 99m HSA
        t. Tc 99m medronate
            sodium
        t. Tc 99m pentetate
            sodium
        t. Tc 99m polyphosphate
        t. Tc 99m pyrophosphate
        t. Tc 99m serum albumin
        t. Tc 99m stannous
            pyrophosphate
        t. Tc 99m sulfur colloid
Technetope II
Tedral
Tegopen
Tegretol
Teldrin
Telepaque
Temaril
temazepam
Tempra
Tenathan
Tenex
Tenoposide
Tenormin
Tensilon
Tepanil
terbutaline sulfate

terfenadine
terpin hydrate
Terra-Cortril
Terramycin
Terrastatin
Teslac
Tessalon
Tes-Tape
Test-Estrin
testolactone
testosterone
    t. cypionate
    t. propionate
Testred
Testryl
Tesuloid
tetracaine hydrochloride
tetrachloroethylene
tetracycline
Tetracyn
tetraethylammonium chloride
tetrahydrozoline hydrochloride
Tetrastatin
tetrazine
Tetrex
Tetrodotoxin
Texacort
6-TG–6-thioguanine
thalidomide
thallous chloride Tl 201
Theelin
Thenfadil
thenyldiamine
Theobid
theobrominal
theobromine
        t. magnesium oleate
Theocalcin
Theoclear L.A.
Theo-Dur
Theolair
Theophyl
theophylline
        t. anhydrous
        t. ethylenediamine
Theovent
Thephorin

Theragran
Theratuss
Theruhistin
thiabendazole
thiamine hydrochloride
thiazide
thiethylperazine
thimerosal
thiocyanate
thioguanine
Thiomerin
thiopental
thiopropazate
thioridazine
thiosemicarbazone
thiosulfate
Thiosulfil
Thio-TEPA
thiothixene
thiouracil
Thiourea
thiphenamil hydrochloride
thonzylamine
Thorazine
thrombin
Thrombostat
Thromboxane
thymol
Thymolin
thymosin
thymulin
thyroglobulin
Thyrolar
D-thyroxine
L-thyroxine
^{201}Ti (titanium)
tiapamil
Ticar
ticarcillin disodium
ticlopidine
Tigan
timolol
Timoptic
Tinactin
tincture of opium
Tindal
Tinver

titanium dioxide
Titralac
^{201}Tl (thallium)
tobramycin
    t. sulfate
Tobrex
tocainide
tocamphyl
Toclase
Tocosamine
Tofranil
tolazamide
tolazoline hydrochloride
tolbutamide
Tolectin
Tolinase
Tolmetin sodium
tolnaftate
Tolserol
Topicort
Topsyn
Torecan
TP–testosterone propionate
Tral
Trancopal
Trandate
Transact
transaminase
Tranxene
tranylcypromine sulfate
Trasentine
Travase ointment
Travasol
trazodone
Trecator
Trest
triacetyloleandomycin
triamcinolone
    t. acetonide
    t. diacetate
    t. hexacetonide
Triaminic
triamterene
Triavil
triazolam
tribromoethanol
Triburon

trichlormethiazide
triclobisonium
Tricoloid
Tri-Cone
tricyclamol chloride
Tridesilon
tridihexethyl chloride
Tridione
trientine
triethylenemelamine (TEM)
trifluoperazine hydrochloride
triflupromazine hydrochloride
trifluridine
trihexyphenidyl hydrochloride
Tri-Immunol
triiodothyronine
Trilafon
Trilene
Trilisate
trimazosin
trimeprazine tartrate
trimethadione
trimethaphan camsylate
trimethobenzamide
      hydrochloride
trimethoprim – sulfamethoxazole
Trimeton
trimipramine maleate
Trimox
Trimpex
Tri-Norinyl
Trinsicon
triolein I 131
      t. (glyceryl trioleate) I 131
trioxsalen
tripelennamine citrate
      t. hydrochloride
triprolidine hydrochloride
Trisoralen
trisulfapyrimidine
Triton WR-1339
Tri-Vi-Sol
Trobicin
Trocinate
Trofan
troleandomycin
trolnitrate

Tronothane Hydrochloride
tropicamide
trypsin
L-tryptophan
tubocurarine chloride
Tuinal
Tusquelin
Tussar
Tusscapine
Tussend
Tuss-Ornade
Twiston
tybamate
Tylenol
Tylox
tyloxapol
Tympagesic
Tyramine
tyrosinase
Tyvid
Tyzine
U-Gencin
Ulo
Ultandren
Ultracef
Ultralente Iletin
Ultran
Ultratard
Ultra-TechneKow
Unguentum Bossi
Unipen
Unitensen
Uracid
Ureaphil
Urecholine
Urex
uricosuric
Urised
Urisedamine
Urispas
Uristix
Uritone
Urobiotic-250
urokinase
Uro-Phosphate
Uroqid-acid
Urostat

ursodiol
Usanol
Uteracon
Uticillin VK
Uticort
Utrasul
Vagilia
Vagisec
Valadol
Valisone
Valium
Vallestril
Valmid
Valpin
valproate sodium
valproic acid
Vancocin
vancomycin hydrochloride
vanillic acid diethylamide
Vanobid
Vanocyn
Vanoxide
Vansil
Vaponefrin
Vapo-N-Iso
Vasocidin
Vasodilan
vasopressin
Vasospan
Vasoxyl
V-Cillin K
Veetids
Velban
Velosef
Velosulin
VePesid
Veralba
verapamil
Vergo
Veriloid
Vermox
Versapen
Vesprin
Vibramycin
Vicodin
vidarabine
Vi-Daylin

vimentin
Vinactane
vinblastine sulfate
vincristine
    v. sulfate
Viocin
Vioform
Viokase
viomycin sulfate
Vio-Thene
Vira A
Virazole
Viroptic
Visine
Vistaril
Vistrax
Vita-Metrazol
Vitron-C
Vivactil
Vivonex
Vleminckx' solution
Voltaren
Vontrol
Voranil
Voxin-Pg
Vytone
WANS
warfarin
Wart-Off
Wellbutrin
Westcort cream
white precipitate
Wigraine
WinGel
Winstrol
Wyamine
Wyamycin E
Wycillin
Wydase
Wygesic
Wymox
Wynestron
Wytensin
Xamoterol
Xanax
^{133}Xe (xenon)
Xeneisol Xe 133

Xenon Xe 133
      s. Xe 133 V.S.S.
         (Ventilation Study
         System)
Xerac
Xeroform
Xseb shampoo
Xylocaine
Xylometazoline
Xylo-Pfan
Xylose
^{169}Yb (ytterbium)
Yocon
Yodoxin
Yohimex
ytterbium Yb 169 DTPA
      y. Yb 169 pentetate
         sodium
Yutopar
Zactirin
Zanchol

Zantac
Zarontin
Zaroxolyn
Zephiran Chloride
Zestoretic
Zestril
Zetar
Zidovudine
Zinchlorundesal
Zincon
zinc sulfate
Ziradryl
Zolyse
Zomax
zomepirac sodium
Zorprin
zorubicin
Zovirax
Zyloprim
Zypan

Laboratory Terminology

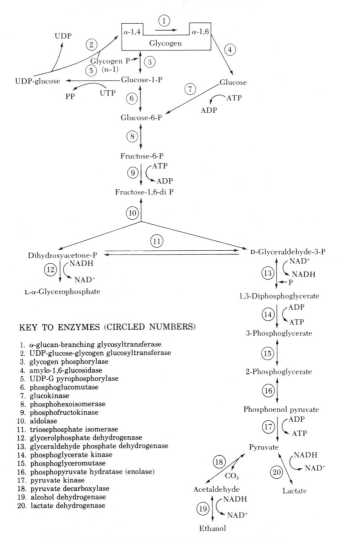

KEY TO ENZYMES (CIRCLED NUMBERS)

1. α-glucan-branching glycosyltransferase
2. UDP-glucose-glycogen glucosyltransferase
3. glycogen phosphorylase
4. amylo-1,6-glucosidase
5. UDP-G pyrophosphorylase
6. phosphoglucomutase
7. glucokinase
8. phosphohexoisomerase
9. phosphofructokinase
10. aldolase
11. triosephosphate isomerase
12. glycerolphosphate dehydrogenase
13. glyceraldehyde phosphate dehydrogenase
14. phosphoglycerate kinase
15. phosphoglyceromutase
16. phosphopyruvate hydratase (enolase)
17. pyruvate kinase
18. pyruvate decarboxylase
19. alcohol dehydrogenase
20. lactate dehydrogenase

EMBDEN-MEYERHOF PATHWAY OF GLUCOSE METABOLISM

(Courtesy of Dorland's Illustrated Medical Dictionary, 26th ed. Plate XLI. Philadelphia, W. B. Saunders Company, 1981.)

Laboratory Terminology
Normal Laboratory Values*

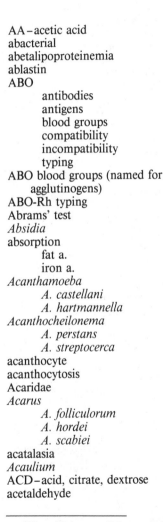

AA – acetic acid
abacterial
abetalipoproteinemia
ablastin
ABO
    antibodies
    antigens
    blood groups
    compatibility
    incompatibility
    typing
ABO blood groups (named for
    agglutinogens)
ABO-Rh typing
Abrams' test
Absidia
absorption
    fat a.
    iron a.
Acanthamoeba
    A. castellani
    A. hartmannella
Acanthocheilonema
    A. perstans
    A. streptocerca
acanthocyte
acanthocytosis
Acaridae
Acarus
    A. folliculorum
    A. hordei
    A. scabiei
acatalasia
Acaulium
ACD – acid, citrate, dextrose
acetaldehyde

acetaminophen
Acetest
Acetobacter
    A. aceti
    A. melanogenus
    A. oxydans
    A. rancens
    A. roseus
    A. suboxydans
    A. xylinus
acetone
acetonemia
acetophenetidin
acetylcholine
acetylcholinesterase
acetyl-CoA
acetylcoenzyme A
acetylcysteine
Acholeplasma laidlawii
Achorion
achroacyte
achromia
Achromobacter
Achromobacteraceae
acid
    acetoacetic a.
    acetylsalicylic a.
    amino a.
    aminolevulinic a.
    argininosuccinic a.
    ascorbic a.
    chloranilic a.
    deoxyribonucleic a.
    diacetic a.
    ethacrynic a.
    folic a.

---

*Normal Laboratory Values section begins on page 198.

acid (continued)
    formiminoglutamic a.
    glucuronic a.
    glutamic a.
    hippuric a.
    homogentisic a.
    homovanillic a.
    hydrochloric a.
    5-hydroxyindoleacetic a.
    lactic a.
    nalidixic a.
    phenylpyruvic a.
    pyruvic a.
    ribonucleic a.
    teichoic a.
    tricarboxylic a.
    trichloroacetic a.
    uric a.
    valproic a.
    vanillylmandelic a.
    xanthurenic a.
acidemia
acid-fast
acidifiable
acidifier
acidify
acidimetry
acidity
acidocyte
acidocytopenia
acidocytosis
acidogenic
acidophil
acidophilic
acidosis
acid phosphatase
acid-Schiff stain
Acinetobacter
    A. anitratum
    A. calcoacceticus
    A. parapertussis
Acladium
Acremonium
Acrotheca pedrosoi
Acrothesium floccosum
ACTH – adrenocorticotropic
    hormone

ACTH test
actin
Actinobacillus
    A. actinomycetem-
        comitans
    A. lignieresii
    A. mallei
    A. pseudomallei
actinochemistry
Actinomadura
    A. madurae
    A. pelletierii
actinomyces
Actinomyces
    A. bovis
    A. israelii
    A. muris
    A. naeslundii
Actinomycetaceae
Actinomycetales
actinomycete
actinomycetic
actinomycin
actinomycosis
actinomycotic
Actinoplanaceae
Actinoplanes
Actinopoda
Actonia
Adamkiewicz's test
ADCC – antibody-dependent
    cell-mediated cytotoxicity
Addis count
adenasthenia
adenine
adenosine
    a. deaminase
    a. diphosphate
adenovirus
adenyl
ADH – alcohol dehydrogenase
    antidiuretic hormone
adjuvant
    Freund a.
Adler's test
ADP – adenosine diphosphate

Aedes
    A. aegypti
    A. albopictus
    A. cinereus
    A. flavescens
    A. leucocelaenus
    A. scutellaris
      pseudoscutellaris
    A. sollicitans
    A. spencerii
    A. taeniorhynchus
Aerobacter
    A. aerogenes
    A. cloacae
    A. lipolyticus
    A. liquefaciens
    A. subgroup A, B, C
aerobe
aerobia
aerobian
aerobic
aerobiotic
Aerococcus
    A. viridans
aerogenic
aerogenous
Aeromonas
    A. hydrophila
    A. liquefaciens
    A. punctata
    A. salmonicida
    A. shigelloides
AFB – acid-fast bacillus
agammaglobulinemia
    Bruton's a.
    Swiss-type a.
Agamodistomum
    A. ophthalmobium
Agamonema
Agamonematodum migrans
A/G ratio test – albumin-globulin
    ratio test
agar
    bile-esculin a.
    bird seed a.
    brain-heart infusion a.
    chocolate a.

agar (continued)
    Columbia blood a.
    corn meal a.
    deoxyribonuclease a.
    DNase a.
    Hektoen a.
    inhibitory mold a.
    lysine iron a.
    mycobiotic a.
    MacConkey a.
    Middlebrook's a.
    nitrate a.
    nutrient a.
    phenylethyl alcohol a.
    potato dextrose a.
    rabbit blood a.
    Sabhi a.
    Sabouraud's dextrose a.
    Salmonella-Shigella a.
    Schaedler blood a.
    Simmons' citrate a.
    thistle seed a.
    trichophyton a.
    triple sugar iron a.
    tryptic soy a.
    urea a.
    Wilkins-Chilgren a.
    xylose-lysine-
          deoxycholate a.
Agarbacterium
agent
    adrenergic blocking a.
    alkylating a.
agglutination
    acid a.
    alpha a.
    bacteriogenic a.
    beta a.
    cold a.
    flagellar a.
    H a.
    immune a.
    intravascular a.
    latex a.
    macroscopic a.
    mediate a.
    microscopic a.

agglutination (continued)
  O a.
  platelet a.
  Rh a.
  salt a.
  spontaneous a.
  T-a.
  Vi a.
  warm a.
agglutinator
agglutinin
  alpha a.
  anti-Rh a.
  beta a.
  chief a.
  cold a.
  febrile a.
  flagellar a.
  group a.
  H a.
  haupt-a.
  immune a.
  latex a.
  leukocyte a.
  Mg a.
  O a.
  platelet a.
  Rh a.
  somatic a.
  warm a.
agglutinogen
aglobulia
aglobuliosis
aglobulism
aglycemia
aglycogenosis
agranulocyte
agranuloplastic
Agrobacterium
ahaptoglobinemia
AHF – antihemophilic
  factor
AHG – antihemophilic globulin
  antihuman globulin
AHT – antihyaluronidase titer
AIDS – acquired immune
  deficiency syndrome. See

Immunology and AIDS
  section.
AIHA – autoimmune hemolytic
  anemia
akaryocyte
akoreon. See *Achorion.*
akro-. See words beginning
  achro-.
ALA – aminolevulinic acid
alamecin
alangine
alanine
albumin
  a. A
  acetosoluble a.
  acid a.
  alkali a.
  a. of Bence Jones
  caseiniform a.
  coagulated a.
  derived a.
  hematin a.
  iodinated serum a.
  normal human serum a.
  Patein's a.
  radio-iodinated serum a.
  serum a.
  a. tannate a.
  triphenyl a.
albuminuria
albumosuria
  Bence Jones a.
  Bradshaw's a.
  enterogenic a.
  pyogenic a.
Alcaligenes
  A. bookeri
  A. bronchosepticus
  A. faecalis
  A. marshallii
  A. metalcaligenes
  A. recti
  A. viscolactis
alcohol
ALD – aldolase
Alder-Reilly anomaly
aldolase

aldosterone
aldosteronism
aleukocytosis
Alginobacter
Alginomonas
alkalemia
alkalescence
alkali
alkaline
    a. phosphatase
alkalosis
    compensated a.
    hypokalemic a.
    metabolic a.
allele
allergen
Allescheria
    A. boydii
alloantibody
Allodermanyssus
    A. sanguineus
allogenic
allotype
alpha
    a. acid glycoprotein
    a.-adrenergic receptor
    a. amino acids
    a. amino nitrogen
    a.-amylase
    a.-amylose
    a. antichymotrypsin
    a. antiplasmin
    a. antitrypsin
    a. band
    a.-beta variation
    a. cells
    a. chain
    a. decay
    a. dinitrophenol
    a.-estradiol
    a.-fetoglobin
    a.-fetoprotein
    a. globulin antibodies
    a.$_1$ globulins
    a.$_2$ globulins
    a. 1,4 glucosidase
    a.-hypophamine

alpha (continued)
    a. ketoglutarate
    a. lipoproteins
    a. macroglobulin
    a. melanocytic-stimulating
        hormone
    a. methyldopa
    a.-naphthol thiourea
    a.-nephthyl acetate
        esterase reaction
    a. particles
    a. protease inhibitor
    a. receptors
    a. seromucoid
    a. streptococcus
    a. thalassemia
    a. trypsin
alpha$_1$
alpha$_2$
alphavirus
Alternaria
Amanita
    A. muscaria
    A. pantherina
    A. phalloides
    A. rubescens
    A. verna
ameba
    coprozoic a.
amebiasis
ameboflagellate
Ames Lab-Tek cryostat
amino
    a. acid
aminoaciduria
aminopeptidase
    leucine a.
aminotransferase
Amoeba
    A. buccalis
    A. cachexica
    A. coli
    A. coli mitis
    A. dentalis
    A. dysenteriae
    A. histolytica
    A. limax

Amoeba (continued)
  A. *meleagridis*
  A. *urinae granulata*
  A. *urogenitalis*
  A. *verrucosa*
amorphous
AMP—adenosine
  monophosphate
amylase
  pancreatic a.
  salivary a.
  serum a.
  urinary a.
amylocast
amyloid
amyloidosis
ANA–antinuclear antibody
anaerobe
  facultative a.
  obligate a.
anaerobia
anaerobian
anaerobiase
anaerobic
anaerogenic
analbuminemia
Anaplasma
Anaplasmataceae
Ancylostoma
  A. *braziliense*
  A. *duodenale*
androgen
androstanedione
androstene
anemia
  aplastic a.
  autoimmune hemolytic a.
  Cooley's a.
  hemolytic a.
  hypochromic a.
  leukoerythroblastic a.
  macrocytic a.
  microcytic a.
  normochromic a.
  normocytic a.
  pernicious a.
  sickle cell a.

anergy
aneuploidy
Angiostrongylus
  A. *cantonensis*
angiotensin I, II, III
angiotensinase
anion
anisocytosis
anisohypercytosis
anisohypocytosis
anisokaryosis
anisoleukocytosis
anomaly
  Alder-Reilly a.
  Pelger-Huët nuclear a.
Anopheles
  A. *maculipennis*
Anoplura
anoxemia
anoxemic
Anthomyia
  A. *canicularis*
  A. *incisura*
  A. *manicata*
  A. *saltatrix*
  A. *scalaris*
Anthomyiidae
  Fannia
  Hydrotaea
  Hylemyia
anthrax
antibiotic
  bactericidal a.
  bacteriostatic a.
  broad-spectrum a.
  oral a.
antibody
  ABO a's
  alloantin-D a.
  anti-acetylcholine
   receptor a.
  antimicrosomal a's
  antimitochondrial a.
  antinuclear a.
  antitubular basement
   membrane a's
  Donath-Landsteiner a.

antibody (continued)
    Duffy a's: Fy^a, Fy^b
    Lewis a's: Le^a, Le^b
anticholinesterase
anticoagulant
anticoagulative
anticoagulin
anticolibacillary
anticollagenase
anticolloidoclastic
anti-DNA
antigen
    ABO a's
    Australia a.
    carcinoembryonic a.
    Diego a.
    E a.
    erythrocyte a.
    H a.
    HLA a's
    Ia a.
    Kell a's
    Kveim a.
    Rh a.
    SD a.
    Vi a.
    von Willebrand's a.
antigen-antibody reaction
antigenic
antigenicity
antigenotherapy
antiglobulin
antihemagglutinin
antihemolysin
antihemolytic
antihemophilic
antiheterolysin
antihyaluronidase
    a. titer
anti-invasin
    a. I
    a. II
anti-isolysin
antilewisite
    British a.
antimicrobial
antinuclear

antistaphylococcic
antistaphylolysin
antistreptococcic
antistreptococcin
antistreptokinase
antistreptolysin
    a. O
antithrombin III
antithromboplastin
antitoxin
aplasmic
aplastic
apoenzyme
apolipoprotein
appliqué form
Apt test
Arachis
    A. hypogaea
Arachnia
    A. propionica
Arachnida
arbovirus
arenavirus
Argas
    A. reflexus
arginine
argininosuccinicaciduria
Argo corn starch test
Arizona
    A. hinshawii
Armanni-Ebstein cell
Arneth count
Arthrographis
    A. langeroni
Arthropoda
arthrospore
arylamine
ASA – acetylsalicylic acid
        argininosuccinic acid
ascariasis
ascaricidal
ascaricide
ascarid
ascarides
Ascaris
    A. lumbricoides
Aschheim-Zondek test

Ascomycetes
ascorbate
ascospore
ascotrophosome
ascus
ASO titer – antistreptolysin O titer
aspartate
aspergillosis
Aspergillus
 A. auricularis
 A. barbae
 A. bouffardi
 A. clavatus
 A. concentricus
 A. flavus
 A. fumigatus
 A. giganteus
 A. glaucus
 A. gliocladium
 A. mucoroides
 A. nidulans
 A. niger
 A. ochraceus
 A. pictor
 A. repens
assay
 biologic a.
 ELISA (enzyme-linked
  immunosorbent a.)
 hemagglutination a.
 immune a.
 immunofluorescent a.
 leukotactic a.
AST – aspartate aminotransferase
Asterococcus
astrocyte
Atelosaccharomyces
ATP – adenosine triphosphate
ATPase stain
atypia
atypical
Auer's bodies
aurococcus
Australia antigen
Australian X disease virus
autoagglutination
autoagglutinin

autoantibody
autoanticomplement
autoantigen
autoantitoxin
autoerythrophagocytosis
autohemolysin
autohemolysis
autoimmune
autoimmunity
autosensitization
aviadenovirus
avipexvirus
AZ test – Aschheim-Zondek test
B cells
Babesia
 B. microti
bacilli
 acid-fast b.
 Battey
bacillus
 b. abortivus equinus
 Bang's b.
 Boas-Oppler b.
 Bordet-Gengou b.
 Calmette-Guérin b.
 Döderlein's b.
 Ducrey's b.
 Escherich's b.
 Fick's b.
 Flexner-Strong b.
 Flexner's b.
 Friedländer's b.
 Gärtner's b.
 Ghon-Sachs b.
 glanders b.
 Hansen's b.
 Hofmann's b.
 Johne's b.
 Klebs-Löffler b.
 Klein's b.
 Koch-Weeks b.
 Morax-Axenfeld b.
 Morgan's b.
 Newcastle-Manchester b.
 Nocard's b.
 paracolon b.
 Pfeiffer's b.

bacillus (continued)
    Preisz-Nocard b.
    rhinoscleroma b.
    Schmitz's b.
    Schmorl's b.
    Shiga's b.
    smegma b.
    Sonne-Duval b.
    Strong's b.
    swine rotlauf b.
    timothy b.
    tubercle b.
    typhoid b.
    vole b.
    Welch's b.
    Whitmore's b.
Bacillus
    B. acidi lactici
    B. aerogenes capsulatus
    B. aertrycke
    B. alvei
    B. anthracis
    B. botulinus
    B. brevis
    B. bronchisepticus
    B. cereus
    B. circulans
    B. coli
    B. diphtheriae
    B. dysenteriae
    B. enteritidis
    B. faecalis alcaligenes
    B. influenzae
    B. larvae
    B. leprae
    B. mallei
    B. oedematiens
    B. oedematis maligni No.
        II
    B. pertussis
    B. pestis
    B. pneumoniae
    B. polymyxa
    B. proteus
    B. pseudomallei
    B. pumilus
    B. pyocyaneus

Bacillus (continued)
    B. stearothermophilus
    B. subtilis
    B. suipestifer
    B. tetani
    B. tuberculosis
    B. tularense
    B. typhi
    B. typhosus
    B. welchii
    B. whitmori
bacteremia
bacteria
    gram-negative b.
bacterioagglutinin
bacteriology
bacteriophage
Bacterium
    B. aerogenes
    B. aeruginosum
    B. anitratum
    B. cholerae suis
    B. cloacae
    B. coli
    B. dysenteriae
    B. pestis bubonicae
    B. sonnei
    B. tularense
    B. typhosum
bacteriuria
Bacteroides
    B. corrodens
    B. fragilis
    B. funduliformis
    B. melaninogenicus
bacteroides
Bactometer
Balantidium
    B. coli
bands
Bang's bacillus
Bargen's streptococcus
Barr bodies
Bartonella
    B. bacilliformis
Bartonellaceae
basal metabolic rate

Baso – basophil
basophil
basophilia
basophilic
basophilism
    Cushing's b.
    pituitary b.
Battey bacilli
BEI-butanol extractable iodine
Bence Jones
    albumin
    albumosuria
    protein test
    proteinuria
    reaction
Benedict's test
bentonite flocculation test
benzidine
Bessey-Lowry unit
Beta 1, 2, 2A, 2M, 3
Beta-endorphin
Beta-lactamase
Bethesda-Ballerup Citrobacter
BFP – biologic false positive
BFT – bentonite flocculation
    test
Bifidobacterium
    B. eriksonii
bile
bilirubin
bilirubinemia
bioassay
biosynthesis
biuret
Blastocystis
    B. hominis
Blastomyces
    B. brasiliensis
    B. coccidioides
    B. dermatitidis
blastomycin
blastomycosis
bleeding time
    Duke's method b.t.
    Ivy's method b.t.
blood
    cord b.

blood serum
    Löffler's b.s.
blood urea nitrogen
Bloor's test
Bloxam's test
BMR – basal metabolic rate
Boas' test
Boas-Oppler
    bacillus
    lactobacillus
Bodansky unit
Bodo
    B. caudatus
    B. saltans
    B. urinaria
Bodonidae
body
    Auer's b's
    Barr b's
    Cabot's ring b's
    chromatin b's
    Donovan's b's
    Heinz b's
    Heinz-Ehrlich b's
    Howell-Jolly b's
    Howell's b's
    inclusion b's
    Jolly's b's
    ketone b's
    Leishman-Donovan b's
    Mallory's b's
    Maragiliano b.
    Negri b's
    psammoma b.
    Todd's b.
    X chromatin b's
Bombay phenotype
Bonanno's test
bone marrow
Bordet-Gengou bacillus
Bordetella
    B. bronchiseptica
    B. parapertussis
    B. pertussis
Borrelia
    B. anserina
    B. berbera

Borrelia (continued)
    B. buccalis
    B. carteri
    B. caucasica
    B. duttonii
    B. hermsii
    B. hispanica
    B. kochii
    B. parkeri
    B. persica
    B. recurrentis
    B. refringens
    B. turicatae
    B. venezuelensis
    B. vincentii
Bowie's stain
Bradshaw's albumosuria
bradykinin
Branhamella
    B. catarrhalis
British antilewisite
bromsulphalein
broth
    brain-heart infusion b.
    hippurate b.
    indole-nitrate b.
    Middlebrook's b.
    Mueller-Hinton b.
    nutrient b.
    selenite b.
    thioglycollate b.
    Todd-Hewitt b.
    Voges-Proskauer b.
Brucella
    B. abortus
    B. bronchiseptica
    B. canis
    B. melitensis
    B. suis
Brucellaceae
brucellosis
Brugia
    B. malayi
    B. microfilariae
Brunhilde virus
Bruton's agammaglobulinemia
BSP–bromsulphalein

BUN–blood urea nitrogen
Bunyamwera virus
Busse's saccharomyces
Butyribacterium
Bwamba fever virus
C–centigrade
C_{alb}–albumin clearance
C_{am}–amylase clearance
C_{cr}–creatinine clearance
C_{in}–insulin clearance
C_{pah}–para-aminohippurate
    clearance
C_u–urea clearance
Cabot's ring bodies
Cache valley virus
calcium
calicivirus
California virus
Calliphora
    C. vomitoria
Calmette-Guérin bacillus
calorimetry
Calymmatobacterium
    C. granulomatis
Campylobacter
    C. fetus
Candida
    C. albicans
    C. albidus
    C. guilliermondi
    C. krusei
    C. laurentii
    C. luteolus
    C. parakrusei
    C. parapsilosis
    C. pseudotropicalis
    C. stellatoidea
    C. tropicalis
candidiasis
candidosis
carbon
    c. dioxide
    c. monoxide
carboxyhemoglobin
carboxypeptidase
carcinoembryonic antigen

CANNABINOIDS- Drug testing

Cardiobacterium
    C. hominis
cardiolipin
carotene
carotenoid
Carpoglyphus
    C. passularum
carrier
Casoni's intradermal test
cast
    granular c.
    hyaline c.
    waxy c.
Castellanella
    C. castellani
Castellani's test
CAT – computed axial
   tomography
   – computerized axial
   tomography
Catalpa
catalysis
cataphylaxis
catecholamine
Catenabacterium
CA virus – croup-associated virus
CBC – complete blood count
C cells
CEA – carcinoembryonic antigen
Celebes' vibrio
cell
    acanthoid c's
    alpha c's
    aneuploid c's
    argentaffin c's
    Armanni-Ebstein c.
    B c's
    band c's
    beta c's
    buffy-coated c's
    burr c.
    C c's
    chromaffin c's
    columnar c.
    comet c.
    crenated c's
    delta c's

cell (continued)
    c. differentiation
    c. division
    endothelial c's
    ependymal c's
    epithelial c's
    erythroid c's
    Ferrata's c's
    gamma c's
    Gaucher's c's
    granulosa c's
    H-2^b mouse c's
    HeLa c's
    hilar c's
    Hürthle's c's
    interstitial c's
    islet c's
    Kupffer's c's
    lacunar c's
    Leydig's c's
    lutein c's
    lymphoid c's
    mast c's
    c.-mediated immunity
    mesothelial c's
    metallophil c's
    migratory c's
    monosomic c's
    null c's
    packed c's
    parafollicular c's
    plasma c's
    progenitor c's
    reticulum c's
    sarcogenic c's
    serous c's
    sickle c.
    stem c's
    suppressor c's
    T c's
    target c.
    tart c.
    theca c's
    trisomic c's
    Türk's c.
    zymogenic c's
cellular

Cellvibrio
   C. flavescens
   C. fulvus
   C. ochraceus
   C. vulgaris
centrifugation
cephalin
Cephalosporium
   C. falciforme
   C. granulomatis
Ceph floc – cephalin flocculation
cercaria
ceruloplasmin
cestode
cestodiasis
CF – complement fixation
CF antibody titer
Chagas' disease
Charcot-Leyden crystals
Chediak's test
chemoluminescence
chemotactic
chemotaxis
chemstrip
Cheyletiella
   C. parasitovorax
Chikungunya virus
Chilomastix
   C. mesnili
Chlamydia
   C. oculogenitalis
   C. psittaci
   C. trachomatis
Chlamydiaceae
Chlamydobacteriaceae
Chlamydobacteriales
Chlamydophrys
chlamydospore
Chlamydozoaceae
Chlamydozoon
chloride
chloroleukemia
cholecystokinin
Choleraesuis
   C. salmonella
cholesterol
cholinesterase

chorionic gonadotropin
chromatin
chromatography
chromoblastomycosis
chromomycosis
chromosomal
chromosome
   gametic c.
   Philadelphia c.
   X, Y c.
Chrysops
CHS – cholinesterase
chylomicron
chymotrypsin
CI – colloidal iron
   crystalline insulin
circadian
Citrobacter
   Bethesda-Ballerup C.
   C. diversus
   C. freundii
Cladosporium
   C. carrionii
   C. werneckii
clasmatocyte
Clathrochloris
Clathrocystis
clearance
   blood urea c.
   creatinine c.
   urea c.
Clinitest
clonorchiasis
Clonorchis
   C. endemicus
   C. sinensis
clostridia
Clostridium
   C. acetobutylicum
   C. aerofoetidum
   C. agni
   C. bifermentans
   C. botulinum
   C. butylicum
   C. chauvoei
   C. cochlearium
   C. fallax

Clostridium (continued)
  C. feseri
  C. haemolyticum
  C. histolyticum
  C. kluyveri
  C. multifermentans
  C. nigrificans
  C. novyi
  C. oedematiens
  C. ovitoxicus
  C. paludis
  C. parabotulinum
  C. parabotulinum equi
  C. pasteurianum
  C. pastorianum
  C. perfringens
  C. ramosum
  C. septicum
  C. sordellii
  C. sporogenes
  C. sticklandii
  C. tertium
  C. tetani
  C. tetanomorphum
  C. thermosaccharolyticum
  C. tyrosinogenes
  C. welchii
clotting time
clumping
CMV – cytomegalovirus
CO_2 – carbon dioxide
coagulant
coagulase
coagulate
coagulation
coagulin
coagulogram
cocci
  gram-negative c.
  gram-positive c.
coccidia
Coccidioides
  C. immitis
coccidioidin
coccidioidomycosis
coccidium
coccobacillus

coccobacteria
coccus
Coe virus
colibacillary
coliform
collagen
collagenase
colloid
colloidal gold
colony
Colorado tick fever virus
Columbia blood agar
compatibility
  ABO c.
complement
  c. activation
  c. fixation
complex
  Ghon c.
ConA – concanavalin A
condenser
conglutination
Congo red
  stain
  test
contagium
  c. animatum
  c. vivum
contaminant
conversion
  Mantoux c.
Cooley's anemia
Coombs' test
  direct
  indirect
coprohematology
Copromastix
  C. prowazeki
Copromonas
  C. subtilis
coproporphyria
coproporphyrin
coproporphyrinogen
Cordylobia
  C. anthropophaga
coronavirus
corpuscle

corticosteroid
cortisol
Cortrosyn
Corynebacteriaceae
Corynebacterium
    C. acnes
    C. belfantii
    C. diphtheriae
    C. enzymicum
    C. equi
    C. hemolyticum
    C. hofmannii
    C. infantisepticum
    C. minutissimum
    C. murisepticum
    C. mycetoides
    C. necrophorum
    C. ovis
    C. parvulum
    C. pseudodiphtheriticum
    C. pseudotuberculosis
    C. pyogenes
    C. renale
    C. tenuis
    C. ulcerans
    C. vaginale
    C. xerosis
Coulter counter
count
    Addis c.
    Arneth c.
    reticulocyte c.
    Schilling blood c.
counter
    Coulter c.
counterimmunoelectrophoresis
Coxiella
    C. burnetii
Coxsackie virus
CPK – creatine phosphokinase
C-reactive protein test
creatinase
creatine
    c. kinase
    c. phosphate
    c. phosphokinase
creatininase

creatinine
crenation
CRF – corticotropin-releasing
    factor
crossmatching
CRP – C-reactive protein
cryocrit
cryofibrinogen
cryogammaglobulin
cryoglobulin
cryoglobulinemia
cryoprecipitate
cryostat
    Ames Lab-Tek c.
cryptococcal
cryptococci
cryptococcosis
Cryptococcus
    C. albidus/albidus
    C. albidus/diffluens
    C. capsulatus
    C. epidermidis
    C. gilchristi
    C. histolyticus
    C. hominis
    C. laurentii
    C. luteolus
    C. meningitidis
    C. neoformans
    C. terreus
Cryptostroma
    C. corticale
cryptozoite
crystal
    Charcot-Leyden c's
C & S – culture and sensitivity
CSF – cerebrospinal fluid
CT. See *CAT.*
Ctenocephalides
    C. canis
Culex
Culicoides
culture
    attenuated c.
    blood c.
    chorioallantoic c.
    direct c.

culture (continued)
    flask c.
    hanging-block c.
    hanging-drop c.
    needle c.
    plate c.
    sensitized c.
    shake c.
    slant c.
    smear c.
    stab c.
    stock c.
    streak c.
    stroke c.
    thrust c.
    tissue c.
    tube c.
    type c.
Cushing's basophilism
C virus – Coxsackie virus
cyclase
    adenyl c.
    adenylate c.
cyclic
    c. adenosine
      monophosphate
      (cAMP)
    c. guanosine
      monophosphate
      (cGMP)
    c. nucleotides
cylindroid
cysticerci
Cysticercus
    C. acanthrotrias
    C. bovis
    C. cellulosae
    C. fasciolaris
    C. ovis
    C. tenuicollis
cysticercus
cystine
cytocentrifugation
cytocentrifuge
cytochemistry
cytofluorography
cytogenetics

cytology
cytolysate
    blood c.
cytolysis
cytomegalovirus
cytoplasm
cytotoxicity
DAGT – direct antiglobulin
    test
Dale-Laidlaw's clotting time
    method
dehydrogenase
    isocitric d.
    lactate d. (LDH)
dehydropeptidase
Dematium
Demodex
    D. folliculorum
dengue
deoxyribonuclease
Dermacentor
    D. andersoni
    D. occidentalis
    D. variabilis
Dermacentroxenus
Dermanyssus
    D. avium et gallinae
Dermatobia
    D. hominis
dermatomycosis
Dermatophagoides
    D. pteronyssinus
    D. scheremetewskyi
Dermatophilus
    D. penetrans
Dermatophytin "O"
dermatophytosis
diacetate
Diagnex Blue test
Dialister
    D. pneumosintes
diastase
Dick test
Dicrocoelium
    D. dendriticum
Diego antigen

Dientamoeba
    D. fragilis
differential
difilo-. See words beginning
    diphyllo-.
dilution
dilutor
Dimastigamoeba
p-dimethylaminoazobenzene
dimethyl sulfoxide
dinitrochlorobenzene
Dipetalonema
    D. perstans
diphtheroid
diphyllobothriasis
Diphyllobothrium
    D. latum
    D. parvum
    D. taenioides
diplobacillus
diplobacterium
diplococcus
    d. of Morax-Axenfeld
    d. of Neisser
    Weichselbaum's d.
Diplococcus
    D. pneumoniae
Diplogonoporus
    D. brauni
    D. grandis
dipstick
Dipylidium
    D. caninum
Dirofilaria
    D. immitis
    D. tenuis
dis-. See also words beginning
    dys-.
disease
    Chagas' d.
    Gaisböck's d.
    Gaucher's d.
    Osler's d.
    Schottmüller's d.
    Vaquez-Osler d.
    Vaquez d.

dish
    Petri's d.
Distoma
distomiasis
DIT – diiodotyrosine
DMSO – dimethylsulfoxide
DNA – deoxyribonucleic acid
DNase – deoxyribonuclease
DNase agar
Döderlein's bacillus
Dolichos
    D. biflorus
Donath-Landsteiner
    antibody
    test
Donovania
    D. granulomatis
Donovan's bodies
Downey-type lymphocyte
Dracunculus
    D. medinensis
drepanocyte
drepanocytemia
drepanocytic
Drepanospira
drumstick
Ducrey's bacillus
Duffy antibodies: Fy^a, Fy^b
Duke's method bleeding time
duovirus
D-xylose tolerance test
dye
    aniline d.
dyscrasia
    blood d.
    lymphatic d.
dysdiemorrhysis
dysemia
dysentery
    amebic d.
    bacillary d.
    balantidial d.
    bilharzial d.
    catarrhal d.
    ciliary d.
    ciliate d.
    flagellate d.

dysentery (continued)
    Flexner's d.
    fulminant d.
    malarial d.
    protozoal d.
    scorbutic d.
    Sonne d.
    spirillar d.
    sporadic d.
    viral d.
dysgammaglobulinemia
dyskaryosis
E antigen
eastern equine encephalomyelitis
    virus
Eberthella
EBV – Epstein-Barr virus
ECBO virus – enteric
    cytopathogenic bovine
    orphan virus
ECDO virus – enteric
    cytopathogenic dog orphan
    virus
ECF – extracellular fluid
ECFA – eosinophil chemotactic
    factor of anaphylaxis
ECG – electrocardiogram
echinococcosis
Echinococcus
    E. granulosus
    E. multilocularis
Echinorhynchus
echinosis
Echinostoma
ECHO virus – enteric
    cytopathogenic human
    orphan virus
ECHO 28 virus
ECMO virus – enteric
    cytopathogenic monkey
    orphan virus
E. coli – *Escherichia coli*
ECSO virus – enteric
    cytopathogenic swine
    orphan virus
ectoplasm
EDTA – ethylenediamino-

    tetraacetate
Edwardsielleae
Edwardsiella
    E. tarda
EEE virus – eastern equine
    encephalomyelitis virus
EEG – electroencephalogram
eelworm
Ehrlich's
    reaction
    test
Eikenella
    E. corrodens
EKG – electrocardiogram
ekino-. See words beginning
    echino-.
elastase
electrocardiogram
electrocardiograph
electrochemistry
electroencephalogram
electroimmunoassay
electrolyte
    amphoteric e.
    colloidal e.
    protein e.
    serum e.
electrophoresis
    serum protein e.
ELISA – enzyme-linked
    immunosorbent assay
Ellsworth-Howard test
El Tor's vibrios
eluate
elution
EMC virus –
    encephalomyocarditis
    virus
Endamoeba
    E. blattae
Endolimax
    E. nana
Endomyces
    E. albicans
    E. capsulatus
    E. epidermatidis
    E. epidermidis

endomycosis
endoplasm
endotheliocyte
endotoxin
Entamoeba
    E. buccalis
    E. buetschlii
    E. coli
    E. gingivalis
    E. hartmanni
    E. histolytica
    E. kartulisi
    E. nana
    E. nipponica
    E. polecki
    E. tetragena
    E. tropicalis
    E. undulans
Enteritidis
    E. salmonella
Enterobacter
    E. aerogenes
    E. agglomerans
    E. alvei
    E. cloacae
    E. gergoviae
    E. hafniae
    E. liquefaciens
    E. sakazakii
Enterobacteriaceae
enterobiasis
Enterobius
    E. vermicularis
enterococcus
enteroglucagon
Enteromonas
    E. hominis
enterovirus
enzyme
    serum e.
Eos–eosinophils
eosinopenia
eosinophil
    polymorphonuclear e.
eosinophilia
epidemiology
Epidermophyton

Epidermophyton (continued)
    E. floccosum
    E. inguinale
    E. rubrum
epithelium
Epstein-Barr virus
eratirus. See *Eratyrus.*
Eratyrus
erisip-. See words beginning
    Erysip-.
erithremea. See *erythremia.*
erithro-. See words beginning
    erythro-.
Erwinia
    E. amylovora
Erwinieae
Erysipelothrix
    E. insidiosa
    E. rhusiopathiae
erythremia
Erythrobacillus
erythroblast
erythroblastoma
erythroblastosis
    e. fetalis
    e. neonatorum
erythrocyte
erythrocythemia
erythrocytophagy
erythrocytosis
    leukemic e.
    e. megalosplenica
erythrogenesis
erythroid
erythrokinetics
erythron
erythroneocytosis
erythropenia
erythrophagocytosis
erythropoiesis
erythropoietin
Escherichia
    E. aerogenes
    E. alkalescens
    E. aurescens
    E. coli
    E. dispar

Escherichia (continued)
    E. dispar var. *ceylonensis*
    E. dispar var.
      madampensis
    E. freundii
    E. intermedia
Escherichieae
Escherich's bacillus
esherikea. See *Escherichia.*
esherikiee. See *Escherichieae.*
ESR – erythrocyte sedimentation
    rate
ester
esterase
estradiol
estrogen
estrus. See *Oestrus.*
ethosuximide
etiocholanolone
Eubacteriales
Eubacterium
    E. alactolyticum
    E. lentum
    E. limosum
Euglena
    E. gracilis
euglobulin
eugonic
eumycotic
Euproctis
    E. chrysorrhoea
Eurotium
    E. malignum
Eusimulium
Eutriatoma
Eutrombicula
    E. alfreddugesi
exfoliative
exocrine
exopeptidase
Exophiala
    E. jeanselmei
    E. mycetoma
    E. werneckii
extracellular
extracorpuscular
exudate

F – Fahrenheit
factor
    coagulation f's: I, II, III,
      IV, V, VII, VIII, IX, X,
      XI, XII
    Hageman f.
fago-. See words beginning
    phago-.
FANA – fluorescent antinuclear
    antibody
faneroplazm. See *phaneroplasm.*
Fannia
    F. canicularis
Fasciola
    F. gigantica
    F. hepatica
Fasciolopsis
    F. buski
FBS – fasting blood sugar
Fehleisen's streptococcus
Fehling's test
fenilketonurea. See
    phenylketonuria.
fenistiks. See *Phenistix.*
feno-. See words beginning
    pheno-.
feo-. See words beginning *pheo-.*
fermentation
    mannitol f.
Ferrata's cells
Ferribacterium
ferritin
ferroflocculation
ferrokinetics
Feulgen test
fibrin
fibrinogen
fibrinogenase
fibrinolysin
    seminal f.
Fick's bacillus
Ficoll-Hypaque technique
fiferz. See *Pfeiffer's.*
Filaria
    F. bancrofti
    F. conjunctivae
    F. hominis oris

Filaria (continued)
    F. juncea
    F. labialis
    F. lentis
    F. lymphatica
    F. palpebralis
    F. philippinensis
filariasis
Filarioidea
fisaloptera. See *Physaloptera*.
Fishberg's concentration test
fixative
    Heidenhain's Susa f.
    Zenker's f.
Flagellata
flagellate
flagellum
flavivirus
Flavobacterium
    F. meningosepticum
flebotomus. See *Phlebotomus*.
Flexner-Strong bacillus
Flexner's
    bacillus
    dysentery
flocculation
    cephalin f.
    Ramon f.
floccule
    toxoid-antitoxin f.
flocculoreaction
flora
fluke
    blood f.
fluorescence
fluorometry
Fonsecaea
    F. compactum
    F. pedrosoi
formalin
forme
    f. fruste
fos-. See words beginning *phos-*.
fractionation
fragility
    erythrocyte f.
    f. test

fragility (continued)
    osmotic f.
    red cell f.
Francisella
    F. tularensis
Frei test
Freund adjuvant
Friedländer's
    bacillus
    pneumobacillus
Friedman's test
fructose
FSH – follicle-stimulating
    hormone
FTA – fluorescent treponemal
    antibody
FTI – free thyroxine index
function
    liver f.
Fungi Imperfecti
fungus
furosemide
Fusarium
Fusiformis
Fusobacterium
    F. fusiforme
    F. mortiferum
    F. necrophorum
    F. nucleatum
    F. plautivincenti
    F. varium
fusocellular
fusospirillary
fusospirillosis
fusospirochetal
fusospirochetosis
fusostreptococcicosis
FVC – forced vital capacity
Gaffkya
    G. tetragena
Gaisböck's disease
galactin
galactose
galactosylceramidase
gallium
gamma A, D, E, G, M
gamma globulin

gamma glutamyl transferase
Gärtner's bacillus
gastrin
Gastrodiscoides
Gaucher's
    cell
    disease
GC – gonococcus
    gonorrhea
    granular casts
gemistocyte
gemistocytic
genestatic
genetic
genotype
geotrichosis
Geotrichum
    G. candidum
Gerhardt's test
GFR – glomerular filtration
    rate
GG – gamma globulin
GGT – gamma glutamyl
    transferase
Ghon complex
Ghon-Sachs bacillus
Giardia
    G. lamblia
giardiasis
Giemsa's stain
GLC – gas-liquid chromatography
globulin
    alpha$_1$ g's
    alpha$_2$ g's
    alpha g's
    beta g's
    gamma g's
    immune serum g.
    g. X
Glossina
glucocorticosteroid
glucose
glucosuria
glutamate
glutaminase
glutamine
glutaraldehyde

glycerolization
glycine
Glyciphagus
    G. buski
    G. domesticus
glycogen
glycoprotein
glycosuria
GMP – guanosine
    monophosphate
Gomori's stain
gonadotropin
    chorionic g.
Gongylonema
    G. pulchrum
gongylonemiasis
gonococcus
gonorrhea
G6PD – glucose-6-phosphate
    dehydrogenase
GPT – glutamic pyruvic
    transaminase
gram-negative
gram-positive
Gram's stain
Gram-Weigert stain
granulocyte
granulocytosis
Gravindex test
gravity
    specific g.
Gruber-Widal reaction
GTT – glucose tolerance test
guaiac
Guaroa virus
Guthrie test
Gutman unit
Haemonchus
    H. contortus
Haemophilus
    H. aegyptius
    H. aphrophilus
    H. bovis
    H. bronchisepticus
    H. ducreyi
    H. duplex
    H. haemolyticus

Haemophilus (continued)
    H. hemoglobinophilus
    H. influenzae
    H. parahaemolyticus
    H. parainfluenzae
    H. parapertussis
    H. paraphrophilus
    H. pertussis
    H. suis
    H. vaginalis
Haemosporidia
Hageman factor
H agglutination
H agglutinin
H antigen
half-life
Ham's test
Hanger's test
Hansen's bacillus
haploid
haplophase
haplotype
hapten
    group A h.
haptoglobin: Hp^1, Hp^2
Harrison's test
Hartmanella
    H. hyalina
Haverhillia
    H. moniliformis
    H. multiformis
$H-2^b$ mouse cells
Hb – hemoglobin
HBD – hydroxybutyrate
    dehydrogenase
HCG – human chorionic
    gonadotropin
HCT – hematocrit
HDL – high-density lipoprotein
H & E – hematoxylin and eosin
Heidenhain's Susa fixative
Heinz bodies
Heinz-Ehrlich bodies
Hektoen agar
HeLa cells
helminth
helminthic

Helminthosporium
Helophilus
Helvella
    H. esculenta
hemadsorption
hemagglutination
hemagglutinin
Hemastix
Hematest
hematocrit
hematocrystallin
hematogen
hematogenesis
hematogenous
hematohyaloid
hematologist
hematology
hematopoiesis
    extramedullary h.
heme
Hemispora stellata
hemizygosity
hemoccult
hemochromogen
hemochromometry
hemocytoblast
hemocytometer
hemoflagellate
Hemofilus. See *Haemophilus.*
hemoglobin
hemoglobinemia
hemoglobinometry
hemoglobinuria
hemogram
hemohistioblast
hemolysin
hemolysis
hemolytic
hemolyze
Hemonkus. See *Haemonchus.*
hemophil
hemophilia
hemophilus
    h. of Koch-Weeks
    h. of Morax-Axenfeld
Hemophilus. See *Haemophilus.*
hemosiderin

hemosiderinuria
hemosiderosis
Hemosporidea. See
  Haemosporidia.
hemostasis
Hemostix
hemotherapy
heparin
hepatocellular
hepatogram
hepatotoxicity
Herellea
  H. vaginicola
Hermetia illucens
herpesvirus
Heterodera
  H. marioni
heterophil
Heterophyes
  H. heterophyes
  H. katsuradai
Heterophyes/Metagonimus
heterophyiasis
heterozygous
HF – Hageman factor
HGF – hyperglycemic-
  glycogenolytic factor
HIAA – hydroxyindoleacetic acid
Hicks-Pitney thromboplastin
  generation test
Hinton test
Histalog test
histamine
histiocyte
histiocytosis
histocompatibility
  h. complex
histology
histopathology
Histoplasma
  H. capsulatum
  H. duboisii
histoplasmin
histoplasmosis
HIV – human immunodeficiency
  virus
HLA – human leukocyte antigen

HLDH – heat-stable lactic
  dehydrogenase
Hofmann's bacillus
Hogben test
Homalomyia
homogentisuria
homozygous
hookworm
Hormodendrum
  H. carrionii
  H. compactum
  H. pedrosoi
Howard test
Howell-Jolly bodies
Howell's bodies
HPF – high-power field
HPL – human placental
  lactogen
5-HT – 5-hydroxytryptamine
HTLV – human T-cell leukemia/
  lymphoma virus
Huebener-Thomsen-Friedenreich
  phenomenon
human chorionic gonadotropin
humoral
Hürthle's cells
hyaline
hyalinization
Hycel-17
Hydatigera
  H. infantis
Hydrotaea
17-hydroxycorticosteroid
17-hydroxycorticosterone
5-hydroxyindoleacetic acid
3-hydroxyisobutyrate
  dehydrogenase
hydroxyketone dye
21-hydroxylase
hydroxy-mercurichlorophenol
hydroxyphenamate
hydroxyproline
17-hydroxysteroid
5-hydroxytryptamine
Hylemyia
hymenolepiasis

Hymenolepis
  H. diminuta
  H. murina
  H. nana
hyperaldosteronism
hyperbetalipoproteinemia
hyperbilirubinemia
hypercalcemia
hypercalciuria
hypercapnia
hypercholesterolemia
hyperchromasia
hyperchromatism
hyperchromemia
hyperchromia
hypercortisolism
hypercupremia
hypergammaglobulinemia
hyperglobulinemia
hyperglycemia
hyperimmunoglobulinemia
hyperkalemia
hyperlipemia
hyperlipidemia
hyperlipoproteinemia
hypernatremia
hyperphosphatemia
hyperprolactinemia
hyperthermia
hyperuricemia
hyperviscosity
hypha
hypoalbuminemia
hypobetalipoproteinemia
hypocalcemia
hypocapnia
hypochromasia
hypochromemia
  idiopathic h.
hypochromia
hypochromic
hypochrosis
Hypoderma
  H. bovis
hypogammaglobulinemia
hypoglycemia
hypokalemia

hyponatremia
hypophosphatasia
hypophosphatemia
hypoplastic
hypoproteinemia
hypothermia
hypotransferrinemia
hypovolemia
hypoxemia
Ia antigen
IBC – iron-binding capacity
ICD – isocitric dehydrogenase
icteric index
^{131}I (radioactive iodine) uptake
  test
Ig – immunoglobulin
IgA – gamma A immunoglobulin
IgD – gamma D immunoglobulin
IgE – gamma E immunoglobulin
IgG – gamma G immunoglobulin
IgM – gamma M
  immunoglobulin
ikso-. See words beginning *ixo-*.
iksodez. See *Ixodes.*
iksodiasis. See *ixodiasis.*
Ilheus virus
immune
  adherence
  complex
  response
  surveillance
  system
immunity
immunization
immunize
immunoadsorbent
immunoassay
immunoblast
immunocatalysis
immunochemistry
immunocompetence
immunocompromised
immunocyte
immunodeficiency
immunodiagnostic
immunodiffusion
immunoelectrophoresis

immunoelectrophoresis (continued)
    countercurrent i.
immunoferritin
immunofiltration
immunofixation
immunofluorescence
immunoglobulin
    gamma A i. (IgA)
    gamma D i. (IgD)
    gamma E i. (IgE)
    gamma G i. (IgG)
    gamma M i. (IgM)
immunohematology
immunohistochemical
immunohistofluorescence
immunoincompetent
immunology. See *Immunology and AIDS* section.
immunoperoxidase
immunosuppression
immunotherapy
incompatibility
    ABO i.
index
    acidophilic i.
    hematopneic i.
    hemolytic i.
    icteric i.
    Krebs' leukocyte i.
    maturation i.
    phagocytic i.
    pyknotic i.
    sedimentation i.
indican
indices
indole
Infusoria
INH – isonicotinic acid hydrazide
inhibitor
    inter-alpha-trypsin i.
inoculum
insulin
intracellular
iodameba. See *Iodamoeba.*
Iodamoeba
    I. büetschlii
    I. williamsi

iodine
iontophoresis
iron-binding capacity
irovirus
ISG – immune serum globulin
isochromosome
isoenzyme
isohemagglutination
isohemagglutinin
isoimmunization
isolation
Isoparorchis
    I. trisimilitubis
Isospora
    I. belli
    I. hominis
isosporiasis
isotope
Ivy's method bleeding time
Ixodes
    I. bicornis
    I. cavipalpus
    I. frequens
    I. pacificus
    I. persulcatus
    I. scapularis
ixodiasis
Ixodoidea
Japanese B encephalitis virus
jaundice
Jenner-Giemsa stain
JH virus
Johne's bacillus
Jolly's bodies
Jones-Cantarow test
Junin virus
K – potassium
Kahn test
kallikrein
Karmen units
karyocyte
karyotype
Katayama's test
KAU – King-Armstrong unit
Kell antigen
ketoacidosis
ketogenic

ketone
ketonemia
ketonuria
ketosis
17-ketosteroid
Ketostix
kilomastiks. See *Chilomastix.*
kimotripsin. See *chymotrypsin.*
kinase
kinetocyte
kinetoplast
King-Armstrong unit
klahmidea. See *Chlamydia.*
klahmideasee. See
    Chlamydiaceae.
klahmid-. See words beginning
    Chlamyd-.
Klebs-Löffler bacillus
Klebsiella
    K. friedländeri
    K. oxytoca
    K. ozaenae
    K. pneumoniae
    K. rhinoscleromatis
Klebsielleae
Klein's bacillus
klorid. See *chloride.*
klor-. See words beginning
    chlor-.
Koch-Weeks
    bacillus
    hemophilus
KOH–potassium hydroxide
koksakee. See *Coxsackie.*
kokseela. See *Coxiella.*
koksidi-. See words beginning
    coccidi-.
kol-. See words beginning *chol-.*
Kolmer's test
koreonik. See *chorionic.*
korinee-. See words beginning
    Coryne-.
Krebs' leukocyte index
kromatin. See *chromatin.*
krom-. See words beginning
    chrom-.
Kumba virus
Kunkel's test

Kupffer's cells
Kveim antigen
Kyasanur Forest disease virus
label
    radioactive l.
Lactobacillaceae
Lactobacilleae
lactobacillus
    l. of Boas-Oppler
Lactobacillus
    L. acidophilus
    L. arabinosus
    L. bifidus
    L. bulgaricus
    L. casei
    L. catenaforme
    L. fermentans
    L. fermenti
    L. leichmannii
    L. plantarum
Lactobacteriaceae
lactogen
lactoglobulin
    immune l.
lactose
Ladendorff's test
Laelaps
LAL–limulus amebocyte
    lysate
Lange's colloidal gold test
Lansing virus
larva
Lassa virus
LD–lymphocyte defined
LDH–lactic dehydrogenase
LE–lupus erythematosus
LE test
lecithin
lecithinase
lectin
Lee-White clotting time method
Legionella
    L. pneumophila
Leishman-Donovan bodies
Leishmania
    L. braziliensis
    L. donovani
    L. infantum

Leishmania (continued)
    L. tropica
    L. tropica mexicana
leishmaniasis
    cutaneous l.
    mucocutaneous l.
    naso-ora! l.
    nasopharyngeal l.
    visceral l.
Leishman's stain
Lelaps. See *Laelaps.*
Leon virus
leptocyte
leptocytosis
Leptomitus
    L. epidermidis
    L. urophilus
    L. vaginae
Leptospira
    L. australis
    L. autumnalis
    L. biflexa
    L. canicola
    L. grippotyphosa
    L. hebdomidis
    L. hyos
    L. icterohaemorrhagiae
    L. interrogans
    L. pomona
leptospirosis
    l. icterohemorrhagica
Leptothrix
Leptotrichia
    L. buccalis
    L. placoides
Leptotrombidium
    L. akamushi
    L. deliense
lesithin. See *lecithin.*
lesithinas. See *lecithinase.*
leucine
leukapheresis
leukemia
    lymphoblastic l.
    lymphocytic l.
    monocytic l.
    myeloblastic l.

leukemia (continued)
    myelocytic l.
    myelogenous l.
    reticuloendothelial cell l.
leukoagglutinins
leukocyte
leukocytosis
    eosinophilic l.
    lymphocytic l.
leukogram
leukopenia
leukotaxis
level
    barbiturate l.
    ethanol l.
    isoelectric l.
    lead l.
Levinson test
Lewis antibodies: Le^a, Le^b
Leydig's cells
Lichtheimia corymbifera
likthimea korimbifera. See
    Lichtheimia corymbifera.
Limnatis
    L. granulosa
    L. mysomelas
    L. nilotica
Limulus
    L. polyphemus
lipase
lipid
lipidase
lipocyte
lipoid
Liponisus. See *Lyponyssus.*
lipoprotein
liquefaction
Lissoflagellata
Listeria
    L. monocytogenes
Loa
    L. loa
Löffler's blood serum
Loxosceles
    L. reclusa
LPF – low-power field
    lymphocytosis-

promoting factor
lukemea. See *leukemia.*
luk-. See words beginning *leuk-.*
Lunyo virus
lupus
    l. erythematosus
lusin. See *leucine.*
lutein
lymphoblast
lymphoblastomid
lymphoblastosis
lymphocyte
    atypical l.
    Downey-type l.
    plasmacytoid l.
lymphocytopenia
lymphocytosis
    neutrophilic l.
    l.-promoting factor
lymphs – lymphocytes
Lyponyssus
lysin
lysine
lysing
lysis
lysokinase
lysolecithin
lysosome
lysozyme
MacConkey agar
Macracanthorhynchus
    M. hirudinaceus
macroaleuriospore
Macrobdella
macroblast
macrocyte
macrocythemia
    hyperchromatic m.
macrocytic
macroglobulin
macroglobulinemia
    Waldenström's m.
Macromonas
    M. bipunctata
    M. mobilis
macromonocyte
macromyeloblast

macronormoblast
macrophage
Macrophoma
macropolycyte
Macrostoma mesnili
Madurella
    M. grisea
    M. mycetomi
maedivirus
magnesium
malabsorption
malaria
malasezeah. See *Malassezia.*
Malassezia
    M. furfur
    M. macfadyani
    M. tropica
mallein
Malleomyces
    M. mallei
    M. pseudomallei
    M. whitmori
Mallory's bodies
Malmejde's test
Mansonella
    M. ozzardi
    M. streptocerca
Mantoux
    conversion
    skin test
Maragiliano body
marrow
    bone m.
Masson stain
mastadenovirus
Mastigophora
materia
maturation
Mayaro virus
May-Grünwald-Giemsa stain
MBC – minimal bactericidal
    concentration
MCD – mean cell diameter
    mean corpuscular
    diameter
MCH – mean corpuscular
    hemoglobin

MCHC–mean corpuscular
    hemoglobin concentration
MCV–mean corpuscular volume
mean cell diameter
mean corpuscular diameter
mean corpuscular hemoglobin
mean corpuscular hemoglobin
    concentration
mean corpuscular volume
MEG–megakaryocytes
megakaryoblast
megakaryocyte
megaloblast
meiosis
melanin
Melanolestes
    M. picipes
Meloidogyne
Mengo virus
meningococci
meningococcin
meningococcus
meningocyte
meniscocyte
Merulius
    M. lacrimans
mesangial
mesangium
mesobacterium
metachromatic
metagglutinin
metaglobulin
metagonimiasis
Metagonimus
    M. ovatus
    M. yokogawai
metamorphosis
metamyelocyte
metanephrine
metaphase
Methanobacterium
Methanococcus
methemalbumin
methemalbuminemia
methemoglobin
methemoglobinemia
methemoglobinuria

method
    chromolytic (dyed-starch)
      m.
    Dale-Laidlaw's clotting
      time m.
    Lee-White clotting time
      m.
methyl
    m. methacrylate
Metopirone test
Mg agglutinin
mico-. See words beginning
    myco-.
Microbacterium
microbiology
microbroth
microchemistry
Micrococcaceae
Micrococcus
    M. pyogenes var. *aureus*
microcyte
microcytic
Microfilaria
    M. bancrofti
    M. streptocerca
microne
microorganism
microphage
microprotein
microscope
microscopic
microscopy
    electron m.
microspherocyte
Microsporon furfur
Microsporum
    M. audouini
    M. canis
    M. felineum
    M. fulvum
    M. furfur
    M. gypseum
    M. lanosum
Middlebrook-Dubos
    hemagglutination test
Middlebrook's
    agar

Middlebrook's (continued)
 broth
MIF – migration-inhibition factor
mikso-. See words beginning
 myxo-.
miksopod. See *myxopod*.
miksosporidea. See
 Myxosporidia.
Mima
  M. polymorpha
minimal bactericidal
 concentration
miosis. See *meiosis*.
mitochondria
mitogen
mitogillin
mitokinetic
mitomalcin
mitoplasm
mitosis
Miyagawanella
  M. illinii
  M. louisianae
  M. lymphogranulomatosis
  M. ornithosis
  M. pneumoniae
  M. psittaci
MLC – minimal lethal
 concentration
moiety
molality
molar
molarity
Monadina
Monas
Monilia
monilial
moniliasis
Moniliformis
monoblast
monochromator
monoclonal
monocyte
monocytopenia
monocytosis
mononuclear
monos – monocytes

monosaccharide
monosomic
monosomy G, X
Monosporium
  M. apiospermum
Monospot test
Monotricha
Morax-Axenfeld
 bacillus
 diplococcus
 hemophilus
Moraxella
  M. lacunata
  M. liquefaciens
morbillivirus
Morgan's bacillus
morococcus
morphology
mosaicism
Mosenthal's test
motile
motility
Motulsky dye reduction test
mouse unit
MU – mouse unit
mucicarmine stain
mucopolysaccharidase
mucopolysaccharide
mucoprotein
Mucor
  M. corymbifer
  M. mucedo
  M. pusillus
  M. racemosus
  M. ramosus
  M. rhizopodiformis
mucormycosis
mucus
Mueller-Hinton broth
muramidase
Murphy-Pattee test
Murray Valley encephalitis virus
murtofilum. See *Myrtophyllum*.
mycoagglutinin
mycobacteria
Mycobacteriaceae
mycobacteriosus

Mycobacterium
    M. avium-intracellulare
    M. balnei
    M. berolinenis
    M. bovis
    M. butyricum
    M. chelonei
    M. flavescens
    M. fortuitum
    M. gastri
    M. gordonae
    M. habana
    M. intracellularis
    M. kansasii
    M. leprae
    M. lepraemurium
    M. luciflavum
    M. marinum
    M. microti
    M. paratuberculosis
    M. phlei
    M. scrofulaceum
    M. simiae
    M. smegmatis
    M. szulgai
    M. terrea-nonchromogenicum-triviale
    M. tuberculosis
    M. tuberculosis var. *avium*
    M. tuberculosis var. *bovis*
    M. tuberculosis var. *hominis*
    M. ulcerans
    M. xenopi
Mycocandida
Mycococcus
Mycoderma
    M. aceti
    M. dermatitis
    M. immite
mycology
Myconostoc
    M. gregarium
Mycoplana
    M. bullata
    M. dimorpha

Mycoplasma
    M. buccale
    M. faucium
    M. fermentans
    M. hominis
    M. orale
    M. pharyngis
    M. pneumoniae
    M. salivarium
Mycoplasmataceae
Mycoplasmatales
mycosis
    m. fungoides
mycotic
myeloblast
myeloclast
myelocyte
myiasis
myoglobin
Myriapoda
Myrtophyllum
    M. hepatis
myxopod
Myxosporidia
myxovirus
NAD—nicotinamide adenine dinucleotide
Naegleria
NANA—N-acetylneuraminic acid
NBT—nitroblue tetrazolium
Necator
    N. americanus
Negri bodies
Neisseria
    N. catarrhalis
    N. caviae
    N. flava
    N. flavescens
    N. gonorrhoeae
    N. intracellularis
    N. lactamicus
    N. meningitidis
    N. mucosa
    N. ovis
    N. perflava
    N. pharyngis
    N. sicca

Neisseria (continued)
    N. subflava
Neisseriaceae
Neisser's diplococcus
Nematoda
nematode
neocyte
neocytosis
Neotestudina
nephelometry
neuraminidase
neutropenia
neutrophil
    band n.
    juvenile n.
    mature n.
    polymorphonuclear n.
    segmented n.
neutrophilia
Newcastle disease virus
Newcastle-Manchester
    bacillus
Nitrobacter
Nitrobacteraceae
Nitrocystis
Nocardia
    N. asteroides
    N. brasiliensis
    N. caviae
    N. madurae
    N. minutissima
    N. pelletieri
    N. tenuis
nocardiosis
Nocard's bacillus
norepinephrine
normoblast
    acidophilic n.
    basophilic n.
    intermediate n.
    orthochromatophilic n.
    polychromatophilic n.
normoblastosis
normocyte
normocytic
normocytosis
normo-orthocytosis

nosomycosis
NPDL – nodular, poorly
    differentiated lymphocytes
NPN – nonprotein nitrogen
NSQ – not sufficient quantity
nuclear
    n. aggregate
    n. cytoplasmic ratio
        alteration
    n. inclusion body
    n. pore alteration
    n. vacuolization
nucleoprotein
nucleus
numo-. See words beginning
    pneumo-.
O agglutination
O agglutinin
O antistreptolysin
Obermayer's test
Obermeier's spirillum
Obermüller's test
occult blood
Ochromyia
    O. anthropophaga
OCT – ornithine carbamyl
    transferase
Octomitus
    O. hominis
Octomyces
    O. etiennei
Oestrus
    O. hominis
    O. ovis
OHCS – hydroxycorticosteroid
Oidiomycetes
oidiomycosis
oligemia
oligocythemia
Onchocherca
    O. caecutiens
    O. volvulus
onchocerciasis
O'nyong-nyong virus
Oospora
opisthorchiasis

Opisthorchis
    O. felineus
    O. noverca
    O. viverrini
orbivirus
organic
organism
    Arizona o.
    Rickett's o.
    Vincent's o.
Ornithodoros
    O. coriaceus
Oropouche virus
orthopoxvirus
Osler's disease
osmolality
osmometry
osmosis
Ostertag
    streptococcus of O.
Otomyces
    O. hageni
    O. purpureus
otomycosis
    o. aspergillina
ova
ovum
oxalate
oxygen
oxyhemoglobin
oxyhemogram
oxyhemograph
oxysteroid
Oxyuris
    O. incognita
    O. vermicularis
PAH – para-aminohippurate
pancytopenia
Pandy's test
panhematopoietic
panhemocytophthisis
Panstrongylus
Papanicolaou's
    smear
    stain
    test
papillomavirus

Papovaviridae
papovavirus
Pappenheim's stain
Parachordodes
Paracoccidioides
    P. brasiliensis
paracoccidioidomycosis
Paracolobactrum
    P. aerogenoides
    P. arizonae
    P. coliforme
    P. intermedium
paraffin
Parafossarulus
Paragonimus
    P. westermani
Paragordius
    P. cinctus
    P. tricuspidatus
    P. varius
parahormone
Paramecium
    P. coli
paramyxovirus
Parasaccharomyces
    P. ashfordi
parasite
parasitic
parasitology
parathormone
paratyphi. See
    Salmonella p. A, B, C
paratyphoid
paravirus
Parvobacteriaceae
Parvoviridae
parvovirus
PAS – para-aminosalicylic acid
    periodic acid – Schiff stain
Pasteurella
    P. haemolytica
    P. multocida
    P. pestis
    P. pneumotropica
    P. pseudotuberculosis
    P. septica
    P. tularensis

Pasteurella (continued)
 P. ureae
Patein's albumin
pathogen
Paul-Bunnell-Barrett test
Paul-Bunnell test
PBG – porphobilinogen
PBI – protein-bound iodine
PCE – pseudocholinesterase
pCO_2 – partial pressure of carbon dioxide
PCV – packed cell volume
Pectobacterium
 P. carotovorum
Pediculoides
 P. ventricosus
Pediculus
 P. humanus var. *capitis*
 P. humanus var. *corporis*
 P. inguinalis
 P. pubis
Pelger-Huët nuclear anomaly
pellicle
Penicillium
 P. barbae
 P. bouffardi
 P. minimum
 P. montoyai
 P. notatum
 P. patulum
 P. spinulosum
Pentastoma
 P. constrictum
 P. denticulatum
 P. taenioides
pentastomiasis
Pentatrichomonas
 P. ardin delteili
pentatrichomoniasis
pentolysis
pentosan
pentosazon
pentose
pepsin
peptidase
 leucine amino p.

Peptococcus
 P. anaerobius
 P. asaccharolyticus
 P. constellatus
 P. magnus
 P. prevotii
Peptostreptococcus
 P. anaerobius
 P. intermedius
 P. lanceolatus
 P. micros
 P. productus
pericyte
periodic acid – Schiff stain
peroxidase
Petriellidium
Petri's
 dish
 test
Pfeiffer's bacillus
pH – hydrogen ion concentration
phagocyte
phagocytic
phagocytoblast
phagocytolysis
phagocytosis
phaneroplasm
Phenistix
phenol
 p. liquefactum
 p. red
 p. salicylate
phenolphthalein
phenolsulfonphthalein
phenothiazine
phenomenon
 Huebener-Thomsen-
  Friedenreich p.
 prozone p.
phenotype
 Bombay p.
phenylalanine
phenylketonuria
pheochromocyte
pheochromocytoma
pheresis
Phialophora

Phialophora (continued)
    P. jeanselmi
    P. verrucosa
Philadelphia chromosome
Phlebotomus
    P. argentipes
    P. chinensis
    P. intermedius
    P. macedonicum
    P. noguchi
    P. papatasii
    P. sergenti
    P. verrucarum
    P. vexator
phosphatase
    acid p.
    alkaline p.
    serum p.
phosphate
phosphatidylethanolamine
phosphocreatine
phosphofructokinase
phospholipase
phospholipid
phosphorus
phosphorylase
Phthirus
    P. pubis
Phycomycetes
phycomycosis
Physaloptera
    P. caucasica
    P. mordens
phytanic acid
phytohemagglutination
Piazza's test
picogram
piedra
Piedraia
    P. hortae
pigment
pinworm
Pityrosporon
    P. orbiculare
    P. ovale
    P. versicolor
PKU – phenylketonuria

plasma
plasmablast
plasmacyte
plasmacytoma
plasmacytosis
plasmagene
plasmahaut
plasmalogen
plasmapheresis
plasmarrhexis
plasmid
plasmin
plasminogen
plasmocyte
Plasmodium
    P. falciparum
    P. malariae
    P. ovale
    P. pleurodyniae
    P. vivax
    P. vivax minuta
plasmodium
    exoerythrocytic p.
platelet
plateletpheresis
pleokaryocyte
pleomorphic
pneumobacillus
    Friedländer's p.
pneumococcal
pneumococcus
Pneumocystis
    P. carinii
pneumovirus
pO_2 – partial pressure of oxygen
poikiloblast
poikilocyte
poikilocytosis
polarography
poly – polymorphonuclear
    leukocyte
polychromasia
polychromatic
polychromatophilia
polychromatosis
polychromemia
polyclonal

polycyte
polycythemia
    p. hypertonica
    myelopathic p.
    p. rubra
    splenomegalic p.
    p. vera
polycytosis
polyemia
    p. aquosa
    p. hyperalbuminosa
    p. polycythaemica
    p. serosa
polymorphocyte
polymorphonuclear
    p. basophil
    p. eosinophil
    p. leukocyte
    p. neutrophil
polynuclear
polyomavirus
polyploid
polyploidy
polyribosome
polysaccharide
polysomaty
polysomy X
Porges-Meier test
Porges-Salomon test
Porocephalus
    P. armillatus
    P. clavatus
    P. constrictus
    P. denticulatus
porphobilinogen
porphyria
porphyrin
postprandial
potassium
potentiometry
Powassan virus
poxvirus
PP–postprandial
PPD–purified protein derivative
prealbumin
pregnanediol
pregnanetriol

Preisz-Nocard bacillus
premyeloblast
premyelocyte
proerythroblast
proerythrocyte
profibrinolysin
profile
    liver p.
prolactin
proliferate
proliferation
prolymphocyte
promegaloblast
promoblast
promonocyte
promyelocyte
pronormoblast
Propionibacterium
    P. acnes
proplasmacyte
Proteeae
proteidin
    pyocyanase p.
protein
    C-reactive p.
proteinemia
proteinosis
proteinuria
    Bence Jones p.
proteoclastic
proteolipid
proteolytic
Proteomyces
proteose
proteosuria
Proteus
    P. inconstans
    P. mirabilis
    P. morganii
    P. OX-K
    P. OX-2
    P. OX-19
    P. rettgeri
    P. vulgaris
prothrombin
prothrombinase
prothrombinogen

prothrombinokinase
prothrombinopenia
protoanemonin
Protobacterieae
protocoproporphyria
protoporphyrin
Protozoa
protozoan
protozoon
protozoophage
Providencia
    P. alcalifaciens
    P. stuartii
Prowazekia
prozone
psammoma
PSD-peptone-starch-dextrose
Pseudamphistomum
    P. truncatum
pseudocholinesterase
Pseudomonadaceae
Pseudomonadales
Pseudomonadineae
Pseudomonas
    P. acidovorans
    P. aeruginosa
    P. alcaligenes
    P. cepacia
    P. diminuta
    P. eisenbergii
    P. fluorescens
    P. fragi
    P. maltophilia
    P. multivorans
    P. non-liquefaciens
    P. paucimobilis
    P. pseudoalcaligenes
    P. pseudomallei
    P. putida
    P. pyocyanea
    P. stutzeri
    P. syncyanea
    P. vesicularis
    P. viscosa
Pseudomonilia
PSP-phenolsulfonphthalein

PTA-plasma thromboplastin
    antecedent
PTC-plasma thromboplastin
    component
PTT-partial thromboplastin
    time
Pulex
    P. irritans
Pullicidae
pullorin
Pullularia
purpura
    thrombocytopenic p.
pyknosis
pyknotic
pyocyanase
pyogenic
pyrogen
pyroglobulin
QNS-quantity not sufficient
qualitative
quantitative
Quick's test
RA-rheumatoid arthritis
rabd-. See words beginning
    rhabd-.
radioassay
radioimmunoassay
radioisotope
radiolabeled
radionuclide
radioreceptor
RAI-radioactive iodine
RAI scan uptake
RA latex fixation test
Ramon flocculation
rate
    sedimentation r.
ratio
    myeloid-erythroid r.
RBC-red blood cell
    red blood cell count
RBC/hpf-red blood cells per
    high-power field
RBE-relative biological
    effectiveness

reaction
  Bence Jones r.
  Ehrlich's r.
  glycine-arginine r.
  Gruber-Widal r.
  sigma r.
  Wassermann r.
  Weil-Felix r.
  Widal r.
reagent
  Sickledex r.
receptor
  adrenergic r.
renin
renogram
reovirus
reticulin
reticulocyte
reticuloendothelial
Retortamonas
  R. intestinalis
Rettgerella
  R. rettgeri
Rh – Rhesus (factor)
Rhabditis
  R. hominis
rhabdocyte
Rhabdomonas
Rh agglutinin
Rh antigen
Rhinocladium
Rhizobiaceae
Rhizobium
Rhizoglyphus
  R. parasiticus
Rhizopoda
Rhizopus
  R. equinus
  R. niger
  R. nigricans
  R. rhizopodoformis
Rhodotorula
  R. rubra
RhoGAM vaccine
RIA – radioimmunoassay
riboflavin

Rickett's organism
Rickettsia
  R. akamushi
  R. akari
  R. australis
  R. burnetii
  R. conorii
  R. diaporica
  R. mooseri
  R. muricola
  R. nipponica
  R. orientalis
  R. pediculi
  R. prowazekii
  R. quintana
  R. rickettsii
  R. sibiricus
  R. tsutsugamushi
  R. typhi
  R. wolhynica
Rickettsiaceae
rickettsial
rickettsialpox
Rift Valley fever virus
Ringer's solution
rinokladeum. See *Rhinocladium.*
RISA – radioactive iodinated
  serum albumin
Rizo-. See words beginning
  Rhizo-.
RNA – ribonucleic acid
RNase – ribonuclease
rod-shaped
Romanowsky's stain
roolo. See *rouleau* and *rouleaux.*
Rose's test
Rose-Waaler test
rotavirus
Rothera's test
Rotter's test
rouleau
rouleaux
roundworm
Rourke-Ernstein sedimentation
  rate
Rous test

Rowntree and Geraghty's
   test
RPF – renal plasma flow
RS (respiratory syncytial) virus
rubella
rubivirus
rubrum
Russell unit
Russian spring-summer
   encephalitis virus
Sabhi agar
Sabouraud's dextrose agar
saccharomyces
      Busse's s.
Saccharomyces
      S. albicans
      S. anginae
      S. apiculatus
      S. cantliei
      S. capillitii
      S. carlsbergensis
      S. cerevisiae
      S. coprogenus
      S. epidermica
      S. galacticolus
      S. glutinis
      S. hominis
      S. lemonnieri
      S. mellis
      S. mycoderma
      S. neoformans
      S. pastorianus
Salmonella
      S. choleraesuis
      S. derby
      S. durazzo
      S. enteritidis
      S. gallinarum
      S. hirschfeldii
      S. indiana
      S. minnesota
      S. montevideo
      S. muenchen
      S. newington
      S. oranienburg
      S. paratyphi A, B, C
      S. pullorum

Salmonella (continued)
      S. schottmülleri
      S. sendai
      S. thompson
      S. typhi
      S. typhimurium
      S. typhisuis
      S. typhosa
      S. virginia
Salmonella-Shigella agar
Salmonelleae
Salvia
      S. horminium
      S. sclarea
Sappinia diploidea
Saprospira
Sarcina
Sarcocystis
sarcocyte
Sarcodina
Sarcophaga
      S. carnaria
      S. dux
      S. fuscicauda
      S. haemorrhoidalis
      S. nificornis
      S. rubicornis
Sarcoptes
      S. scabiei
scan
      bilirubin s.
      brain s.
      CAT (computed axial
         tomography) s.
      gallium s.
      kidney s.
      krypton s.
      liver s.
      RAI (radioactive iodine) s.
      risa s.
      spleen s.
      technetium s.
SCG – serum chemistry graph
Schaedler blood agar
Schick test
Schilling
      blood count

Schilling (continued)
    test
schistocyte
Schistosoma
    S. haematobium
    S. intercalatum
    S. japonicum
    S. mansoni
schistosome
schistosomiasis
Schizoblastosporion
schizogony
Schmitz's bacillus
Schmorl's bacillus
Schottmüller's disease
schwannoma
Schwann's white substance
scintiphotograph
scolecoid
scolex
Scopulariopsis
    S. americana
    S. aureus
    S. blochi
    S. brevicaulis
    S. cinereus
    S. koningi
    S. minimus
scopulariopsosis
SD antigen
sediment
sedimentation
    erythrocyte s.
sedimentation rate
    Rourke-Ernstein s.r.
    Westergren's s.r.
    Wintrobe's s.r.
    Zeta s.r.
sefalin. See *cephalin.*
sefalosporeum. See
    Cephalosporium.
seg – segmented (leukocyte)
SEGS – segmented neutrophils
Semliki Forest virus
Sendai virus
sensitivity
septicemia

serine
serkarea. See *cercaria.*
serodiagnosis
serological
serology
serotonin
serotype
serous
Serratia
    S. indica
    S. kiliensis
    S. liquefaciens
    S. marcescens
    S. piscatorum
    S. plymuthica
    S. rubidaea
Serratieae
serum creatinine
sfero-. See words beginning with
    sphero-.
SGOT – serum glutamic
    oxaloacetic transaminase
SGPT – serum glutamic pyruvic
    transaminase
SH – serum hepatitis
shaletela. See *Cheyletiella.*
Shiga's bacillus
Shigella
    S. alkalescens
    S. ambigua
    S. arabinotarda Type A, B
    S. boydii
    S. ceylonensis
    S. dispar
    S. dysenteriae
    S. etousae
    S. flexneri
    S. madampensis
    S. newcastle
    S. paradysenteriae
    S. parashigae
    S. schmitzii
    S. shigae
    S. sonnei
    S. wakefield
Shinowara-Jones-Reinhard unit
Sia test

sickle cell
Sickledex reagent
sickling
Siderobacter
sideroblast
Siderocapsa
Siderocapsaceae
Siderococcus
siderocyte
siderophilin
sifasea. See *Syphacia.*
sigma reaction
sigmavirus
Simbu virus
Simmons' citrate agar
Sims-Huhner test
Sindbis virus
skisto-. See words beginning
    schisto-.
skizo-. See words beginning
    schizo-.
SMA 6/60 (Sequential Multiple
    Analyzer)
SMA 12 profile test (Sequential
    Multiple Analyzer)
SMA 12/6 (Sequential Multiple
    Analyzer)
SMAF – Specific Macrophage
    Arming Factor
smear
        fungi s.
        Papanicolaou's s.
        TB s.
sodium
solution
        formaldehyde s.
        Ringer's s.
somatomedin
somatostatin
Somogyi unit
Sonne-Duval bacillus
Sonne dysentery
sparganosis
sparganum
SPCA – serum prothrombin-
    conversion accelerator
spectrometer

spectrophotometry
SPEP – serum protein
    electrophoresis
SPF – specific pathogen-free
sp. gr. – specific gravity
spherocyte
spherocytosis
sphingomyelin
sphingosine
Spirillaceae
Spirillum
        S. minor
        Obermeier's s.
Spirochaeta
        S. daxensis
        S. eurystrepta
        S. marina
        S. pallida
        S. plicatilis
        S. stenostrepta
        S. vincenti
spirochete
spirochetemia
spirogram
spirometry
Sporothrix
        S. schenckii
sporotrichosis
Sporozoa
sporozoite
sporozoon
sputum
SSKI – saturated solution of
    potassium iodide
stab – stabnuclear neutrophil
staf-. See words beginning *staph-.*
stain
        acid-Schiff s.
        alcian blue s.
        ATPase s.
        Bowie's s.
        carbol fuchsin s.
        chlorazol black E s.
        Congo red s.
        cresyl violet s.
        eosin s.
        Giemsa's s.

Stain (continued)
    Gomori's s.
    Gram's s.
    Gram-Weigert s.
    hematoxylin-eosin s.
    Jenner-Giemsa s.
    Leishman's s.
    Masson s.
    May-Grünwald-Giemsa s.
    methenamine silver s.
    mucicarmine s.
    Papanicolaou's s.
    Pappenheim's s.
    periodic acid–Schiff s.
    polychrome methylene
      blue s.
    quinacrine s.
    Romanowsky's s.
    Truant's s.
    van Gieson's s.
    von Kossa's s.
    Wade-Fite-Faraco s.
    Weigert's s.
    Wright's s.
    Ziehl-Neelsen's s.
staphylocoagulase
staphylococcal
staphylococcemia
staphylococci
staphyloccus
Staphylococcus
    S. albus
    S. aureus
    S. citreus
    S. epidermidis
    S. pyogenes aureus
    S. pyogenes var. *albus*
    S. saprophyticus
staphylolysin
    α s., alpha s.
    β s., beta s.
    δ s., delta s.
    ϵ s., epsilon s.
    γ s., gamma s.
steroid
stippling
    basophilic s.

St. Louis encephalitis
    virus
Stormer viscosimeter
Streptobacillus
    S. moniliformis
streptococcal
Streptococceae
streptococci
streptococcus
    alpha s.
    anhemolytic s.
    Bargen's s.
    beta s.
    Fehleisen's s.
    gamma s.
    hemolytic s.
    nonhemolytic s.
    s. of Ostertag
Streptococcus
    S. agalactiae
    S. anginosus
    S. bovis
    S. cremoris
    S. durans
    S. equi
    S. equisimilis
    S. faecalis
    S. faecium
    S. haemolyticus
    S. lactis
    S. liquefaciens
    S. MG
    S. mitis
    S. pneumoniae
    S. pyogenes
    S. salivarius
    S. uberis
    S. viridans
    S. zooepidemicus
    S. zymogenes
streptolysin
    s. O
Streptomyces
    S. madurae
    S. pelletieri
    S. somaliensis
Streptothrix

Strong's bacillus
Strongyloides
    S. stercoralis
strongyloidiasis
STS – serologic test for syphilis
    standard test for syphilis
STU – skin test unit
study
    erythrokinetic s's
    fat absorption s's
subculture
substance
    white s. of Schwann
    zymoplastic s.
Sudan
    S. black
    S. I
    S. II
    S. G. S. III
    S. IV
    S. yellow G
sudo-. See words beginning
    pseudo-.
sulfhemoglobin
sulfmethemoglobin
sulfobromophthalein
Sulkowitch's test
survival
    red blood cell s.
Swiss-type agammaglobulinemia
syncytial
    s. alteration
    s. trophoblast
Syphacia
    S. obvelata
T_3 – triiodothyronine
T_4 – thyroxine, levothyroxine,
    tetraiodothyronine
tachogram
Taenia
    T. africana
    T. bremneri
    T. brunerri
    T. confusa
    T. echinococcus
    T. philippina
    T. saginata

Taenia (continued)
    T. solium
T agglutination
Takata-Ara test
tapeworm
target cell
TAT – tetanus antitoxin
    toxin-antitoxin
    turn-around time
TB – tubercle bacillus
    tuberculosis
TBC – tuberculosis
TBG – thyroxine-binding globulin
TBI – thyroxine-binding index
T cells
technique
    Ficoll-Hypaque t.
    zinc sulfate centrifugal
      flotation t.
tenea. See *Taenia.*
tenosefalidez. See
    Ctenocephalides.
Teschen virus
test
    Abrams' t.
    acetic acid t.
    acetic acid and potassium
      ferrocyanide t.
    acetoacetic acid t.
    acetone t.
    acidified serum t.
    acidity reduction t.
    acid-lability t.
    acidosis t.
    acid phosphatase t.
    ACTH t.
    Adamkiewicz's t.
    Adler's t.
    adrenalin t.
    adrenocortical inhibition t.
    A/G ratio t.
    agglutination t.
    albumin t.
    adolase t.
    aldosterone t.
    alizarin t.
    alkali t.

test (continued)

   alkali denaturation t.
   alkali tolerance t.
   alkaline phosphatase t.
   alkaloid t.
   alpha amino nitrogen t.
   amylase t.
   antiglobulin t.
   Apt t.
   arginine t.
   Argo corn starch t.
   arylsulfatase t.
   Aschheim-Zondek t.
   ascorbate cyanide t.
   ascorbic acid t.
   automated reagin t.
   AZ (Aschheim-Zondek) t.
   BEI
   Bence Jones protein t.
   Benedict's t.
   bentonite flocculation t.
   bile acid t.
   bile pigment t.
   bile solubility t.
   bilirubin t., direct, indirect
   bilirubin tolerance t.
   biuret t.
   blood urea nitrogen t.
   Bloor's t.
   blot t.
   Bloxam's t.
   Boas' t.
   Bonanno's t.
   bromosulfalein t.
   butanol extractable
      iodine t.
   calcium t.
   capillary fragility t.
   carbon dioxide combining
      power t.
   Casoni's intradermal t.
   Castellani's t.
   catecholamine t.
   cephalin-cholesterol
      flocculation t.
   cephalin flocculation t.
   cetylpyridium chloride t.

test (continued)

   Chediak's t.
   cholesterol t.
   cholesterol-lecithin
      flocculation t.
   cholinesterase t.
   chromogenic
      cephalosporin t.
   coagulation t.
   colloidal gold t.
   complement-fixation
      (CF) t.
   Congo red t.
   Coombs' t., direct, indirect
   coproporphyrin t.
   cortisone-glucose
      tolerance t.
   C-reactive protein t.
   creatine t.
   creatinine clearance t.
   cyanide-nitroprusside t.
   dexamethasone
      suppression t.
   dextrose t.
   Diagnex Blue t.
   Dick t.
   dinitrophenylhydrazine t.
   direct antiglobulin t.
   dithionite t.
   Donath-Landsteiner t.
   edrophonium chloride t.
   Ehrlich's t.
   electrophoresis t.
   Ellsworth-Howard t.
   Fehling's t.
   ferric chloride t.
   Feulgen t.
   fibrinogen t.
   Fishberg's concentration t.
   flocculation t.
   fluorescent treponemal
      antibody t.
   formol-gel t.
   fragility t.
   Frei t.
   Friedman's t.
   frog t.

test (continued)
FTA
galactose tolerance t.
Gerhardt's t.
glucagon t.
glucose tolerance t.
glycogen storage t.
Gravindex t.
guaiac t.
Guthrie t.
Ham's t.
Hanger's t.
Harrison's t.
hemagglutination t.
heterophil antibody t.
Hicks-Pitney
thromboplastin
generation t.
Hinton t.
hippuric acid t.
Histalog t.
histamine t.
HIVAGEN t.
Hogben t.
homogentisic acid t.
Howard t.
17-hydroxycorticosteroid t.
5-hydroxyindoleacetic
acid t.
^{131}I (radioactive iodine)
uptake t.
icterus index t.
immunofluorescent t.
indican t.
indigo-carmine t.
indole t.
insulin clearance t.
insulin tolerance t.
interference t.
iron-binding capacity t.
isoiodeikon t.
isopropanol precipitation t.
Jones-Cantarow t.
Kahn t.
Katayama's t.
17-ketosteroid t.
Kolmer's t.

test (continued)
Kunkel's t.
lactic acid t.
lactic dehydrogenase t.
lactose tolerance t.
Ladendorff's t.
Lange's colloidal gold t.
latex fixation t.
latex slide agglutination t.
LE t.
leucine aminopeptidase t.
Levinson t.
levulose tolerance t.
limulus lysate t.
lipase t.
lipid t.
lymphocyte transfer t.
magnesium t.
malaria film t.
mallein t.
Malmejde's t.
Mantoux skin t.
mastic t.
melanin t.
methylene blue t.
Metopirone t.
Middlebrook-Dubos
hemagglutination t.
monocyte function t.
Monospot t.
Mosenthal's t.
Motulsky dye reduction t.
mucoprotein t.
Murphy-Pattee t.
nitrate utilization t.
nitroblue tetrazolium t.
nitroprusside t.
nonprotein nitrogen t.
Obermayer's t.
Obermüller's t.
occult blood t.
osazone t.
osmotic fragility t.
Pandy's t.
Papanicolaou's t.
partial thromboplastin
time t.

test (continued)
    Paul-Bunnell-Barrett t.
    Paul-Bunnell t.
    Petri's t.
    phenolphthalein t.
    phenolsulfonphthalein t.
    phenylketonuria t.
    phosphatase t.
    phospholipid t.
    phosphoric acid t.
    Piazza's t.
    plasma hemoglobin t.
    Porges-Meier t.
    Porges-Salomon t.
    porphobilinogen t.
    porphyrin t.
    potassium t.
    precipitin t.
    prolactin t.
    protein t.
    protein-bound iodine t.
    prothrombin t.
    pulmonary function t.
    purine bodies t.
    quantitation t.
    Quick's t.
    RA latex fixation t.
    radioactive iodine t.
    reactone red t.
    resorcinol t.
    rose bengal t.
    Rose's t.
    Rose-Waaler t.
    Rothera's t.
    Rotter's t.
    Rous t.
    Rowntree and Geraghty's
      t.
    Schick t.
    Schilling t.
    secretin t.
    sedimentation t.
    serology t.
    serum alkaline
      phosphatase t.
    serum globulin t.
    Sia t.

test (continued)
    sickle cell t.
    sickling t.
    silver nitroprusside t.
    Sims-Huhner t.
    SMA 12 profile t.
    sodium t.
    streptozyme t.
    Sulkowitch's t.
    sweat t.
    T_3 uptake t.
    Takata-Ara t.
    tetrazolium t.
    Thayer-Martin t.
    Thorn t.
    thromboplastin
      generation t.
    thymol turbidity t.
    thyroxine-binding index t.
    tine t.
    tolbutamide tolerance t.
    transaminase (SGOT-
      SGPT) t.
    trypsin t.
    tyrosine t.
    Tzanck t.
    Uffelmann's t.
    urea clearance t.
    urea nitrogen t.
    urease t.
    uric acid t.
    urine acetone t.
    urobilinogen t.
    van den Bergh t.
    vanillylmandelic acid t.
    Van Slyke t.
    VDRL (Venereal Disease
      Research Laboratories)
      t.
    Voges-Proskauer t.
    Volhard's t.
    Wassermann t.
    Watson-Schwartz t.
    western blot t.
    wire loop t.
    xylose concentration t.
    D-xylose tolerance t.

test (continued)
    zinc flocculation t.
    zinc turbidity t.
Tes-Tape
tetraploidy
TGT – thromboplastin generation
   test
    thromboplastin generation
   time
thalassemia
THAM – trihydroxy-
   methylaminomethane
Thayer-Martin test
Theiler's virus
theolin
thermogram
thiocyanate
Thorn test
thread
    mucous t's
thrombasthenia
thrombin
thrombocyte
thrombocytopenia
thrombocytopoiesis
thrombocytosis
thrombometer
thromboplastic
thromboplastin
thromboplastinogen
thrombostasis
thrombosthenin
thrombotest
thymidine
thymol turbidity
thyrocalcitonin
thyrotropin
thyroxine
TIBC – total iron-binding
   capacity
timothy bacillus
titer
    agglutination t.
    antihyaluronidase t.
    CF antibody t.
titration
TLC – thin-layer chromatography

TNTC – too numerous to count
Todd-Hewitt broth
Todd's bodies
Todd unit
toluidine
   t. blue O
Torula
   T. capsulatus
   T. histolytica
Torulopsis
   T. glabrata
toxicology
toxin
Toxocara
   T. canis
   T. cati
   T. mystax
toxocariasis
toxoid
toxoid-antitoxoid
Toxoplasma
   T. gondii
   T. pyrogenes
toxoplasmosis
TPI – *Treponema pallidum*
   immobilization
TPTZ – tripyridyltriazine
Trachybdella bistriata
transaminase
transferase
transferrin
Trematoda
   T. Clonorchis
   T. Dicrocoelium
   T. Echinostoma
   T. Fasciola
   T. Fasciolopsis
   T. Gastrodiscoides
   T. Heterophyes
   T. Metagonimus
   T. Opisthorchis
   T. Paragonimus
   T. Schistosoma
trematode
Treponema
   T. calligyrum
   T. carateum

Treponema (continued)
    T. genitalis
    T. macrodentium
    T. microdentium
    T. mucosum
    T. pallidum
    T. pertenue
    T. pintae
TRF – thyrotropin-releasing
    factor
TRH – thyrotropin-releasing
    hormone
Tricercomonas
Trichinella
    T. spiralis
trichinosis
trichomonad
Trichomonas
    T. buccalis
    T. hominis
    T. intestinalis
    T. pulmonalis
    T. tenax
    T. vaginalis
trichomoniasis
Trichophyton
    T. concentricum
    T. epilans
    T. ferrugineum
    T. mentagrophytes
    T. rosaceum
    T. rubrum
    T. sabouraudi
    T. schoenleini
    T. sulfureum
    T. tonsurans
    T. verrucosum
    T. violaceum
trichophytosis
Trichoptera
Trichosporon
    T. beigelii
    T. cutaneum
    T. pedrosianum
Trichostrongylus
    T. axei
    T. brevis

Trichostrongylus (continued)
    T. colubriformis
    T. instabilis
    T. orientalis
    T. vitrinus
Trichothecium
    T. roseum
Trichuris
    T. trichiura
triglyceride
triiodothyronine
Triodontophorus
    T. diminutus
Triphleps insidiosus
triploidy
trisomies
trisomy C, mosaic
trisomy D
trisomy E
trisomy G
trisomy X
trisomy 8
trisomy 13
trisomy 18
trisomy 21
tritiated
Trombicula
    T. autumnalis
    T. irritans
    T. tsalsahuatl
    T. vandersandi
Trombiculidae
trophoplasm
trophozoite
TRP – tubular reabsorption of
    phosphate
Truant's stain
Trypanosoma
    T. brucei
    T. cruzi
    T. escomeli
    T. gambiense
    T. rangeli
    T. rhodesiense
trypanosomiasis
trypsin
trypsinogen

tryptase
TSH – thyroid-stimulating
   hormone
tularemia
Tunga
     T. penetrans
turbidimetric
turbidimetry
turbidity
Türk's cell
typhoid
typhus
typing
     ABO t.
     ABO-Rh t.
Tyroglyphus
     T. siro
tyrosine
tyrosinosis
Tzanck test
ubakterealez. See *Eubacteriales*.
ubaktereum. See *Eubacterium*.
Uffelmann's test
Uganda S virus
Uglena. See *Euglena*.
uglobulin. See *euglobulin*.
ugonik. See *eugonic*.
ultracentrifugation
unit
     Bessey-Lowry u.
     Bodansky u.
     Gutman u.
     Karmen u's
     King-Armstrong u.
     mouse u.
     rat u.
     Russell u.
     Shinowara-Jones-
       Reinhard u.
     Somogyi u.
     Todd u's
     Wohlgemuth u.
Uproktis. See *Euproctis*.
uptake
     RAI (radioactive iodine) u.
     resin u.
urate

urea
Ureaplasma
     U. urealyticum
urease
uric
urinalysis
urobilin
urobilinogen
Uronema caudatum
uropepsin
uroporphyrin
uroporphyrinogen I, III
uroreaction
Urosheum. See *Eurotium*.
Uruma virus
Usimuleum. See *Eusimulium*.
Utriatoma. See *Eutriatoma*.
Utrombikula. See *Eutrombicula*.
vaccinate
vaccine
vacuolation
vacuole
     autophagic v.
     contractile v.
     plasmocrine v.
     rhagiocrine v.
Vahlkampfia
valine
van den Bergh test
van Gieson's stain
Van Slyke test
Vaquez-Osler disease
Vaquez's disease
VDRL – Venereal Disease
     Research Laboratories
VDRL test
VEE virus – Venezuelan
     equine encephalomyelitis
     virus
Veillonella
     V. alcalescens
     V. discoides
     V. orbiculus
     V. parvula
     V. reniformis
     V. vulvovaginitidis
venipuncture

Verticillium
  V. graphii
Vi agglutination
Vi antigen
vibrio
  Celebes' v.
  cholera v.
  El Tor's v's
  non-agglutinating v's
  paracholera v's
Vibrio
  V. alginolyticus
  V. bulbulus
  V. cholerae
  V. cholerae-asiaticae
  V. coli
  V. comma
  V. danubicus
  V. faecalis
  V. fetus
  V. finkleri
  V. ghinda
  V. jejuni
  V. massauah
  V. metchnikovii
  V. niger
  V. parahaemolyticus
  V. phosphorescens
  V. proteus
  V. septicus
  V. tyrogenus
vibrion
  v. septique
Vicia
  V. graminea
Vincent's organism
viral
virology
viruria
virus
  animal v's
  v. animatum
  arbor v's
  attenuated v.
  Australian X disease v.
  bacterial v.
  Brunhilde v.

virus (continued)
  Bunyamwera v.
  Bwamba fever v.
  C v.
  CA v.
  Cache valley v.
  California v.
  Chikungunya v.
  Coe v.
  Colorado tick fever v.
  coryza v.
  Coxsackie v.
  croup-associated v.
  cytomegalic inclusion
    disease v.
  dengue v.
  eastern equine
    encephalomyelitis v.
  EBV (Epstein-Barr) v.
  ECBO (enteric
    cytopathogenic bovine
    orphan) v.
  ECDO (enteric
    cytopathogenic dog
    orphan) v.
  ECHO (enteric
    cytopathogenic human
    orphan) v.
  ECHO 28 v.
  ECMO (enteric
    cytopathogenic monkey
    orphan) v.
  ECSO (enteric
    cytopathogenic swine
    orphan) v.
  EEE (eastern equine
    encephalomyelitis) v.
  EMC
    (encephalomyocarditis)
    v.
  encephalomyocarditis v.
  enteric orphan v's
  entomopox v.
  epidemic
    keratoconjunctivitis
    v.
  Epstein-Barr v.

virus (continued)

    equine encephalo-
      myelitis v.
    filterable v.
    fixed v.
    Guaroa v.
    hemadsorption v.: types 1
      and 2
    hepatitis v.
    herpangina v.
    herpes v.
    human immunodeficiency
      v.
    human T-cell leukemia/
      lymphoma v.
    Ilheus v.
    inclusion conjunctivitis v.
    influenza v.
    Japanese B encephalitis v.
    JH v.
    Junin v.
    Kumba v.
    Kyasanur Forest disease v.
    Lansing v.
    Lassa v.
    latent v.
    Leon v.
    lepori pox v.
    louping ill v.
    Lunyo v.
    lymphocytic
      choriomeningitis v.
    lymphogranuloma
      venereum v.
    masked v.
    Mayaro v.
    Mengo v.
    Murray Valley
      encephalitis v.
    Newcastle disease v.
    O'nyong-nyong v.
    ornithosis v.
    Oropouche v.
    orphan v's
    pappataci fever v.
    parainfluenza v.
    parapox v.

virus (continued)

    parrot v.
    pharyngoconjunctival
      fever v.
    pneumonitis v.
    poliomyelitis v.
    polyoma v.
    Powassan v.
    poxvirus
    psittacosis v.
    rabies v.
    respiratory syncytial v.
    Rift Valley fever v.
    RS (respiratory syncytial)
      v.
    rubella v.
    Russian spring-summer
      encephalitis v.
    salivary gland v.
    Semliki Forest v.
    Sendai v.
    Simbu v.
    simian v's
    Sindbis v.
    St. Louis encephalitis v.
    street v.
    Teschen v.
    Theiler's v.
    tick-borne v's
    trachoma v.
    2060 v.
    Uganda S v.
    unorganized v.
    Uruma v.
    vaccine v.
    varicella-zoster v.
    variola v.
    VEE (Venezuelan equine
      encephalomyelitis) v.
    WEE (western equine
      encephalomyelitis) v.
    Wesselsbron v.
    western equine
      encephalomyelitis v.
    West Nile v.

viscosimeter

    Stormer v.

viscosity
viscous
VMA – vanillylmandelic acid
Voges-Proskauer
    broth
    test
Volhard's test
volumetric
von Kossa's stain
von Willebrand's antigen
Wade-Fite-Faraco stain
Waldenström's
    macroglobulinemia
washing
    bronchial w.
Wassermann
    reaction
    test
Watson-Schwartz test
WBC – white blood cell
    white blood cell count
WBC/hpf – white blood cells per
    high-power field
WEE virus – western equine
    encephalomyelitis virus
Weichselbaum's diplococcus
Weigert's stain
Weil-Felix reaction
Wesselsbron virus
Westergren's sedimentation rate
western equine
    encephalomyelitis virus
West Nile virus
whipworm
Whitmore's bacillus
Widal reaction
Wilkins-Chilgren agar
Wintrobe's sedimentation rate

Wohlgemuth unit
Wright's stain
Wuchereria
    W. bancrofti
    W. malayi
wuchereriasis
xanthochromatic
xanthocyte
xanthomatous
Xanthomonas
X chromosome
X chromatin bodies
Xenopsylla
    X. cheopis
Xenopus
    X. laevis
xeroradiography
D-xylose tolerance test

Y chromosome
Yersinia
    Y. enterocolitica
    Y. pestis
    Y. pseudotuberculosis
Yersinieae

zantho-. See words beginning
    xantho-.
Zenker's fixative
Zeta sedimentation rate
Ziehl-Neelsen's stain
Zoogloea
Zuberella
Zygomyces
Zygomycetes
zygomycosis
Zymobacterium
zymogen

Reference Values in Hematology

	Conventional Units		S.I. Units		Notes
Acid hemolysis test (Ham)	No hemolysis		No hemolysis		a
Alkaline phosphatase, leukocyte	Total score 14–100		Total score 14–100		
Carboxyhemoglobin	Up to 5% of total		0.05 of total		
Cell counts					
Erythrocytes					
Males	4.6–6.2 million/cu mm		$4.6–6.2 \times 10^{12}$/l		
Females	4.2–5.4 million/cu mm		$4.2–5.4 \times 10^{12}$/l		
Children (varies with age)	4.5–5.1 million/cu mm		$4.5–5.1 \times 10^{12}$/l		
Leukocytes					
Total	4500–11,000/cu mm		$4.5–11.0 \times 10^{9}$/l		
Differential	*Percentage*	*Absolute*			b
	0	0/cu mm	0/l		
Myelocytes	3–5	150–400/cu mm	$150–400 \times 10^{6}$/l		
Band neutrophils	54–62	3000–5800/cu mm	$3000–5800 \times 10^{6}$/l		
Segmented neutrophils	25–33	1500–3000/cu mm	$1500–3000 \times 10^{6}$/l		
Lymphocytes	3–7	300–500/cu mm	$300–500 \times 10^{6}$/l		
Monocytes	1–3	50–250/cu mm	$50–250 \times 10^{6}$/l		
Eosinophils	0–0.75	15–50/cu mm	$15–50 \times 10^{6}$/l		
Basophils					
Platelets	150,000–350,000/cu mm		$150–350 \times 10^{9}$/l		b
Reticulocytes	0.5–1.5% of erythrocytes		$25–75 \times 10^{9}$/l		
Bone marrow, differential cell count					a
	Range	*Average*	*Range*	*Average*	
Myeloblasts	0.3–5.0%	2.0%	0.003–0.05	0.02	
Promyelocytes	1.0–8.0%	5.0%	0.01–0.08	0.05	

Myelocytes: Neutrophilic	5.0–19.0%	12.0%	0.05–0.19	0.12
Eosinophilic	0.5–3.0%	1.5%	0.005–0.03	0.015
Basophilic	0.0–0.5%	0.3%	0.00–0.005	0.003
Metamyelocytes	13.0–32.0%	22.0%	0.13–0.32	0.22
Polymorphonuclear neutrophils	7.0–30.0%	20.0%	0.07–0.30	0.20
Polymorphonuclear eosinophils	0.5–4.0%	2.0%	0.005–0.04	0.02
Polymorphonuclear basophils	0.0–0.7%	0.2%	0.00–0.007	0.002
Lymphocytes	3.0–17.0%	10.0%	0.03–0.17	0.10
Plasma cells	0.0–2.0%	0.4%	0.00–0.02	0.004
Monocytes	0.5–5.0%	2.0%	0.005–0.05	0.02
Reticulum cells	0.1–2.0%	0.2%	0.001–0.02	0.002
Megakaryocytes	0.3–3.0%	0.4%	0.003–0.03	0.004
Pronormoblasts	1.0–8.0%	4.0%	0.01–0.08	0.04
Normoblasts	7.0–32.0%	18.0%	0.07–0.32	0.18

Coagulation tests

Antithrombin III (synthetic substrate)

Bleeding time (Duke)	80–120% of normal	0.8–1.2 of normal
Bleeding time (Ivy)	1–5 min	1–5 min
Bleeding time (template)	Less than 5 min	Less than 5 min
Clot retraction, qualitative	2.5–9.5 min	2.5–9.5 min
	Begins in 30–60 min	Begins in 30–60 min
	Complete in 24 hrs	Complete in 24 h
Coagulation time (Lee-White)	5–15 min (glass tubes)	5–15 min (glass tubes)
	19–60 min (siliconized tubes)	19–60 min (siliconized tubes)
Euglobulin lysis time	2–6 hrs at 37°C	2–6 h at 37°C
Factor VIII and other coagulation factors	50–150% of normal	0.50–1.5 of normal

a

Table continued on following page

Reference Values in Hematology *Continued*

	Conventional Units	S.I. Units	Notes
Fibrin split products (Thrombo-Wellco test)	Less than 10 mcg/ml	Less than 10 mg/l	
Fibrinogen	200–400 mg/dl	5.9–11.7 μmol/l	c
Fibrinolysins	0	0	
Partial thromboplastin time, activated (APTT)	20–35 sec	20–35 sec	
Prothrombin consumption	Over 80% consumed in 1 hr	Over 0.80 consumed in 1 h	a
Prothrombin content	100% (calculated from prothrombin time)	1.0 (calculated from prothrombin time)	a
	12.0–14.0 sec	12.0–14.0 sec	
Prothrombin time (one stage)			
Tourniquet test	Ten or fewer petechiae in a 2.5-cm circle after 5 min	Ten or fewer petechiae in a 2.5-cm circle after 5 min	
Cold hemolysin test (Donath-Landsteiner)	No hemolysis	No hemolysis	
Coombs' test			
Direct	Negative	Negative	
Indirect	Negative	Negative	
Corpuscular values of erythrocytes (values are for adults; in children, values vary with age)			
MCH (mean corpuscular hemoglobin)	27–31 picogm	0.42–0.48 fmol	d

Test	Conventional	SI units	
MCV (mean corpuscular volume)	80–96 cu micra	80–96 fl	
MCHC (mean corpuscular hemoglobin concentration)	32–36%	0.32–0.36	a
Haptoglobin (as hemoglobin binding capacity)	100–200 mg/dl	16–31 μmol/l	d
Hematocrit			a
Males	40–54 ml/dl	0.40–0.54	
Females	37–47 ml/dl	0.37–0.47	
Newborn	49–54 ml/dl	0.49–0.54	
Children (varies with age)	35–49 ml/dl	0.35–0.49	
Hemoglobin			d
Males	14.0–18.0 grams/dl	2.17–2.79 mmol/l	
Females	12.0–16.0 grams/dl	1.86–2.48 mmol/l	
Newborn	16.5–19.5 grams/dl	2.56–3.02 mmol/l	
Children (varies with age)	11.2–16.5 grams/dl	1.74–2.56 mmol/l	
Hemoglobin, fetal	Less than 1% of total	Less than 0.01 of total	a
Hemoglobin A$_{1c}$	3–5% of total	0.03–0.05 of total	a
Hemoglobin A$_2$	1.5–3.0% of total	0.015–0.03 of total	a
Hemoglobin, plasma	0–5.0 mg/dl	0–0.8 μmol/l	d
Methemoglobin	0–130 mg/dl	4.7–20 μmol/l	e
Osmotic fragility of erythrocytes	Begins in 0.45–0.39% NaCl	Begins in 77–67 mmol/NaCl NaCl	
	Complete in 0.33–0.30% NaCl	Complete in 56–51 mmol/l NaCl	
Sedimentation rate			
Wintrobe: Males	0–5 mm in 1 hr	0–5 mm/h	
Females	0–15 mm in 1 hr	0–15 mm/h	
Westergren: Male	0–15 mm in 1 hr	0–15 mm/h	
Females	0–20 mm in 1 hr	0–20 mm/h	
(May be slightly higher in children and during pregnancy)			

Reference Values for Blood, Plasma, and Serum

(For some procedures the reference values may vary depending upon the method used)

	Conventional Units	S.I. Units	Notes
Acetoacetate plus acetone, serum			
Qualitative	Negative	Negative	
Quantitative	0.3–2.0 mg/dl	3–20 mg/l	
Adrenocorticotropin (ACTH), plasma			
6 AM	10–80 picogm/ml	10–80 ng/l	
6 PM	Less than 50 picogm/ml	Less than 50 ng/l	
Alanine aminotransferase: *see*			
Transaminase			
Aldolase, serum	0–11 milliunits/ml (30°C)	0–11 units/1 (30°C)	f
Aldosterone			
Adult, supine	3–10 nanogm/dl	0.08–0.3 nmol/l	
standing			
male	6–22 nanogm/dl	0.17–0.61 nmol/l	
female	5–30 nanogm/dl	0.14–0.8 nmol/l	
Alpha amino nitrogen, serum	3.0–5.5 mg/dl	2.1–3.9 mmol/l	
Ammonia (nitrogen), plasma	15–49 mcg/dl	11–35 μmol/l	
Amylase, serum	25–125 milliunits/ml	25–125 units/l	
Anion gap	8–16 mEq/liter	8–16 mmol/l	
Ascorbic acid, blood	0.4–1.5 mg/dl	23–85 μmol/l	
Aspartate aminotransferase: *see*			
Transaminase			
Base excess, blood	0 ± 2 mEq/liter	0 ± 2 mmol/l	
Bicarbonate, serum	23–29 mEq/liter	23–29 mmol/l	
Bile acids, serum	0.3–3.0 mg/dl	3.0–30.0 mg/l	
Bilirubin, serum			

Direct	0.1–0.4 mg/dl	1.7–6.8 μmol/l	
Indirect	0.2–0.7 mg/dl (total minus direct)	3.4–12 μmol/l (total minus direct)	
Total	0.3–1.1 mg/dl	5.1–19 μmol/l	a
Calcium, serum	4.5–5.5 mEq/liter	2.25–2.75 mmol/l	
	9.0–11.0 mg/dl		
	(Slightly higher in children)	(Slightly higher in children)	
Calcium, ionized, serum	2.1–2.6 mEq/liter	(Varies with protein concentration)	
	4.25–5.25 mg/dl	1.05–1.30 mmol/l	
Carbon dioxide content, serum			
Adults	24–30 mEq/liter	24–30 mmol/l	
Infants	20–28 mEq/liter	20–28 mmol/l	
Carbon dioxide tension (Pco₂), blood	35–45 mm Hg	35–45 mm Hg	g
Carotene, serum	40–200 mcg/dl	0.74–3.72 μmol/l	
Ceruloplasmin, serum	23–44 mg/dl	230–440 mg/l	h
Chloride, serum	96–106 mEq/liter	96–106 mmol/l	
Cholesterol, serum			
Total	150–250 mg/dl	3.9–6.5 mmol/l	a
Esters	68–76% of total cholesterol	0.68–0.76 of total cholesterol	
Cholinesterase			
Serum	0.5–1.3 pH units	0.5–1.3 pH units	f
Erythrocytes	0.5–1.0 pH unit	0.5–1.0 pH unit	f
Copper, serum			
Males	70–140 mcg/dl	11–22 μmol/l	
Females	85–155 mcg/dl	13–24 μmol/l	
Cortisol, plasma			
8 AM	6–23 mcg/dl	170–635 nmol/l	
4 PM	3–15 mcg/dl	82–413 nmol/l	
10 PM	Less than 50% of 8 AM value	Less than 0.5 of 8 AM value	
Creatine, serum	0.2–0.8 mg/dl	15–61 μmol/l	

Table continued on following page

Reference Values for Blood, Plasma, and Serum *Continued*

	Conventional Units	S.I. Units	Notes
Creatine kinase, serum (CK, CPK)			
Males	12–80 milliunits/ml (30°C)	12–80 units/l (30°C)	f
	55–170 milliunits/ml (37°C)	55–170 units/l (37°C)	f
Females	10–55 milliunits/ml (30°C)	10–55 units/l (30°C)	f
	30–135 milliunits/ml (37°C)	30–135 units/l (37°C)	f
Creatine kinase isoenzymes, serum			
CK-MM	Present	Present	
CK-MB	Absent	Absent	
CK-BB	Absent	Absent	
Creatinine, serum	0.6–1.2 mg/dl	53–106 μmol/l	
Cryoglobulins, serum	0	0	
Fatty acids, serum			
Total	190–420 mg/dl	7–15 mmol/l	i
Nonesterified	8–25 mg/dl	0.30–0.90 mmol/l	
Ferritin, serum	20–200 nanogm/ml	20–200 μg/l	
Fibrinogen, plasma	200–400 mg/100 ml	5.9–11.7 μmol/l	c
Folate, serum	1.8–9.0 nanogm/ml	4.1–20.4 nmol/l	
Erythrocytes	150–450 nanogm/ml	340–1020 nmol/l	
Follicle-stimulating hormone (FSH), plasma			
Males	4–25 milliunits/ml (I.U.)	4–25 IU/l	
Females	4–30 milliunits/ml (I.U.)	4–30 IU/l	
Postmenopausal	40–250 milliunits/ml (I.U.)	40–250 IU/l	
Gamma glutamyltransferase			
Males	6–32 milliunits/ml (30°C)	6–32 units/l (30°C)	f
Females	4–18 milliunits/ml (30°C)	4–18 units/l (30°C)	f

	Conventional units	SI units	
Gastrin, serum	0–200 picogm/ml	0–200 ng/l	
Glucose (fasting)			
Blood	60–100 mg/dl	3.33–5.55 mmol/l	
Plasma or serum	70–115 mg/dl	3.89–6.38 mmol/l	
Growth hormone, serum	0–10 nanogm/ml	0.10 µg/l	
Haptoglobin, serum	100–200 mg/dl	16–31 µmol/l	d
	(As hemoglobin binding capacity)	(As hemoglobin binding capacity)	
Hydroxybutyric dehydrogenase, serum (HBD)	0–180 milliunits/ml (30°C)	0–180 units/l (30°C)	f
17-Hydroxycorticosteroids, plasma	8–18 mcg/dl	0.22–0.50 µmol/l	j
Immunoglobulins, serum			
IgG	550–1900 mg/dl	5.5–19.0 g/l	
IgA	60–333 mg/dl	0.60–3.3 g/l	
IgM	45–145 mg/dl	0.45–1.5 g/l	
IgD	0.5–3.0 mg/dl	5–30 mg/l	
IgE	<500 nanogm/ml	<500 µg/l	
	(Varies with age in children)	(Varies with age in children)	
Insulin, plasma (fasting)	5–25 microunits/ml	36–179 pmol/l	k
Iodine, protein bound, serum	3.5–8.0 mcg/dl	0.28–0.63 µmol/l	
Iron, serum	75–175 mcg/dl	13–31 µmol/l	
Iron-binding capacity, serum			
Total	250–410 mcg/dl	45–73 µmol/l	a
Saturation	20–55%	0.20–0.55	
Lactate, blood, venous	4.5–19.8 mg/dl	0.5–2.2 mmol/l	
arterial	4.5–14.4 mg/dl	0.5–1.6 mmol/l	
Lactate dehydrogenase, serum (LD, LDH)	45–90 milliunits/ml (I.U.) (30°C)	45–90 units/l (30°C)	f
	100–190 milliunits/ml (37°C)	100–190 units/l (37°C)	
LDH$_1$	22–37% of total	0.22–0.37 of total	
LDH$_2$	30–46% of total	0.30–0.46 of total	a
LDH$_3$	14–29% of total	0.14–0.29 of total	

Table continued on following page

205

Reference Values for Blood, Plasma, and Serum *Continued*

	Conventional Units	S.I. Units	Notes
LDH$_4$	5–11% of total	0.05–0.11 of total	
LDH$_5$	2–11% of total	0.02–0.11 of total	
Leucine aminopeptidase, serum	14–40 milliunits/ml (30°C)	14–40 units/l (30°C)	f
Lipase, serum	0–1.5 units (Cherry-Crandall)	0–1.5 units (Cherry-Crandall)	f
Lipids, total, serum	450–850 mg/dl	4.5–8.5 g/l	m
Lipoprotein cholesterol, serum			
LDL cholesterol	60–180 mg/dl	600–1800 mg/l	
HDL cholesterol	30–80 mg/dl	300–800 mg/l	
Luteinizing hormone (LH), serum			
Males	6–18 milliunits/ml (I.U.)	6–18 IU/l	
Females, premenopausal	5–22 milliunits/ml (I.U.)	5–22 IU/l	
midcycle	3 times baseline	3 times baseline	
postmenopausal	Greater than 30 milliunits/ml (I.U.)	Greater than 30 IU/l	
Magnesium, serum	1.5–2.5 mEq/liter	0.75–1.25 mmol/l	
	1.8–3.0 mg/dl		
5'-Nucleotidase, serum	3.5–12.7 milliunits/ml (37°C)	3.5–12.5 units/l (37°C)	f
Nitrogen, nonprotein, serum	15–35 mg/dl	10.7–25.0 mmol/l	
Osmolality, serum	285–295 mOsm/kg serum water	285–295 mmol/kg serum water	n
Oxygen, blood			
Capacity	16–24 vol % (varies with hemoglobin)	7.14–10.7 mmol/l (varies with hemoglobin)	o
Content Arterial	15–23 vol %	6.69–10.3 mmol/l	o
Venous	10–16 vol %	4.46–7.14 mmol/l	o

Saturation Arterial	94–100% of capacity	0.94–1.00 of capacity	a
Venous	60–85% of capacity	0.60–0.85 of capacity	a
Tension, P_{O_2} Arterial	75–100 mm Hg	75–100 mm Hg	g
P_{50}, blood	26–27 mm Hg	26–27 mm Hg	g
pH, arterial, blood	7.35–7.45	7.35–7.45	p
Phenylalanine, serum	Less than 3 mg/dl	Less than 0.18 mmol/l	f
Phosphatase, acid serum	0.11–0.60 milliunit/ml (37°C)	0.11–0.60 units/l	
	(Roy, Brower, Hayden)		
Phosphatase, alkaline, serum (ALP)	20–90 milliunits/ml (30°C)	20–90 units/l (30°C)	f
	(Values are higher in children)	(Values are higher in children)	
Phosphate, inorganic, serum			
Adults	3.0–4.5 mg/dl	1.0–1.5 mmol/l	
Children	4.0–7.0 mg/dl	1.3–2.3 mmol/l	
Phospholipids, serum	6–12 mg/dl	1.9–3.9 mmol/l	
	(As lipid phosphorus)	(As lipid phosphorus)	
Potassium, serum	3.5–5.0 mEq/liter	3.5–5.0 mmol/l	
Prolactin, serum			
Males	1–20 nanogm/ml	1–20 µg/l	
Females	1–25 nanogm/ml	1–25 µg/l	
Protein, serum			
Total	6.0–8.0 grams/dl	60–80 g/l	m
Albumin	3.5–5.5 grams/dl	35–55 g/l	q
	52–68% of total	0.52–0.68 of total	a
Globulin			
Alpha$_1$	0.2–0.4 gram/dl	2–4 g/l	m
	2–5% of total	0.02–0.05 of total	a
Alpha$_2$	0.5–0.9 gram/dl	5–9 g/l	m
	7–14% of total	0.07–0.14 of total	a
Beta	0.6–1.1 grams/dl	6–11 g/l	m
	9–15% of total	0.09–0.15 of total	a

Table continued on following page

207

Reference Values for Blood, Plasma, and Serum *Continued*

	Conventional Units	S.I. Units	Notes
Gamma	0.7–1.7 grams/dl	7–17 g/l	m
	11–21% of total	0.11–0.21 of total	a
Protoporphyrin, erythrocyte	27–61 mcg/dl packed RBC	0.48–1.09 μmol/l packed RBC	
Pyruvate, blood	0.3–0.9 mg/dl	0.03–0.10 mmol/l	
Sodium, serum	136–145 mEq/liter	136–145 mmol/l	
Sulfates, inorganic, serum	0.8–1.2 mg/dl	83–125 μmol/l	
Testosterone, plasma			
Males	275–875 nanogm/dl	9.5–30 nmol/l	
Females	23–75 nanogm/dl	0.8–2.6 nmol/l	
Pregnant	38–190 nanogm/dl	1.3–6.6 nmol/l	
Thyroid-stimulating hormone (TSH), serum	0–7 microunits/ml	0–7 milliunits/ml	
Thyroxine, free, serum	1.0–2.1 nanogm/dl	13–27 pmol/l	
Thyroxine (T_4), serum	4.4–9.9 mcg/dl	57–128 nmol/l	
Thyroxine-binding globulin (TBG), serum (as thyroxine)	10–26 mcg/dl	129–335 nmol/l	
Thyroxine iodine, serum	2.9–6.4 mcg/dl	229–504 nmol/l	k
Triiodothyronine (T_3), serum	150–250 nanogm/dl	2.3–3.9 nmol/l	
Triiodothyronine (T_3) uptake, resin (T_3RU)	25–38% uptake	0.25–0.38 uptake	a

Transaminase, serum			
SGOT (aspartate aminotransferase, AST)	8–20 milliunits/ml (30°C)	8–20 units/l (30 C)	f
	7–40 milliunits/ml (37°C)	7–40 units/l (37 C)	f
SGPT (alanine aminotransferase, ALT)	8–20 milliunits/ml (30°C)	8–20 units/l (30 C)	
	5–35 milliunits/ml (37°C)	5–35 units/l (37 C)	
Triglycerides, serum	40–150 mg/dl	0.4–1.5 g/l	r
		0.45–1.71 mmol/l	
Urate, serum			
Males	2.5–8.0 mg/dl	0.15–0.48 mmol/l	
Females	1.5–7.0 mg/dl	0.09–0.42 mmol/l	
Urea			
Blood	21–43 mg/dl	3.5–7.3 mmol/l	
Plasma or serum	24–49 mg/dl	4.0–8.3 mmol/l	
Urea nitrogen			
Blood	10–20 mg/dl	7.1–14.3 mmol/l	
Plasma or serum	11–23 mg/dl	7.9–16.4 mmol/l	
Viscosity, serum	1.4–1.8 times water	1.4–1.8 times water	k
Vitamin A, serum	20–80 mcg/dl	0.70–2.8 μmol/l	
Vitamin B$_{12}$, serum	180–900 picogm/ml	133–664 pmol/l	

Reference Values for Urine

(For some procedures the reference values may vary depending upon the method used)

	Conventional Units	S.I. Units	Notes
Acetone and acetoacetate, qualitative	Negative	Negative	
Albumin			
Qualitative	Negative	Negative	
Quantitative	10–100 mg/24 hrs	10–100 mg/24 h	q
		0.15–1.5 μmol/24 h	
Aldosterone	3–20 mcg/24 hrs	8.3–55 nmol/24 h	
Alpha amino nitrogen	50–200 mg/24 hrs	3.6–14.3 mmol/24 h	
Ammonia nitrogen	20–70 mEq/24 hrs	20–70 mmol/24 h	
Amylase	1–17 units/hr	1–17 units/h	f
Amylase/creatinine clearance ratio	1–4%	0.01–0.04	
Bilirubin, qualitative	Negative	Negative	
Calcium			
Low Ca diet	Less than 150 mg/24 hrs	Less than 3.8 mmol/24 h	
Usual diet	Less than 250 mg/24 hrs	Less than 6.3 mmol/24 h	
Catecholamines			
Epinephrine	Less than 10 mcg/24 hrs	Less than 55 nmol/24 h	
Norepinephrine	Less than 100 mcg/24 hrs	Less than 590 nmol/24 h	
Total free catecholamines	4–126 mcg/24 hrs	24–745 nmol/24 h	s
Total metanephrines	0.1–1.6 mg/24 hrs	0.5–8.1 μmol/24 h	t
Chloride	110–250 mEq/24 hrs	110–250 mmol/24 h	
	(Varies with intake)	(Varies with intake)	
Chorionic gonadotropin	0	0	
Copper	0–50 mcg/24 hrs	0–0.80 μmol/24 h	
Cortisol, free	10–100 mcg/24 hrs	27.6–276 mmol/24 h	
Creatine			

Males	0–40 mg/24 hrs	0–0.30 mmol/24 h
Females	0–100 mg/24 hrs	0–0.76 mmol/24 h
	(Higher in children and during pregnancy)	(Higher in children and during pregnancy)
Creatinine	15–25 mg/kg body weight/24 hrs	0.13–0.22 mmol·kg⁻¹ body weight/24 h
Creatinine clearance		
Males	110–150 ml/min	110–150 ml/min
Females	105–132 ml/min	105–132 ml/min
	(1.73 sq meter surface area)	(1.73 m² surface area)
Cystine or cysteine, qualitative	Negative	Negative
Dehydroepiandrosterone	Less than 15% of total 17-ketosteroids	Less than 0.15 of total 17-ketosteroids [a]
Males	0.2–2.0 mg/24 hrs	0.7–6.9 µmol/24 h
Females	0.2–1.8 mg/24 hrs	0.7–6.2 µmol/24 h
Delta aminolevulinic acid	1.3–7.0 mg/24 hrs	10–53 µmol/24 h
Estrogens		
Males		
Estrone	3–8 µg/24 hrs	11–30 nmol/24 h
Estradiol	0–6 µg/24 hrs	0–22 nmol/24 h
Estriol	1–11 µg/24 hrs	3–38 nmol/24 h
Total	4–25 µg/24 hrs	14–90 nmol/24 h [u]
Females		
Estrone	4–31 µg/24 hrs	15–115 nmol/24 h
Estradiol	0–14 µg/24 hrs	0–51 nmol/24 h
Estriol	0–72 µg/24 hrs	0–250 nmol/24 h
Total	5–100 µg/24 hrs	18–360 nmol/24 h [u]
	(Markedly increased during pregnancy)	(Markedly increased during pregnancy)
Glucose (as reducing substance)	Less than 250 mg/24 hrs	Less than 250 mg/24 h
Hemoglobin and myoglobin, qualitative	Negative	Negative

Table continued on following page

211

Reference Values for Urine *Continued*

	Conventional Units	S.I. Units	Notes
Homogentisic acid, qualitative	Negative	Negative	
17-Hydroxycorticosteroids			j
Males	3–9 mg/24 hrs	8.3–25 μmol/24 h	
Females	2–8 mg/24 hrs	5.5–22 μmol/24 h	
5-Hydroxyindoleacetic acid			
Qualitative	Negative	Negative	
Quantitative	Less than 9 mg/24 hrs	Less than 47 μmol/24 h	
17-Ketosteroids			l
Males	6–18 mg/24 hrs	21–62 μmol/24 h	
Females	4–13 mg/24 hrs	14–45 μmol/24 h	
	(Varies with age)	(Varies with age)	
Magnesium	6.0–8.5 mEq/24 hrs	3.0–4.3 mmol/24 h	
Metanephrines (see Catecholamines)			
Osmolality	38–1400 mOsm/kg water	38–1400 mmol/kg water	n
pH	4.6–8.0, average 6.0	4.6–8.0, average 6.0	p
	(Depends on diet)	(Depends on diet)	
Phenolsulfonphthalein excretion (PSP)	25% or more in 15 min	0.25 or more in 15 min	a
	40% or more in 30 min	0.40 or more in 30 min	
	55% or more in 2 hrs	0.55 or more in 2 h	
	(After injection of 1 ml PSP intravenously)	(After injection of 1 ml PSP intravenously)	
Phenylpyruvic acid, qualitative	Negative	Negative	
Phosphorus	0.9–1.3 grams/24 hrs	29–42 mmol/24 h	
Porphobilinogen			
Qualitative	Negative	Negative	
Quantitative	0–0.2 mg/dl	0–0.9 μmol/l	
	Less than 2.0 mg/24 hrs	Less than 9 μmol/24 h	

		m
Porphyrins		
Coproporphyrin	50–250 mcg/24 hrs	77–380 nmol/24 h
Uroporphyrin	10–30 mcg/24 hrs	12–36 nmol/24 h
Potassium	25–100 mEq/24 hrs	25–100 mmol/24 h
	(Varies with intake)	(Varies with intake)
Pregnanediol		
Males	0.4–1.4 mg/24 hrs	1.2–4.4 μmol/24 h
Females		
Proliferative phase	0.5–1.5 mg/24 hrs	1.6–4.7 μmol/24 h
Luteal phase	2.0–7.0 mg/24 hrs	6.2–22 μmol/24 h
Postmenopausal phase	0.2–1.0 mg/24 hrs	0.6–3.1 μmol/24 h
Pregnanetriol	Less than 2.5 mg/24 hrs in adults	Less than 7.4 μmol/24 h in adults
Protein		
Qualitative	Negative	Negative
Quantitative	10–150 mg/24 hrs	10–150 mg/24 h
Sodium	130–260 mEq/24 hrs	130–260 mmol/24 h
	(Varies with intake)	(Varies with intake)
Specific gravity	1.003–1.030	1.003–1.030
Titratable acidity	20–40 mEq/24 hrs	20–40 mmol/24 h
Urate	200–500 mg/24 hrs	1.2–3.0 mmol/24 h
	(With normal diet)	(With normal diet)
Urobilinogen	Up to 1.0 Ehrlich unit/2 hrs	Up to 1.0 Ehrlich unit/2 h
	(1–3 PM)	(1–3 PM)
Vanillylmandelic acid (VMA)	0–4.0 mg/24 hrs	0–6.8 μmol/24 h
(4-hydroxy-3-methoxymandelic acid)	1–8 mg/24 hrs	5–40 μmol/24 h

Reference Values for Therapeutic Drug Monitoring

Drug	Therapeutic Range	Toxic Levels	Proprietary Names
Antibiotics			
Amikacin, serum	15–25 mcg/ml	Peak: >35 mcg/ml Trough: >5–8 mcg/ml	Amikin
Chloramphenicol, serum	10–20 mcg/ml	>25 mcg/ml	Chloromycetin
Gentamicin, serum	5–10 mcg/ml	Peak: >12 mcg/ml Trough: >2 mcg/ml	Garamycin
Tobramycin, serum	5–10 mcg/ml	Peak: >12 mcg/ml Trough: >2 mcg/ml	Nebcin
Anticonvulsants			
Carbamazepine, serum	5–12 mcg/ml	>12 mcg/ml	Tegretol
Ethosuximide, serum	40–100 mcg/ml	>100 mcg/ml	Zarontin
Phenobarbital, serum	10–30 mcg/ml	Vary widely because of developed tolerance	
Phenytoin, serum (diphenylhydantoin)	10–20 mcg/ml	>20 mcg/ml	Dilantin
Primidone, serum	5–12 mcg/ml	>15 mcg/ml	Mysoline
Valproic acid, serum	50–100 mcg/ml	>100 mcg/ml	Depakene
Analgesics			
Acetaminophen, serum	10–20 mcg/ml	>250 mcg/ml	Tylenol Datril
Salicylate, serum	100–250 mcg/ml	>300 mcg/ml	
Bronchodilator			
Theophylline (aminophylline)	10–20 mcg/ml	>20 mcg/ml	
Cardiovascular Drugs			
Digitoxin, serum	15–25 nanogm/ml (Specimen obtained 12–24 hrs after last dose)	>25 nanogm/ml	Crystodigin
Digoxin, serum	0.8–2 nanogm/ml (Specimen obtained 12–24 hrs	>2.4 nanogm/ml	Lanoxin

Drug	Therapeutic Range	Alert Level	Trade Names
Disopyramide, serum	2–5 mcg/ml	>5 mcg/ml	Norpace
Lidocaine, serum	1.5–5 mcg/ml	>5 nanogm/ml	Anestacon Xylocaine
	(after last dose)		Pronestyl
Procainamide, serum	4–10 mcg/ml	>16 mcg/ml	
	*10–30 mcg/ml (*Procainamide + N-Acetyl Procainamide)	*>30 mcg/ml	
Propranolol, serum	50–100 nanogm/ml	Variable	Inderal
Quinidine, serum	2–5 mcg/ml	>10 mcg/ml	Cardioquin Quinaglute Quinidex Quinora

Psychopharmacologic Drugs

Drug	Therapeutic Range	Alert Level	Trade Names
Amitriptyline, serum	*120–150 nanogm/ml (*Amitriptyline + Nortriptyline)	*>500 nanogm/ml	Amitril Elavil Endep Etrafon Limbitrol Triavil
Desipramine, serum	*150–300 nanogm/ml (*Desipramine + Imipramine)	*>500 nanogm/ml	Norpramin Pertofrane
Imipramine, serum	*150–300 nanogm/ml (*Imipramine + Desipramine)	*>500 nanogm/ml	Antipress Imavate Janimine Presamine Tofranil
Lithium, serum	0.8–1.2 mEq/liter (Specimen obtained 12 hrs after last dose)	>2.0 mEq/liter	Lithobid Lithotabs
Nortriptyline, serum	50–150 nanogm/ml	>500 nanogm/ml	Aventyl Pamelor

Reference Values in Toxicology

	Conventional Units	S.I. Units	Notes
Arsenic, blood	3.5–7.2 mcg/dl	0.47–0.96 μmol/l	
Arsenic, urine	Less than 100 mcg/24 hrs	Less than 1.3 μmol/24 h	
Bromides, serum	0	0	
Carbon monoxide, blood	Toxic levels: Above 17 mmol/l	Toxic levels: Above 17 mmol/l	[a]
	Up to 5% saturation	Up to 0.5 saturation	
	Symptoms occur with 20% saturation	Symptoms occur with 0.20 saturation	
Ethanol, blood	Less than 0.005%	Less than 1 mmol/l	
Marked intoxication	0.3–0.4%	65–87 mmol/l	
Alcoholic stupor	0.4–0.5% mcg/dl	87–109 mmol/l	
Coma	Above 0.5%	Above 109 mmol/l	
Lead, blood	0–40 mcg/dl	0–2 μmol/l	
Lead, urine	Less than 100 mcg/24 hrs	Less than 0.48 μmol/24 h	
Mercury, urine	Less than 100 mcg/24 hrs	Less than 50 nmol/24 h	

Reference Values for Cerebrospinal Fluid

	Conventional Units	S.I. Units	Notes
Cells	Fewer than 5/cu mm; all mononuclear	Fewer than 5/µl; all mononuclear	
Chloride	120–130 mEq/liter	120–130 mmol/l	
	(20 mEq/liter higher than serum)	(20 mmol/l higher than serum)	
Electrophoresis	Predominantly albumin	Predominantly albumin	
Glucose	50–75 mg/dl	2.8–4.2 mmol/l	
	(20 mg/dl less than serum)	(1.1 mmol/less than serum)	
IgG			a,m
Children under 14	Less than 8% of total protein	Less than 0.08 of total protein	
Adults	Less than 14% of total protein	Less than 0.14 of total protein	
Pressure	70–180 mm water	70–180 mm water	g
Protein, total	15–45 mg/dl	0.150–0.450 g/l	m
	(Higher, up to 70 mg/dl, in elderly adults and children)	(Higher, up to 0.70 g/l, in elderly adults and children)	

Reference Values for Gastric Analysis

	Conventional Units	S.I. Units	Notes
Basal gastric secretion (1 hour)			
Concentration	(Mean ± 1 S.D.)	(Mean ± 1 S.D.)	
Males	25.8 ± 1.8 mEq/liter	25.8 ± 1.8 mmol/l	
Females	20.3 ± 3.0 mEq/liter	20.3 ± 3.0 mmol/l	
Output	(Mean ± 1 S.D.)	(Mean ± 1 S.D.)	
Males	2.57 ± 0.16 mEq/hr	2.57 ± 0.16 mmol/h	
Females	1.61 ± 0.18 mEq/hr	1.61 ± 0.18 mmol/h	
After histamine stimulation			
Normal	Mean output 11.8 mEq/hr	Mean output 11.8 mmol/h	
Duodenal ulcer	Mean output 15.2 mEq/hr	Mean output 15.2 mmol/h	
After maximal histamine stimulation			
Normal	Mean output 22.6 mEq/hr	Mean output 22.6 mmol/h	
Duodenal ulcer	Mean output 44.6 mEq/hr	Mean output 44.6 mmol/h	
Volume, fasting stomach content	50–100 ml	50–100 ml	
Emptying time	3–6 hrs	3–6 h	
Color	Opalescent or colorless	Opalescent or colorless	
Specific gravity	1.006–1.009	1.006–1.009	
pH (adults)	0.9–1.5	0.9–1.5	

Reference Values for Gastrointestinal Absorption Tests

	Conventional Units	S.I. Units
D-Xylose absorption test	After an 8-hour fast, 10 ml/kg body weight of a 0.05 solution of D-xylose is given by mouth. Nothing further by mouth is given until the test has been completed. All urine voided during the following 5 hours is pooled, and blood samples are taken at 0, 60, and 120 minutes. Normally 0.26 (range 0.16–0.33) of ingested xylose is excreted within 5 hours, and the serum xylose reaches a level between 25 and 40 mg/100 dl after 1 hour and is maintained at this level for another 60 minutes.	No change
Vitamin A absorption	A fasting blood specimen is obtained and 200,000 units of vitamin A in oil is given by mouth. Serum vitamin A level should rise to twice fasting level in 3 to 5 hours.	No change

Reference Values for Feces

	Conventional Units	S.I. Units	Notes
Bulk	100–200 grams/24 hrs	100–200 g/24 h	
Dry matter	23–32 grams/24 hrs	23–32 g/24 h	
Fat, total	Less than 6.0 grams/24 hrs	Less than 6.0 g/24 h	
Nitrogen, total	Less than 2.0 grams/24 hrs	Less than 2.0 g/24 h	
Urobilinogen	40–280 mg/24 hrs	40–280 mg/24 h	
Water	Approximately 65%	Approximately 0.65	a

Reference Values for Immunologic Procedures

	Conventional Units
Lymphocyte subsets	
T cells	60–85%
B cells	1–20%
T-helper cells	35–60%
T-suppressor cells	15–30%
T-H/S ratio	1.5–2.5
Complement	
C3	85–175 mg/dl
C4	15–45 mg/dl
CH_{50}	25–55 H_{50} units/ml
Tumor markers	
Carcinoembryonic antigen (CEA)	
(Roche)	Less than 5 nanogm/ml
(Abbott)	Less than 4.1 nanogm/ml
Alpha-fetoprotein (AFP)	Less than 10–30 nanogm/ml
	(depends on method)

Reference Values for Semen Analysis

	Conventional Units	S.I. Units	Notes
Volume	2–5 ml; usually 3–4 ml	2–5 ml; usually 3–4 ml	
Liquefaction	Complete in 15 min	Complete in 15 min	
pH	7.2–8.0; average 7.8	7.2–8.0; average 7.8	p
Leukocytes	Occasional or absent	Occasional or absent	
Count	60–150 million/ml	60–150 million/ml	
	Below 60 million/ml is abnormal	Below 60 million/ml is abnormal	
Motility	80% or more motile	0.80 or more motile	a
Morphology	80–90% normal forms	0.80–0.90 normal forms	a

Normal Laboratory Values*

NOTES KEYED TO TABLES

a. Percentage is expressed as a decimal fraction.
b. Percentage may be expressed as a decimal fraction; however, when the result expressed is itself a variable fraction of another variable, the absolute value is more meaningful. There is no reason, other than custom, for expressing reticulocyte counts and differential leukocyte counts in percentages or decimal fractions rather than in absolute numbers.
c. Molecular weight of fibrinogen = 341,000 daltons.
d. Molecular weight of hemoglobin = 64,500 daltons. Because of disagreement as to whether the monomer or tetramer of hemoglobin should be used in the conversion, it has been recommended that the conventional grams per deciliter be retained. The tetramer is used in the table; values given should be multiplied by 4 to obtain concentration of the monomer.
e. Molecular weight of methemoglobin = 64,500 daltons. See note d above.
f. Enzyme units have not been changed in these tables because the proposed enzyme unit, the katal, has not been universally adopted (1 International Unit = 16.7 nkat).
g. It has been proposed that pressure be expressed in the pascal (1 mm Hg = 0.133 kPa); however, this convention has not been universally accepted.
h. Molecular weight of ceruloplasmin = 151,000 daltons.
i. "Fatty acids" includes a mixture of different aliphatic acids of varying molecular weight. A mean molecular weight of 284 daltons has been assumed in calculating the conversion factor.
j. Based upon molecular weight of cortisol 362.47 daltons.
k. The practice of expressing concentration of an organic molecule in terms of one of its constituent elements originated when measurements included a heterogeneous class of compounds (nonprotein nitrogenous compounds, iodine-containing compounds bound to serum proteins). It was carried over to expressing measurements of specific substances (urea, thyroxine), but the practice should be discarded. For iodine and nitrogen 1 mole is taken as the monoatomic form, although they occur as diatomic molecules.

---

*Most of the reference values shown in the preceding tables are reproduced courtesy of Rakel, R. E. (ed.): Conn's Current Therapy 1990, Philadelphia, W. B. Saunders Company, 1990.

223

l. Based upon molecular weight of dehydroepiandrosterone 288.41 daltons.

m. Weight per volume is retained as the unit because of the heterogeneous nature of the material measured.

n. The proposal that osmolality be reported as freezing point depression using the millikelvin as the unit has not been received with universal enthusiasm. The milliosmole is not an S.I. unit, and the unit used here is the millimole.

o. Volumes per cent might be converted to a decimal fraction; however, this would not permit direct correlation with hemoglobin content, which is possible when oxygen content and capacity are expressed in molar quantities. One millimole of hemoglobin combines with 4 millimoles of oxygen.

p. Hydrogen ion concentration in S.I. units would be expressed in nanomoles per liter; however, this change has not received general approval. Conversion can be calculated as antilog $(-pH)$.

q. Albumin is expressed in grams per liter to be consistent with units used for other proteins. Concentration of albumin may be expressed in mmol/l also, an expression that permits assessment of binding capacity of albumin for substances such as bilirubin. Molecular weight of albumin is 65,000 daltons.

r. Most techniques for quantitating triglycerides measure the glycerol moiety, and the total mass is calculated using an average molecular weight. The factor given assumes a mean molecular weight of 875 daltons for triglycerides.

s. Calculated as norepinephrine, molecular weight 169.18 daltons.

t. Calculated as metanephrine, molecular weight 197.23 daltons.

u. Conversion factor calculated from molecular weights of estrone, estradiol, and estriol in proportions of 2 : 1 : 2 daltons.

References

1. AMA Drug Evaluations, 6th ed. Chicago, American Medical Association, 1986.
2. AMA Council on Scientific Affairs: J.A.M.A. *253*:2552, 1985.
3. Goodman, A. G., Gilman, L. S., Rall, T. W., and Murad, F.: Goodman and Gilman's The Pharmacological Basis of Therapeutics, 7th ed. New York, Macmillan, 1985.
4. Henry, J. B.: Clinical Diagnosis and Management by Laboratory Methods, 17th ed. Philadelphia, W. B. Saunders Company, 1984.
5. Henry, R. J., Cannon, D. C., and Winkleman, J. W.: Clinical Chemistry–Principles and Techniques, 2nd ed. New York, Harper & Row, 1974.
6. International Committee for Standardization in Hematology, International Federation of Clinical Chemistry and World Association of Pathology Societies: Clin. Chem. *19*:135, 1973.
7. Lundberg, G. D., Iverson, C., and Radulescu, G.: J.A.M.A. *255*:2247, 1986.

8. Miale, J. B.: Laboratory Medicine–Hematology, 6th ed. St. Louis, C. V. Mosby, 1982.

9. National Diabetes Data Group: Diabetes 28:1039, 1979.

10. Page, C. H., and Vigourex, P.: The International System of Units (S.I.). U.S. Department of Commerce, National Bureau of Standards, Special Publication 330, 1974.

11. Physicians' Desk Reference, 43rd ed. Oradell, N.J., Medical Economics Company, 1989.

12. Scully, R. E., McNeely, B. U., and Mark, E. J.: N. Engl. J. Med. 314:39, 1986.

13. Tietz, N. W.: Clinical Guide to Laboratory Tests. Philadelphia, W. B. Saunders Company, 1983.

14. Tietz, N. W.: Textbook of Clinical Chemistry. Philadelphia, W. B. Saunders Company, 1986.

15. Williams, W. J., Beutler, E., Erslev, A. J., and Lichtman, M. A.: Hematology, 3rd ed. New York, McGraw-Hill Book Company, 1983.

Some of the values have been established by the Clinical Pathology Laboratories, Emory University Hospital, Atlanta, Georgia, or by the Clinical Laboratories, Thomas Jefferson University Hospital, Philadelphia, Pennsylvania, and have not been published elsewhere.

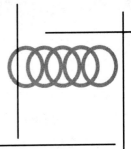

Part Two

Systems and Specialties

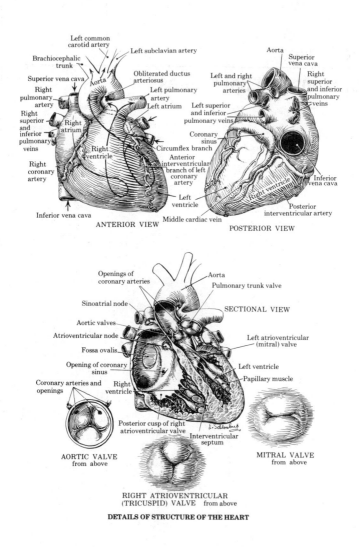

ANTERIOR VIEW

Left common carotid artery
Left subclavian artery
Brachiocephalic trunk
Obliterated ductus arteriosus
Superior vena cava
Aorta
Right pulmonary artery
Left pulmonary artery
Left atrium
Right superior and inferior pulmonary veins
Right atrium
Right ventricle
Circumflex branch
Anterior interventricular branch of left coronary artery
Right coronary artery
Left ventricle
Inferior vena cava
Middle cardiac vein

POSTERIOR VIEW

Aorta
Superior vena cava
Left and right pulmonary arteries
Right superior and inferior pulmonary veins
Left superior and inferior pulmonary veins
Coronary sinus
Inferior vena cava
Right ventricle
Posterior interventricular artery

SECTIONAL VIEW

Openings of coronary arteries
Aorta
Pulmonary trunk valve
Sinoatrial node
Aortic valves
Atrioventricular node
Fossa ovalis
Opening of coronary sinus
Coronary arteries and openings
Right ventricle
Left atrioventricular (mitral) valve
Left ventricle
Papillary muscle
Posterior cusp of right atrioventricular valve
Interventricular septum

AORTIC VALVE from above

MITRAL VALVE from above

RIGHT ATRIOVENTRICULAR (TRICUSPID) VALVE from above

DETAILS OF STRUCTURE OF THE HEART

(Courtesy of Dorland's Illustrated Medical Dictionary, 27th ed. Plate 19. Philadelphia, W. B. Saunders Company, 1988.)

Cardiovascular System

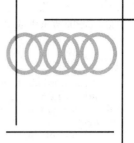

A$_2$–aortic second sound
AA–ascending aorta
A band
abdomino-jugular reflux
ABE–acute bacterial
    endocarditis
Abée's support
aberrancy
aberrant
abetalipoproteinemia
Abrams' heart reflex
abscess
    myocardial a.
absorbed dose
AC–anodal closure
    anterior chamber
    aortic closure
ACC–anodal closing contraction
accelerans
accretio
    a. cordis
    a. pericardii
ACD–absolute cardiac dullness
achalasia
acid-base imbalance
acidemia
acidosis
Acinetobacter
acoustic imaging
acquired immunodeficiency
    syndrome
acromegaly
acromioclavicular
Actinobacillus
    *A. actinomycetemcom-
        itans*
Actinomyces
    A. israelii

actinomycosis
acyl coenzyme
Adams-DeWeese device
Adams' disease
Adams-Stokes
    disease
    syncope
    syndrome
ADC–analog-to-digital
    conversion
Addison's disease
adenovirus
ADG–atrial diastolic gallop
ADH–antidiuretic hormone
adipositas
    a. cordis
adrenal
    a. adenoma
    a. cortex
    a. gland
    a. hyperplasia
    a. medulla
adrenergic
    a. antagonist
    a. nervous system
    a. stimulant
adrenoceptor
adrenogenital syndrome
Adson's
    forceps
    hook
    needle
    retractor
adult respiratory distress
    syndrome
adventitia
adventitious
aerendocardia

229

Aerococcus
AF – aortic flow
    atrial fibrillation
    atrial flutter
afterdepolarization
afterload
    a. matching
    a. mismatching
    a. reduction
AG – atrial gallop
AHD – arteriosclerotic
    heart disease
    atherosclerotic
    heart disease
A-H interval
AI – aortic incompetence
    aortic insufficiency
    apical impulse
AICD – automatic implanted
    cardioverter difibrillator
AIDS – acquired
    immunodeficiency
    syndrome
akinesia
akinesis
aldosteronism
Alexander-Farabeuf
    periosteotome
Alfred M. Large's clamp
ALG – antilymphocyte globulin
aliasing
alkalosis
alkaptonuria
Allen's test
Allison's retractor
allorhythmia
allorhythmic
all or none law
Allport-Babcock searcher
alternans
    a. of the heart
Alvarez' prosthesis
alveolar
    a. capillary membrane
    a. hypoventilation
    a. proteinosis

AMI – acute myocardial
    infarction
aminoglycoside
A-mode
Amplatz' coronary catheter
amplitude image
Amtech-Killeen pacemaker
amyloid
amyloidosis
analog-to-digital conversion
anaphylaxis
anastomosis
anesthesia. See *General Surgical
    Terms section.*
aneurysm
    abdominal a.
    aortic arch a.
    aortic sinusal a.
    arteriovenous a.
    axial a.
    Bérard's a.
    cardiac a.
    cylindroid a.
    cystogenic a.
    dissecting a.
    ectatic a.
    embolic a.
    embolomycotic a.
    endogenous a.
    erosive a.
    exogenous a.
    fusiform a.
    luetic a.
    mycotic a.
    Park's a.
    popliteal a.
    Pott's a.
    Richet's a.
    Rodrigues' a.
    saccular a.
    syphilitic a.
    thoracic a.
    traumatic a.
    ventricular a.
aneurysmal
aneurysmectomy

aneurysmogram
aneurysmoplasty
aneurysmorrhaphy
aneurysmotomy
Anger camera
angialgia
angiasthenia
angiectasis
angiectatic
angiectid
angiectomy
angiectopia
angiemphraxis
angiitis
angileucitis
angina
    a. cordis
    a. decubitus
    a. dyspeptica
    exertional a.
    hysteric a.
    a. inversa
    a. pectoris
    a. pectoris vasomotoria
    Prinzmetal's a.
    a. sine dolore
    variant a. pectoris
anginal equivalent
anginiform
anginoid
anginose
anginosis
angioataxia
angioblast
angioblastic
angioblastoma
angiocardiogram
angiocardiography
angiocardiokinetic
angiocardiopathy
angiocarditis
angioclast
angiodiascopy
angiodiathermy
angioedema
angiogenesis

angiogenic
angiogram
angiograph
angiography
    digital subtraction a.
angiohypertonia
angiohypotonia
angioinvasive
angiokeratoma corporis diffusum
angiokinesis
angiokinetic
angiolipoma
angiolith
angiolithic
angiologia
angiology
angioma
angiomatosis
angiometer
angiomyocardiac
angioneoplasm
angioneumography
angioneurosis
angioneurotomy
angionoma
angioparalysis
angioparesis
angiopathology
angiopathy
angioplasty
    laser a.
    percutaneous
      transluminal a.
angiopressure
angiorrhaphy
angiosarcoma
angiosclerosis
angiosclerotic
angioscopy
    fiberoptic a.
angiospasm
angiostomy
angiotelectasis
angiotensin
angiotribe
angloid

ankylosing spondylitis
annuloaortic ectasia
annuloplasty
    DeVega a.
annulus
anomalous
anomaly
    Ebstein's a.
anorexia
    a. nervosa
anoxemia
anoxia
    myocardial a.
    stagnant a.
anoxic
"Anrep effect"
antagonism
anteroposterior
anteroseptal
anthracycline
anthraquinone
antiarrhythmic
antibodies
    B cell a.
anticoagulant
anticoagulation
antidiuretic hormone
anti-DNase B
antidromic
antimony
antinuclear
antiplatelet
antistreptolysin O
antistreptozyme test
antithrombin III
AO–anodal opening
    aorta
    aortic opening
    opening of the
      atrioventricular
    valves
AOC–anodal opening
    contraction
aorta(ae)
    abdominal a.
    a. abdominalis
    a. ascendens
    ascending a.

aorta(ae) (continued)
    a. chlorotica
    a. descendens
    descending a.
    dextropositioned a.
    dynamic a.
    overriding a.
    palpable a.
    primitive a.
    a. sacrococcygea
    straddling a.
    a. thoracalis
    thoracic a.
    a. thoracica
    throbbing a.
    ventral a.
aortal
aortalgia
aortarctia
aortectasia
aortectasis
aortectomy
aortic
    a. aneurysm
    a. arch
    a. arteritis
    a. cross clamp
    a. dissection
    a. embolism
    a. impedance
    a. insufficiency
    a. knob
    a. prosthesis
    a. regurgitation
    a. septal defect
    a. sinus
    a. stenosis
    a. thrombosis
    a. valve
    a. valvulitis
    a. valvuloplasty
aorticopulmonary
aorticorenal
aortism
aortismus
    a. abdominalis

aortitis
  Dohle-Heller a.
  luetic a.
  nummular a.
  rheumatic a.
  syphilitic a.
  a. syphilitica
  a. syphilitica obliterans
aortoclasia
aortogram
  transbrachial arch a.
  translumbar a.
aortography
  retrograde a.
  translumbar a.
aortolith
aortomalacia
aortopathy
aortoptosia
aortorrhaphy
aortosclerosis
aortostenosis
aortotomy
AOS – anodal opening sound
AOT – anodal opening tetanus
AP – angina pectoris
  anteroposterior
  arterial pressure
apathetic
APB – atrial premature beat
  auricular premature
  beat
APC – atrial premature
  contraction
apex
  a. cordis
apexcardiogram
apexcardiography
apical
apices
apnea
apneic
apolipoprotein
  A-I
  B
  C-II
  D
  E

appendage
  atrial a.
  auricular a.
aprotinin
AR – aortic regurgitation
  artificial respiration
arch
  aortic a.
Arco pacemaker
arcus
  a. aortae
ARDS – adult respiratory distress
  syndrome
area
  Bamberger's a.
ARF – acute rheumatic
  fever
Argyle's catheter
arrest
  cardiac a.
  sinus a.
arrhythmia
  inotropic a.
  nodal a.
  phasic a.
  respiratory a.
  sinus a.
  vagus a.
  ventricular a.
arrhythmic
arrhythmogenesis
arrhythmogenic
arterial
  a. blood flow
  a. calcification
  a. coupling
  a. pressure
  a. pulse
  a. thrombosis
arterialization
arteriarctia
arteriasis
arteriectasis
arteriectomy
arterioatony
arteriocapillary

arteriodilating
arteriofibrosia
arteriogram
    femoral a.
    subclavian a.
arteriograph
arteriography
    digital subtraction a.
arteriohepatic
arteriolae
arteriolar
arteriole
arteriolith
arteriolitis
arteriolonecrosis
arteriolosclerosis
arteriolosclerotic
arteriomalacia
arteriometer
arteriomotor
arteriomyomatosis
arterionecrosis
arteriopalmus
arteriopathy
    hypertensive a.
arteriophlebotomy
arterioplania
arterioplasty
arteriorenal
arteriorrhagia
arteriorrhaphy
arteriorrhexis
arteriosclerosis
    cerebral a.
    coronary a.
    decrescent a.
    diffuse a.
    hyaline a.
    hypertensive a.
    infantile a.
    intimal a.
    Mönckeberg's a.
    nodose a.
    nodular a.
    a. obliterans
    peripheral a.
    presenile a.

arteriosclerosis (continued)
    senile a.
arteriosclerotic
arteriospasm
arteriostenosis
arteriosteogenesis
arteriostosis
arteriostrepsis
arteriosus
    patent ductus a.
    truncus a.
arteriosympathectomy
arteriotome
arteriotomy
arteriotony
arteriovenous
    a. fistula
    a. oxygen difference
    a. shunt
arterioversion
arteritis
    brachiocephalic a.
    a. deformans
    giant cell a.
    a. hyperplastica
    necrosing a.
    a. nodosa
    a. obliterans
    temporal a.
    a. umbilicalis
    a. verrucosa
artery
    brachial a.
    brachiocephalic a.
    carotid a.
    celiac a.
    circumflex a.
    coronary a.
    epicardial coronary a.
    esophageal a.
    femoral a.
    iliac a.
    innominate a.
    intercostal a.
    interventricular a.
    marginal a.
    peroneal a.

artery (continued)
    preventricular a.
    pulmonary a.
    renal a.
    subclavian a.
    tibial a.
arthritis
    Jaccoud's a.
    rheumatoid a.
artifact
AS – aortic stenosis
    arteriosclerosis
Aschoff and Tawara node
Aschoff's
    bodies
    node
ascites
ASCVD – arteriosclerotic
    cardiovascular
    disease
    atherosclerotic
    cardiovascular
    disease
ASD – atrial septal defect
asequence
ASH – asymmetrical septal
    hypertrophy
ASHD – arteriosclerotic heart
    disease
Ashman's phenomenon
Ask-Upmark syndrome
ASMI – anteroseptal myocardial
    infarct
ASO – arteriosclerosis obliterans
aspergillosis
Aspergillus
asphygmia
asplenia
AST – aspartate aminotransferase
asthenia
    neurocirculatory a.
asthma
    cardiac a.
    Elsner's a.
    Heberden's a.
    Rostan's a.
ASTZ – antistreptozyme

asynchronism
asynchrony
asystole
asystolic arrest
atelocardia
atherogenesis
atheroma
atheromatous
atheronecrosis
atherosclerosis
ATPase
atresia
    aortic a.
    tricuspid a.
atria
atrial
    a. fibrillation
    a. flutter
    a. infarction
    a. "kick"
    a. myocardial cell
    a. natriuretic peptide
    a. pacing
    a. premature contraction
    a. rhythm
    a. septal defect
    a. septum
    a. standstill
    a. tachycardia
Atricor pacemaker
atriocommissuropexy
atriohisian tract
atriomegaly
atrionector
atrioseptopexy
atriotome
atriotomy
atrioventricular
    a. block
    a. bundle
    a. canal defect
    a. conduction
    a. dissociation
    a. flow rumbling murmurs
    a. junction
    a. junctional escape beat
    a. junctional rhythm

atrioventricular (continued)
    a. nodal reentrant
      tachycardia
    a. nodal reentry
    a. node artery
    a. septal defect
    a. valve
atrium
    common a.
    a. cordis
    a. dextrum
    a. pulmonale
    pulmonary a.
    a. sinistrum
Auenbrugger's sign
auricle
auricula
    a. atrii
    a. atrii dextri
    a. atrii sinistri
    a. cordis
    a. dextra cordis
    a. sinistra cordis
auricular
auriculoventricular
auscultation
auscultatory
Austin Flint murmur
automaticity
autoregulation
AV or A-V – arteriovenous
              atrioventricular
AV or A-V
    dissociation
    heart block
avascular
AVR – aortic valve replacement
AVRP – atrioventricular
    refractory period
A wave
awbooshma. See *embouchment.*
AWI – anterior wall infarction
awl
    Rochester's a.
    Wangensteen's a.
AWMI – anterior wall
    myocardial infarction

axis
Ayerza's syndrome
azotemia
azygography
azygos vein
Babinski's syndrome
Bachmann's bundle
bacteremia
bacterial
    b. endocarditis
    b. myocarditis
    b. pericarditis
Bahnson's clamp
Bailey-Gibbon rib contractor
Bailey-Glover-O'Neil knife
Bailey-Morse knife
Bailey's
    clamp
    rib contractor
Bainbridge's reflex
Balke-Ware test
ballistocardiogram
ballistocardiograph
ballistocardiography
balloon
    b. angioplasty
    b. atrial septostomy
    b. atrial septotomy
    b. tuboplasty
    b. valvuloplasty
ballooning mitral cusp syndrome
ball-valve thrombus
Bamberger's
    area
    bulbar pulse
    sign
Bardic's cannula
Barlow's syndrome
Barraya's forceps
Bayes' theorem
Bayliss' theory
Baylor's sump
B cell antibody
BE – bacterial endocarditis
Beardsley's dilator
beat
    capture b's

beat (continued)
    ectopic b's
    nodal b's
    premature auricular b's
Beau's
    disease
    syndrome
Beck I operation
Beck II operation
Beck's
    clamp
    rasp
    triad
Béhier-Hardy sign
Bengolea's forceps
Bérard's aneurysm
beriberi
Bernheim's syndrome
Bernouilli's theorem
beta
    b. adrenoceptor
    b. ray
    b. thromboglobulin
Bethune's rib shears
Bezold-Jarisch reflex
bicuspid
bifurcation
bigeminal
bigeminy
    nodal b.
billowing mitral valve syndrome
bioptome
    Stanford b.
Biotronik pacemaker
bipolar
bisferious
Bishop's sphygmoscope
biventricular
Björk-Shiley
    prosthesis
    valve
blade
    Cooley-Pontius b.
    DeBakey's b.
Blalock-Hanlen operation
Blalock-Taussig operation
Blastomyces

blastomycosis
Block. See *heart block.*
blocker
    alpha-adrenergic b.
    alpha-adrenoceptor b's
    beta b.
    calcium channel b.
    renin-angiotensin b's
blood
    deoxygenated b.
blow
    diastolic b.
"blue toe" syndrome
body
    Aschoff's b's
Boettcher's forceps
Borg scale
Bosher's knife
Botallo's duct
Bouillaud's
    sign
    syndrome
    tinkle
Bouveret's
    disease
    syndrome
BP – blood pressure
brachial artery
brachiocephalic
Bradshaw-O'Neill clamp
bradyarrhythmia
bradyarrhythmic arrest
bradycardia
    Branham's b.
    cardiomuscular b.
    clinostatic b.
    essential b.
    nodal b.
    postinfective b.
    sinoatrial b.
    sinus b.
    vagal b.
bradycardiac
bradycrotic
bradydiastole
bradydiastolia
bradykinin

bradytachycardia
Branham's
    bradycardia
    sign
Brauer's operation
Braunwald's
    prosthesis
    sign
bridging
    myocardial b.
Bright's murmur
Broadbent's sign
Brockenbrough's
    catheter
    sign
Brock's
    knife
    operation
    punch
bronchiectasis
bronchodilator
Bruce treadmill protocol
bruit (*brwe*)
    aneurysmal b.
    b. de canon (*brwe duh kahnaw*)
    b. de choc (*brwe duh shawk*)
    b. de craquement (*brwe duh krak maw*)
    b. de cuir neuf (*brwe duh kwer nuf*)
    b. de diable (*brwe duh de ahbl*)
    b. de frolement (*brwe duh frolmaw*)
    b. de lime (*brwe duh lem*)
    b. de moulin (*brwe duh moola*)
    b. de parchemin (*brwe duh parshmaw*)
    b. de piaulement (*brwe duh pyolmaw*)
    b. de rape (*brwe duh rahp*)
    b. de rappel (*brwe duh rahpel*)

bruit (*brwe*) (continued)
    b. de Roger (*brwe duh rozha*)
    b. de scie (*brwe duh se*)
    Roger's b.
    systolic b.
brwe. See *bruit*.
Buerger's disease
bulbus
    b. aortae
    b. arteriosus
    b. caroticus
    b. cordis
    b. venae jugularis
bundle
    atrioventricular b.
    a-v. b.
    Bachmann's b.
    b. branch block
    b. branch reentry
    b. of His
    Keith's b.
    Kent-His b.
    Kent's b.
    sinoatrial b.
    b. of Stanley-Kent
    Thorel's b.
Burford's rib spreader
Burger's triangle
bypass
    aortocoronary vein b.
    aortoiliac b.
    cardiopulmonary b.
    coronary artery b.
    femoropopliteal b.
    saphenous vein b.
CA – cardiac arrest
    coronary artery
CAB – coronary artery bypass
CABG – coronary artery bypass graft
cachexia
CAD – coronary artery disease
café coronary
caged-ball valve
calcium
    c. antagonist

calcium (continued)
    c. channel blocker
    c. ions
    c. paradox
    "c. sign"
    c. transient
camera
    Anger c.
    gamma c.
Cameron-Haight elevator
Campylobacter
canalization
Candida
candidiasis
Cannon's endarterectomy
    loop
cannula
    Bardic's c.
    Floyd's c.
    Mayo's c.
    Morris' c.
    Rockey's c.
    Silastic coronary artery c.
    Soresi's c.
    venous c.
cannulate
cannulation
Cape Town prosthesis
capillary
    Meigs' c's
capture beats
carbomethoxyisopropyl
    isonitrile
carcinoid
    c. heart disease
    c. plaque
    c. syndrome
    c. tumor
    c. valve disease
cardiac
cardialgia
cardianastrophe
cardiasthenia
cardiasthma
cardiectasis
cardiectomy
cardioaccelerator

cardioaortic
cardioarterial
cardiocairograph
cardiocele
cardiocentesis
cardiocirrhosis
cardioclasis
cardiodiaphragmatic
cardiodilator
cardiodiosis
cardiogenic
cardiogram
cardiograph
cardiography
Cardio-green
cardiohepatic
cardiohepatomegaly
cardioinhibitory
cardiokinetic
cardiolith
cardiologist
cardiology
cardiolysis
cardiomalacia
cardiomegalia
    c. glycogenica
      circumscripta
cardiomegaly
cardiomelanosis
cardiometer
cardiometry
cardiomotility
cardiomyoliposis
cardiomyopathy
    alcoholic c.
    cobalt c.
    dilated c.
    hypertrophic c.
    idiopathic dilated c.
    infiltrative c.
    restrictive c.
cardiomyopexy
cardiomyotomy
cardionecrosis
cardionector
cardionephric
cardioneural

cardioneuropathy
cardioneurosis
cardio-omentopexy
cardiopalmus
cardiopaludism
cardiopathy
    endocrine c.
cardiopericardiopexy
cardiopericarditis
cardiophone
cardioplegia
cardioplegic
cardiopneumograph
cardiopneumonopexy
cardioptosis
cardiopulmonary
cardiorrhaphy
cardiorrhexis
cardioschisis
cardiosclerosis
cardioscope
cardioselectivity
cardiospasm
cardiosphygmogram
cardiosphygmograph
cardiosplenopexy
cardiosymphysis
cardiotachometer
cardiothoracic
cardiothymic
cardiotomy
cardiotoxic
cardiotoxicity
cardiovalvular
cardiovalvulitis
cardiovalvulotomy
cardiovascular
cardioversion
cardioverter-defibrillator
carditis
    rheumatic c.
    Sterges' c.
Carey-Coombs murmur
Carmalt's forceps
carotid
    c. artery
    c. endarterectomy

carotid (continued)
    c. pulse
    c. shudder
    c. sinus
Carpentier-Edwards valve
Carpentier's
    rings
    stent
Carter's retractor
Cartwright's prosthesis
Carvallo's sign
CAST – cardiac arrhythmia
    suppression trial
catecholamine
catheter
    Amplatz' coronary c.
    Argyle's c.
    Brockenbrough's c.
    Cournand's c.
    Edwards' c.
    Fogarty's c.
    Goodale-Lubin c.
    Gruentzig's c.
    Lehman's c.
    NIH c.
    Nycore pigtail c.
    pigtail c.
    Sones' coronary c.
    Swan-Ganz c.
    Teflon c.
    thermodilution c.
catheterization
    cardiac c.
    hepatic vein c.
CC – cardiac cycle
CCU – coronary care unit
CD – cardiac disease
    cardiac dullness
    cardiovascular disease
CE – cardiac enlargement
Cegka's sign
cell
    B c.
    P c.
    T c.
cerebral
cerebrocardiac

cerebrovascular
CESD—cholesteryl ester storage
    disease
CF–cardiac failure
change
       QRS c's
       QRS-T c's
       ST segment c's
       T wave c's
Chardak-Greatbatch pacemaker
CHB–complete heart block
CHD–congenital heart disease
    coronary heart disease
chemoreceptor
Cheyne-Stokes respiration
CHF–congestive heart failure
Chlamydia
       C. psittaci
       C. trachomatis
chloride ion
choc
       bruit de c.
       c. en dome
cholesterol
cholesteryl ester storage disease
chorda
       c. tendineae cordis
Chromobacterium
Chromosporinum
chylomicron
chylomicronemia
chylopericardium
CI–cardiac index
    cardiac insufficiency
    coronary insufficiency
CICU–cardiology intensive
    care unit
    coronary intensive care
    unit
cineangiocardiography
cineangiography
cineradiography
circadian
circle
       c. of Willis
circulation
       extracorporeal c.

circulation (continued)
    systemic c.
circulatory
circulus
       c. arteriosus
       c. arteriosus cerebri
       c. articuli vasculosus
circumflex artery
Citrobacter
CK–creatine kinase
clamp
       Alfred M. Large's c.
       Bahnson's c.
       Bailey's c.
       Beck's c.
       Bradshaw-O'Neill c.
       bulldog c.
       Cooley's c.
       Crafoord's c.
       Crutchfield's c.
       Davis' c.
       DeBakey's c.
       Derra's c.
       Diethrich's shunt c.
       Edwards' c.
       Glover's c.
       Gross' c.
       Herbert-Adams c.
       Hopkins' c.
       Hufnagel's c.
       Hume's c.
       Humphries' c.
       Jacobson's c.
       Javid's bypass c.
       Johns Hopkins c.
       Juevenell's c.
       Kantrowicz's c.
       Kapp-Beck c.
       Kelly's c.
       McDonald's c.
       Nichols' c.
       Poppen-Blalock c.
       Poppen's c.
       Potts' c.
       Potts-Niedner c.
       Potts-Smith c.
       Reich-Nechtow c.

clamp (continued)
    Rienhoff's c.
    Rumel's c.
    Salibi's c.
    Satinsky's c.
    Selverstone's c.
    Shoemaker's c.
    Trendelenburg-
        Craafoord c.
classification
    Killip's c.
claudication
    intermittent c.
    venous c.
click
    midsystolic c.
click-murmur syndrome
clip
    Scoville-Lewis c.
    Smith's c.
    Sugar's c.
Clostridium
    C. perfringens
clubbing
CO_2–carbon dioxide
coagulation
coarctation
    c. of the aorta
cobalt
Coccidiodes
coccidioidomycosis
coenzyme
    A
    Q
    Q 10
coeur
    c. en sabot
collagen
collapse
    hemodynamic c.
collateral
collimator
columnae
    c. carneae cordis
commissure
commissurorrhaphy

commissurotomy
communis
    atrioventricularis c.
compensation
complex
    Eisenmenger's c.
    Lutembacher's c.
    QRS c.
    QS c.
    ventricular c. (Q,R,S,T
        waves)
computed tomography
concretio
    c. cordis
conduction
    decremental c.
    ventricular c.
congenital
congestion
congestive heart failure
contractile
contractility
contraction
    anodal closure c.
    anodal opening c.
    atrial premature c.
    automatic ventricular c.
    isometric c.
    isotonic c.
    nodal premature c.
    supraventricular
        premature c.
conus
    c. arteriosus
conversion
convertin
Cooley-Pontius blade
Cooley's
    clamp
    dilator
    forceps
    prosthesis
    retractor
    scissors
COPD–chronic obstructive
    pulmonary disease

cor
    c. adiposum
    c. arteriosum
    c. biloculare
    c. bovinum
    c. dextrum
    c. hirsutum
    c. juvenum
    c. mobile
    c. pendulum
    c. pseudotriloculare
        biatriatum
    c. pulmonale
    c. sinistrum
    c. taurinum
    c. tomentosum
    c. triatriatum
    c. triloculare biatriatum
    c. triloculare
        biventriculare
    c. venosum
    c. villosum
Coratomic pacemaker
Cordis' pacemaker
Cordis Atricor pacemaker
Cordis-Ectocor pacemaker
Cordis' fixed-rate pacemaker
Cordis Ventricor pacemaker
coronarism
coronaritis
coronary
    c. angiography
    c. angioplasty
    c. arterial reserve
    c. arteriography
    c. artery ectasia
    c. artery occlusion
    c. atherosclerosis
    c. bifurcation
    c. bypass surgery
    c. insufficiency
    c. ostial stenosis
    c. sinus
    c. steal
    c. stenosis
    c. thrombolysis

coronary (continued)
    c. thrombosis
    c. vascular resistance
Corrigan's
    disease
    pulse
    respiration
    sign
corticosteroid
Corvisart's
    disease
    facies
Coryllos'
    raspatory
    retractor
Corynebacterium
costochondritis
costosternal
costotome
    Tudor-Edwards c.
counterpulsation
    intra-aortic balloon c.
countershock
Cournand's
    catheter
    needle
Coxiella
    C. burnetii
CPB – cardiopulmonary
    bypass
CPI Maxilith pacemaker
CPI Minilith pacemaker
cpm – counts per minute
CPR – cardiopulmonary
    resuscitation
C protein
Crafoord's
    clamp
    forceps
Crawford-Cooley tunneler
Crawford's retractor
creatine kinase
Creech's technique
crista
    c. supraventricularis
    c. terminalis atrii dextri

criteria
      Jones' c.
crus
      c. fasciculi
          atrioventricularis
          dextrum
      c. fasciculi
          atrioventricularis
          sinistrum
Crutchfield's clamp
Cruveilhier-Baumgarten murmur
crux
      c. of heart
cryoblation
cryocardioplegia
cryoprecipitate
cryptococcosis
Cryptococcus
      C. neoformans
CT – cardiothoracic (ratio)
      carotid tracing
CTR – cardiothoracic ratio
current
      K c's
Curry's needle
curve
      Traube's c's
Cushing's
      forceps
      needle
cusp
cuspis
      c. anterior valvae
          atrioventricularis
          dextrae
      c. anterior valvae
          atrioventricularis
          sinistrae
      c. anterior valvulae
          bicuspidalis
      c. anterior valvulae
          tricuspidalis
      c. medialis valvulae
          tricuspidalis
      c. posterior valvae
          atrioventricularis
          dextrae

cuspis (continued)
      c. posterior valvae
          atrioventricularis
          sinistrae
      c. posterior valvulae
          bicuspidalis
      c. posterior valvulae
          tricuspidalis
      c. septalis valvae
          atrioventricularis
          dextrae
Cutter-SCDK prosthesis
Cutter-Smeloff prosthesis
CVA – cardiovascular accident
      cerebrovascular accident
CVS – cardiovascular surgery
      cardiovascular system
C wave
cyanosis
      shunt c.
      tardive c.
cyanotic
cyst
      pericardial c.
cytomegalovirus
Dacron
      graft
      prosthesis
DAH – disordered action of
      the heart
Davidson's retractor
Davis' clamp
DeBakey-Bahnson forceps
DeBakey-Bainbridge forceps
DeBakey-Balfour retractor
DeBakey-Cooley
      dilator
      forceps
      retractor
DeBakey-Metzenbaum scissors
DeBakey's
      blade
      clamp
      forceps
      graft
      prosthesis
      scissors

DeBakey's (continued)
    tunneler
decannulation
"declamping shock"
decompensation
deconditioning
decortication
    arterial d.
decremental conduction
defect
    aortic septal d.
    aorticopulmonary d.
    atrial septal d.
    atrioseptal d.
    endocardial cushion d.
    ostium primum d.
    ostium secundum d.
    septal d.
    ventricular septal d.
defibrillated
defibrillation
defibrillator
deflection
    Q-S d's
degeneration
    Mönckeberg's d.
    Quain's d.
deglutition syncope
Dehio's test
Delorme's operation
delta wave
de Musset's sign
deoxygenated
depolarization
depressant
    cardiac d.
depression
    ST d.
    systolic d.
dermatomyositis
Derra's
    clamp
    dilator
    knife
Desault's ligation
devasation
    senile cortical d.

devascularization
DeVega annuloplasty
deviation
    right axis d.
    ST-T d's
device
    Adams-DeWeese d.
dextrocardia
    mirror-image d.
dextrocardiogram
dextro-transposition
dextroversion
DG – diastolic gallop
D gate
diaphoresis
diaphragm
diastasis
    d. cordis
diastole
diastolic
    d. filling
    d. function
    d. motion
    d. overload
    d. pressure-time index
    d. pressure-volume
        relation
    d. reserve
    d. stiffness
DIC – diffuse intravascular
    coagulation
    disseminated
    intravascular
    coagulation
Dick's dilator
dicliditis
diclidostosis
dicrotic wave
diet
    Karell's d.
    Kempner's d.
Diethrich's shunt clamp
Dieuaide's sign
digitalis
digitalism
digitalization
digitalized

dilatation
dilator
    Beardsley's d.
    Cooley's d.
    DeBakey-Cooley d.
    Derra's d.
    Dick's d.
    Gohrbrand's d.
    Jackson-Mosher d.
    Tubbs' d.
    Tucker's d.
diplocardia
dipyridamole
disease
    Adams' d.
    Adams-Stokes d.
    Addison's d.
    Beau's d.
    Bouveret's d.
    Buerger's d.
    coronary artery d.
    Corrigan's d.
    Corvisart's d.
    Duroziez's d.
    Eisenmenger's d.
    eosinophilic
      endomyocardial d.
    Hamman's d.
    Heller-Döhle d.
    Hodgson's d.
    Lenegre's d.
    Lev's d.
    Libman-Sacks d.
    Lutembacher's d.
    Lyme d.
    Pick's d.
    pulseless d.
    Raynaud's d.
    rheumatic heart d.
    Roger's d.
    Rummo's d.
    thyrotoxic heart d.
    von Willebrand's d.
    Wenckebach's d.
dissecting
    d. aortic aneurysm
    d. hematoma

dissociation
    auriculoventricular d.
    A-V d.
    electromechanical d.
distensibility
Dittrich's stenosis
diuresis
diuretic
DM – diastolic murmur
DOE – dyspnea on exercise
    dyspnea on exertion
Dohle-Heller aortitis
Doppler
    d. echocardiography
    d. ultrasonography
Doyen's elevator
DPTI – diastolic pressure-time
    index
dressing. See *General Surgical
    Terms section.*
Dressler's syndrome
DRGs – diagnosis related groups
drugs. See *Drugs and Chemistry*
    section.
Drummond's sign
duct
    d. of Botallo
ductus
    d. arteriosus
Duromedics
    prosthesis
    valve
Duroziez's
    disease
    murmur
    sign
dyskinesia
dyskinesis
dyskinetic
dysphagia
dyspnea
    cardiac d.
    exertional d.
    orthostatic d.
    paroxysmal d.
dyspneic
dyspneoneurosis

dyssynchrony
dyssynergia
dyssystole
Ebstein's anomaly
ECG–electrocardiogram
Echinococcus
echo
    e. delay time
    ventricular e's
echocardiogram
echocardiography
    Doppler e.
echophonocardiography
echovirus
Eck's fistula
Ectocor pacemaker
ectopia
    e. cordis
    e. cordis abdominalis
    e. cordis pectoral
ectopic
edema
    alveolar e.
    angioneurotic e.
    cardiac e.
    interstitial e.
    pulmonary e.
    subpleural e.
EDP–end-diastolic pressure
Edwards'
    catheter
    clamp
    patch
    prosthesis
EF–ejection fraction
effect
    "Anrep e."
    Venturi e.
efficacy
Effler's ring
effusion
    pericardial e.
Eikenella
    E. corrodens
Einthoven's
    law
    triangle

Eisenmenger's
    complex
    disease
    syndrome
ejection
    e. fraction
    e. phase indices
    e. shell image
    e. sound
EKG–electrocardiogram
elasticity
electrocardiogram
electrocardiograph
electrocardiography
    precordial e.
electrocardiophonogram
electrocardiophonograph
electrocardioscopy
electrocardioversion
electrode
    esophageal pill e.
Electrodyne pacemaker
electrofluoroscopy
electrokymography
electrolytes
electromechanical
    e. coupling
    e. dissociation
    e. interval
electron volt
electrophoresis
electrophysiological
electrophysiology
    cardiac e.
electrostethograph
elevation
    ST segment e.
elevator
    Cameron-Haight e.
    Doyen's e.
    Hedblom's e.
    Matson's e.
    Overholt's e.
    Phemister's e.
    Sedillot's e.
elimination half-life
elongation

Elsner's asthma
EM – ejection murmur
embolectomy
emboli
embolic
embolism
 air e.
 coronary e.
 paradoxical e.
 plasmodium e.
 pulmonary e.
 venous e.
embolization
embolus
embouchment
EMD – electromechanical
 dissociation
Emerson's pump
emphysema
empyema
 e. of pericardium
 pulsating e.
encephalopathy
endaortic
endaortitis
 bacterial e.
endarterectomize
endarterectomy
endarterial
endarteritis
 e. deformans
 Heubner's specific e.
 e. obliterans
 e. proliferans
endarterium
endarteropathy
endartery
end-diastolic
endoaneurysmorrhaphy
endocardial
 e. cushion defect
 e. fibroelastosis
 e. fibrosis
 e. resection
 e. sclerosis
endocarditis
 acute bacterial e.

endocarditis (continued)
 e. benigna
 e. chordalis
 constrictive e.
 fungal e.
 infective e.
 e. lenta
 Libman-Sacks e.
 Löffler's e.
 malignant e.
 "marantic" e.
 mural e.
 mycotic e.
 nonbacterial thrombotic e.
 noninfective e.
 parietal e.
 e. parietalis fibroplastica
 plastic e.
 polypous e.
 prosthetic valve e.
 pulmonic e.
 pustulous e.
 rheumatic e.
 rickettsial e.
 septic e.
 subacute bacterial e.
 syphilitic e.
 tuberculous e.
 ulcerative e.
 valvular e.
 vegetative e.
 verrucous e.
 viridans e.
endocardium
endocytosis
endomyocardial
 e. biopsy
 e. fibrosis
endoperoxide steal
endophlebitis
 e. hepatica obliterans
 proliferative e.
endostethoscope
endothelial
endothelium
endovasculitis

end-systolic
 e.-s. counts
 e.-s. pressure-volume
  relation
 e.-s. stress-dimension
  relation
 e.-s. volume
engorgement
Engström respirator
enzyme(s)
eosinophilia
eparterial
epicardia
epicardiectomy
epicardiolysis
epicardium
equation
 Nernst's e.
 Starling's e.
Erben's reflex
Erb's point
ergocardiogram
ergocardiography
ergonovine test
Erlanger's sphygmomanometer
Erysipelothrix
erythema marginatum
erythrocyte sedimentation rate
erythrocytosis
erythromelalgia
Escherichia
 E. coli
ESM – ejection systolic murmur
esophageal
ESR – erythrocyte sedimentation
 rate
estrogen(s)
ethmocarditis
E to F slope
Eustace Smith's murmur
Evans' forceps
Ewart's sign
excitation
 anomalous
  atrioventricular e.
exit block
extracorporeal

extrasystole
 auricular e.
 auriculoventricular e.
 infranodal e.
 interpolated e.
 nodal e.
 retrograde e.
 ventricular e.
Fab fragments
facies
 Corvisart's f.
factor
 Hageman's f.
Fallot
 pentalogy of F.
 tetralogy of F.
 trilogy of F.
fascicle
fascicular block
Faught's sphygmomanometer
FDG – 2-fluoro-2-deoxyglucose
femoral artery
fenestration
 aortopulmonary f.
feokromositoma. See
 pheochromocytoma.
fever
 rheumatic f.
F gates
fiber
 Purkinje's f's
fiberoptic
fibrillation
 atrial f.
 auricular f.
 ventricular f.
fibrinogen
fibrinoid
fibrinolytic
fibroelastosis
 endocardial f.
fibrosarcoma
fibrosis
 arteriocapillary f.
Fick's principle
Fiedler's myocarditis

filter
> Kimray-Greenfield f.
> Mobin-Uddin umbrella f.

Finochietto's rib spreader
first-order kinetics
Fisher's murmur
fissure
> Henle's f's

fistula
> arteriovenous f.
> congenital coronary f.
> coronary artery f.
> Eck's f.

Fitzgerald's forceps
Flack's node
FLASH – fast low-angle shot
fleb-. See words beginning *phleb-*.
Flint's murmur
floppy valve syndrome
flowmeter
flow tract
Floyd's cannula
fluoroscopy
flutter
> atrial f.
> auricular f.
> impure f.
> pure f.
> ventricular f.

flutter-fibrillation
Flynt's needle
Fogarty's catheter
Fontan procedure
foramen
> Galen's f.
> f. ovale cordis
> f. venae cavae

foramina venarum minimarum
> cordis

force
> Starling's f's

force-frequency relation
force-length relation
force-velocity relation
forceps
> Adson's f.
> Barraya's f.

forceps (continued)
> Bengolea's f.
> Boettcher's f.
> Carmalt's f.
> Cooley's f.
> Crafoord's f.
> Cushing's f.
> DeBakey-Bahnson f.
> DeBakey-Bainbridge f.
> DeBakey-Cooley f.
> DeBakey's f.
> Evans' f.
> Fitzgerald's f.
> Foss' f.
> Glover's f.
> Harken's f.
> Harrington's f.
> Hendren's f.
> Horsley's f.
> Jacobson's f.
> Johns Hopkins f.
> Julian's f.
> Lebsche's f.
> Lcland-Jones f.
> Leriche's f.
> Liston-Stille f.
> Love-Gruenwald f.
> McNealy-Glassman-
>   Mixter f.
> Mixter's f.
> Mount-Mayfield f.
> O'Shaughnessy's f.
> Potts-Smith f.
> Rienhoff's f.
> Rumel's f.
> Ruskin's f.
> Satinsky's f.
> Sauerbruch's f.
> Selman's f.
> Semb's f.
> Stille-Luer f.
> Stille's f.
> Vanderbilt's f.

Foss' forceps
fossa
> f. ovalis cordis

F & R – force and rhythm

Fraentzel's murmur
fragmentation
    f. of myocardium
Framingham Heart Study
Fränkel's treatment
Frank-Starling mechanism
fremitus
    pericardial f.
fren-. See words beginning *phren-.*
friction rub
Friedreich's sign
frolement
fulguration
functional
    f. image
    f. imaging
    f. subtraction
fundus
fungus
furrow
    atrioventricular f.
fusion beats
F waves
Galen's foramen
gallium-62
gallop
    atrial g.
    protodiastolic g.
    S_3 g.
gamma
    g. camera
    g. ray
ganglia
    cardiac g.
    g. cardiaca
    Wrisberg's g.
ganglion
gasendarterectomy
gated system
gating
General Electric pacemaker
George Lewis technique
Gibbon-Landis test
Gibson's
    murmur
    vestibule
Giertz-Shoemaker rib shears

glomera
    g. aortica
glomus
    g. carotideum
Glover's
    clamp
    forceps
Gluck's rib shears
glucocorticoids
glucocorticosteroids
glycolysis
glycosides
glycosuria
Gohrbrand's dilator
Goldberg-MPC mediastinoscope
Goodale-Lubin catheter
"gooseneck deformity"
Gore-Tex graft
Gott's prosthesis
Gower's syndrome
gradient
    ventricular g.
graft
    autogenous vein g.
    cross-leg g.
    Dacron g.
    DeBakey's g.
    femoropopliteal bypass g.
    Gore-Tex g.
    saphenous vein bypass g.
    Weavenit patch g.
Graham Steell murmur
granular cell tumor
granulocytopenia
granulomatosis
GRASS – gradient recalled
    acquisition in a steady state
groove
    deltopectoral g.
Gross'
    clamp
    retractor
Gross-Pomeranz-Watkins
    retractor
Gruentzig's
    catheter
    technique

Haemophilus
  H. haemolyticus
  H. influenzae
Hageman's factor
Hamman's
  disease
  murmur
  sign
Hampton's hump
Hancock's valve
Harken's
  forceps
  prosthesis
  rib spreader
Harrington-Pemberton retractor
Harrington's
  forceps
  operation
  retractor
HB – heart block
HCVD – hypertensive
  cardiovascular disease
HD – heart disease
HDH – heart disease history
HDL – high-density
  lipoproteins
heart
  armored h.
  athletic h.
  beriberi h.
  h. block
  bovine h.
  chaotic h.
  encased h.
  extracorporeal h.
  h. failure
  fibroid h.
  flask-shaped h.
  frosted h.
  hyperthyroid h.
  hypoplastic h.
  intracorporeal h.
  irritable h.
  luxus h.
  h. murmur
  myxedema h.
  paracorporeal h.

heart (continued)
  Quain's fatty h.
  tabby cat h.
  Traube's h.
  triatrial h.
  triocular h.
  h. valve
  vertical h.
  wandering h.
  wooden-shoe h.
heart block
  arborization h.b.
  atrioventricular h.b.
  AV h.b.
  bifascicular h.b.
  bundle-branch h.b.
  complete h.b.
  congenital h.b.
  divisional h.b.
  entrance h.b.
  exit h.b.
  fascicular h.b.
  incomplete h.b.
  interventricular h.b.
  intraventricular h.b.
  Mobitz' h.b.
  partial h.b.
  periinfarction h.b.
  sinoauricular h.b.
  subjunctional h.b.
  Wenckebach's h.b.
heart failure
  backward h.f.
  congestive h.f.
  forward h.f.
  high output h.f.
  left ventricular h.f.
  right ventricular h.f.
heart-lung machine
heave
Heberden's asthma
Hedblom's
  elevator
  retractor
Heller-Döhle disease
hemangioma
hemangiosarcoma

hemartoma
hemithorax
hemochromatosis
hemodynamic
hemopericardium
Hemophilus. See *Haemophilus.*
hemopneumopericardium
hemoptysis
> cardiac h.

hemorrhage
hemosiderosis
Hendren's forceps
Henle's
> fissure
> membrane

heparinize
hepatic
hepatitis
hepatomegaly
Herbert-Adams clamp
hertz
heterograft
> porcine h.

heterophyiasis
heterozygosity
heterozygote
Heubner's specific endarteritis
H gates
HHD – hypertensive heart disease
hiatus
> aortic h.

Hibbs' retractor
hibernating myocardium
Hill's sign
His
> bundle of H.

His-Purkinje
> system
> tissue

His-Tawara node
histocompatibility
histogram mode
Hodgson's disease
holodiastolic
holosystolic
Holter monitor
Holt-Oram syndrome

homeometric autoregulation
homocystinuria
homozygosity
homozygote
hook
> Adson's h.

Hope's sign
Hopkins' clamp
Horsley's forceps
Hufnagel's
> clamp
> knife
> operation
> prosthesis

human immunodeficiency virus
Hume's clamp
hump
> Hampton's h.

Humphries' clamp
H-V interval
HVD – hypertensive vascular
> disease

hydropericarditis
hydropericardium
hydropneumopericardium
hydrothorax
hypercalcemia
hypercholesterolemia
hyperchylomicronemia
hypercontractility
hyperemia
hypergammaglobulinemia
hyperkalemia
hyperkinesia
hyperkinesis
hyperkinetic
hyperlipidemia
hyperlipoproteinemia
hypermagnesemia
hypernatremia
hyperplastic
hyperproteinemia
hypersensitivity
hypertension
> arterial h.
> essential h.
> portal h.

hypertension (continued)
    pulmonary h.
    renovascular h.
    secondary h.
    vascular h.
hypertensive
    h. crisis
    h. encephalopathy
    h. pulmonary vascular
      disease
hyperthermia
hypertriglyceridemia
hypertrophy
    ventricular h.
hyperventilation
hypocalcemia
hypokalemia
hypokinemia
hypokinesia
hypokinesis
hypolipidemia
hypolipoproteinemia
hyponatremia
hypoplastic
hypoproteinemia
hypoprothrombinemia
hypotension
    orthostatic h.
hypothermia
hypothyroidism
hypoventilation
hypovolemia
hypoxemia
hypoxia
hysterosystole
hz – hertz
IA – intra-aortic
    intra-arterial
IABP – intra-aortic balloon
    pump
IAS – interatrial septum
IASD – interatrial septal defect
I band
ICC – intensive coronary care
ICCU – intensive coronary care
    unit
ictometer

ictus
    i. cordis
ICU – intensive care unit
idiopathic
idioventricular
IDL – intermediate-density
    lipoproteins
IHD – ischemic heart disease
IHSS – idiopathic hypertrophic
    subaortic stenosis
imaging
imbalance
    electrolyte i.
IMH – idiopathic myocardial
    hypertrophy
immunodeficiency virus
immunoglobulin
immunotherapy
impedance
    i. plethysmography
implantation
impressio
    i. cardiaca pulmonis
impulse
    apex i.
    apical i.
    i. conduction
    episternal i.
incision. See *General Surgical
    Terms section.*
incisura
    i. apicis cordis
incompetence
indium-111
infarct
infarction
    anteroinferior myo-
      cardial i.
    anterolateral myocardial i.
    anteroseptal myocardial i.
    atrial i.
    cardiac i.
    diaphragmatic i.
    inferolateral myocardial i
    lateral myocardial i.
    myocardial i.
    posterior myocardial i.
    Roesler-Dressler i.

infarction (continued)
    septal myocardial i.
    subendocardial i.
    transmural myocardial i.
infectious mononucleosis
infective
inferolateral
"inflammatory reaction"
infundibular
infundibulum
    i. of heart
inotropic
inotropy
insufficiency
    aortic i.
    cardiac i.
    coronary i.
    mitral i.
    myocardial i.
    myovascular i.
    pseudoaortic i.
    tricuspid i.
    valvular i.
    venous i.
interatrial
intercalated
intercostal
interosseous
interval
    A-H i
    atriocarotid i.
    atrioventricular i.
    auriculocarotid i.
    auriculoventricular i.
    a.-v. i.
    c.-a. i.
    cardioarterial i.
    H-V i.
    P-A i.
    P-Q i.
    P-R i.
    Q-M i.
    QRST i.
    QT i.
    QU i.
    RS-T i.
    T-P i.
interventricular

intimal
intima-pia
intimectomy
intimitis
intra-aortic balloon pump
intra-arterial
intra-atrial
intra-auricular
intracardiac
intracaval
intracoronary
intramural
intramyocardial
intrapericardial
intrathoracic
intravascular
intraventricular
intrinsicoid deflection
intrinsic sympathomimetic
    activity
inversion
    T-wave i.
Ionescu-Shiley
    prosthesis
    valve
IPPB – intermittent positive
    pressure breathing
irregularity
    luminal i.
    i. of pulse
ISA – intrinsic sympathomimetic
    activity
ischemia
    i. cordis intermittens
    myocardial i.
ischemic
isoelectric point
isoenzymes
isometric handgrip
isotopes
isovolumetric
isovolumic
isozyme
IVC – inferior vena cava
IVCD – intraventricular
    conduction defect
IVSD – interventricular septal
    defect

IWMI – inferior wall myocardial
    infarction
Jaccoud's arthritis
Jackson-Mosher dilator
Jacobson's
    clamp
    forceps
    scissors
    spatula
Janeway's
    lesion
    sphygmomanometer
Javid's
    bypass clamp
    shunt
Jenkins Activity survey
jeopardy score
Jervell and Lange-Nielson
    syndrome
jet effect
Johns Hopkins
    clamp
    forceps
Jones' criteria
J point
Jorgenson's scissors
Judkin's technique
Juevenell's clamp
jugular
    j. venous distention
    j. venous pressure
    j. venous pulse
Julian's forceps
junctional
    j. escape rhythm
juxtaductal
    j. coarctation
JV – jugular vein jugular
    venous
JVP – jugular venous pulse
kahkekseah. See *cachexia.*
Kantrowicz's clamp
Kapp-Beck clamp
Karell's
    diet
    treatment
Katz-Wachtel phenomenon

Kay-Shiley prosthesis
Kay-Suzuki prosthesis
K currents
Keith's bundle
Kelly's clamp
Kempner's diet
Kent-His bundle
Kent's bundle
Kerley
    A lines
    B lines
ker-on-sabo. See *coeur en sabot.*
KeV – electron volts
Killip's classification
Kimray-Greenfield filter
kinetics
kinking
kissing balloon technique
knife
    Bailey-Glover-O'Neill k.
    Bailey-Morse k.
    Bosher's k.
    Brock's k.
    Derra's k.
    Hufnagel's k.
    Lebsche's k.
    Niedner's k.
    Nunez-Nunez k.
    Rochester's k.
    Sellor's k.
Korotkoff's
    method
    sounds
    test
Krasky's retractor
Kronecker's
    needle
    puncture
Krönig's steps
Kussmaul's
    pulse
    sign
LA – left atrial left atrium
lactic dehydrogenase
Lactobacillus
LAE – left atrial enlargement
LAH – left atrial hypertrophy

LAP – left atrial pressure
Laplace's law
laser angioplasty
law
    all or none l.
    Einthoven's l.
    Laplace's l.
    Ohm's l.
    Starling's l.
LBBB – left bundle branch
  block
LD – lactic dehydrogenase
LDH – lactic dehydrogenase
LDL – low-density lipoprotein
lead
    precordial l's
    sternal l.
    V l's: 1 through 6
    Wilson's l's
leaflet
Lebsche's
    forceps
    knife
    shears
Lehman's catheter
Leksell's rongeur
Leland-Jones forceps
Lemmon's rib spreader
Lenegre's disease
leptospirosis
Leptotrichia
    L. buccalis
Leriche's
    forceps
    operation
    syndrome
lesion
    Janeway's l.
Levine's sign
levocardia
levo-transposition
levoversion
Lev's disease
Libman-Sacks
    disease
    endocarditis
    syndrome

ligamentum
    l. arteriosum
ligation
    Desault's l.
    proximal l.
ligature
    Woodbridge's l.
Lilienthal-Sauerbruch rib
  spreader
Lillehei-Kaster
    prosthesis
    valve
limbus
    l. fossae ovalis
line
    midclavicular l.
    Z l.
lipid
lipocardiac
lipoma
lipoprotein
    high-density l.
    intermediate-density l.
    low-density l.
    very-low-density l.
liposarcoma
Liston-Stille forceps
Litten's sign
Litwak's scissors
Livierato's
    reflex
    test
Löffler's endocarditis
loop
    Cannon's endarter-
      ectomy l.
    P l.
Love-Gruenwald forceps
Lown-Ganong-Levine syndrome
LSM – late systolic murmur
LSV – left subclavian vein
lubb
lubb-dupp
Luken's retractor
lumen
luminal
lupus erythematosus

Lutembacher's
    complex
    disease
    syndrome
luxus
LV – left ventricle
LVAD – left ventricular assist
    device
LVET – left ventricular ejection
    time
LVH – left ventricular
    hypertrophy
Lyme disease
lymphadenopathy
lymphangioma
Lyon-Horgan operation
lysosomal enzyme
M₂ – mitral second sound
MABP – mean arterial blood
    pressure
machine
    heart-lung m.
magnetic
    m. moment
    m. relaxation time
    m. resonance imaging
    m. resonance signal
    m. resonance spectroscopy
Magovern's prosthesis
Makins' murmur
malformation
mammary artery
maneuver
    Mueller's m.
    Valsalva's m.
manometric
manubrium
MAOI – monoamine oxidase
    inhibitor
Marfan's syndrome
mask node subtraction
Mason-Likar limb lead
    modification
Master's "2-step" exercise test
Master's two-step test
matrix mode
Matson's elevator

Mayo's cannula
McCallum's patch
McDonald's clamp
McDowall's reflex
McGinn-White sign
MCI – mean cardiac index
MCL – midclavicular line
McNealy-Glassman-Mixter
    forceps
mechanism
    Frank-Starling m.
    Starling's m.
mediastinal
mediastinitis
mediastinopericarditis
mediastinoscope
    Goldberg-MPC m.
mediastinum
medications. See *Drugs and
    Chemistry* section.
Medtronic-Hall valve
Meigs' capillaries
membrane
    Henle's m.
mesaortitis
mesarteritis
mesoaortitis
    m. syphilitica
mesocardia
mesocardium
mesothelioma
MET – metabolic equivalents
    system
metarterioles
method
    Korotkoff's m.
    Orsi-Grocco m.
Meyerding's retractor
M gates
MI – mitral incompetence
    mitral insufficiency
    myocardial infarction
microembolism
microparticle
microsphere
microvascular
midsystolic click

MILIS–Multicenter
Investigation for the
Limitation of Infarct Size
Minitran
mitochondria
mitochondrial
mitogen
mitral
    m. annulus
    m. incompetence
    m. insufficiency
    m. opening snaps
    m. prolapse
    m. prosthesis
    m. regurgitation
    m. stenosis
    m. valve
    m. valve prolapse
    m. valvulitis
    m. valvuloplasty
mitrale
    P m.
mitralization
mitroarterial
Mixter's forceps
M line protein
M mode echocardiography
Mobin-Uddin umbrella filter
Mobitz' heart block
modification
    Mason-Likar limb lead m.
Mönckeberg's
    arteriosclerosis
    degeneration
monitor
    Holter m.
Monneret's pulse
monoamine oxidase inhibitor(s)
monocardiogram
Moore's operation
Morgagni's sinus
Morris' cannula
Morse's scissors
Mount-Mayfield forceps
Moure-Coryllos rib shears
M protein serotype
MR–mitral reflux

MR–(continued)
    mitral regurgitation
MRF–mitral regurgitant flow
MRFIT–Multiple-Risk Factor
    Intervention Trial
MRI–magnetic resonance
    imaging
MS–mitral stenosis
MSL–midsternal line
Mucor
Mueller's maneuver
Müller's sign
multifocal
multivalvular
mural
murmur
    amphoric m.
    aneurysmal m.
    aortic m.
    apex m.
    apical diastolic m.
    arterial m.
    attrition m.
    Austin Flint m.
    basal diastolic m.
    bellows m.
    blowing m.
    Bright's m.
    cardiac m.
    cardiopulmonary m.
    cardiorespiratory m.
    Carey-Coombs m.
    continuous m.
    cooing m.
    crescendo m.
    Cruveilhier-Baum-
      garten m.
    decrescendo m.
    deglutition m.
    diamond-shaped m.
    diastolic m.
    Duroziez's m.
    dynamic m.
    ejection m.
    endocardial m.
    Eustace Smith's m.
    exocardial m.

murmur (continued)
- expiratory m.
- Fisher's m.
- Flint's m.
- Fraentzel's m.
- friction m.
- functional m.
- Gibson's m.
- grade 1, 2, 3, 4, 5, or 6 m.
- Graham Steell m.
- Hamman's m.
- harsh m.
- hemic m.
- holosystolic m.
- hour-glass m.
- humming-top m.
- inorganic m.
- inspiratory m.
- lapping m.
- machinery m.
- Makins' m.
- mitral m.
- musical m.
- nun's m.
- obstructive m.
- organic m.
- pansystolic m.
- Parrot's m.
- pericardial m.
- pleuropericardial m.
- prediastolic m.
- presystolic m.
- pulmonic m.
- reduplication m.
- regurgitant m.
- respiratory m.
- Roger's m.
- sea-gull m.
- seesaw m.
- Steell's m.
- stenosal m.
- Still's m.
- subclavicular m.
- systolic m.
- to-and-fro m.
- Traube's m.
- tricuspid m.

murmur (continued)
- vascular m.
- venous m.
- vesicular m.
- water-wheel m.

muscle
- papillary m.
- pectinate m.

musculoskeletal
Mustard's operation
mutation
MV – mitral valve
MVP – mitral valve prolapse
Mycoplasma
    M. pneumoniae
Myer's stripper
myocardial
- m. bridging
- m. concussion
- m. contractility
- m. depolarization
- m. disease
- m. edema
- m. failure
- m. fiber shortening
- m. function
- m. hibernation
- m. hypertrophy
- m. imaging
- m. infarction
- m. ischemia
- m. metabolism
- m. necrosis
- m. oxygen consumption
- m. perfusion imaging
- m. perfusion scintigraphy
- m. perfusion study
- m. rupture
- m. stiffness
- m. stunning
- m. tension
- m. tissue

myocardiogram
myocardiograph
myocardiopathy
- idiopathic m.

myocardiorrhaphy

myocarditis
    acute bacterial m.
    Fiedler's m.
    fragmentation m.
    giant cell m.
    indurative m.
    infectious m.
    interstitial m.
    parenchymatous m.
    protozoal m.
    rickettsial m.
    m. scarlatinosa
    toxic m.
    viral m.
myocardium
myocardosis
    Riesman's m.
myocytolysis
    coagulative m.
myofibrosis
    m. cordis
myofilaments
myoglobin
myomalacia
    m. cordis
myopathia
    m. cordis
myositis
myotomy-myectomy-septal
   resection
myxedema
myxoma
myxomatous
Nathan's pacemaker
Naughton's treadmill protocol
necrosis
needle
    Adson's n.
    Cournand's n.
    Curry's n.
    Cushing's n.
    Flynt's n.
    Kronecker's n.
    Parhad-Poppen n.
    Retter's n.
    Rochester's n.
    Sanders-Brown-Shaw n.

needle (continued)
    Seldinger's n.
    Sheldon-Spatz n.
    Smiley-Williams n.
    Tuohy's n.
    Wood's n.
Neisseria
    N. meningitides
neoplasm
nephrectomy
nephritis
nephron
Nernst's equation
nerve
    parasympathetic n.
    sympathetic n.
    vagus n.
network
    Purkinje's n.
NH region
Nichols' clamp
Niedner's knife
NIH catheter
nitrate(s)
nitroglycerin
nocturia
nodal
node
    Aschoff's n.
    n. of Aschoff and Tawara
    atrioventricular n.
    Flack's n.
    His-Tawara n.
    Osler's n's
    sinoatrial n.
nodule
Noonan's syndrome
notch
    Sibson's n.
notching
NPB – nodal premature beat
N region
NSR – normal sinus rhythm
nuclear
nucleus
Nunez-Nunez knife
Nycore-pigtail catheter

obesity
obesity-hypoventilation
　　syndrome
obstruction
　　　　vena cava o.
occlusion
　　　　coronary o.
　　　　thrombotic o.
occlusive
ochronosis
Oertel's treatment
Ohm's law
Öhnell
　　　　X wave of O.
oliguria
omentopexy
OMI – old myocardial infarction
Omni-Atricor pacemaker
Omnicarbon valve
Omni-Ectocor pacemaker
Omniscience valve
Omni-Stanicor pacemaker
operation
　　　　Beck I o.
　　　　Beck II o.
　　　　Blalock-Hanlen o.
　　　　Blalock-Taussig o.
　　　　Brauer's o.
　　　　Brock's o.
　　　　Delorme's o.
　　　　Harrington's o.
　　　　Hufnagel's o.
　　　　Leriche's o.
　　　　Lyon-Horgan o.
　　　　Moore's o.
　　　　Mustard's o.
　　　　Potts' o.
　　　　Potts-Smith-Gibson o.
　　　　Rastelli's o.
　　　　Vineberg's o.
Orsi-Grocco method
orthopnea
orthopneic
orthostatic
Osborne wave
oscillation

oscillometer
oscillometric
oscillometry
oscilloscope
O'Shaughnessy's forceps
Osler's
　　　　nodes
　　　　sign
osmometer
ostium (ostia)
　　　　o. aortae
　　　　o. arteriosum cordis
　　　　o. atrioventriculare
　　　　　　dextrum
　　　　o. atrioventriculare
　　　　　　sinistrum
　　　　o. cardiacum
　　　　o. primum
　　　　o. secundum
　　　　sinusoidal o.
　　　　o. trunci pulmonalis
　　　　o. venarum pulmonalium
　　　　o. venosum cordis
Overholt's elevator
oximetry
oxygen
oxygenate
oxygenator
P_2 – pulmonic second sound
PAC – premature auricular
　　contraction
pacemaker
　　　　Amtech-Killeen p.
　　　　Arco p.
　　　　artificial p.
　　　　asynchronous p.
　　　　Atricor p.
　　　　bifocal demand p.
　　　　Biotronik p.
　　　　bipolar p.
　　　　Chardak-Greatbatch p.
　　　　Coratomic p.
　　　　Cordis' p.
　　　　Cordis Atricor p.
　　　　Cordis-Ectocor p.
　　　　Cordis' fixed rate p.

pacemaker (continued)
    Cordis Ventricor p.
    CPI Maxilith p.
    CPI Minilith p.
    demand p.
    Ectocor p.
    Electrodyne p.
    endocardial bipolar p.
    epicardial p.
    General Electric p.
    implantable p.
    lithium p.
    Nathan's p.
    nuclear p.
    Omni-Atricor p.
    Omni-Ectocor p.
    Omni-Stanicor p.
    radio frequency p.
    Stanicor p.
    Starr-Edwards p.
    Telectronic p.
    transvenous p.
    unipolar p.
    Ventricor p.
    wandering p.
    Zoll's p.
    Zyrel's p.
    Zytron p.
pacemapping
pacing
PAH – pulmonary artery
    hypertension
P-A interval
palmitic acid
palpitation
panangiitis
    diffuse necrotizing p.
panarteritis
pansphygmograph
papillary
paracentesis
    p. cordis
    p. pericardii
paradox image
paradoxical
paraganglioma

paramagnetic
parametric
parasternal
parasympathetic
parasystole
Parhad-Poppen needle
paries
    p. caroticus cavi tympani
Park's aneurysm
paroxysmal
Parrot's murmur
Pasteurella
    P. multocida
PAT – paroxysmal atrial
    tachycardia
patch
    Edwards' p.
    McCallum's p.
    Teflon p.
patent
    p. ductus arteriosus
    p. foramen ovale
paulocardia
P cell
PDA – patent ductus arteriosus
pectoral
pectoralis
pectus
    p. carinatum
    p. excavatum
PEEP – positive end-expiratory
    pressure
Penicillium
pentalogy
    p. of Fallot
PEP – preejection period
percussion
percutaneous
    p. transluminal coronary
      angioplasty
perfusion
periaortitis
periarteritis
    p. nodosa
periatrial
periauricular

pericardial
>   p. calcification
>   p. cyst
>   p. effusion
>   p. fluid
>   p. friction
>   p. knock
>   p. peel
>   p. window

pericardicentesis
pericardiectomy
pericardiocentesis
pericardiolysis
pericardiomediastinitis
pericardiophrenic
pericardiopleural
pericardiorrhaphy
pericardiostomy
pericardiosymphysis
pericardiotomy
pericarditis
>   acute fibrinous p.
>   adhesive p.
>   amebic p.
>   bacterial p.
>   p. calculosa
>   p. callosa
>   carcinomatous p.
>   constrictive p.
>   p. epistenocardiaca
>   p. externa et interna
>   fibrous p.
>   hemorrhagic p.
>   idiopathic p.
>   localized p.
>   mediastinal p.
>   neoplastic p.
>   p. obliterans
>   obliterating p.
>   purulent p.
>   rheumatic p.
>   serofibrinous p.
>   p. sicca
>   suppurative p.
>   tuberculous p.
>   uremic p.
>   p. villosa

pericarditis (continued)
>   viral p.
>   p. with effusion

pericardium
>   adherent p.
>   bread-and-butter p.
>   calcified p.
>   p. fibrosum
>   fibrous p.
>   parietal p.
>   p. serosum
>   serous p.
>   shaggy p.
>   visceral p.

pericardosis
pericardotomy
periinfarction block
perimuscular plexus
perimysial plexus
period
>   Wenckebach's p.

periosteotome
>   Alexander-Farabeuf p.

peripericarditis
peripheral
periphlebitis
PET – positron-emission
>   tomography

petechia
Phemister's elevator
phenomenon
>   Ashman's p.
>   Katz-Wachtel p.
>   Raynaud's p.
>   "R" on "T" p.

pheochromocytoma
Phialophora
phlebangioma
phlebarteriectasia
phlebarteriodialysis
phlebasthenia
phlebectasia
phlebectomy
phlebectopia
phlebemphraxis
phlebexairesis
phlebismus

phlebitis
phlebocarcinoma
phlebocholosis
phlebogram
phlebography
phlebolith
phlebolithiasis
phlebomanometer
phlebomyomatosis
phlebophlebostomy
phlebopiezometry
phleboplasty
phleborrhagia
phleborrhaphy
phleborrhexis
phlebosclerosis
phlebosis
phlebostasis
phlebostenosis
phlebostrepsis
phlebothrombosis
phlebotome
phlebotomy
phonocardiogram
phonocardiograph
phonocardiographic
phonocardiography
    intracardiac p.
phonoelectrocardioscope
phonogram
phosphodiesterase
phosphofructokinase
phospholamban
phosphomonoesterase
phosphorus
phrenocardia
phrenopericarditis
Pick's
    disease
    syndrome
piezoelectric crystal
pigtail catheter
pixel
plasmalemma
plasmin
plasminogen
plethora

plethysmograph
plethysmography
plethysmometer
plethysmometry
pleuropericardial
pleuropericarditis
plexogenic
plexus
    cardiac p.
    p. cardiacus profundus
    p. cardiacus superficialis
    p. caroticus communis
    p. caroticus externus
    p. caroticus internus
    p. coronarius cordis
    perimuscular p.
    perimysial p.
    vascular p.
    p. venosus caroticus
      internus
    venous p.
P loop
PMI–point of maximal impulse
P mitrale
PND–paroxysmal nocturnal
    dyspnea
pneumatocardia
pneumocardial
pneumohemia
pneumohemopericardium
pneumohydropericardium
pneumomediastinum
pneumopericardium
pneumoprecordium
pneumopyopericardium
point
    Erb's p.
    isoelectric p.
    J p.
polarity
polyarteritis
    p. nodosa
polycythemia
    p. hypertonica
    p. vera
polyunsaturated fat
poodrazh. See *poudrage.*

Poppen-Blalock clamp
Poppen's clamp
porcine
    p. heterograft
    p. xenograft
position. See *General Surgical Terms section.*
positron-emission tomography
postmyocardial infarction
postpump syndrome
potassium
Pott's aneurysm
Potts'
    clamp
    operation
    rib shears
    scissors
Potts-Niedner clamp
Potts-Smith
    clamp
    forceps
    scissors
Potts-Smith-Gibson operation
poudrage
P pulmonale
P-Q interval
P-Q segment
precardiac
precordial
precordium
preejection period
preexcitation syndrome
prekallikrein
premature
preponderance
    ventricular p.
presbycardia
presystolic
preventriculosis
preventriculus
principle
    Fick's p.
P-R interval
Prinzmetal's angina
proarrhythmic
procedure
    Fontan p.

procedure (continued)
    Senning's p.
prolapse
    mitral valve p.
propranolol
prosthesis (valves and grafts)
    Alvarez' p.
    Björk-Shiley p.
    Braunwald's p.
    caged-ball p.
    Cape Town p.
    Cartwright's p.
    Cooley's p.
    Cutter-SCDK p.
    Cutter-Smeloff p.
    Dacron p.
    DeBakey's p.
    discoid aortic p.
    Duromedics p.
    Edwards' p.
    Gott's p.
    Harken's p.
    Hufnagel's p.
    Ionescu-Shiley p.
    Kay-Shiley p.
    Kay-Suzuki p.
    Lillehei-Kaster p.
    Magovern's p.
    Smeloff-Cutter p.
    Starr-Edwards p.
    tilting disk p.
    tri-leaflet aortic p.
    Wada's p.
    Weavenit's p.
    Wesolowski's p.
prosthetic
prothrombin time
protocol
    Bruce treadmill p.
    Naughton's treadmill p.
protodiastolic
P-R segment
pseudoanemia
    p. angiospastica
pseudoaneurysm
pseudoangina
pseudoangioma

pseudocoarctation
Pseudomonas
    P. aeruginosa
pseudotruncus arteriosus
pseudoxanthoma elasticum
PSS – progressive systemic
    sclerosis
PTAV – percutaneous
    transluminal atrial
    valvuloplasty
PTCA – percutaneous
    transluminal coronary
    angioplasty
PTMV – percutaneous
    transluminal mitral
    valvuloplasty
PTRA – percutaneous
    transluminal renal
    angioplasty
pulmonale
    cor p.
pulmonary
pulmonic
    p. atresia
    p. stenosis
pulsate
pulsatile
pulsation
    expansile p.
    suprasternal p.
pulse
    allorhythmic p.
    anacrotic p.
    anadicrotic p.
    anatricrotic p.
    arachnoid p.
    auriculovenous p.
    Bamberger's bulbar p.
    bigeminal p.
    bisferious p.
    cannon ball p.
    catacrotic p.
    catadicrotic p.
    catatricrotic p.
    centripetal venous p.
    collapsing p.
    cordy p.

pulse (continued)
    Corrigan's p.
    coupled p.
    decurtate p.
    dicrotic p.
    digitalate p.
    elastic p.
    entopic p.
    filiform p.
    formicant p.
    gaseous p.
    guttural p.
    high-tension p.
    hyperdicrotic p.
    jugular p.
    Kussmaul's p.
    Monneret's p.
    monocrotic p.
    mouse tail p.
    paradoxical p.
    pedal p.
    pistol-shot p.
    plateau p.
    polycrotic p.
    pulmonary p.
    quadrigeminal p.
    Quincke's p.
    Riegel's p.
    thready p.
    tremulous p.
    tricrotic p.
    trigeminal p.
    undulating p.
    vagus p.
    ventricular venous p.
    vermicular p.
    vibrating p.
    water-hammer p.
pulsus
    p. alternans
    p. bigeminus
    p. bisferiens
    p. celer
    p. contractus
    p. cordis
    p. debilis
    p. deficiens

pulsus (continued)
    p. deletus
    p. differens
    p. duplex
    p. durus
    p. filiformis
    p. formicans
    p. frequens
    p. heterochronicus
    p. intercurrens
    p. irregularis perpetuus
    p. magnus et celer
    p. mollis
    p. monocrotus
    p. oppressus
    p. paradoxus
    p. parvus et tardus
    p. plenus
    p. pseudo-intermittens
    p. rarus
    p. tardus
    p. trigeminus
    p. undulosus
    p. vacuus
    p. venosus
    p. vibrans
pump
    Emerson's p.
"pump lung"
punch
    Brock's p.
puncture
    Kronecker's p.
Purkinje's
    fibers
    network
purpura
    p. fulminans
purulent
PVC – premature ventricular
    contraction
P vector
PVS – premature ventricular
    systole
PVT – paroxysmal ventricular
    tachycardia
P wave

pyelophlebitis
pyemia
    arterial p.
    portal p.
pyopneumopericardium
pyrogen
pyrophosphate
pyruvic acid
Q fever
Q-M interval
QRS
    alternans
    axis
    changes
    complex
    loop
    vector
QRS-ST junction
QRS-T changes
QRST interval
QRS wave
QS complex
Q-S deflections
Q-T interval
quadrigeminy
Quain's
    degeneration
    fatty heart
Quénu-Muret sign
Quincke's
    pulse
    sign
Q-U interval
Q wave
RA – right atrial
    right atrium
radicle
radioimmunoassay
radioisotopic
radionuclide
radiotracer
rales
ramus
rankenangioma
raphe
rasp
    Beck's r.

raspatory
  Coryllos' r.
Rastelli's operation
ratio
  R/S r.
ray
  gamma r.
Raynaud's
  disease
  phenomenon
RBBB – right bundle branch
  block
RCD – relative cardiac
  dullness
reanastomosis
reciprocal beat
reflex
  Abrams' heart r.
  Bainbridge's r.
  Bezold-Jarisch r.
  bregmocardiac r.
  carotid-sinus r.
  Erben's r.
  Livierato's r.
  McDowall's r.
  oculocardiac r.
  psychocardiac r.
  pulmonocoronary r.
  viscerocardiac r.
reflux
  abdomino-jugular r.
regurgitant
regurgitation
  aortic r.
  mitral r.
  pulmonic r.
  tricuspid r.
Reich-Nechtow clamp
repolarization
respiration
  Cheyne-Stokes r.
  Corrigan's r.
respirator
  Engström r.
respiratory distress
resuscitation
  cardiopulmonary r.

rete
  r. arteriosum
  r. mirabile
  r. vasculosum
  r. venosum
retractor
  Adson's r.
  Allison's r.
  Carter's r.
  Cooley's r.
  Coryllos' r.
  Crawford's r.
  Davidson's r.
  DeBakey-Balfour r.
  DeBakey-Cooley r.
  Gross' r.
  Gross-Pomeranz-
    Watkins r.
  Harrington-Pemberton r.
  Harrington's r.
  Hedblom's r.
  Hibbs' r.
  Krasky's r.
  Lukens' r.
  Meyerding's r.
  Richardson's r.
  Ross' r.
  Sauerbruch's r.
  Semb's r.
  Walter-Deaver r.
Retter's needle
revascularization
  myocardial r.
RF – rheumatic fever
rhabdomyoma
rhabdomyosarcoma
RHD – rheumatic heart disease
rheumapyra
rheumatic
  r. fever
  r. heart disease
rheumatoid arthritis
rhythm
  atrial r.
  auriculoventricular r.
  cantering r.
  coupled r.

rhythm (continued)
    gallop r.
    idioventricular r.
    nodal r.
    pendulum r.
    reversed r.
    sinus r.
    triple r.
    ventricular r.
rhythmophone
rib contractor
    Bailey-Gibbon r.c.
    Bailey's r.c.
    Sellor's r.c.
rib shears
    Bethune's r.s.
    Giertz-Shoemaker r.s.
    Gluck's r.s.
    Moure-Coryllos r.s.
    Potts' r.s.
    Sauerbruch's r.s.
    Shoemaker's r.s.
rib spreader
    Burford's r.s.
    Finochietto's r.s.
    Harken's r.s.
    Lemmon's r.s.
    Lilienthal-Sauerbruch r.s.
    Rienhoff-Finochietto r.s.
    Tuffier's r.s.
    Wilson's r.s.
Richardson's retractor
Richet's aneurysm
Riegel's pulse
Rienhoff-Finochietto rib
    spreader
Rienhoff's
    clamp
    forceps
Riesman's myocardosis
ring
    atrial r.
    Carpentier's r's
    Effler's r.
    vascular r.
Riva-Rocci sphygmomanometer
Rivero-Carvello's sign

Rochester's
    awl
    knife
    needle
Rockey's cannula
Rodrigues' aneurysm
roentgenocardiogram
roentgenography
Roesler-Dressler infarction
Roger's
    bruit
    disease
    murmur
    sphygmomanometer
rongeur
    Leksell's r.
"R on T" phenomenon
rooma-. See words beginning
    rheuma-.
Rose's tamponade
Ross' retractor
Rostan's asthma
Rotch's sign
Roth's spots
RSR – regular sinus rhythm
R/S ratio
R/S-T interval
rubella
rubeola
rumble
    diastolic r.
Rumel's
    clamp
    forceps
    tourniquet
Rummo's disease
Ruskin's forceps
RV – right ventricle
RVE – right ventricular
    enlargement
RVH – right ventricular
    hypertrophy
R wave
Saccharomyces
"saddle emboli"
St. Jude valve

Salibi's clamp
Salmonella
Sanders-Brown-Shaw needle
sanguis
Sansom's sign
saphenofemoral
saphenous
sarcoid
sarcoidosis
    s. cordis
sarcolemma
sarcoma
sarcomere
Satinsky's
    clamp
    forceps
    scissors
saturated fat
Sauerbruch's
    forceps
    retractor
    rib shears
SBE – subacute bacterial
    endocarditis
scale
    Borg s.
scan
    cardiac s.
    thallium-201 scan
scanner
scavenger cell pathway
schistosomiasis
scintigram
scintigraphy
scintillation
    s. camera
    s. probe
    s. scan
scissors
    Cooley's s.
    DeBakey-Metzenbaum s.
    DeBakey's s.
    Jacobson's s.
    Jorgenson's s.
    Litwak's s.
    Morse's s.

scissors (continued)
    Potts' s.
    Potts-Smith s.
    Satinsky's s.
    Thorek-Feldman s.
    Thorek's s.
    Toennis' s.
scleroderma
sclerosis
    arterial s.
sclerotic
Scoville-Lewis clip
Scribner's shunt
scurvy
searcher
    Allport-Babcock s.
Sedillot's elevator
segment
    P-Q s.
    P-R s.
    S-T s.
    T-P s.
    T-P-Q s.
Seldinger's needle
selenium
Sellor's
    knife
    rib contractor
Selman's forceps
Selverstone's clamp
Semb's
    forceps
    retractor
semilunar
Senning's procedure
septa
septal
    s. defect
    s. resection
septic
    s. embolization
    s. shock
septum
    s. atriorum cordis
    s. atrioventriculare cordis
    interatrial s.
    s. interatriale cordis

septum (continued)
    interauricular s.
    interventricular s.
    s. interventriculare cordis
    s. membranaceum
        ventriculorum cordis
    s. musculare
        ventriculorum cordis
    s. primum
    s. secundum
    s. ventriculorum cordis
serotonin
Serratia
serrefine
sfigmo-. See words beginning
    sphygmo-.
SGOT – serum glutamic-oxalic
        transaminase
        serum glutamic-
        oxaloacetic transaminase
Shaw's stripper
shears
    Lebsche's s.
Sheehan Dodge technique
Sheldon-Spatz needle
"shock lung"
Shoemaker's
    clamp
    rib shears
shunt
    aortopulmonary s.
    arteriovenous s.
    cardiovascular s.
    cavamesenteric s.
    intracardia s.
    Javid's s.
    left-to-right s.
    portacaval s.
    portarenal s.
    postcaval s.
    right-to-left s.
    Scribner's s.
    ventriculoatrial s.
    ventriculoperitoneal s.
    Warren's s.
    Waterson's s.

Sibson's
    notch
    vestibule
sick sinus syndrome
siderosis
sign
    Auenbrugger's s.
    Bamberger's s.
    Béhier-Hardy s.
    Bouillaud's s.
    Branham's s.
    Braunwald's s.
    Broadbent's s.
    Brockenbrough's s.
    Carvallo's s.
    Cegka's s.
    Corrigan's s.
    de Musset's s.
    Dieuaide's s.
    Drummond's s.
    Duroziez's s.
    Ewart's s.
    Friedreich's s.
    Hamman's s.
    Hill's s.
    Hope's s.
    Kussmaul's s.
    Levine's s.
    Litten's s.
    McGinn-White s.
    Müller's s.
    Osler's s.
    Quénu-Muret s.
    Quincke's s.
    Rivero-Carvello's s.
    Rotch's s.
    Sansom's s.
    Sterles' s.
    Traube's s.
    vital s's
    Wenckebach's s.
Silastic coronary artery cannula
silhouette
    cardiovascular s.
silicone
sinistrocardia

sinoatrial
sinoauricular
sinospiral
sinoventricular
sinus
    s. arrest
    s. arrhythmia
    s. bradycardia
    s. caroticus
    carotid s.
    coronary s.
    s. of Morgagni
    s. nodal cell
    s. nodal reentrant
    s. node
    s. pause
    s. rhythm
    s. tachycardia
    s. transversus pericardii
    s. of Valsalva
    s. venous defect
sinusoid
    myocardial s's
SLE – systemic lupus
    erythematosus
sleep apnea syndrome
slope
    E to F s.
Smeloff-Cutter prosthesis
Smiley-Williams needle
Smith's clip
somatostatin
Sones' coronary catheter
Soresi's cannula
soroche
souffle
    cardiac s.
sound
    bellows s.
    flapping s.
    heart s's: first s., second s.
    Korotkoff's s's
    pistol-shot s.
    tick-tack s's
Southey-Leech tubes

spasm
    coronary-artery s.
spatula
    Jacobson's s.
SPECT – single-photon emission
    computed tomography
spectroscopy
    proton s.
sphygmobologram
sphygmobolometer
sphygmocardiogram
sphygmocardiograph
sphygmocardioscope
sphygmodynamometer
sphygmogram
sphygmography
sphygmomanometer
    Erlanger's s.
    Faught's s.
    Janeway's s.
    Riva-Rocci s.
    Rogers' s.
    Staunton's s.
    Tycos' s.
sphygmomanometroscope
sphygmometer
sphygmometrograph
sphygmometroscope
sphygmo-oscillometer
sphygmopalpation
sphygmophone
sphygmoplethysmograph
sphygmoscope
    Bishop's s.
sphygmosignal
sphygmosystole
sphygmotonogram
sphygmotonograph
sphygmotonometer
sphygmoviscosimetry
spin-echo imaging
splenomegaly
splenosis
    pericardial s.
spot
    Roth's s's

SPTI – systolic pressure-time
   index
squatting
standstill
     atrial s.
     auricular s.
     cardiac s.
     respiratory s.
     ventricular s.
Stanford bioptome
Stanicor pacemaker
Stanley-Kent bundle
staphylococci
Staphylococcus
     S. aureus
Starling's
     equation
     forces
     law
     mechanism
Starr-Edwards
     pacemaker
     prosthesis
     valve
stasis
     venous s.
Staunton's
     sphygmomanometer
ST depression
steal
     subclavian s.
Steell's murmur
stellectomy
stenocardia
stenosis
     aortic s.
     Dittrich's s.
     mitral s.
     preventricular s.
     pulmonary s.
     pulmonic s.
     subaortic s.
     tricuspid s.
stenotic
stent
     Carpentier's s.

step
     Krönig's s's
Sterges' carditis
Sterles' sign
steroid
sternopericardial
sternotomy
sternum
stethoscope
Stille-Luer forceps
Stille's forceps
Still's murmur
stimulation
     vagus s.
Stomatococcus
"stone heart"
Streptobacillus
     S. moniliformis
Streptococcus
     S. pneumoniae
stress test
stress thallium-201
striation
     tabby cat s.
     tigroid s.
stripper
     Myer's s.
     Shaw's s.
     Wylie's s.
ST segment
     alterans
     changes
     elevation
S-T segment
ST-T deviations
study
     opacification s.
stylet
subaortic
subclavian
subclavicular
sublingual
subpulmonic
subvalvular
suffusion
Sugar's clip

sulcus
> s. aorticus
> atrioventricular s.
> s. coronarius cordis
> interventricular s. of heart
> longitudinal s. of heart
> s. of subclavian artery
> transverse s. of heart

sump
> Baylor's s.

support
> Abée's s.

supraclavicular
supravalvular
supraventricular
surgical procedures. See *operation.*

survey
> Jenkins Activity s.

suture. See *General Surgical Terms section.*

SVC – superior vena cava
Swan-Ganz catheter
S wave
sympathectomy
sympathetic
> s. ganglia
> s. nervous system

sympathoadrenal
sympathomimetic
symphysis
> cardiac s.

synanastomosis
synchronous
syncopal
syncope
> Adams-Stokes s.
> s. anginosa
> carotid s.
> deglutition s.
> vasovagal s.

syndrome
> acquired immunodeficiency s.
> Adams-Stokes s.
> adrenogenital s.
> adult respiratory distress s.

syndrome (continued)
> Ask-Upmark s.
> Ayerza's s.
> Babinski's s.
> Barlow's s.
> Beau's s.
> Bernheim's s.
> Bouillaud's s.
> Bouveret's s.
> bradycardia-tachycardia s.
> cardiofacial s.
> click-murmur s.
> Dressler's s.
> Eisenmenger's s.
> floppy valve s.
> Gower's s.
> Holt-Oram s.
> Jervell and Lange-Nielson s.
> Leriche's s.
> Libman-Sacks s.
> Lown-Ganong-Levine s.
> Lutembacher's s.
> Marfan's s.
> Noonan's s.
> Pick's s.
> sick sinus s.
> "stiff-heart" s.
> straight back s.
> Takayasu's s.
> Taussig-Bing s.
> Wolff-Parkinson-White s.
> XO s.
> XXXX s.
> XXXY s.

system
> cardiovascular s.
> conduction s.
> His-Purkinje s.
> vascular s.

systemic
> s. lupus erythematosus

systole
> aborted s.
> arterial s.
> atrial s.
> auricular s.

systole (continued)
    catalectic s.
    extra s.
    frustrate s.
    hemic s.
    ventricular s.
systolic
    s. apical impulse
    s. click-murmur syndrome
    s. current
    s. function
    s. motion
    s. murmur
    s. pressure time index
    s. reserve
    s. time interval
systolometer
tachyarrhythmia
tachycardia
    antidromic t.
    atrial t.
    alternating bidirectional t.
    atrioventricular t.
    auricular t.
    nodal t.
    nonparoxysmal t.
    orthostatic t.
    paroxysmal ventricular t.
    reciprocating t.
    sinus t.
    supraventricular t.
    ventricular t.
tachycardiac
tachypnea
tachysystole
    atrial t.
    auricular t.
taeni
    t. terminalis
Takayasu's syndrome
takipnea. See *tachypnea.*
TAMI – thrombolysis and angioplasty in myocardial infarction trial
tamponade
    cardiac t.
    pericardial t.

tamponade (continued)
    Rose's t.
TAR – thrombocytopenia with absence of radius
TA segment
Taussig-Bing syndrome
T cell
technetium-99m
technique
    Creech's t.
    George Lewis t.
    Gruentzig's t.
    Judkin's t.
    Sheehan Dodge t.
Teflon
    catheter
    patch
telangiectasia
telangiectasis
telangiosis
telecardiogram
telecardiography
Telectronic pacemaker
telelectrocardiogram
telelectrocardiograph
teratoma
test
    Allen's t.
    antistreptozyme t.
    Balke-Ware t.
    Dehio's t.
    ergonovine t.
    Gibbon-Landis t.
    Korotkoff's t.
    lipid t.
    Livierato's t.
    Master's "2-step" exercise t.
    radioactive fibrinogen uptake t.
    regitine t.
    serum enzyme t.
    stress t.
    thallium stress t.
    treadmill t.
    Trendelenburg's t.
tetrad

tetralogy
    t. of Fallot
TGF-beta – transforming growth
    factor – beta
thallium-201 scan
thebesian
theca
    t. cordis
theorem
    Bayes' t.
    Bernouilli's t.
theory
    Bayliss' t.
thermodilution
    t. catheter
    t. technique
thoracentesis
thoracic outlet syndrome
thoracotomy
Thorek-Feldman scissors
Thorek's scissors
Thorel's bundle
thrill
    aneurysmal t.
    aortic t.
    diastolic t.
    presystolic t.
    systolic t.
thrombasthenia
thrombectomy
thromboangiitis
    t. obliterans
thromboaortopathy
    occlusive t.
thromboarteritis
    t. purulenta
thromboclasis
thrombocytopenia
    t. with absence of radius
thrombocytosis
thromboembolic
thromboembolism
thromboendarterectomy
thromboendarteritis
thromboendocarditis
thrombokinesis
thrombolymphangitis

thrombolysis
thrombolytic
thrombomodulin
thrombophlebitis
    iliofemoral t.
    t. migrans
    t. purulenta
    t. saltans
thrombopoiesis
thrombosis
    coronary t.
thrombotic
thrombus
thumpversion
thyroid storm
thyrotoxic
thyrotoxicosis
TI – tricuspid incompetence
    tricuspid insufficiency
TIA – transient ischemic attack
TIMII – Thrombolysis in
    Myocardial Infarction Trial
    II
tinkle
    Bouillaud's t.
tissue
    His-Purkinje t.
T loop
Toennis' scissors
tomography
tortuosity
tourniquet
    Rumel's t.
TPA – tissue plasminogen
    activator
T-P interval
T-P segment
T-P-Q segment
trabeculae
    t. carneae cordis
    flesh t. of heart
trabecular
tract
    atriohisian t.
transducer
transforming growth factor – beta
transient

transplant
transposition
    t. of great vessels
transseptal
transvenous
transventricular
Traube-Hering waves
Traube's
    curves
    heart
    murmur
    sign
treadmill test
treatment
    Fränkel's t.
    Karell's t.
    Oertel's t.
Trendelenburg-Crafoord
    clamp
Trendelenburg's test
triad
    Beck's t.
triangle
    Burger's t.
    cardiohepatic t.
    Einthoven's t.
trichinosis
Trichosporon
tricuspid
    t. atresia
    t. opening snaps
    t. regurgitation
    t. stenosis
    t. valve
trifascicular
trigeminy
triglyceride
trigona
    t. fibrosa cordis
trilogy
    t. of Fallot
trisomy
    13
    18
    21
tropomyosin

troponin
    C
    I
    T
truncus
    t. arteriosus
    t. brachiocephalicus
    t. fasciculi
        atrioventricularis
trunk
    brachiocephalic t.
Trypanosoma
    T. cruzi
    t. rhodesiense
trypanosomiasis
T system
Tubbs' dilator
tube
    nasogastric t.
    Southey-Leech t's
tubular
    t. necrosis
Tucker's dilator
Tudor-Edwards costotome
Tuffier's rib spreader
tumor plop
tunica
    t. adventitia vasorum
    t. externa vasorum
    t. intima vasorum
    t. media vasorum
    t. vasculosa
tunneler
    Crawford-Cooley t.
    DeBakey's t.
Tuohy's needle
turgescent
turgid
turgor
    t. vitalis
T vector
T wave
    changes
    inversion
Tycos' sphygmomanometer
ultrasonography
    Doppler u.

ultrasonoscope
ultrasound
unipolar
univentricular
uremia
U wave
vagal
Valsalva's
    maneuver
    sinus
valve
    aortic v.
    atrioventricular v.
    auriculoventricular v.
    ball-type v.
    bicuspid v.
    Björk-Shiley v.
    caged-ball v.
    cardiac v's
    Carpentier-Edwards v.
    caval v.
    v. of coronary sinus
    Duromedics v.
    eustachian v.
    Hancock's v.
    Ionescu-Shiley v.
    Lillehei-Kaster v.
    Medtronic-Hall v.
    mitral v.
    Omnicarbon v.
    Omniscience v.
    porcine v.
    pulmonary v.
    semilunar v's
    St. Jude v.
    Starr-Edwards v.
    thebesian v.
    tricuspid v.
valvotome
valvotomy
    mitral v.
valvula
    v. bicuspidalis
    v. semilunaris dextra
        aortae
    v. semilunaris posterior
        aortae

valvula (continued)
    v. semilunaris sinistra
        aortae
    v. sinus coronarii
    v. tricuspidalis
    v. venae cavae inferioris
    v. venosa
    v. vestibuli
valvulae semilunares aortae
valvular
    v. aortic stenosis
    v. stenosis
valvulitis
    rheumatic v.
valvuloplasty
    percutaneous
        transluminal atrial v.
    percutaneous
        transluminal mitral v.
valvulotome
valvulotomy
Vanderbilt's forceps
variant angina
variceal
varices
varicose
    v. vein
varicosity
varix
    aneurysmal v.
    arterial v.
vascular
    v. impedance
    v. resistance
    v. ring
    v. stenosis
vascularity
vascularization
vasculature
vasculitis
vasoactive
vasoconstriction
vasoconstrictor
vasodepression
vasodepressor
vasodilation
vasodilator

vasoinhibitor
vasomotor
vasopressor
vasospasm
    refractory ergonovine-
        induced v.
VCG – vectorcardiogram-
    vectorcardiography
VDG – ventricular diastolic gallop
vector
    P v.
    T v.
vectorcardiogram
vectorcardiography
    spatial v.
vegetation
    bacterial v's
    verrucous v's
vein
    azygos v.
    cephalic v.
    portal v.
    pulmonary v.
    saphenous v.
    varicose v.
velocardiofacial
velocity
vena cava
    inferior v.c.
    superior v.c.
vena cavagram
venae cavae
venipuncture
venoauricular
venoconstriction
venofibrosis
venogram
venography
veno-occlusive
venosinal
venostasis
venotomy
venous
    v. hum
    v. pressure
    v. pulse
    v. resistance

venous (continued)
    v. return curve
    v. smooth muscle
    v. thromboembolism
    v. thrombosis
ventilation
    arterial v.
    v.-perfusion ratio
    v. scintigraphy
    v. threshold
ventricle
Ventricor pacemaker
ventricular
    v. arrhythmia
    v. assist device
    v. contour
    v. dilatation
    v. ectopy
    v. end-diastolic volume
    v. end-systolic pressure
    v. fibrillation
    v. filling
    v. flutter
    v. function
    v. fusion
    v. gradient
    v. hypertrophy
    v. interdependence
    v. mapping
    v. pacing
    v. performance
    v. premature beat
    v. premature contractions
    v. pressure-volume loop
    v. reentry
    v. relaxation
    v. rhythm
    v. septal defect
    v. septum
    v. systole
    v. tachyarrhythmia
    v. tachycardia
    v. wall motion
    v. wall shortening
ventriculoarterial
    v. coupling
ventriculography

ventriculomyotomy
ventriculonector
ventriculotomy
ventriculus
 v. cordis
 v. dexter cordis
 v. sinister cordis
Venturi effect
venule
vessel
vestibule
 Gibson's v.
 Sibson's v.
videodensitometry
Vineberg's operation
virus
 ECHO (enteric
  cytopathogenic human
  orphan) v.
 immunodeficiency v.
vitium
 v. cordis
VLDL – very low-density
 lipoprotein
V leads: 1 through 6
volume load hypertrophy
von Willebrand's disease
VPB – ventricular premature beat
VPC – ventricular premature
 contraction
VSD – ventricular septal defect
Wada's prosthesis
Walter-Deaver retractor
Wangensteen's awl
Warren's shunt
water-hammer pulse
Waterson's shunt
wave
 A w.
 arterial w.
 C w.
 delta w.
 dicrotic w.
 F w's
 fibrillary w's
 Osborne w.
 oscillation w.

wave (continued)
 overflow w.
 P w.
 percussion w.
 peridicrotic w.
 predicrotic w.
 pre-excitation w.
 Q w.
 QRS w.
 R w.
 recoil w.
 respiratory w.
 S w.
 T w.
 tidal w.
 transverse w.
 Traube-Hering w's
 tricrotic w.
 U w.
 vasomotor w.
 ventricular w.
 X w. of Öhnell
Weavenit's
 patch graft
 prosthesis
Wenckebach's
 cycle
 disease
 heart block
 period
 sign
Wesolowski's prosthesis
Willis' circle
Wilson's
 leads
 rib spreader
Wolff-Parkinson-White
 syndrome
Woodbridge's ligature
Wood's needle
WPW – Wolff-Parkinson-White
 (syndrome)
Wrisberg's ganglia
Wylie's stripper
xanthelasma
xanthoma
 x. tendinosum

xenograft
xenon
    127
    133
xiphoid process
XO syndrome
X wave of Öhnell
XXXX syndrome
XXXY syndrome

yeast
Yersinia
zenograft. See *xenograft.*
zero-order kinetics
Z line
Zoll's pacemaker
Zyrel's pacemaker
Zytron pacemaker

Dermatology and Allergy

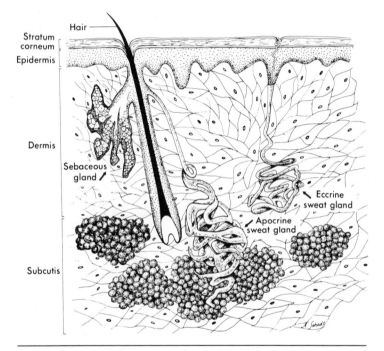

(Courtesy of Prior, J. A., Silberstein, J. S., and Stang, J. M.: Physical Diagnosis, 6th ed. St. Louis, C. V. Mosby Company, 1981.)

Dermatology and Allergy

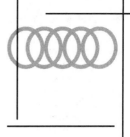

A-alpha nerve fibers
Abernethy's sarcoma
abscess
    Monro's a.
    Paget's a.
Absidia
absorbed dose
Abt-Letterer-Siwe syndrome
acanthocheilonemiasis
acanthokeratodermia
acantholysis
    a. bullosa
acanthoma
    a. adenoides cysticum
    a. inguinale
    a. tropicum
    a. verrucosa seborrhoeica
acanthosis
    a. nigricans
    a. papulosa nigra
    a. seborrhoeica
    a. verrucosa
acanthotic
acariasis
    chorioptic a.
    demodectic a.
    psoroptic a.
    sarcoptic a.
acarodermatitis
    a. urticarioides
acarophobia
Acarus
    A. folliculorum
    A. gallinae
    A. hordei
    A. rhyzoglypticus
        hyacinthi
    A. scabiei

Acarus (continued)
    A. tritici
acclimatization
acetonasthma
achor
achromatosis
achromia
    congenital a.
    a. parasitica
achromic
    a. nevus
achromoderma
achromotrichia
aciduria
acladiosis
acne
    adenoid a.
    a. aggregata seu
        conglobata
    a. agminata
    a. albida
    a. artificialis
    a. atrophica
    bromine a.
    a. cachecticorum
    a. cheloidique
    a. ciliaris
    common a.
    a. conglobata
    cystic a.
    a. decalvans
    a. disseminata
    a. dorsalis
    epileptic a.
    a. erythematosa
    a. excoriée des jeunes filles
    a. frontalis
    a. generalis

acne (continued)
    halogen a.
    halowax a.
    a. hordeolaris
    a. hypertrophica
    a. indurata
    iodine a.
    a. keloid
    lupoid a.
    a. mentagra
    a. necrotica miliaris
    a. necroticans et
      exulcerans serpiginosa
      nasi
    a. neonatorum
    pancreatic a.
    a. papulosa
    petroleum a.
    a. picealis
    a. punctata
    a. pustulosa
    a. rodens
    a. rosacea
    a. scorbutica
    a. scrofulosorum
    a. seborrhoeica
    a. simplex
    a. syphilitica
    tar a.
    a. tarsi
    a. tropicalis
    a. urticata polycythemica
    a. varioliformis
    a. vermoulante
    a. vulgaris
acnegenic
acneiform
acquired immunodeficiency
    syndrome
acrochordon
acrocyanosis
acrodermatitis
    a. chronica atrophicans
    a. continua
    a. enteropathica
    Hallopeau's a.
    a. hiemalis

acrodermatitis (continued)
    a. papulosa infantum
    a. perstans
    a. vesiculosa tropica
acrodermatoses
acrodermatosis
acrodynia
acrokeratosis
    paraneoplastic a.
    a. verruciformis
acromegaly
acropachy
acropustulosis
acroscleroderma
acrosclerosis
actinic
    a. elastosis
    a. keratosis
    a. porokeratosis
    a. reticuloid
    a. telangiectasis
actinocutitis
actinodermatitis
actinomycosis
adamantinoma
Addison-Gull disease
Addison's
    disease
    keloid
adenocarcinoma
adenoma
    a. sebaceum
adenomatosis
    a. oris
adermia
adermogenesis
adipocyte
adipogenesis
adiponecrosis
adipose
adjuvant
    Freund's a.
    mycobacterial a.
adventitial
    a. dermis
afibrinogenemia
aftha. See *aphtha.*

agammaglobulinemia
agglutination
agglutinin
agglutinogen
agranulocytosis
agria
agrius
AIDS—acquired
   immunodeficiency
   syndrome
ainhum
alastrim
albinism
albinismus
    a. conscriptus
    a. totalis
    a. universalis
albino
Albright's syndrome
alcian blue stain
Alibert-Bazin syndrome
Alibert's
    disease
    mentagra
alkaptonuria
allergen
allergenic
allergic
    a. contact dermatitis
    a. granuloma
    a. purpura
    a. urticaria
allergy
alopecia
    androgenetic a.
    a. areata
    a. capitis totalis
    cicatricial a.
    a. cicatrisata
    a. circumscripta
    congenital a.
    a. congenitalis
    a. disseminata
    drug a.
    female pattern a.
    follicular a.
    a. follicularis

alopecia (continued)
    a. hereditaria
    hereditary a.
    a. liminaris
    male pattern a.
    marginal a.
    a. marginalis
    a. medicamentosa
    a. mucinosa
    a. orbicularis
    a. perinevica
    physiologic a.
    postpartum a.
    a. prematura
    a. presenilis
    pressure a.
    roentgen a.
    a. seborrhoeica
    senile a.
    a. senilis
    symptomatic a.
    a. symptomatica
    syphilitic a.
    a. syphilitica
    a. totalis
    toxic a.
    a. toxica
    traction a.
    traumatic a.
    a. traumatica
    a. triangularis congenitalis
    a. universalis
    x-ray a.
alopecic
alphodermia
alphos
altauna
alymphoplasia
amboceptor
amebiasis
amelanotic
ameloblastoma
Amico's
    drill
    extractor
    nail nipper
    skin lifter

amyloid
amyloidosis
    cutaneous a.
      a. cutis
anaerobic
anagen
anagen to telogen ratio
anaphylactic
anaphylactoid
anaphylaxis
Andrews' disease
androgenetic
anergy
anesthesia. See *General Surgical Terms.*
anetoderma
    Jadassohn-Pellizari a.
    Schweninger-Buzzi a.
angiocavernous
angiodermatitis
angioedema
angioendotheliomatosis
angiofibroma
angioid streaks
angiokeratoma
angioleiomyoma
angiolipoma
angiolupoid
angioma
    cherry a.
    a. pigmentosum
    plexiform a.
    a. serpiginosum
angioneurotic
    a. edema
angiosarcoma
anhidrosis
anogenital
anonychia
anthema
anthracia
anthracoid
anthrax
antibody
    antinuclear a's
antifungal

antifungoid
antigen
antihistamine
antiserum
    Reenstierna a.
antitoxigen
antitoxin
antitoxinogen
aphtha
aphthoid
aphthous
apiotherapy
apisination
aplasia cutis congenita
apocrine
    a. chromhidrosis
    a. cystadenoma
    a. gland(s)
aponeurotic
appendage
areatus
areola
    Chaussier's a.
    vaccinal a.
areolitis
arevareva
argininosuccinicaciduria
argon laser
argyria
ariboflavinosis
Arndt-Gottron disease
arterial spider
Arthus phenomenon
Asboe-Hansen's disease
aspergillosis
asteatosis
    a. cutis
asthma
    Millar's a.
asthmatic
Asturian leprosy
atheroma
    a. cutis
atheromasia
atheromatosis
    a. cutis

atheromatous
athlete's foot
atopen
atopic
atopy
atrichia
atrichosis
atrophic
    a. striae
atrophie
    a. blanche
    a. noire
atrophoderma
    a. vermicularis
atrophodermatosis
atrophy
aurantiasis
aurid
Auspitz's dermatosis
autoantibody
autoantigen
autodermic
autodesensitization
autoeczematization
autoimmunization
autoinoculation
autosensitization
Aveeno bath
avulsion
bacille Calmette-Guérin vaccine
bacillus
    Ducrey's b.
    Hansen's b.
bacterial
bacterid
    pustular b.
Baerensprung's erythrasma
balanitis
    b. xerotica obliterans
bandage. See *General Surgical Terms.*
Barber's dermatosis
Bard-Parker dermatome
Barker Vacu-tome dermatome
bartonellosis
basal layer

bath
    Aveeno b.
Bazex's syndrome
Bazin's disease
BCG – bacille Calmette-Guérin (vaccine)
Beau's lines
Becker's nevus
bejel
Besnier-Boeck disease
Besnier's prurigo
Biett's collar
biopsy
    punch b.
biotripsis
black-dot ringworm
blastomycosis
    cutaneous b.
    systemic b.
bleb
blef-. See words beginning *bleph-.*
blennorrhagia
blennorrhea
blepharitis
blepharochalasis
blister
Bloch's reaction
Bloch-Siemens-Sulzberger syndrome
blotch
    palpebral b.
"blueberry muffin" lesion
Bockhart's impetigo
body
    Leishman-Donovan b's
    Lipschütz's b's
Boeck's
    disease
    itch
    sarcoid
    scabies
boil
boot
    Unna's b.
botryomycosis

Bowen's
    disease
    precancerous dermatosis
Brocq's
    erythrose péribuccale
       pigmentaire
    pseudopelade
bromhidrosis
bromoderma
Brooke's disease
Brown-Brenn stain
Brown's dermatome
brucellosis
Bruck's test
bubo
    Frei's b.
bubon
    b. d'emblée
bubonic plague
Buerger's disease
bulla(e)
bullous
    b. erythema multiforme
    b. impetigo
    b. pemphigoid
Burkitt's lymphoma
Buschke-Ollendorff syndrome
Buschke's scleredema
butterfly rash
cachexia
cactus granuloma
café-au-lait spot
calcification
calcinosis
    c. circumscripta
    c. cutis
calciphylaxis
callosity
callous
callus
calor
    c. mordax
    c. mordicans
calva
calvities
calvitium

Calymmatobacterium
    C. granulomatis
canceroderm
cancroid
cancrum oris
Candida
    C. albicans
candidiasis
canities
canker
Cantlie's foot tetter
capillary
caprolactams
carboxyhemoglobinuria
carbuncle
carbuncular
carbunculosis
carcinelcosis
carcinogenesis
carcinoid
carcinoma
carcinomelcosis
carotenemia
carotenodermia
Carrión's disease
caruncle
caruncula
Casal's necklace
caseation
caseous
    c. necrosis
Castellani's paint
cativi
cat-scratch disease
causalgia
cavernous
    c. hemangioma
    c. lymphangioma
Cazenave's
    disease
    lupus
    vitiligo
cell
    basal c.
    horny c.
    keratinized c.

cell (continued)
    Langhans' c's
    Lipschütz's c.
    malpighian c's
    mast c.
    c.-mediated
        immunity
    Merkel's c's
    Paget's c.
    prickle c.
    Schwann c.
    squamous c.
    Touton giant c's
    Tzank c.
cellulitis
    clostridial c.
    eosinophilic c.
    gangrenous c.
    streptococcus c.
cellulocutaneous
Celsus'
    kerion
    papules
    vitiligo
centrocyte
cervicofacial
cestode
chalazia
chalazion
chancre
    fungating c.
    indurated c.
    Ricord's c.
    Rollet's c.
    sporotrichotic c.
    sulcus c.
chancriform
chancroid
chapped
Chaussier's areola
cheilitis
    actinic c.
    c. actinica
    apostematous c.
    commissural c.
    exfoliativa c.

cheilitis (continued)
    glandularis aposte-
        matosa c.
    c. granulomatosa
    impetiginous c.
    migrating c.
    c. venenata
cheiropompholyx
chemocautery
chemosurgery
chicken pox
chigger
chigoe
chilblain
    necrotized c.
Chlamydia
    C. trachomatis
chloasma
    c. hepaticum
    c. periorale virginium
    c. phthisicorum
    c. traumaticum
chloracne
chloroma
chlorosis
cholesterosis
    c. cutis
chondrodermatitis
    c. nodularis chronica
        helicis
chondrodysplasia
    c. punctata
chondroid
    c. syringoma
chromate
chromatophore
chromatosis
chromhidrosis
chromoblastomycosis
chromomycosis
chromophytosis
chrotoplast
chrysiasis
chrysotherapy
Ciarrocchi's disease

cicatricial
    c. alopecia
cicatrix
cimicosis
circinate
Civatte's poikiloderma
Cladosporium
    C. carrionii
    C. mansonii
    C. werneckii
clavus
    c. syphiliticus
clostridial
clubbing
CMI – cell-mediated immunity
Coccidioides
    C. immitis
coccidioidomycosis
Cole's herpetiform lesion
collagen
collagenosis
collagenous
    c. plaques
collar
    Biett's c.
    c. of pearls
    c. of Venus
collarette
Collins' dynamometer
comedo
comedones
complex
    EAHF (eczema, asthma,
      hay fever) c.
condyloma
    c. acuminatum
    c. latum
    c. subcutaneum
confluent
congelation
congenital
Conidiobolus
    C. coronatus
conjunctivitis
contracture
    Dupuytren's c.
coproporphyria

corium
Corlett's pyosis
corneum
cornification
cornified
cornu
    c. cutaneum
corona
    c. seborrhoeica
    c. veneris
corticosteroids
Corynebacterium
    C. diphtheriae
Coxiella
    C. burnetii
coxsackievirus
cradle cap
craw-craw
croup
crusta
crustosus
cryocautery
cryofibrinogenemia
cryoglobulinemia
cryoslush
cryosurgery
cryotherapy
cryptococcosis
cuniculus
curet
    Fox's c.
    Piffard's c.
    Walsh's c.
curettage
cutaneous
cuticle
cuticularization
cutireaction
cutis
    c. anserina
    c. elastica
    c. hyperelastica
    c. laxa
    c. marmorata
     telangiectatica
     congenita

cutis (continued)
    c. pendula
    c. pensilis
    c. rhomboidalis nuchae
    c. testacea
    c. unctuosa
    c. vera
    c. verticis gyrata
cutisector
cutitis
cutization
cyanosis
cyasma
cylindroma
cyst
    dermoid c.
    epidermal c.
    epithelial c.
    hydatid c.
    mucous c.
    myxoid c.
    pheomycotic c.
    pilonidal c.
    popliteal c.
    sebaceous c.
    thyroglossal c.
    trichilemmal c.
cytolysis
cytomegalovirus
cytophagic
dactylitis
    d. strumosa
    d. syphilitica
    d. tuberculosa
dander
dandruff
Danielssen's disease
Danlos' syndrome
Darier-Roussy sarcoid
Darier's
    disease
    sign
Darier-White disease
dartre
dartrous
deallergization
debride

debridement
    enzymatic d.
    surgical d.
decalvant
decongestant
decongestive
decubital
decubitus
deficiency
    C2 d.
    C4 d.
    C5 d.
    C6 d.
    C7 d.
    C8 d.
    C9 d.
    riboflavin d.
deflorescence
defluxio
    d. capillorum
    d. ciliorum
defurfuration
Degos-Delort-Tricot
    syndrome
Degos' disease
degranulation
"degreaser's flush"
dehydration
demarcation
Demodex
    D. folliculorum
dengue
depigmentation
depilate
depilation
depilatory
derma
dermabrader
    Iverson's d.
    sandpaper d.
dermabrasion
dermad
dermadrome
dermagen
dermal
dermalaxia
dermametropathism

dermamyiasis
    d. linearis migrans
       oestrosa
dermanaplasty
dermapostasis
dermatalgia
dermataneuria
dermatauxe
dermatergosis
dermathemia
dermatic
dermatitides
dermatitis
    actinic d.
    d. aestivalis
    allergic d.
    d. ambustionis
    ancylostome d.
    arsphenamine d.
    d. artefacta
    atopic d.
    d. atrophicans
    avian mite d.
    berlock d.
    berloque d.
    bhiwanol d.
    blastomycetic d.
    brucella d.
    d. bullosa
    d. calorica
    cement d.
    cercarial d.
    chromate d.
    d. combustionis
    d. congelationis
    contact d.
    d. contusiformis
    copra mite d.
    cosmetic d.
    d. cruris pustulosa et
      atrophicans
    dhobie mark d.
    diaper d.
    d. dysmenorrhoeica
    eczematous d.
    d. epidemica
    d. erythematosa

dermatitis (continued)
    d. escharotica
    d. excoriativa infantum
    d. exfoliativa epidemica
    d. exfoliativa infantum
    d. exfoliative
    exudative discoid and
      lichenoid d.
    factitial d.
    d. gangrenosa
    d. gangrenosa infantum
    d. hemostatica
    d. herpetiformis
    d. hiemalis
    d. hypostatica
    d. infectiosa eczematoides
    Jacquet's d.
    Leiner's d.
    livedoid d.
    d. medicamentosa
    d. multiformis
    mycotic d.
    d. nodosa
    d. nodularis necrotica
    nummular d.
    d. papillaris capillitii
    papular d.
    d. pediculoides ventricosus
    periocular d.
    perioral d.
    pigmented purpuric
      lichenoid d.
    poison ivy d.
    poison oak d.
    poison sumac d.
    precancerous d.
    d. psoriasiformis nodularis
    purpuric pigmented
      lichenoid d.
    radiation d.
    d. repens
    rhus d.
    roentgen-ray d.
    schistosome d.
    seborrheic d.
    d. seborrhoeica
    d. simplex

dermatitis (continued)
    d. skiagraphica
    d. solaris
    d. striata pratensis bullosa
    stasis d.
    d. traumatica
    uncinarial d.
    d. vegetans
    d. venenata
    d. verrucosa
    weeping d.
dermatoarthritis
dermatoautoplasty
dermatobiasis
dermatocandidiasis
dermatocele
dermatocellulitis
dermatochalasis
dermatoconiosis
dermatoconjunctivitis
dermatocyst
dermatodysplasia
    d. verruciformis
dermatofibroma
    d. protuberans
dermatofibrosarcoma
    d. protuberans
dermatofibrosis
    d. lenticularis disseminata
dermatogen
dermatogenous
dermatoglyphic
dermatograph
dermatographia
dermatoheteroplasty
dermatoid
dermatokelidosis
dermatologic
dermatologist
dermatology
dermatolysis
    d. palpebrarum
dermatoma
dermatome
    Bard-Parker d.
    Barker Vacu-tome d.
    Brown's d.

dermatome (continued)
    Hall's d.
    Hood's d.
    Meek-Wall d.
    Padgett's d.
    Reese's d.
    Stryker's d.
dermatomegaly
dermatomucosomyositis
dermatomycosis
    blastomycetic d.
    d. furfuracea
    d. microsporina
    d. trichophytina
dermatomyiasis
dermatomyoma
dermatomyositis
dermatoneurology
dermato-ophthalmitis
dermatopathic
dermatopathy
dermatophiliasis
Dermatophilus
    D. penetrans
dermatophylaxis
dermatophyte
dermatophytid
dermatophytosis
    d. furfuracea
dermatoplastic
dermatoplasty
dermatopolyneuritis
dermatorrhagia
dermatorrhea
dermatorrhexis
dermatoscopy
dermatosis
    acarine d.
    angioneurotic d.
    ashy d.
    Auspitz's d.
    Barber's d.
    Bowen's precancerous d.
    d. cinecienta
    lichenoid d.
    meadow grass d.
    neutrophilic d.

dermatosis (continued)
    palmoplantar d.
    d. papulosa nigra
    precancerous d.
    progressive pigmentary d.
    purpuric d.
    "rhythmical" d.
    Schamberg's d.
    stasis d.
    subcorneal pustular d.
    Unna's d.
dermatostomatitis
dermatotherapy
dermatotome
dermatotropic
dermatozoonosus
dermis
dermitis
dermoanergy
dermoblast
dermoepidermal junction
dermograph
dermographia
dermographism
dermohemia
dermoid
dermoidectomy
dermolipoma
dermolysis
dermomycosis
dermopathy
dermophlebitis
dermostenosis
dermostosis
dermosynovitis
dermosyphilography
dermosyphilopathy
dermotactile
dermotropic
dermovaccine
dermovascular
desensitization
desensitize
desiccation
    electric d.
desmoid

desmoplastic
    d. trichoepithelioma
desmosome
desquamation
    furfuraceous d.
    membranous d.
    siliquose d.
desquamative
Devergie's disease
DGI – disseminated gonococcal
    infection
dialysis
diamonds
diaphoresis
diascope
diascopy
diathermy
Dick test
digital
    d. fibromatosis
digitate
    d. warts
dinitrochlorobenzene
discoid
    d. lupus erythematosus
disease
    Addison-Gull d.
    Addison's d.
    Alibert's d.
    Andrews' d.
    Arndt-Gottron d.
    Asboe-Hansen's d.
    Bazin's d.
    Besnier-Boeck d.
    Boeck's d.
    Bowen's d.
    Brooke's d.
    Buerger's d.
    Carrión's d.
    Cazenave's d.
    Ciarrocchi's d.
    Danielssen's d.
    Darier's d.
    Darier-White d.
    Degos' d.
    Devergie's d.
    Duhring's d.

disease (continued)
> Fordyce's d.
> Fox-Fordyce d.
> Frei's d.
> Gaucher's d.
> Gibert's d.
> Gilchrist's d.
> Hailey and Hailey d.
> Hallopeau's d.
> Hand-Schüller-Christian d.
> Hansen's d.
> Hartnup's d.
> Hebra's d.
> Hodgkin's d.
> Hutchinson's d.
> Hyde's d.
> Jadassohn's d.
> Kaposi's d.
> Kawasaki d.
> Köbner's d.
> Landouzy's d.
> Leiner's d.
> Leloir's d.
> Letterer-Siwe d.
> Lipschütz's d.
> Lortat-Jacobs d.
> Lutz-Miescher d.
> Majocchi's d.
> Mibelli's d.
> Mucha-Habermann d.
> Neumann's d.
> Nicolas-Favre d.
> Niemann-Pick d.
> Osler's d.
> Osler-Vaquez d.
> Pollitzer's d.
> Puente's d.
> Quincke's d.
> Quinquaud's d.
> Rayer's d.
> Raynaud's d.
> Recklinghausen's d.
> Reiter's d.
> Robinson's d.
> Schamberg's d.
> Senear-Usher d.

disease (continued)
> Sticker's d.
> Sutton's d.
> Taenzer's d.
> Urbach-Oppenheim d.
> vagabonds' d.
> Weber-Christian d.
> Weber's d.
> White's d.
> Woringer-Kolopp d.

dissecting
> d. cellulitis

disseminated
> d. lupus erythematosus
> d. granuloma annulare
> d. rosacea
> d. porokeratosis
> d. xanthoma

distichia

DLE – discoid lupus erythematosus

donovaniasis

dopaoxidase

dracunculiasis

Draize's test

dressing. See *General Surgical Terms.*

drill
> Amico's d.
> Ralks' d.

drugs. See *Drugs and Chemistry* section.

D & S – dermatology and syphilology

Ducrey's bacillus

Duhring's
> disease
> pruritus

Dupuytren's contracture

dynamometer
> Collins' d.

dysautonomia

dyschromia

dyshidrosis
> trichophytic d.

dyskeratoma

dyskeratosis
    d. congenita
    d. follicularis
dyspigmentation
dysplasia
dysplastic
dyssebacia
dystrophic
    d. epidermolysis bullosa
    d. palmoplantar
        hyperkeratosis
dystrophy
        median canaliform d. of
            the nail
EAHF–eczema, asthma, hay
    fever
ecchymosis
eccrine
echinococcosis
Echinodermata
ECHO (enteric cytopathogenic
    human orphan) virus
ecthyma
    e. contagiosum
    e. gangrenosum
    e. syphiliticum
ectoderm
ectodermal
    e. dysplasia
ectodermosis
    e. erosiva pluriorificialis
ectopic
ectothrix
Ectotrichophyton
ectropion
ectylotic
eczema
    allergic e.
    e. articulorum
    atopic e.
    e. barbae
    e. capitis
    e. craquelé
    e. crustosum
    e. diabeticorum
    dyshidrotic e.
    e. epilans

eczema (continued)
    e. epizootica
    e. erythematosum
    flexural e.
    follicular e.
    e. herpeticum
    e. hypertrophicum
    infantile e.
    e. intertrigo
    lichenoid e.
    linear e.
    e. madidans
    e. marginatum
    e. neuriticum
    e. nummulare
    e. papulosum
    e. parasiticum
    e. pustulosum
    e. rubrum
    e. scrofuloderma
    e. seborrhoeicum
    e. siccum
    solar e.
    e. solare
    e. squamosum
    stasis e.
    e. tyloticum
    e. vaccinatum
    e. verrucosum
    e. vesiculosum
    weeping e.
eczematid
eczematization
eczematoid
eczematosis
eczematous
edema
        angioneurotic e.
        cyclic e.
        epidermal e.
        periorbital e.
efelis. See *ephelis.*
effluvium
        anagen e.
        telogen e.
efidrosis. See *ephidrosis.*
Ehlers-Danlos syndrome

eksan-. See words beginning
   exan-.
ekzema. See *eczema*.
elastin
elastocytic
elastolysis
elastosis
      actinic e.
      e. senilis
electrocautery
electrocoagulation
electrode
electrodermogram
electrodermography
electrodesiccation
electrofulguration
electrolysis
electromagnetic
      e. radiation
electron
      e. beam therapy
      e. microscopy
electrosection
electrosurgery
elephantiasis
      e. arabicum
      e. asturiensis
      e. filariensis
      e. graecorum
      e. leishmaniana
      lymphangiectatic e.
      e. neuromatosa
      e. nostras
      e. telangiectodes
elevator
      Ralks' e.
emaculation
emollient
emphlysis
emphractic
emulsion
      Pusey's e.
enanthema
encrusted
endothelioma
      e. capitis
      e. cutis

endothelium
endothrix
endotoxin
Entamoeba
      E. histolytica
enterobiasis
enteropathy
entomophthoromycosis
enzymatic
enzyme
eosinophilia
eosinophilic
      e. cellulitis
      e. fasciitis
      e. granuloma
      e. spongiosis
ephelis
ephidrosis
      e. cruenta
epidermal
epidermatitis
epidermatoplasty
epidermicula
epidermidosis
epidermis
epidermitis
epidermization
epidermodysplasia
      e. verruciformis
epidermoid
epidermolysis
      e. acquisita
      e. bullosa
      e. bullosa dystrophica,
         polydysplastic
      e. bullosa, junctional
      e. bullosa simplex
      toxic bullous e.
epidermolytic
      e. hyperkeratosis
epidermoma
epidermomycosis
epidermophytid
Epidermophyton
      E. floccosum
epidermophytosis
      e. cruris

epidermophytosis (continued)
    e. interdigitale
epidermosis
epidermotropic
    e. reticulosis
epidermotropism
epilation
epilatory
epiparonychia
epithelial
epithelialization
epithelioid
epithelioma
    e. adenoides cysticum
    e. capitis
    Malherbe's calcifying e.
    e. molluscum
epitheliomatosis
epitheliomatous
epithelium
epithelization
eponychia
eponychium
epulis
ergodermatosis
erisipelas. See *erysipelas.*
erosio
    e. interdigitalis
        blastomycetica
erosion
erubescence
eruption
    bullous e.
    creeping e.
    crustaceous e.
    erythematous e.
    Kaposi's varicelliform e.
    maculopapular e.
    papulosquamous e.
    petechial e.
    pustular e.
    serum e.
    squamous e.
    tubercular e.
    vesicular e.
    vesiculopustular e.
eruptive

erysipelas
    ambulant e.
    coast e.
    gangrenous e.
    e. grave internum
    idiopathic e.
    migrant e.
    e. perstans
    phlegmonous e.
    e. pustulosum
    e. verrucosum
    e. vesiculosum
    zoonotic e.
erysipelatous
erysipeloid
erythema
    e. ab igne
    acrodynic e.
    e. annulare
    e. annulare centrifugum
    e. annulare rheumaticum
    e. arthriticum
    e. bullosum
    e. caloricum
    e. circinatum
    e. chromicum figuratum
        melanodermicum
    e. chronicum migrans
    e. contusiformis
    e. dyschromicum perstans
    e. elevatum diutinum
    e. exudativum
    e. figuratum
    e. fugax
    e. gyratum repens
    e. induratum
    e. infectiosum
    e. intertrigo
    e. iris
    Jacquet's e.
    e. marginatum
        rheumaticum
    migratory e.
    Milian's e.
    e. multiforme
    e. neonatorum
    e. neonatorum toxicum

erythema (continued)
   e. nodosum
   e. nodosum leprosum
   e. nodosum migrans
   e. nodosum syphiliticum
   palmar e.
   e. paratrimma
   e. pernio
   e. perstans
   e. pudicitiae
   e. punctatum
   e. scarlatiniforme
   e. simplex
   e. solare
   e. streptogenes
   e. toxicum neonatorum
   e. traumaticum
   e. venenatum
erythematosus
   discoid lupus e.
   systemic lupus e.
erythematous
erythermalgia
erythra
erythralgia
erythrasma
   Baerensprung's e.
erythredema polyneuropathy
erythrocyanosis
   e. crurum puellaris
   e. frigida crurum
      puellarum
   e. supramalleolaris
erythroderma
   atopic e.
   congenital ichthyosiform
      e.
   e. desquamativum
   exfoliative e.
   e. ichthyosiforme
      congenitum
   lymphomatous e.
   e. psoriaticum
   Sézary e.
   e. squamosum
erythrodermatitis

erythrokeratodermia
   e. variabilis
erythromelia
erythroplasia
   e. of Queyrat
erythropoiesis
erythrose
   e. péribuccale pigmentaire
      of Brocq
eschar
escharotics
eskar. See *eschar.*
esthiomene
evanescent
exanthem
   vesicular e.
exanthema
   e. subitum
exanthematous
excoriation
   necrotic e.
excrescence
excrescent
exfoliation
exfoliative
exocrine
exocytosis
Exophiala
   E. jeanselmi
extractor
   Amico's e.
   comedo e.
   Saalfield's e.
   Schamberg's e.
   Unna's e.
   Walton's e.
exudate
exudation
exulceratio
   e. simplex
exuviae
fajedenah. See *phagedena.*
FANA – fluorescent antinuclear
   antibody
fasciitis
   exudative f.
   necrotizing f.

fasciitis (continued)
    nodular f.
    proliferative f.
    pseudosarcomatous f.
favid
favus
    f. circinatus
    f. herpeticus
    f. herpetiformis
    f. pilaris
felon
Felty's syndrome
fester
fever
    Mediterranean f.
    Q f.
    Rocky Mountain
        spotted f.
    scarlet f.
fiber
    A-alpha nerve f's
    Herxheimer's f's
fibroblast
fibroepithelial
fibrokeratoma
fibroma
    f. cutis
    f. lipomatodes
    f. pendulum
    perifollicular f.
    telangiectatic f.
    f. xanthoma
fibromatosis
    f. colli
fibronoid
    f. necrosis
fibrosclerosis
fibrosis
fibrous
    f. histiocytoma
    f. papule
fibroxanthoma
filariasis
filiform
    f. tumor
    f. wart
filtration

fissure
fistula
fitofotodermatitis. See
    phytophotodermatitis.
flare
flexural
flexure
flumen
flumina pilorum
fluorescence
fogo selvagem
follicle
    sebaceous f.
follicular
    f. eczema
    f. lichen planus
    f. mucinosis
    f. psoriasis
folliculitis
    f. abscedens et suffodiens
    agminate f.
    f. barbae
    f. cheloidalis
    f. decalvans
    f. decalvans et lichen
        spinulosus
    f. gonorrhoeica
    f. keloidalis
    f. nares perforans
    f. ulerythematosa
        reticulata
    f. varioliformis
Fonsecaea
    F. compacta
    F. pedrosoi
foot tetter
    Cantlie's f.t.
Fordyce's
    disease
    spots
formication
formiciasis
Forschheimer's spots
Foshay's test
Fournier's gangrene
Fox-Fordyce disease
Fox's
    curet

Fox's (continued)
    impetigo
fragilitas
    f. crinium
    f. unguium
frambesia
frambesioma
freckle
    melanotic f. of Hutchison
Frei's
    bubo
    disease
    test
frenulum
frenum
Freund's adjuvant
frostbite
FTA-ABS test – fluorescent
    treponemal antibody
    absorption test
fucosidosis
fulguration
fulgurize
fungal
fungate
fungous
fungus
furfur
furfuraceous
furuncle
furuncular
furunculoid
furunculosis
furunculus
    f. vulgaris
fusospirochetal
Futcher's lines
galvanic
    g. epilator
galvanism
ganglion
gangosa
gangrene
    cutaneous g.
    disseminated cutaneous g.
    Fournier's g.
    gaseous g.

gangrene (continued)
    Raynaud's g.
gangrenous
Gaucher's disease
geniculate
Gennerich's treatment
genodermatology
genodermatosis
German measles
Gianotti-Crosti syndrome
giant cell
    g.c. arteritis
    g.c. epulis
    g.c. granuloma
Gibert's
    disease
    pityriasis
Giemsa stain
Gilchrist's disease
gingivitis
gingivoglossitis
gingivosis
gingivostomatitis
glabrous
gland
    apocrine g.
    sebaceous g.
    sweat g.
glioma
globulin
    antidiphtheritic g.
    antitoxic g.
    gamma g's
    immune serum g.
glomus
    g. body
    g. cell
    cutaneous g.
    digital g.
    neuromyoarterial g.
    g. tumor
glossitis
    g. areata exfoliativa
    g. dissecans
    Hunter's g.
    g. migrans
    Moeller's g.

glossitis (continued)
    g. parasitica
    parenchymatous g.
    rhomboid g.
    g. rhomboidea mediana
glossodynia
glossopyrosis
glucagonoma
glycoprotein
glycosaminoglycans
gnathostomiasis
goatpox
Goeckerman treatment
gonitis
    fungous g.
gonococcal
gonococcemia
gonococcus
gonorrhea
gonorrheal
Gottron's papule(s)
Gougerot's syndrome
Gowers' panatrophy
granular
granulation
granuloma
    g. annulare
    g. endemicum
    eosinophilic g.
    g. fissuratum
    g. fungoides
    g. gangraenescens
    Hodgkin's g.
    g. inguinale
    lipoid g.
    lycopodium g.
    Majocchi's g.
    g. malignum
    g. multiforme
    g. pyogenicum
    g. sarcomatodes
    g. telangiectaticum
    g. trichophyticum
    g. venereum
granulomatosis
    Miescher-Leder g.
    Wegener's g.

granulomatous
    g. reaction
    g. rosacea
    g. vasculitis
granulosis rubra nasi
grenz ray therapy
gumma
gummatous
gustatory
gutta
    g. rosacea
guttate
gyrate
Haemophilus
    H. ducreyi
    H. influenzae
Hailey and Hailey disease
hairy
    h. nevus
    h. tongue
Hallopeau's
    acrodermatitis
    disease
Hall's dermatome
hamartoma
hamartomatosis
hamartomatous
Hand-Schüller-Christian disease
"hanging groin"
Hansen's
    bacillus
    disease
haplodermatitis
Hartnup's disease
Hebra's
    disease
    ointment
    pityriasis
helix
helminthiasis
    h. elastica
helminthic
hemangioendothelioma
hemangioma
    capillary h.
    cavernous h.
    h. congenitale

hemangioma (continued)
   h. hypertrophicum cutis
   sclerosing h.
   h. simplex
   strawberry h.
   h.-thrombocytopenia
      syndrome
   verrucous h.
hemangiomatosis
hemangiopericytoma
hemangiosarcoma
hematid
hematidrosis
hemochromatosis
hemorrhage
hemorrhagic
heparin
"herald plaque"
heredodegenerative
herpangina
herpes
   h. catarrhalis
   h. digitalis
   h. facialis
   h. farinosus
   h. febrilis
   h. generalisatus
   h. genitalis
   h. gestationis
   h. gladiatorum
   h. iris
   h. labialis
   h. menstrualis
   h. mentalis
   nasal h.
   h. oticus
   h. phlyctaenodes
   h. praeputialis
   h. progenitalis
   h. recurrens
   h. simplex
   h. simplex recurrens
   h. tonsurans
   h. tonsurans maculosus
   h. vegetans
   wrestler's h.
   h. zoster

herpes (continued)
   h. zoster ophthalmicus
   h. zoster oticus
   h. zoster varicellosus
herpesvirus
herpetic
herpetiform
Herxheimer's
   fibers
   reaction
   spirals
heterochromia
heterodermic
heterophil
heterophilic
heterotrichosis
   h. superciliorum
hidradenitis
   h. suppurativa
hidradenoma
   h. papilliferum
hidrocystoma
hidromeiosis
hidrorrhea
hidrosadenitis
   h. axillaris
   h. destruens suppurativa
hidroschesis
hidrosis
hidrotic
hirsuties
hirsutism
histaminase
histamine
histaminia
histiocyte
histiocytic
   h. lymphoma
   h. panniculitis
   h. reticulosis
histiocytoma
   h. cutis
   eruptive h.
   fibrous h.
   lipoid h.
histiocytomatosis

histiocytosis
    atypical h.
    cephalic h.
    h. X
histoplasmosis
Hodgkin's
    disease
    granuloma
hodi-potsy
holocrine
homme
    h. rouge
homograft
homologous
Hood's dermatome
hookworm infection
hordeolum
hornification
horny
horripilation
Hotchkiss-McManus stain
hot quartz lamp
Hunter's glossitis
Hutchinson's
    disease
    freckle
    mask
    triad
hyalin
hyaline
hyalinization
hyalinosis cutis et mucosae
hydatid
Hyde's disease
hydration
hydroa
    h. aestivale
    h. febrile
    h. gestationis
    h. gravidarum
    h. puerorum
    h. vacciniforme
    h. vesiculosum
hydrocystoma
hydrotherapy
hygroma
    h. colli

hygroma (continued)
    cystic h.
    h. cysticum
hyperbaric oxygen therapy
hyperergia
hyperergy
hypergammaglobulinemia
hyperhidrosis
hyperimmunoglobulin
hyperirritability
hyperkeratosis
    h. congenitalis palmaris et
        plantaris
    epidermolytic h.
    h. excentrica
    h. figurata centrifuga
        atrophica
    h. follicularis in cutem
        penetrans
    h. follicularis vegetans
    h. linguae
    palmoplantar h.
    h. penetrans
    h. subungualis
    h. universalis congenita
hyperkeratotic
hypermelanosis
hyperpigmentation
hyperpituitarism
hyperplasia
hypersarcosis
hypersecretion
hypersensibility
hypersensitiveness
hypersensitivity
hypersensitization
hypertrichiasis
hypertrichophrydia
hypertrichosis
    h. lanuginosa
    h. universalis
hypertrophic
hypertrophy
hypha
hyphomycetic
hyphomycosis
hypochromotrichia

hypodermis
hypodermolithiasis
hypoergia
hypogammaglobulin
hypogammaglobulinemia
hypohidrosis
hypohidrotic
hypomelanosis
hyponychium
hyponychon
hypopigmentation
hyposensitive
hyposensitization
hypothermia
Ia antigen
ichthyismus
 i. exanthematicus
ichthyosiform
 i. erythroderma
ichthyosis
 i. congenita
 i. cornea
 follicular i.
 i. follicularis
 i. hystrix
 i. intrauterina
 lamellar i.
 linear i.
 i. linguae
 nacreous i.
 i. palmaris
 i. palmaris et plantaris
 i. plantaris
 i. sauroderma
 i. scutulata
 i. sebacea cornea
 i. serpentina
 i. simplex
 i. spinosa
 i. thysanotrichica
 i. uteri
 i. vulgaris
icterus
I & D—incision and drainage
"id"
 erysipelas-like i's
 papular i's

"id" (continued)
 vesicular i's
idiopathic
 i. thrombocytopenic
  purpura
idiosyncrasy
iksodiahsis. See *ixodiasis.*
ikthe-. See words beginning
 ichthy-.
immune
immunity
immunization
immunochemical
immunodeficiency
immunodiagnosis
immunoelectrophoresis
immunofluorescence
immunofluorescent
immunoglobulin
immunohistochemical
immunology
immunomodulatory
immunoperoxidase staining
immunoreaction
immunosuppression
immunotherapy
impetiginization
impetiginous
impetigo
 Bockhart's i.
 i. bullosa
 bullous i.
 i. contagiosa
 i. eczematodes
 follicular i.
 Fox's i.
 furfuraceous i.
 i. herpetiformis
 i. neonatorum
 i. simplex
 i. staphylogenes
 i. syphilitica
 i. variolosa
incontinentia
 i. pigmenti
 i. pigmenti achromians

indurated
>i. cellulitis
>i. lymphangitis

induration
infectious
infestation
infiltrate
infiltration
>adipose i.
>cellular i.
>inflammatory i.
>lymphocytic i.

inflammation
inflammatory tinea barbae
infrared radiation
infundibulo-folliculitis
infundibulum
inoculation
integument
integumentary
integumentum
>i. commune

interstitial
intertriginous
intertrigo
>i. labialis
>i. saccharomycetica

intimitis
>proliferative i.

intracutaneous
intradermal
intradermoreaction
intraepidermal
intraepithelial
intralesional
ionizing radiation
isomorphic
isthmus
itch
>Boeck's i.
>dhobie i.
>grain i.
>Moeller's i.
>seven-year i.
>swimmers' i.

itching
Ito's nevus

Ito-Reenstierna test
Iverson's dermabrader
ixodiasis
Jacquet's
>dermatitis
>erythema

Jadassohn-Bloch test
Jadassohn-Lewandosky law
Jadassohn-Pellizari anetoderma
Jadassohn's
>disease
>nevus

Janeway's lesion
Jarisch-Herxheimer reaction
Jarisch's ointment
jaundice
jigger
Jones-Mote reaction
junctional
>j. epidermolysis bullosa
>j. nevus

juvenile
>j. hyaline fibromatosis
>j. lentigo
>j. melanoma
>j. rheumatoid arthritis
>j. xanthogranuloma

kala-azar
kalazea. See *chalazia.*
kalazeon. See *chalazion.*
Kaposi's
>disease
>sarcoma
>varicelliform eruption
>xeroderma

Kasabach-Merritt syndrome
Kawasaki disease
Keller's ultraviolet test
keloid
>Addison's k.

keloidal blastomycosis
keloidosis
keratiasis
keratin
keratinization
keratinocyte
keratinous

keratitis
  amebic k.
  interstitial k.
keratoacanthoma
keratoderma
  k. blennorrhagica
  k. palmaris et plantaris
keratodermatitis
keratohyalin
keratohyaline
keratolysis
  k. exfoliativa
  k. neonatorum
keratoma
  k. diffusum
  k. hereditaria mutilans
  k. malignum congenitale
  k. palmare et plantare
  k. plantare sulcatum
  k. senile
keratomycosis
  k. linguae
keratonosis
keratoprotein
keratosis(es)
  actinic k.
  arsenical k.
  k. blennorrhagica
  k. diffusa fetalis
  k. follicularis
  k. follicularis contagiosa
  gonorrheal k.
  k. labialis
  k. linguae
  nevoid k.
  k. nigricans
  k. obturans
  k. palmaris et plantaris
  k. pilaris
  k. punctata
  seborrheic k.
  k. seborrhoeica
  senile k.
  k. senilis
  "stucco" k.
  k. suprafollicularis
  k. vegetans

keratotic
kerion
  k. celsi
  Celsus' k.
Keyes' dermal punch
kilitis. See *cheilitis.*
kiropomfoliks. See
  cheiropompholyx.
kloazma. See *chloasma.*
klor-. See words beginning *chlor-.*
Köbner's disease
Koebner's phenomenon
KOH – potassium hydroxide
koilonychia
Kolmer's test
kondro-. See words beginning
  chondro-.
Koplik's spots
kraurosis
  k. penis
  k. vulvae
Kveim test
lacuna
lamellar
  l. exfoliation
  l. granules
  l. ichthyosis
lamp
  black light fluorescent l.
  black ray l.
  carbon arc l.
  cold quartz l.
  fluorescent sun l.
  hot quartz l.
  quartz-iodine l.
  xenon arc l.
Landouzy's
  disease
  purpura
Langhans'
  cells
  layer
lanugo
larva
  l. migrans
laser
  argon l.

Lassar's paste
law
    Jadassohn-Lewandosky l.
layer
    Langhans' l.
    malpighian l.
LE – lupus erythematosus
Leiner's
    dermatitis
    disease
leiodermia
leiomyoma
    l. cutis
leiomyosarcoma
Leishman-Donovan bodies
leishmaniasis
    l. recidivans
Leloir's disease
lenticula
lentigines
lentigo
    l. maligna
lentigomelanosis
Lepidoptera
lepidosis
lepothrix
lepra
    l. alba
    l. alphoides
    l. alphos
    l. anaesthetica
    l. arabum
    l. conjunctivae
    l. graecorum
    l. maculosa
    l. mutilans
    l. nervorum
    l. nervosa
    l. tuberculoides
    Willan's l.
leprid
leproma
lepromatous
leprosy
    Asturian l.
    borderline l.
    cutaneous l.

leprosy (continued)
    dimorphous l.
    lazarine l.
    lepromatous l.
    Lombardy l.
    macular l.
    maculoanesthetic l.
    neural l.
    nodular l.
    trophoneurotic l.
    tuberculoid l.
leprotic
leprous
leptochroa
Leser-Trélat sign
lesion
    "blueberry muffin" l.
    Cole's herpetiform l.
    disseminated l.
    initial syphilitic l.
    Janeway's l.
Letterer-Siwe disease
leukemia
    l. cutis
leukocytosis
leukoderma
    l. acquisitum centrifugum
    l. colli
leukodermatous
leukonychia
leukopenia
leukoplakia
Lewandowsky's nevus elasticus
Libman-Sacks syndrome
lichen
    l. albus
    l. amyloidosus
    l. annularis
    l. aureus
    l. chronicus simplex
    l. corneus hypertrophicus
    l. fibromucinoidosus
    l. frambesianus
    l. leprosus
    l. myxedematosus
    l. nitidus
    l. obtusus corneus

lichen (continued)
    l. pilaris
    l. planopilaris
    l. planus
    l. planus, acute bullous
    l. planus et acuminatus
        atrophicans
    l. planus, hypertrophic
    l. planus hypertrophicus
    l. ruber acuminatus
    l. ruber moniliformis
    l. ruber planus
    l. sclerosus et atrophicus
    l. scrofulosorum
    l. simplex chronicus
    l. spinulosus
    l. striatus
    l. urticatus
licheniasis
lichenificatio
    l. gigantea
lichenification
lichenization
lichenoid
    l. amyloidosis
    l. dermatosis
    l. phase
light
    Wood's l.
line
    Beau's l's
    Futcher's l's
    Voigt's l's
lingua
    l. fissurata
    l. nigra
lipedema
lipoatrophy
lipoblast
lipocyte
lipogranulomatosis
lipoidosis
lipoidproteinosis
lipoma
lipomatosis
liposarcoma

Lipschütz's
    bodies
    cell
    disease
    ulcer
lipsotrichia
livedo
    l. annularis
    l. racemosa
    l. reticularis
    l. reticularis idiopathica
    l. reticularis symptomatica
    l. telangiectatica
livedoid
livid
lobomycosis
Lombardy leprosy
Lortat-Jacob's disease
louse
lues
    l. nervosa
    l. tarda
    l. venerea
lunula
    l. of nail
    l. unguis
lupoid
lupus
    Cazenave's l.
    l. erythematodes
    l. erythematosus
    l. erythematosus discoides
    l. erythematosus
        disseminatus
    l. livido
    l. miliaris disseminatus
        faciei
    l. pernio
    l. profundus
    l. tuberculosus
    l. tumidus
    l. verrucosus
    l. vorax
    l. vulgaris
Lutz-Miescher disease
Lutz-Splendore-de Almeida
    syndrome

Lyell's syndrome
lymphadenitis
lymphadenopathy
lymphangioma
    l. cavernosum
    l. circumscriptum
    l. cysticum
    l. tuberosum multiplex
    l. xanthelasmoideum
lymphangiosarcoma
lymphangitic
    l. sporotrichosis
lymphangitis
    l. carcinomatosa
lymphedema
    l. praecox
    l. tarda
lymphocutaneous
lymphocytoma
    l. cutis
lymphocytosis
lymphodermia
lymphogranuloma
    l. benignum
    l. inguinale
    l. venereum
lymphogranulomatosis
    l. cutis
    l. inguinalis
    l. maligna
lymphoid
lymphokine
lymphoma
    Burkitt's l.
    l. cutis
lymphomatoid
    l. granulomatosis
    l. papulosis
    l. vasculitis
lymphoreticular
lymphosarcoma
lymphosarcomatosis
maceration
macroglobulinemia
macula
    m. solaris

maculae
    m. atrophicae
    m. caeruleae
macular
maculate
maculation
macule
maculopapular
maculopapule
maduromycosis
Majocchi's
    disease
    granuloma
    purpura
mal de Meleda
Malherbe's calcifying epithelioma
mal morado
Malpighi rete
malpighian
    m. cells
    m. layer
mange
    demodectic m.
    follicular m.
Mantoux test
mask
    Hutchinson's m.
Masson trichrome stain
mastocytoma
mastocytosis
    diffuse cutaneous m.
matrix
    nail m.
    m. unguis
matrixitis
Mauriac's syndrome
measles
medications. See *Drugs and Chemistry* section.
Mediterranean fever
Meek-Wall dermatome
melanin
melanism
melanization
melanocyte
melanocytic

melanoderma
    m. cachecticorum
    senile m.
melanodermatitis
melanoleukoderma
    m. colli
melanoma
    acral lentiginous m.
    malignant m.
    nodular m.
    subungual m.
melanomatosis
melanomatous
melanonychia
melanopathy
melanosis
    addisonian m.
    m. cachecticorum
    m. circumscripta
      precancerosa
    m. lenticularis progressiva
    periorbital m.
    pustular m.
    Riehl's m.
melanotic
melanotrichia
melasma
    m. universale
melioidosis
Melkersson-Rosenthal syndrome
membrane
    basement m.
meningococcemia
mentagra
    Alibert's m.
Merkel's cell
Mibelli's disease
microabscess
microsporosis
    m. capitis
Microsporum
    M. audouini
    M. canis
    M. ferrugineum
    M. furfur
    M. gypseum

Microsporum (continued)
    M. lanosum
Miescher-Leder granulomatosis
milia
Milian's
    erythema
    sign
    syndrome
miliaria
    m. crystallina
    m. profunda
    m. pustulosa
    m. rubra
miliary
milium
    colloid m.
Millar's asthma
Milton's urticaria
Mitsuda test
Moeller's
    glossitis
    itch
Mohs' procedure
mole
molluscoid
molluscum
    cholesterinic m.
    m. contagiosum
    m. epitheliale
    m. fibrosum
    m. lipomatodes
    m. pendulum
    m. sebaceum
    m. simplex
    m. varioliformis
    m. verrucosum
monilethrix
Monilia
moniliasis
Monro's abscess
morbilliform
morphea
    acroteric m.
    m. alba
    m. atrophica
    m. flammea

morphea (continued)
    m. guttata
    herpetiform m.
    m. linearis
    m. nigra
M-plasty
Mucha-Habermann
    disease
mucinosis
    follicular m.
    papular m.
mucocele
mucocutaneous
mucodermal
mucopolysaccharidosis
mucormycosis
mucosa
mucous
mycetoma
    actinomycotic m.
    eumycotic m.
mycid
Mycobacterium
    M. avium
    M. balnei
    M. bovis
    M. chelonei
    M. fortuitum
    M. kansasii
    M. leprae
    M. marinum
    M. scrofulaceum
    M. simiae
    M. szulgai
    M. tuberculosis
    M. ulcerans
    M. xenopi
mycoderma
mycodermatitis
mycology
mycosis
    cutaneous m.
    m. cutis chronica
    m. favosa
    m. framboesioides
    m. fungoides
    m. interdigitalis

mycotic
myeloma
myiasis
myoblastoma
myoepithelium
myositis
myringodermatitis
myxedema
myxodermia
myxoid
myxoma
nail
    double-edge n's
    eggshell n.
    hang n.
    ingrown n.
    parrot beak n.
    reedy n.
    spoon n.
    turtle-back n.
nail nipper
    Amico's n.n.
necklace
    Casal's n.
necrobiosis
    n. lipoidica diabeticorum
necrobiotic
    n. xanthogranuloma
necrolysis
necrosis
    caseous n.
    coagulative n.
    cold-induced n.
    enzymatic n.
    fibrinoid n.
    gangrenous n.
    gummatous n.
    liquefactive n.
necrotic
necrotizing
    n. fasciitis
    n. gingivitis
    n. sialometaplasia
    n. vasculitis
Neisseria
    N. gonorrhoeae
    N. meningitidis

neoplasm
Neumann's disease
neurilemoma
neurodermatitis
    n. disseminata
neurodermatosis
neurodermite
neurofibroma
neurofibromatosis
neurofibrosarcoma
neurogenic
neuroma
nevi
    epithelial n.
nevocarcinoma
nevoid
    n. lentigo
    n. telangiectasia
nevose
nevoxanthoendothelioma
nevus
    amelanotic n.
    n. anemicus
    n. angiectodes
    n. angiomatodes
    n. arachnoideus
    n. araneosus
    n. araneus
    n. avasculosus
    bathing trunk n.
    Becker's n.
    blue n.
    n. cavernosus
    cellular blue n.
    n. cerebelliformis
    n. comedonicus
    compound n.
    connective-tissue n.
    n. depigmentosus
    dermoepidermal n.
    n. elasticus of
      Lewandowsky
    epidermal n.
    epithelial n.
    n. fibrosus
    n. flammeus
    n. follicularis

nevus (continued)
    n. fuscoceruleus
      acromiodeltoideus
    n. fuscoceruleus
      ophthalmomaxillaris
    giant pigmented n.
    hairy n.
    halo n.
    Ito's n.
    Jadassohn's n.
    junctional n.
    linear n.
    n. lipomatosus
    n. lymphaticus
    n. maternus
    melanocytic n.
    n. mollusciformis
    n. morus
    multiplex n.
    n. nervosus
    nevocytic n.
    nonpigmented n.
    Ota's n.
    n. papillaris
    n. papillomatosus
    n. pigmentosus
    n. pilosus
    polyploid n.
    n. sanguineus
    sebaceous n. of Jadassohn
    n. spilus
    n. spilus tardus
    spindle cell n.
    Spitz' n.
    n. spongiosus albus
      mucosae
    strawberry n.
    n. syringocystadenosus
      papilliferus
    n. unius lateralis
    Unna's n.
    n. vasculosus
    n. venosus
    n. verrucosus
    n. vinosus
Nicolas-Favre disease
Niemann-Pick disease

Nikolsky's sign
nitric acid
Nocardia
 N. madurae
nocardiosis
nodose
nodosity
nodular
nodule
nodulus
noli-me-tangere
noma
nonallergic
Norwegian scabies
nummular
oasthouse urine disease
ochronosis
 exogenous o.
 ocular o.
oidiomycosis
ointment
 Hebra's o.
 Jarisch's o.
 Whitfield's o.
onchocerciasis
onchocercoma
onikalja. See *onychalgia.*
onikatrofea. See *onychatrophia.*
onikawksis. See *onychauxis*
onikea. See *onychia.*
onikeksalaksis. See
 onychexallaxis.
onikektome. See *onychectomy.*
onikitis. See *onychitis.*
oniko-. See words beginning
 onycho-.
onychalgia
onychatrophia
onychauxis
onychectomy
onychexallaxis
onychia
 o. lateralis
 o. maligna
 o. parasitica
 o. periungualis
 o. sicca

onychitis
onychoclasis
onychocryptosis
onychodynia
onychodystrophy
onychogenic
onychograph
onychogryphosis
onychogryposis
onychohelcosis
onycholysis
onychoma
onychomadesis
onychomalacia
onychomycosis
onychonosus
onychopathic
onychopathology
onychopathy
onychophagia
onychophagist
onychophyma
onychophysis
onychoptosis
onychorrhexis
onychoschizia
onychosis
onychotillomania
onychotomy
ophryitis
orf
Osler's disease
Osler-Vaquez disease
osmidrosis
osseous
 o. syphilis
 o. yaws
ossification
osteogenesis
 o. imperfecta
osteoma cutis
Ota's nevus
otitis externa
Otomyces
 O. hageni
 O. purpureus
otomycosis

otopathy
oxyuriasis
pachyderma
    p. lymphangiectatica
pachydermatocele
pachydermatosis
pachydermatous
pachydermic
pachydermoperiostosis
    p. plicata
pachyhymenic
pachylosis
pachymenia
pachymenic
pachyonychia
Padgett's dermatome
Paget's
    abscess
    cell
paint
    Castellani's p.
palate
pallor
palmoplantar
panatrophy
    Gower's p.
panniculitis
    nodular nonsuppurative p.
panniculus
    p. adiposus
papilla
papillary
papillocarcinoma
papilloma
    p. diffusum
    intracanalicular p.
    p. lineare
papular
papule
    Celsus' p's
    Gottron's p's
    pearly penile p.
    piezogenic p's
    prurigo p.
    split p's
papuliferous
papuloerythematous

papuloid
papulonecrotic
papulopustular
papulopustule
papulosis
    bowenoid p.
    lymphomatoid p.
papulosquamous
papulovesicular
paracanthosis
paracoccidioidomycosis
paraeponychia
parakeratosis
    p. ostracea
    p. papulosa
    p. psoriasiformis
    p. scutularis
    p. variegata
paraneoplastic
parapsoriasis
    p. atrophicans
    p. variegata
    p. varioliformis
parasite
parasitic
paronychia
    p. tendinosa
paronychial
paronychosis
paste
    Lassar's p.
    Veiel's p.
Pasteurella
    P. multocida
patch
    shagreen p.
    p. test
peau
    p. d'orange
pediculation
Pediculoides
    P. ventricosus
pediculosis
    p. capillitii
    p. capitis
    p. corporis
    p. inguinalis

pediculosis (continued)
    p. palpebrarum
    p. pubis
    p. vestimenti
    p. vestimentorum
Pediculus
    P. humanus capitis
    P. humanus corporis
    P. inguinalis
    P. pubis
pedunculated
pellagra
pemphigoid
    bullous p.
pemphigus
    p. acutus
    p. erythematosus
    p. foliaceus
    p. gangrenosus
    p. hemorrhagicus
    p. malignus
    p. neonatorum
    p. syphiliticus
    p. vegetans
    p. vulgaris
perforating
perforation
periadenitis
    p. mucosa necrotica
      recurrens
periadnexal
    p. dermis
periarteritis
    p. gummosa
    p. nodosa
periderm
perifollicular
perifolliculitis
    p. capitis abscedens et
      suffodiens
    superficial pustular p.
perionychia
perionychium
perionyx
perionyxis
periorificial
    p. lentiginosis

periostitis
periphery
periporitis
periungual
perlèche
perlesh. See *perlèche.*
permeability
perna
pernio
petechia
petechial
petechiasis
peteke-. See words beginning
    petechi-.
Petriellidium
    P. boydii
phacoanaphylaxis
phagedena
    sloughing p.
    tropical p.
phagedenic
phakomatoses
phenomenon
    p. of Arthus
    Koebner's p.
    Raynaud's p.
Phialophora
    P. verrucosa
phlebothrombosis
phlebotomy
phlegmasia cerulea dolens
photoallergic
photochemotherapy
photodermatitis
photosensitive
photosensitization
phthiriasis
    p. inguinalis
    pubic p.
Phthirus
    P. pubis
phthisic
phycomycosis
phytophotodermatitis
piebaldism
piedra
piezogenic

Piffard's curet
pigment
pigmentary
pigmentation
pilar
pili
    p. annulati
    p. incarnati
    p. multigemini
    p. torti
pilomatricoma
pilonidal
pilosebaceous
pilus
    p. annulatus
    p. cuniculatus
    p. incarnatus recurvus
    p. tortus
pimple
pinta
pintado
pintid
pinworm
pityriasic
pityriasis
    p. alba
    p. amiantacea
    p. capitis
    p. circinata
    p. circinata et marginata
    p. furfuracea
    Gibert's p.
    Hebra's p.
    p. lichenoides
    p. lichenoides et
      varioliformis acuta
    p. linguae
    p. maculata
    p. pilaris
    p. rosea
    p. rotunda
    p. rubra
    p. rubra pilaris
    p. sicca
    p. simplex
    p. steatoides
    p. versicolor

pityroid
Pityrosporon
    P. orbiculare
    P. ovale
planar
    p. xanthoma
plantar
    p. fibromatosis
    p. hyperkeratosis
    p. inoculum
    p. nevi
    p. wart
plaque
    herald p.
Plasmodium
plexiform
plexus
po dorahnj. See *peau d'orange.*
poikiloderma
    p. atrophicans vasculare
    Civatte's p.
    p. congenitale
poikilodermatomyositis
poliosis
    p. eccentrica
pollen
pollinosis
Pollitzer's disease
polyarteritis
    p. nodosa
polyclonal
polycythemia
polymorphic
polymyositis
polyonychia
polyp
pomphoid
pompholyx
pomphus
porokeratosis
poroma
porphyria
    p. cutanea tarda
      hereditaria
    p. variegata
PPD—purified protein
    derivative

PPD test
prairie itch
pressure ring
    Walsh's p. r.
procedure
    Mohs' p.
progeria
prophylaxis
Propionibacterium
    P. acnes
protoporphyria
    erythropoietic p.
protothecosis
prurigo
    p. agria
    Besnier's p.
    p. chronica multiformis
    p. estivalis
    p. ferox
    p. gestationis
    p. mitis
    p. nodularis
    polymorphic p.
    p. simplex
    p. universalis
pruritic
pruritus
    p. ani
    Duhring's p.
    p. gravidarum
    p. hiemalis
    p. scroti
    p. senilis
    p. vulvae
pseudocarcinomatous
pseudofolliculitis
    p. barbae
pseudohypopigmentation
Pseudomonas
    P. aeruginosa
    P. mallei
    P. pseudomallei
pseudoscleroderma
pseudoxanthoma
    p. elasticum
psora
psoralen

psorelcosis
psoriasiform
psoriasis
    p. annularis
    p. arthropathica
    p. buccalis
    p. circinata
    p. diffusa
    p. discoides
    p. figurata
    flexural p.
    p. follicularis
    p. guttata
    p. gyrata
    inverse p.
    p. inveterata
    p. linguae
    p. nummularis
    p. ostracea
    p. palmaris et plantaris
    p. punctata
    pustular p.
    p. rupioides
    p. universalis
    volar p.
psoriatic
psoric
psorospermosis
    p. follicularis
psorous
psydracium
PTA—plasma thromboplastin
    antecedent
PTC—plasma thromboplastin
    component
pterygium
    p. unguis
Puente's disease
Pulex
    P. irritans
pulicosis
punch
    Keyes' dermal p.
punctate
punctiform
punctum

purpura
- allergic p.
- anaphylactoid p.
- p. angioneurotica
- p. annularis telangiectodes
- p. bullosa
- p. cachectica
- p. fulminans
- p. hemorrhagica
- p. hyperglobulinemica
- p. iodica
- Landouzy's p.
- p. maculosa
- Majocchi's p.
- orthostatic p.
- p. pigmentosa chronica
- p. pulicosa
- p. rheumatica
- Schönlein-Henoch p.
- Schönlein's p.
- p. senilis
- p. simplex
- p. symptomatica
- thrombocytopenic p.
- p. urticans
- p. variolosa

purpuric
purulent
purupuru
pus
Pusey's emulsion
pustula
- p. maligna

pustular
pustulation
pustule
pustulocrustaceous
pustulosis
- p. palmaris
- p. vacciniformis acuta

pyemia
pyoderma
- p. chancriforme faciei
- p. faciale
- p. gangrenosum
- p. ulcerosum tropicalum
- p. vegetans

pyoderma (continued)
- p. verrucosum

pyodermatitis
- p. vegetans

pyodermatosis
pyodermitis
- p. vegetans

pyogenic
pyonychia
pyosis
- Corlett's p.

Q fever
Queyrat's erythroplasia
Quincke's disease
Quinquaud's disease
racemose
radiation
- r. dermatitis
- electromagnetic r.
- r. erythema
- r. spectrum

radioallergosorbent test
radiodermatitis
radioepidermitis
radionuclide
radiotherapy
ragadez. See rhagades.
rakoma. See rhacoma.
Ralks'
- drill
- elevator

ranula
rash
rat-bite fever
Rayer's disease
Raynaud's
- disease
- gangrene
- phenomenon

reaction
- Bloch's r.
- dopa r.
- Herxheimer's r.
- Jarisch-Herxheimer r.
- Jones-Mote r.
- Sanarelli-Shwartzman r.
- Schultz-Charlton r.

reaction (continued)
    Schultz-Dale r.
Recklinghausen's disease
Reenstierna antiserum
Reese's dermatome
Reiter's disease
renocutaneous
replication
rete
    dermal r.
    malpighian rete
reticular
    r. dermis
    r. erythematous mucinosis
reticulate
reticulosis
    epidermotropic r.
    lipomelanotic r.
    medullary r.
    pagetoid r.
retiform
    r. parapsoriasis
rhacoma
rhagades
rhinophyma
rhinoscleroma
rhinosporidiosis
Rhus
    R. diversiloba L.
    R. radicans L.
    R. vernix L.
rhus dermatitis
Ricord's chancre
Riehl's melanosis
ringworm
rino-. See words beginning *rhino-*.
Robinson's disease
Rocky Mountain spotted fever
Rollet's chancre
rosacea
roseola
    r. infantum
rosette
Rothmund-Thomson syndrome
RPR-CT – rapid plasma reagin
    circle card test
rubefacient

rubella
rubeola
rubeosis
ruber
rubescent
rupia
    r. escharotica
Saalfield's extractor
Saccharomyces
saccharomycosis
Salmonella
    S. typhi
Sanarelli-Shwartzman reaction
sarcoid
    Boeck's s.
    Darier-Roussy s.
    Spiegler-Fendt s.
sarcoidosis
sarcoma
    Abernethy's s.
    adipose s.
    Kaposi's s.
sarcomagenic
sarcomatosis
    s. cutis
satellite
sauriasis
sauriderma
sauriosis
scabetic
scabicide
scabies
    Boeck's s.
    Norwegian s.
scabrities
    s. unguium
scale
scaling
    s. nodule
    s. plaque
scaly
scanning
scarification
scarlatiniform
scarlet fever
Schamberg's
    dermatosis

Schamberg's (continued)
    disease
    extractor
Schick test
schistosomiasis
Schönlein-Henoch purpura
Schönlein's purpura
Schultz-Charlton reaction
Schultz-Dale reaction
Schwann's cells
schwannoma
Schweninger-Buzzi
    anetoderma
scleredema
    Buschke's s.
    s. neonatorum
sclerema
    s. neonatorum
sclerodactylia
    s. annularis ainhumoides
sclerodactyly
scleroderma
sclerodermatitis
scleromyxedema
scleronychia
sclerosing
sclerosis
Scopulariopsis
    S. brevicaulis
scrofuloderma
    s. gummosa
    papular s.
    pustular s.
    tuberculous s.
    ulcerative s.
    verrucous s.
scrofulophyma
scrotal tongue
scrotum
scurf
scurvy
scutulum
sebaceous
seborrhea
    s. adiposa
    s. capitis
    s. congestiva

seborrhea (continued)
    s. corporis
    eczematoid s.
    s. faciei
    s. furfuracea
    s. generalis
    s. nigricans
    s. oleosa
    s. sicca
    s. squamo neonatorum
seborrheic
sebum
Senear-Usher disease
senile
    s. keratosis
    s. lentigines
    s. purpura
sensibilisinogen
sensitinogen
sensitization
sepsis
septal
septicemia
serpiginous
serum prothrombin conversion
    accelerator
sessile
Sézary
    erythroderma
    reticulosis
    syndrome
shagreen patch
shanker. See *chancre.*
shankreform. See *chancriform.*
shankroid. See *chancroid.*
shingles
shock
    anaphylactic s.
siazma. See *cyasma.*
sidraseum. See *psydracium.*
sign
    Darier's s.
    Leser-Trélat s.
    Milian's s.
    Nikolsky's s.
    Silex's s.
Silex's sign

silicone
    s. granuloma
Sjögren's syndrome
skin lifter
    Amico's s.l.
SLE – systemic lupus
    erythematosus
slough
sluf. See *slough.*
smallpox
solenonychia
solum
    s. unguis
sora. See *psora.*
soreatik. See *psoriatic.*
sorelkosis. See *psorelcosis.*
soriasis. See *psoriasis.*
sorik. See *psoric.*
sorospermosis. See
    psorospermosis.
sorus. See *psorous.*
SPCA – serum prothrombin
    conversion accelerator
sparganosis
spherocytosis
Spiegler-Fendt sarcoid
spiloplania
spiloplaxia
spiradenoma
spiral
    Herxheimer's s's
Spirillum
    S. minus
Spitz' nevus
spongiosis
spooning
sporotrichosis
Sporotrichum
    S. schenckii
spot
    café au laits's
    Fordyce's s's
    Forschheimer's s's
    Koplik's s's
squamous
stain
    alcian blue s.

stain (continued)
    Brown-Brenn s.
    Giemsa s.
    Hotchkiss-McManus s.
    Masson trichrome s.
staining
    immunoperoxidase s.
Staphylococcus
    S. epidermidis
staphyloderma
staphylodermatitis
stasis
steatocystoma
    s. multiplex
steatoma
steatomatosis
steroid
Stevens-Johnson syndrome
Sticker's disease
stigmatosis
stomatitis
    aphthous s.
    s. medicamentosa
    s. venenata
strata
stratified
stratum
    s. basale epidermidis
    s. corneum epidermidis
    s. corneum unguis
    s. filamentosum
    s. germinativum
        epidermidis
    s. germinativum unguis
    s. granulosum epidermidis
    s. malpighii
streak
    angioid s.
Streptobacillus
    S. moniliformis
streptocerciasis
Streptothrix
streptotrichosis
stria
striae
    s. distensae
    Wickham's s.

Stryker-Halbeisen syndrome
Stryker's dermatome
STS – serologic test for syphilis
"stucco" keratosis
stye
subcutaneous
subcuticular
subungual
sudamen
sudoriferous
sudorrhea
sudozanthoma. See
  pseudoxanthoma.
sulfonamide
sumac
    swamp s.
suppurative
Sutton's disease
Sweet's syndrome
sycoma
sycosiform
    s. tinea barbae
sycosis
    bacillogenic s.
    s. barbae
    coccogenic s.
    s. contagiosa
    s. framboesia
    s. framboesiaeformis
    hyphomycotic c.
    lupoid s.
    nonparasitic s.
    s. nuchae necrotisans
    parasitic s.
    s. staphylogenes
    s. vulgaris
synanthema
syndrome
    Abt-Letterer-Siwe s.
    Albright's s.
    Alibert-Bazin s.
    antibody deficiency s.
    Bazex's s.
    Bloch-Siemens-
      Sulzberger s.
    Buschke-Ollendorff s.
    Danlos' s.

syndrome (continued)
    Degos-Delort-Tricot s.
    Ehlers-Danlos s.
    Felty's s.
    Gianotti-Crosti s.
    Gougerot's s.
    Kasabach-Merritt s.
    Libman-Sacks s.
    Lutz-Splendore-
      de Almeida s.
    Lyell's s.
    Mauriac's s.
    Melkersson-Rosenthal s.
    Milian's s.
    Rothmund-Thomson s.
    Sézary s.
    Sjögren's s.
    Stevens-Johnson s.
    Stryker-Halbeisen s.
    Sweet's s.
    Touraine-Solente-Golé s.
    Waterhouse-Friderichsen
      s.
    Weber-Christian s.
    Weber-Cockayne s.
synergistic
synovitis
syphilid
syphilis
syphilitic
syphiloderm
syphilophyma
syringadenoma
syringocystadenoma
    s. papilliferum
syringocystoma
syringoma
syringometaplasia
syringomyelia
system
    integumentary s.
systemic
tabes
    t. dorsalis
tache
    t's bleuâtres
tachetic

Taenzer's disease
T cell(s)
    T. c. antibody labeling
    T. c. lymphoma
    T. c. marker(s)
tegument
telangiectasia
telangiectasis
telangiectatic
teleroentgen
telogen
teratoma
terijeum. See *pterygium.*
test
    agglutination t.
    basophil degranulation t.
    Bruck's t.
    coccidioidin skin t.
    complement-fixation t.
    Dick t.
    Draize's t.
    fluorescent antinuclear
      antibody t.
    fluorescent treponemal
      antibody absorption t.
    Foshay's t.
    Frei's t.
    in vitro t.
    Ito-Reenstierna t.
    Jadassohn-Bloch t.
    Keller's ultraviolet t.
    Kolmer's t.
    Kveim t.
    lepromin t.
    Mantoux t.
    mast cell degranulation t.
    Mitsuda t.
    patch t.
    PPD (purified protein
      derivative) t.
    radioallergosorbent t.
    rapid plasma reagin circle
      card t.
    Schick t.
    scratch t.
    tine t.
    tuberculin t.

test (continued)
    Tzank t.
    Vollmer's t.
    Wassermann-fast t.
    Wassermann reaction t.
tetter
    brawny t.
    Cantlies' foot t.
    honeycomb t.
thenar eminence
therapy
    grenz ray t.
thiriasis. See *phthiriasis.*
thrush
tinea
    t. amiantacea
    t. axillaris
    t. barbae
    t. capitis
    t. ciliorum
    t. circinata
    t. corporis
    t. cruris
    t. decalvans
    t. favosa
    t. furfuracea
    t. glabrosa
    t. imbricata
    t. inguinalis
    t. kerion
    t. manuum
    t. nigra
    t. nodosa
    t. pedis
    t. profunda
    t. sycosis
    t. tarsi
    t. tonsurans
    t. unguium
    t. versicolor
tizik. See *phthisic.*
tonofibril
tophus
    t. syphiliticus
Torula
toruli
    t. tactiles

toruloma
torulosis
torulus
Touraine-Solente-Golé syndrome
Touton giant cells
toxicity
toxicoderma
toxicodermatitis
treatment
    Gennerich's t.
    Goeckerman t.
Treponema
    T. carateum
    T. pallidum
    T. pertenue
triad
    Hutchinson's t.
trichiasis
trichilemmal
trichilemmoma
trichitis
trichoadenoma
trichoepithelioma
    t. papillosum multiplex
trichofibroacanthoma
trichofibroepithelioma
trichofolliculoma
trichoglossia
trichoid
trichologia
trichomadesis
trichomatosis
Trichomonas
trichomycosis
    t. axillaris
    t. chromatica
    t. favosa
    t. nigra
    t. nodosa
    t. palmellina
    t. pustulosa
    t. rubra
trichonocardiasis
trichonodosis
trichonosis
    t. furfuracea
trichopathic

trichophytic
trichophytid
Trichophyton
    T. concentricum
    T. faviforme
    T. mentagrophytes
    T. rubrum
    T. schoenleinii
    T. tonsurans
    T. verrucosum
    T. violaceum
trichophytosis
    t. barbae
    t. capitis
    t. corporis
    t. cruris
    t. unguium
trichorhinophalangeal
trichorrhea
trichorrhexis
    t. invaginata
    t. nodosa
trichoschisis
Trichosporon
    T. beigelii
    T. cutaneum
trichostasis spinulosa
Trichothecium
    T. roseum
trichotillomania
trichrome
    t. vitiligo
Triphelps insidiosus
trisomy
Trombicula
Trypanosoma
    T. brucei
    T. cruzi
trypanosomiasis
tubercle
tubercular
tuberculid
    papulonecrotic t.
    rosacea-like t.
tuberculoderm
tuberculosis
    t. colliquativa

tuberculosis (continued)
    miliary t.
    orificial t.
    t. papulonecrotica
    t. verrucosa cutis
tuberous
tularemia
tumefaction
tumescence
Tunga
    T. penetrans
tungiasis
turgor
twenty-nail (20-nail)
tylosis
    t. ciliaris
    t. palmaris et plantaris
typhus
Tzank
    cell
    test
ulcer
    chancroid u.
    decubitus u.
    Lipschütz's u.
ulceration
ulcus
    u. ambulans
    u. ambustiforme
    u. durum
    u. interdigitale
    u. molle cutis
    u. scorbuticum
    u. syphiliticum
    u. vulvae acutum
ulerythema
    u. acneiforma
    u. centrifugum
    u. ophryogenes
    u. sycosiforme
ulodermatitis
uloid
ultraviolet radiation
ungual
unguinal
unguis
    u. incarnatus

Unna's
    boot
    dermatosis
    extractor
    nevus
Urbach-Oppenheim disease
uremia
urethritis
    gonorrheal u.
urhidrosis
urtica
urticaria
    aquagenic u.
    u. bullosa
    cholinergic u.
    endemic u.
    u. endemica
    u. epidemica
    u. factitia
    u. gigantea
    u. hemorrhagica
    heredofamilial u.
    u. medicamentosa
    Milton's u.
    papular u.
    u. papulosa
    u. perstans
    u. photogenica
    u. pigmentosa
    solar u.
    u. solaris
    u. subcutanea
    subcutaneous u.
urticarial
urticariogenic
urticate
vaccination
vaccine
    bacille Calmette-Guérin v.
vaccinia
    v. gangrenosa
vagabonds' disease
varicella
    v. gangrenosa
    pustular v.
    v. pustulosa

varicelliform
    Kaposi's v. eruption
variegate porphyria
variola
    v. crystallina
    v. inserta
    v. miliaris
    v. minor
    v. mitigata
    v. pemphigosa
    v. siliquosa
    v. vera
    v. verrucosa
varioloid
vascular
    v. endothelium
    v. hamartoma
    v. hemophilia
    v. nevus
    v. spider
    v. tumor
vasculitis
    granulomatous v.
    livedoid v.
    lymphomatoid v.
    necrotizing v.
    nodular v.
    septic v.
    urticarial v.
vasodilation
Veiel's paste
vellus
    v. hair
Venus
    collar of V.
verruca (verrucae)
    v. acuminata
    v. digitata
    v. filiformis
    v. glabra
    v. necrogenica
    v. peruana
    v. peruviana
    v. plana
    v. plana juvenilis
    v. plantaris
    v. seborrhoeica

verruca (verrucae) (continued)
    v. senilis
    v. simplex
    v. tuberculosa
    v. vulgaris
verrucae
verruciform
verrucose
verrucosis
verruga
    v. peruana
vesicant
vesication
vesicle
vesicular
    v. bullous pemphigoid
    v. dermatophytid
    v. ringworm
    v. stomatitis
vesiculation
vesiculobullous
vesiculopapular
vesiculopustular
vibratory
    v. angioedema
virus
    coxsackievirus
    ECHO v.-enteric
      cytopathogenic human
      orphan v.
visceral
    v. larva migrans
    v. leishmaniasis
    v. schistosomiasis
    v. syphilis
vitiligo
    v. capitis
    Cazenave's v.
    Celsus' v.
    circumscribed v.
    perinevic v.
Voigt's lines
Vollmer's test
vulgaris
vulva
vulvitis
vulvovaginitis

Walsh's
    curet
    pressure ring
Walton's extractor
Wangiella dermatitidis
wart
    anatomical w.
    filiform w.
    mosaic w.
    mucocutaneous w.
    necrogenic w.
    periungual w.
    pitch w.
    plantar w.
    seborrheic w.
    telangiectatic w.
    tuberculous w.
    venereal w.
warty
    w. dyskeratoma
    w. tuberculosis
Wassermann-fast test
Wassermann reaction test
Waterhouse-Friderichsen
    syndrome
Weber-Christian
    disease
    syndrome
Weber-Cockayne syndrome
Weber's disease
Wegener's granulomatosis
wen
wheal
White's disease
whitehead
Whitfield's ointment
whitlow
Wickham's striae
Willan's lepra
Wood's light
Woringer-Kolopp disease
wrestler's herpes
xanthelasma
xanthoderma
xanthogranuloma

xanthoma
    x. diabeticorum
    x. disseminatum
    x. eruptivum
    x. multiplex
    x. planum
    x. striatum palmare
    x. tendinosum
    x. tuberosum
    x. tuberosum multiplex
xanthomatosis
xanthomatous
xanthosiderohistiocytosis
xanthosis
    x. cutis
XDP – xeroderma pigmentosum
xeroderma
    follicular x.
    Kaposi's x.
    x. pigmentosum
xerodermatic
xerodermosteosis
xeroradiography
xerosis
    x. cutis
xerostomia
x-linked
    cutis laxa
    hypogammaglobulinemia
    ichthyosis
    recessive inheritance
XP – xeroderma pigmentosum
yaws
yellow nail syndrome
Yersinia pestis infection
zan-. See words beginning *xan-*.
zero-. See words beginning *xero-*.
zoacanthosis
zona
    z. dermatica
    z. epithelioserosa
    z. facialis
zosteriform
zosteroid
zyderm collagen implant

Gastroenterology

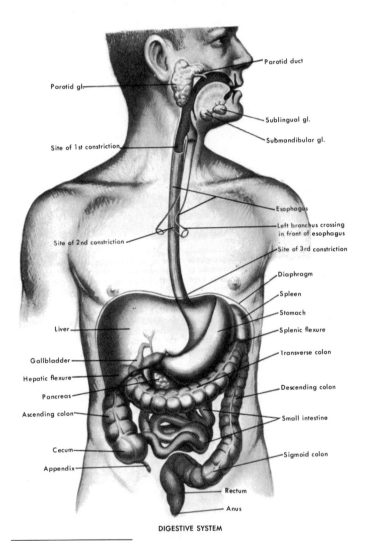

Parotid duct

Parotid gl.

Sublingual gl.

Submandibular gl.

Site of 1st constriction

Esophagus

Left bronchus crossing
in front of esophagus

Site of 2nd constriction

Site of 3rd constriction

Diaphragm

Spleen

Stomach

Splenic flexure

Liver

Transverse colon

Gallbladder

Hepatic flexure

Pancreas

Descending colon

Ascending colon

Small intestine

Cecum

Appendix

Sigmoid colon

Rectum

Anus

DIGESTIVE SYSTEM

(Courtesy of Gardner, W. D., and Osburn, W. A.: Anatomy of the Human Body, 3rd
ed. Copyright 1978, and 1967, by W. B. Saunders, Philadelphia; reprinted by Holt, Rine-
hart, and Winston, New York.)

Gastroenterology

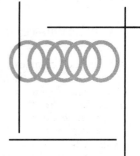

abdominal
    a. abscess
    a. aortic aneurysm
a-beta-lipoproteinemia
abscess
    amebic a.
    anorectal a.
    diaphragmatic a.
    hepatic a.
    intra-abdominal a.
    midabdominal a.
    pancreatic a.
    pericholecystic a.
    perirectal a.
    splenic a.
    subphrenic a
absorption
AC—adenylate cyclase
a.c.—before meals (ante
    cibum)
acanthosis
    a. nigricans
achalasia
achlorhydria
    a. apepsia
acholia
acholic
achylia
    a. gastrica haemorrhagica
    a. pancreatica
achylous
acid
    amino a.
    hydrochloric a.
acidity
acinar
ACMI gastroscope
acquired immunodeficiency
    syndrome

acrodermatitis
    a. enteropathica
adenasthenia
    a. gastrica
adenia
    angibromic a.
adenitis
    mesenteric a.
adenoacanthoma
adenocarcinoma
adenohypersthenia
    a. gastrica
adenoma
    papillary a.
    villous a.
adenomatous
    a. polyposis
adenomyoma
adenomyosis
adenovirus
adhesion
adipolysis
aerenterectasia
aerocoly
aerogastria
aerogastrocolia
aeroperitoneum
aerophagia
aerophagy
aganglionosis
agastroneuria
agenesis
aglutition
agranulocytic
AIDS—acquired
    immunodeficiency
    syndrome. See *Immunology
    with special reference to
    AIDS* section.

AIDS-related complex
akahlazea. See *achalasia.*
akilea. See *achylia.*
akilus. See *achylous.*
aklorhidreah. See
     achlorhydria.
akoleah. See *acholia.*
akolic. See *acholic.*
alimentary tract
alimentation
alkaline
alkalosis
alopecia
ALP – alkaline phosphatase
Althausen's test
amebiasis
     intestinal a.
amebic
American Anorexia/Bulemia
     Association
American Society for
     Gastrointestinal Endoscopy
amino acid
ampulla
     a. hepatopancreatica
     a. of Vater
amylase
amyloidosis
anacidity
anal
     a. canal
     a. manometry
     a. sphincter
analysis
     gastric a.
anapepsia
anaphylactoid
anaphylaxis
anastomosis
     Billroth I a.
     Billroth II a.
     Braun's a.
     enteric a.
     peristaltic a.
     Roux-en-Y a.
Ancylostoma
     A. duodenale

ancylostomiasis
Andresen's diet
anesthesia. See *General Surgical*
     Terms section.
aneurysm
Angelchik's prosthesis
angina
     abdominal a.
     a. abdominalis
     a. dyspeptica
     intestinal a.
angiocholecystitis
angiocholitis
     a. proliferans
angiodysplasia
angiography
angioplasia
angulation
angulus
anisakiasis
anismus
annular
anoplasty
anorectal
anorectum
anorexia
     a. nervosa
anoscopy
anoxia
antacid
anticholagogic
anticholinergic
antidiarrheal
antiemetic
antimesenteric
antimicrobial
antimotility
antiperistalsis
antispasmodic
antral
antrectomy
antrum
anus
     imperforate a.
apepsia
     achlorhydria a.
apepsinia

aperistalsis
apparatus
    Golgi's a.
appendectomy
appendicitis
appendix
    vermiform a.
appetite
arachnogastria
ARC – AIDS-related complex
arch
    Treitz's a.
argentaffinoma
Argyle's tube
arrhythmia
arthritis
ascariasis
ascending
ascites
aspiration
atony
atresia
atrophic
atrophy
    gastric mucosal a.
autoimmune
autonomic
autotransplantation
awbarra. See *embarras.*
Ba – barium
Bacillus
    B. Calmette-Guérin
    B. cereus
bacteremia
bacteria
bacteriocholia
BaE – barium enema
Baker's tube
balantidiasis
balloon
    b. defecation
    b. dilation
    Garren's b.
    b. manometry
    b. tamponade
band
    Ladd's b.'s

band (continued)
    Lane's b.
Banti's syndrome
barium
Barrett's
    esophagus
    syndrome
BCG – bacillus Calmette-Guérin
Behçet's syndrome
belching
Benedict's gastroscope
bentiromide test
Bernstein test
bezoar
bifurcation
bile
biliary
bilidigestive
bilihumin
bilious
biliousness
biliprasin
bilirubin
bilirubinemia
Billroth
    I anastomosis
    II anastomosis
Billroth's hypertrophy
biofeedback
biopsy
Blakemore's tube
blind loop syndrome
bloating
blood
    occult b.
Blumer's shelf
Boas' test meal
Boerhaave's syndrome
bolus
borborygmi
borborygmus
bougie
bowel
    gangrenous b.
    greedy b.
Bowen's disease
Boyden's test meal

bradygastria
bradykinin
bradypepsia
bradystalsis
brash
Braun's anastomosis
Brinton's disease
bronchoscope
Browne-McHardy dilator
bruit
Brunner's glands
brush border digestion
brwe. See *bruit.*
bubble
        Garren-Edwards gastric b.
bulb
        duodenal b.
bulimia
calculi
Calmette-Guérin bacillus
Campylobacter
        C. pyloris
canaliculus
Candida
        C. albicans
candidiasis
Cannon's ring
Cantor's tube
cap
        phrygian c.
capotement
capsule
        Glisson's c.
caput
        c. medusae
carcinoembryonic
carcinoid
carcinoma
        adenoid cystic c.
        bile duct c.
        biliary c.
        colorectal c.
        esophageal c.
        hepatocellular c.
        hilar c.
        oat cell c.
        pancreatic c.

carcinoma (continued)
        peritoneal c.
carcinomatosis
        c. peritonei
cardia
        c. of stomach
cardiac
cardialgia
cardiopulmonary
cardiospasm
cardiovascular
carminative
Carnot's test
carreau
CAT – computerized axial
        tomography
catabolism
cathartic
cecitis
cecocolon
cecocolostomy
cecoileostomy
cecopexy
cecosigmoidostomy
cecostomy
cecotomy
cecum
celiac
celiocentesis
celiomyalgia
celiomyomotomy
celioparacentesis
celiopathy
celiopyosis
celioscope
celitis
cell
        acinar c's
        goblet c's
        Paneth's c's
cestode
Chagas' disease
chemoreceptor
chemotherapy
Chevalier Jackson gastroscope
Chlamydia
        C. trachomatis

cholagogic
cholagogue
cholaligenic
cholaneresis
cholangeitis
cholangiectasis
cholangioadenoma
cholangiocarcinoma
cholangiocholecysto-
    choledochectomy
cholangioenterostomy
cholangiogastrostomy
cholangiogram
cholangiography
    endoscopic c.
    operative c.
    transhepatic c.
cholangiohepatitis
cholangiohepatoma
cholangiojejunostomy
    intrahepatic c.
cholangiole
cholangiolitis
cholangioma
cholangiopancreatography
cholangiostomy
cholangiotomy
cholangitis
    catarrhal c.
    c. lenta
cholecyst
cholecystalgia
cholecystatony
cholecystectasia
cholecystectomy
cholecystenteric
cholecystenteroanastomosis
cholecystenterorrhaphy
cholecystenterostomy
cholecystic
cholecystis
cholecystitis
    acute c.
    chronic c.
    c. emphysematosa
    emphysematous c.
    follicular c.

cholecystitis (continued)
    gaseous c.
    c. glandularis
      proliferans
cholecystocholangiogram
cholecystocolonic
cholecystocolostomy
cholecystocolotomy
cholecystoduodenostomy
cholecystogastric
cholecystogastrostomy
cholecystogram
cholecystography
cholecystoileostomy
cholecystojejunostomy
cholecystokinetic
cholecystokinin
cholecystolithiasis
cholecystolithotripsy
cholecystopathy
cholecystoptosis
cholecystorrhaphy
cholecystosis
    hyperplastic c.
cholecystostomy
cholecystotomy
choledochal
choledochectomy
choledochitis
choledochocele
choledochocholedochostomy
choledochoduodenostomy
choledochoenterostomy
choledochogastrostomy
choledochogram
choledochography
choledochohepatostomy
choledochoileostomy
choledochojejunostomy
choledocholith
choledocholithiasis
choledocholithotomy
choledocholithotripsy
choledochoplasty
choledochorrhaphy
choledochoscope
choledochostomy

choledochotomy
choledochus
cholelithiasis
cholelithotomy
cholelithotripsy
cholemesis
cholemimetry
cholepathia
    c. spastica
choleperitoneum
cholepoiesis
cholepoietic
cholera
    bilious c.
    c. morbus
    c. nostras
choleretic
cholerrhagia
cholestasis
cholesterol
cholesterolosis
cholinergic
choloscopy
chromatography
chromoscopy
    gastric c.
chyle
chylous
chymase
chyme
chymification
chymorrhea
cicatricial
cirrhosis
    biliary c.
    calculus c.
    cardiac c.
    Maixner's c.
claudication
    intermittent c.
Clostridium
    C. perfringens
clysma
clyster
CMV – cytomegalovirus
coccidiosis
colectomy

colic
    biliary c.
    bilious c.
    crapulent c.
    gallstone c.
    gastric c.
    hepatic c.
    intestinal c.
    mucous c.
    pancreatic c.
    pseudomembranous c.
    saburral c.
    stercoral c.
    vermicular c.
    verminous c.
colicky
colicolitis
coliform
colitis
    adaptive c.
    amebic c.
    balantidial c.
    collagenous c.
    c. cystica profunda
    c. cystica superficialis
    diversion c.
    fulminating c.
    granulomatous c.
    c. gravis
    mucous c.
    myxomembranous c.
    c. polyposa
    pseudomembranous c.
    segmental c.
    transmural c.
    ulcerative c.
collagen
collagenous
colloid
coloclyster
colocutaneous
colodyspepsia
coloenteritis
colon
    ascending c.
    descending c.
    distal c.

colon (continued)
    irritable c.
    lead-pipe c.
    proximal c.
    sigmoid c.
    spastic c.
    transverse c.
    unstable c.
colonic
colonorrhea
colonoscope
    fiberoptic c.
colonoscopy
colonotomy
coloproctitis
colorectal
colorectitis
colorectostomy
colorrhea
colostomy
    end-to-side ileotransverse
      c.
complex
    Golgi's c.
congenital
Congo red test
coniasis
constipation
    gastrojejunal c.
contraction
copremia
coprolith
coprostasis
Corner's tampon
corticosteroid
Courvoisier-Terrier syndrome
craigiasis
crater
crepitus
cricopharyngeal
Crohn's disease
crura
Cruveilhier's disease
cryosurgery
cryptosporidia
cryptosporidiosis

curvature
    greater c.
    lesser c.
Cushing's ulcer
cyclic
cystadenocarcinoma
cystadenoma
cystic
cystinuria
cytomegalovirus
cytotoxic
DAN–diabetic autonomic
    neuropathy
defecation
defecography
deglutition
Degos' disease
dehydration
dehydrocholaneresis
dehydrogenase
    lactic d.
demucosatio
    d. intestini
descending
    d. colon
desmoid
diabetes
diabetic
    d. autonomic neuropathy
    d. gastroparesis
    d. ketoacidosis
Diagnex blue test
dialysis
diaphragm
diarrhea
diastalsis
diastase
    pancreatic d.
diathesis
diet
    Andresen's d.
    Giordano-Giovannetti d.
    gluten free d.
    Jarotsky's d.
    Meulengracht's d.
    Sippy d.
Dieulafoy's erosion

digestion
digestive
dilatation
dilation
dilator
    Browne-McHardy d.
    Einhorn's d.
    esophageal d.
Diphyllobothrium
    D. latum
dis-. See also words beginning
    dys-.
disaccharidase
disease
    Bowen's d.
    Brinton's d.
    celiac d.
    Chagas' d.
    Crohn's d.
    Cruveilhier's d.
    Degos' d.
    graft-versus-host d.
    Hanot's d.
    hepatobiliary tract d.
    Hirschsprung's d.
    Hodgkin's d.
    Köhlmeier-Degos d.
    Menetrier's d.
    Myà's d.
    Patella's d.
    Payr's d.
    Reichmann's d.
    Tangier d.
    Whipple's d.
    Wolman d.
distention
distomiasis
    intestinal d.
DIT – diet-induced thermogenesis
diuretic
diversion
    d. colitis
diverticulitis
diverticulosis
    jejunal d.
diverticulum
    epiphrenic d.

diverticulum (continued)
    hepatic d.
    hypopharyngeal d.
diverticula
    jejunal d.
    Meckel's d.
    midesophageal d.
    Zenker's d.
DKA – diabetic ketoacidosis
Dock's test meal
Doppler study
drip
    intragastric d.
drugs. See *Drugs and Chemistry*
    section.
Dubin-Johnson syndrome
duct
    biliary d.
    common bile d.
    extrahepatic bile d.
    hepatic d.
    Wirsung's d.
ductus
    d. choledochus
dumping syndrome
duodenal
    d. atresia
    d. diverticula
    d. drainage
    d. ulcer
duodenectomy
duodenitis
duodenocholangitis
duodenocholecystostomy
duodenocholedochotomy
duodenocolic
duodenocystostomy
duodenoduodenostomy
duodenoenterostomy
duodenogram
duodenohepatic
duodenoileostomy
duodenojejunostomy
duodenolysis
duodenorrhaphy
duodenoscope
duodenoscopy

duodenostomy
duodenotomy
duodenum
duplication
D-xylose absorption test
dyschezia
dysentery
 amebic d.
dysgeusia
dyskinesia
 biliary d.
dyspepsia
dysperistalsis
dysphagia
 d. lusoria
 oropharyngeal d.
 sideropenic d.
dysplasia
dyspragia
 d. intermittens
  angiosclerotica
  intestinalis
dysproteinemia
dysrhythmia
dyssynergia
dystrophic
D-zylose. See D-xylose.
echinococcosis
ectasia
ecterograph
ectocolon
ectoperitonitis
edema
 alimentary e.
edematous
efferent
EGD – esophagogastro-
 duodenoscopy
EGG – electrogastrogram
Ehlers-Danlos syndrome
Ehrmann's alcohol test
 meal
Einhorn's dilator
electrocoagulation
electrogastrogram
electrogastrography
electromyography

embarras
 e. gastrique
embolization
empyema
emulsification
encapsulation
endocolitis
endocrine
endoenteritis
endogastric
endogastritis
endometrioma
endometriosis
 e. of colon
endoscopic
endoscopy
enema
 barium e.
Entamoeba
 E. histolytica
enteraden
enteradenitis
enteral
enteralgia
enterauxe
enterectasis
enterectomy
enterelcosis
enteric
enteritides
enteritis
 choleriform e.
 cicatrizing e.
 e. cystica chronica
 granulomatous e.
 e. gravis
 leishmanial e.
 myxomembranous e.
 e. necroticans
 e. nodularis
 pellicular e.
 phlegmonous e.
 e. polyposa
 protozoan e.
 pseudomembranous e.
 radiation e.
 regional e.

enteritis (continued)
    segmental e.
    streptococcus e.
    ulcerative e.
enteroanastomosis
enteroapokleisis
enterobiasis
enterobiliary
Enterobius
    E. vermicularis
enterocele
enterocentesis
enterochirurgia
enterocholecystostomy
enterocholecystotomy
enterocinesia
enterocinetic
enterocleisis
enteroclysis
enterocoele
enterocolectomy
enterocolitis
    hemorrhagic e.
    necrotizing e.
    pseudomembranous e.
    regional e.
enterocolostomy
enterocutaneous
enterocyst
enterocystocele
enterocystoma
enterodynia
enteroenterostomy
enteroepiplocele
enterogastric
enterogastritis
enterogenous
enteroglucagon
enterogram
enterograph
enterography
enterohepatitis
enterohepatopexy
enteroidea
enterointestinal
enterokinase
enterokinesia

enterokinetic
enterokinin
enterolith
enterolithiasis
enterology
enterolysis
enteromegaly
enteromere
enteromycosis
    e. bacteriaceae
enteromyiasis
enteron
enteroneuritis
enteronitis
    polytropous e.
enteroparesis
enteropathogen
enteropathogenesis
enteropathogenic
enteropathy
    gluten e.
    protein-losing e.
enteropeptidase
enteropexy
enteroplasty
enteroplegia
enteroptosis
enteroptychia
enterorrhagia
enterorrhaphy
enterorrhea
enterorrhexis
enteroscope
enterosepsis
enterosorption
enterospasm
enterostasis
enterostaxis
enterostenosis
enterostomal
enterostomy
    gun-barrel e.
enterotome
enterotomy
enterotoxin
enterovirus
enzyme

eosinophilic
>   e. gastroenteropathy
>   e. granuloma

epidermal
epidermoid
epigastralgia
epigastric
epigastrium
epigastrocele
epiphrenic
epiploon
epithalaxia
epithelium
erepsin
erosion
>   Dieulafoy's e.

eructation
>   nervous e.

erythema
>   e. necrolytica migrans

erythrocytosis
Escherichia
>   *E. coli*

esofa-. See words beginning
>   *esopha-.*

esogastritis
esophagalgia
esophageal
esophagectasia
esophagism
esophagitis
>   e. dissecans superficialis
>   peptic e.
>   reflux e.

esophagocologastrostomy
esophagoduodenostomy
esophagodynia
esophagoenterostomy
esophagofundopexy
esophagogastrectomy
esophagogastric
esophagogastroanastomosis
esophagogastroduodenoscopy
esophagogastromyotomy
esophagogastroplasty
esophagogastroscopy
esophagogastrostomy

esophagogram
esophagography
esophagojejunogastrostomosis
esophagojejunogastrostomy
esophagojejunoplasty
esophagojejunostomy
esophagomyotomy
esophagoscope
>   Jesberg's e.

esophagoscopy
esophagospasm
esophagostenosis
esophagus
>   Barrett's e.

etiology
euchlorhydria
eucholia
euchylia
eupepsia
evacuation
eventration
Ewald's test meal
excrement
excrementitious
excreta
excretion
exocrine
extrahepatic
exudation
fecal
>   f. continence
>   f. fluid
>   f. impaction
>   f. incontinence
>   f. leukocytes

fecalith
feces
feculent
fiberscope
>   Hirschowitz's f.
>   Olympus f.

fibroblast
Finney's pyloroplasty
Fischer's test meal
fissure
fistula
>   enterocolic f.

fistula (continued)
    enteroenteric f.
    gastrojejunocolic f.
    jejunocolic f.
    tracheoesophageal f.
fitobezor. See *phytobezoar.*
flatulence
flatulent
flatus
flexure
    splenic f.
flora
    intestinal f.
fluke
    intestinal f's
flux
    bilious f.
    celiac f.
folate
foramen
    Winslow's f.
fossa
    Treitz's f.
freezing
    gastric f.
fundoplication
fundus
fungal
GA – gastric analysis
Galeati's glands
gall
gallbladder
gallstone
GALT – gastrointestinal-
    associated lymphoid tissue
gamma
    g.-aminobutyric acid
    g. heavy chain disease
    g. interferon
gangrenous
Gardner's syndrome
Garren-Edwards gastric bubble
Garren's balloon
gastradenitis
gastralgia
    appendicular g.
gastralgokenosis

gastraneuria
gastrasthenia
gastratrophia
gastrectasia
gastrectomy
    Roux-en-Y g.
gastric
    g. acid
    g. actinomycosis
    g. adenocarcinoma
    g. anoxia
    g. atrophy
    g. balloon implantation
    g. bubble
    g. by-pass surgery
    g. carcinoma
    g. dilation
    g. duplication
    g. dysfunction
    g. dysrhythmia
    g. emptying
    g. hyperemia
    g. hypersecretion
    g. ileus
    g. inhibitory polypeptides
    g. lavage
    g. mucosal barrier
    g. outlet obstruction
    g. pseudolymphoma
    g. retention
    g. rupture
    g. stasis
    g. teratoma
    g. ulcer
    g. varices
    g. volvulus
gastricism
gastricsin
gastrin
gastrinoma
gastritic
gastritis
    antral g.
    atrophic g.
    catarrhal g.
    cirrhotic g.
    emphysematous g.

gastritis (continued)
    eosinophilic g.
    erosive g.
    exfoliative g.
    follicular g.
    giant hypertrophic g.
    g. granulomatosa
      fibroplastica
    hyperpeptic g.
    hypertrophic g.
    idiopathic g.
    interstitial g.
    mycotic g.
    nonerosive g.
    phlegmonous g.
    polypous g.
    pseudomembranous g.
    purulent g.
    superficial g.
    suppurating g.
    syphilitic g.
    tuberculous g.
gastroalbuminorrhea
gastroatonia
gastroblennorrhea
gastrobrosis
gastrocamera
gastrocardiac
gastrocele
gastrochronorrhea
gastrocolic
gastrocolitis
gastrocoloptosis
gastrocolostomy
gastrocolotomy
gastrocutaneous
gastrodialysis
gastrodiaphane
gastrodiaphany
gastroduodenal
gastroduodenitis
gastroduodenoscopy
gastroduodenostomy
gastrodynia
gastroenteralgia
gastroenteric
gastroenteritis

gastroenteroanastomosis
gastroenterocolic
gastroenterocolitis
gastroenterocolostomy
gastroenterologist
gastroenterology
gastroenteropathy
gastroenteroplasty
gastroenteroptosis
gastroenterostomy
gastroenterotomy
gastroepiploic
gastroesophageal
gastroesophagitis
gastroesophagostomy
gastrogalvanization
gastrogastrostomy
gastrogavage
gastrogenic
Gastrografin
gastrograph
gastrohelcoma
gastrohelcosis
gastrohepatic
gastrohepatitis
gastrohydrorrhea
gastrohyperneuria
gastrohypertonic
gastrohyponeuria
gastroileitis
gastroileostomy
gastrointestinal
    g.-associated lymphoid
      tissue
    g. fistula
    g. fungal balls
    g. immunodeficiency
      syndrome
    g. peptide hormone
    g. reflux
    g. smooth muscle
gastrojejunocolic
gastrojejunostomy
gastrokinesograph
gastrolienal
gastrolith
gastrolithiasis

gastrologist
gastrology
gastrolysis
gastromalacia
gastromegaly
gastromycosis
gastromyotomy
gastromyxorrhea
gastrone
gastronesteostomy
gastropancreatitis
gastroparalysis
gastroparesis
gastropathy
gastroperiodynia
gastroperitonitis
gastropexy
gastrophotography
gastrophrenic
gastrophthisis
gastroplasty
gastroplication
gastroptosis
gastroptyxis
gastropylorectomy
gastropyloric
gastroradiculitis
gastrorrhagia
gastrorrhaphy
gastrorrhea
    g. continua chronica
gastrorrhexis
gastroschisis
gastroscope
    ACMI g.
    Benedict's g.
    Chevalier Jackson g.
    fiberoptic g.
    flexible g.
    Hirschowitz's g.
    Housset Debray g.
    Wolf-Schindler g.
gastroscopic
gastroscopy
gastrosia
    g. fungosa
gastrospasm

gastrosplenic
gastrostaxis
gastrostenosis
gastrostogavage
gastrostolavage
gastrostoma
gastrostomy
    Ssabanejew-Frank g.
    Stamm's g.
gastrosuccorrhea
    digestive g.
    g. mucosa
gastrotome
gastrotomy
gastrotonometer
gastrotoxin
gastroxynsis
    g. fungosa
gavage
genital
geotrichosis
GER – gastroesophageal reflux
GERD – gastroesophageal reflux disease
GERL – Golgi-endoplasmic reticulum lysosomes
GET – gastric emptying time
GET$\frac{1}{2}$ – gastric emptying half-time
GI – gastrointestinal
Giardia
    G. lamblia
giardiasis
Giordano-Giovannetti diet
GIP – gastric inhibitory peptides
gland
    Brunner's g's
    Galeati's g's
    Theile's g's
Glénard's syndrome
gliadin
glioma-polyposis syndrome
Glisson's capsule
globus
    esophageal g.
    g. hystericus
glucagon

glucagonoma
glucose
gluten
    g. enteropathy
    g.-free diet
    g. sensitivity
glycogen
glycogenesis
glycogenolysis
glycolysis
glyconeogenesis
glycoprotein
glycoside
GM – gastric mucosa
Gmelin's test
goblet cell
Goldstein's hematemesis
Golgi's
    apparatus
    complex
gonococcal
    g. proctitis
gonorrhea
Goodsall's rule
graft-versus-host disease
granulation
granule
    zymogen g's
granuloma
GRP – gastrin releasing peptide
granulomatosis
    lipophagic intestinal g.
granulomatous
GU – gastric ulcer
guaiac
gutter
    paracolic g.
GVHD – graft-versus-host
   disease
hamartoma
Hanot-Rössle syndrome
Hanot's disease
Hartmann's pouch
haustra of colon
haustral
haustrum
HBV – hepatitis B virus

HCC – hepatocellular carcinoma
heartburn
Heineke-Mikulicz pyloroplasty
Helicobacter
    H. pylori
helminthemesis
hematemesis
    Goldstein's h.
    h. puellaris
hematobilia
hematochezia
hematoma
hemidiaphragm
hemigastrectomy
hemobilia
hemocholecystitis
hemolysis
hemoperitoneum
hemoptysis
hemorrhage
    petechial h.
hemorrhagic
hemorrhoid
Henoch's purpura
hepar
hepatic
hepatitis
    anicteric h.
    h. B virus
    serum h.
    viral h.
hepatobiliary
hepatocellular
hepatocholangitis
hepatocholangioduodenostomy
hepatocolic
hepatocystic
hepatoenteric
hepatogastric
hepatoid
hepatolithiasis
hepatomegaly
hepatorrhea
hepatosplenomegaly
hernia
    diaphragmatic h.
    hiatal h.

hernia (continued)
    hiatus h.
    Morgagni's h.
    spigelian h.
    Treitz's h.
herniorrhaphy
herniotomy
herpes
    h. pharyngitis
    h. simplex
    h. zoster
heterochylia
hiatus
    esophageal h.
hiccup
Hirschowitz's
    fiberscope
    gastroscope
Hirschsprung's disease
histamine
histocompatibility
Hodgkin's disease
Hoguet's maneuver
hologastroschisis
hookworm
Housset-Debray gastroscope
Hueter's maneuver
hydatid
hydraeroperitoneum
hydragogue
hydrepigastrium
hydrochloric
hydrocholecystis
hydrocholeresis
hydrolysis
hydroperitoneum
hydrops
    h. abdominis
hydrothorax
hyperalimentation
hyperamylasemia
hyperbilirubinemia
hypercalcemia
hyperchlorhydria
hypercholia
hyperemesis
    h. hiemis

hyperemic
hypergastrinemia
hyperglycemia
hyperlipemia
hyperlipidemia
hyperoxaluria
hyperpepsia
hyperpepsinia
hyperperistalsis
hypersalivation
hypersecretion
    gastric h.
hypertrophy
    Billroth's h.
hypocalcemia
hypochloremia
hypochlorhydria
hypochondrium
hypochylia
hypogammaglobulinemia
hypogastric
hypogastrium
hypogastroschisis
hypogeusia
hypoglycemia
hypokalemia
hypomagnesemia
hyponatremia
hypopepsia
hypopepsinia
hypoperistalsis
hypophrenium
hypoplasia
hypoproteinemia
hypoprothrombinemia
hyposteatolysis
hypothalamus
hypothermia
hypothesis
    Keller's h.
hypoxemia
hypoxia
IBD – inflammatory bowel
    disease
IBS – irritable bowel
    syndrome
IC – irritable colon

ichthyismus
    i. exanthematicus
icterus
idiopathic
ileal
ileectomy
ileitis
    prestomal i.
    regional i.
    terminal i.
ileocecal
ileocecum
ileocolitis
    i. ulcerosa chronica
ileocolostomy
ileojejunitis
    granulomatous i.
    nongranulomatous i.
ileoproctostomy
ileorectal
ileosigmoid
ileostomy
ileum
    terminal i.
ileus
    adynamic i.
    gallstone i.
    gastric i.
    meconium i.
    paralytic i.
    spastic i.
iliohypogastric
ilioinguinal
iliopectineal
immunocompromised
immunodeficiency
immunoglobulin
immunoproliferative
impaction
    fecal i.
incision. See *General Surgical Terms* section.
incontinence
    fecal i.
indigestion
inertia
    colonic i.

infarction
inflammation
inflammatory
ingestion
innervation
insufficiency
    pancreatic i.
insulin
insulinoma
interstitial
intestinal
    i. atresia
    i. lymphangiectasia
    i. metaplasia
    i. obstruction
    i. peptides
    i. perfusion
intestine
intestinum
intubated
intubation
intussusception
irritable bowel syndrome
ischemia
    mesenteric i.
    midgut i.
ischemic
ischocholia
ischochymia
isko-. See words beginning *ischo-.*
islet
    Langerhans' i's
isometric
isotonic
isotope
IVC–intravenous cholangiogram
Jarotsky's diet
jaundice
    obstructive j.
jaw wiring
jejunal
jejunitis
jejunoileal
jejunoileitis
jejunoileostomy
jejunojejunostomy
jejunostomy

jejunum
Jesberg's esophagoscope
junction
    esophagogastric j.
juvenile
    j. polyposis
juxtapyloric
kallidin
kallikrein
Kanagawa phenomenon
Kaposi's sarcoma
kapotmaw. See *capotement.*
karro. See *carreau.*
Kehr's sign
Keller's hypothesis
ketogenesis
kil. See *chyle.*
kim. See *chyme.*
kimas. See *chymase.*
kimifikashun. See *chymification.*
kimorea. See *chymorrhea.*
kinin
Klebsiella
Kock's pouch
Köhlmeier-Degos disease
kolange-. See words beginning
    cholangi-.
kole-. See words beginning *chole-.*
kolera. See *cholera.*
lactase deficiency
lactic
    l. acidosis
lactoferrin
lactose
Ladd's bands
lamina
    l. propria
lamp
    Wood's l.
Lane's band
Langerhans' islet
laparoscopy
laparotomy
laser
lavage
    gastric l.
leiomyoma

leiomyosarcoma
leishmanial
LES – lower esophageal sphincter
Leube's test meal
leukocytosis
leukopenia
Levin tube
ligament
    falciform l.
    gastrohepatic l.
    Treitz's l.
linitis
    l. plastica
liomioma. See *leiomyoma.*
liomiosarkoma. See
    leiomyosarcoma.
lipase
lipid
lipodystrophia
    l. intestinalis
lipodystrophy
    intestinal l.
lipoid
lipolysis
lipoma
lipophagia
    l. granulomatosis
lipoprotein
liposarcoma
lithotripsy
liver
    biliary cirrhotic l.
loop
    afferent l.
    efferent l.
    jejunal l.
    terminal ileal l.
lumen
Lundh test
lymphadenitis
lymphadenopathy
lymphangiectasia
lymphangiectasis
lymphenteritis
lymphogranuloma
    l. venereum
lymphoid

lymphokine
lymphoma
lysozyme
lysyl bradykinin
macrogastria
macrophage
Maffucci's syndrome
magnetic resonance imaging. See *Radiology and Nuclear Medicine* section.
Maixner's cirrhosis
malabsorption
malakoplakia
malignant
Mallory-Weiss syndrome
malnutrition
maneuver
    Hoguet's m.
    Hueter's m.
manometry
mastication
McArthur's method
meal
    barium m.
Meckel's diverticulum
meconium
    m. ileus
    m. peritonitis
medications. See *Drugs and Chemistry* section.
megacolon
megadolichocolon
megaduodenum
megaesophagus
megalobulbus
Meigs' syndrome
melanoma
melanosis
    m. coli
melena
melenemesis
melenic
Menetrier's disease
mesenteric
    m. adenitis
    m. fibromatosis
mesenteriolum

mesenteritis
mesenterium
mesentery
mesoappendicitis
mesoappendix
mesocecum
mesocolon
mesothelioma
metabolism
metaduodenum
metadysentery
metaplasia
metastases
meteorism
method
    McArthur's m.
    Nimeh's m.
Meulengracht's diet
micelle
microgastria
microsporidia
microvillous
midgut
mikso-. See words beginning *myxo-*.
Miller-Abbott tube
mitochondria
mittelschmerz
Morgagni's hernia
motility
Moynihan's test
MRI – magnetic resonance imaging
mucin
mucinous
mucopolysaccharide
mucoprotein
mucormycosis
mucosa
    antral m.
    colonic m.
    duodenal m.
    esophageal m.
    gastric m.
    gastroduodenal m.
    jejunal m.
mucosal

mucous
mucus
Murphy's
  sign
  treatment
muscle
  Treitz's m.
muscularis
  m. mucosa
  m. propria
Myà's disease
myasthenia
  m. gastrica
mycobacteria
Mycobacterium
  M. avium intracellulare
  M. tuberculosis
mycogastritis
mycoplasma
mycosis
  m. intestinalis
myenteric plexus
myenteron
myocelialgia
myocelitis
myoelectric
myoneurosis
  colic m.
  intestinal m.
myotomy
myotonic
myxedema
myxoneurosis
  intestinal m.
myxorrhea
  m. intestinalis
narcotic bowel syndrome
nasobiliary
nasogastric
  n. intubation
  n. suction
National Association of
  Anorexia Nervosa and
  Associated Disorders
natural killer cells
nausea
Necator
  N. americanus

necrotizing
nematode
neoplastic
nephrolithiasis
nerve
  splanchnic n.
  vagus n.
neural
  n. pathway
neurectomy
  gastric n.
neurofibromatosis
neurogastric
neurogenic
neurohumoral
neuron
neuronal
neuropathy
neuropeptide Y
neurotensin
neurotransmitter
neutropenia
nexus
NG – nasogastric
NHL – non-Hodgkin's
  lymphoma
Nimeh's method
nitrate
node
  Troisier's n.
  Virchow's n.
nodular
noncholinergic
nongranulomatous
non-Hodgkin's lymphoma
nonocclusive
  n. intestinal infarction
nonsteroidal anti-inflammatory
  drugs
NPO – nothing by mouth (nulla
  per os)
NSAIDs – nonsteroidal anti-
  inflammatory drugs
nucleation
NUD – non-ulcer dyspepsia
numo-. See words beginning
  pneumo-.

nutrition
oat cell carcinoma
obesity
obstipation
obstruction
      biliary tract o.
      intestinal o.
obstructive
occlusion
occult blood
OCG–oral cholecystogram
Ochsner's
      ring
      treatment
Oddi's sphincter
odditis
odynophagia
Ogilvie's syndrome
oil breakfast
Oldfield's syndrome
oligocholia
oligochylia
oligochymia
oligopepsia
oligosaccharidases
Olympus fiberscope
omentum
omphalocele
oncogene
operation. See *General Surgical Terms* section.
oropharyngeal
oscillatory
Osler's syndrome
osmolality
osmotic
pancreas
      p. divisum
pancreatectomy
pancreatic
pancreaticoduodenal
pancreaticoduodenectomy
pancreaticduodenostomy
pancreaticoenterostomy
pancreaticogastrostomy
pancreaticojejunostomy

pancreatitis
pancreatoduodenectomy
pancreatoduodenostomy
pancreatogenic
pancreatography
pancreatolith
pancreatolithectomy
pancreatolithiasis
pancreatolithotomy
pancreatotomy
pancreolithotomy
pancreopathy
pancreotherapy
Paneth's cells
panniculitis
PAO–peak acid output
papilla
      duodenal p.
papilloma
papillomatous
paracentesis
paracholia
paracolitis
parasitic
parasympathetic
parenteral
parepigastric
parietography
      gastric p.
pars
      p. superior duodeni
Patella's disease
Paterson-Brown-Kelly
      syndrome
Payr's disease
p.c.–after meals (post cibum)
pellagra
pepsin
pepsinogen
peptic
peptide
percutaneous
perforation
      pyloroduodenal p.
perianal
pericecal
pericecitis

pericholangitis
pericholecystic
pericholecystitis
    gaseous p.
pericolic
pericolitis
perigastric
perigastritis
perihepatitis
perimolysis
peristalsis
peristaltic
peristole
peristolic
peritoneal
peritoneoscope
peritoneoscopy
peritoneum
    visceral p.
peritonitis
    bacterial p.
    chylous p.
    coccidioidal p.
    fungal p.
    granulomatous p.
    parasitic p.
    sclerosing p.
    tuberculous p.
perityphlitis
    p. actinomycotica
periumbilical
PET – positron emission
    tomography
petechial
Peutz-Jeghers syndrome
pharynx
phenomenon
    Kanagawa p.
pheochromocytoma
phlegmonous
phytobezoar
pleurocholecystitis
plexus
    enteric p.
    myenteric p.
Plummer-Vinson
    syndrome

pneumatosis
    p. cystoides intestinalis
    p. cystoides intestinorum
    p. intestinales
pneumocholecystitis
pneumocolon
pneumoenteritis
pneumogastric
pneumogastrography
pneumogastroscopy
pneumoperitoneum
pneumoperitonitis
PNI – prognostic nutritional
    index
PO – by mouth (per os)
polycholia
polygastria
polyp
    adenomatous p.
    colonic p.
    hyperplastic p.
    mucosal p.
    neoplastic p.
    non-neoplastic p.
    sessile p.
polyphagia
polypoid
polyposis
    p. coli
    p. gastrica
    p. intestinalis
    p. ventriculi
porta
    p. hepatis
portal
postcibal
postprandial
pouch
    Hartmann's p.
    Kock's p.
p.p. – after meals (postprandial)
prepyloric
procedure
    Puestow-Gillesby p.
proctalgia
    p. fugax
proctitis

proctoclysis
proctocolectomy
proctocolitis
proctologist
proctosigmoidoscopy
projectile
prolapse
prosthesis
    Angelchik's p.
    biliary p.
protoduodenitis
protoduodenum
pruritus
    p. ani
pseudocyst
pseudodiverticula
pseudoleukemia
    p. gastrointestinalis
pseudomegacolon
pseudomyxoma
    p. peritonei
pseudopolyp
pseudosarcoma
psorenteria
psychogenic
PTBD – percutaneous biliary
    drainage
PTC – percutaneous transhepatic
    cholangiography
PU – peptic ulcer
Puestow-Gillesby procedure
purpura
    p. abdominalis
    Henoch's p.
    Schönlein-Henoch p.
pylephlebitis
pyloralgia
pyloric
pyloristenosis
pyloritis
pyloroduodenitis
pyloromyotomy
pyloroplasty
    Finney's p.
    Heineke-Mikulicz p.
pyloroptosis
pylorospasm

pylorotomy
pylorus
pyochezia
pyoderma
    p. gangrenosum
pyogenic
pyrosis
qualitative fecal fat test
quantitative stool collection
radioallergosorbent test
radiography
radioimmunoassay
radioimmunoprecipitation
radionuclide scan
radioscintigraphy
rectoanal
rectosigmoid
rectosphincteric
rectostenosis
rectovaginal
rectum
reflex
    epigastric r.
    gastroileac r.
    ileogastric r.
    myenteric r.
reflux
refractory
regurgitation
rehydration
Reichmann's disease
renninogen
rentgenograhfe. See
    roentgenography.
resection
    antral r.
    gastric r.
retching
retrocecal
retroileal
retrovirus
Riegel's test meal
rigidity
ring
    Cannon's r.
    Ochsner's r.
    Schatzki's r.

roentgenography
rotavirus
roundworm
Roux-en-Y
    anastomosis
    gastrectomy
Rubin's tube
ruga(ae)
    r. gastrica
rugitus
rule
    Goodsall's r.
Sahli's test
saliva
salivary
salmonellosis
Salomon's test
Salzer's test meal
sarcoidosis
sarcoma
    Kaposi's s.
satiety
scan
    CAT (computerized axial
      tomography) s.
    radionuclide s.
Schatzki's ring
Schilling test
schistosomiasis
Schönlein-Henoch purpura
scintigraphy
scirrhous
scleroderma
sclerosing
    s. cholangitis
    s. peritonitis
sclerosis
    gastric s.
scoretemia
secretagogue
secretion
Sengstaken's tube
sepsis
    s. intestinalis
serosa
serosal
serosanguineous

serotonin
shelf
    Blumer's s.
shigellosis
short bowel syndrome
sialoaerophagy
sialorrhea
    s. pancreatica
sigmoid
sigmoidoscope
sigmoidoscopic
sigmoidoscopy
sign
    Kehr's s.
    Murphy's s.
    Trousseau's s.
    Zugsmith's s.
sikwa. See *siqua.*
singultus
    s. gastricus nervosus
Sippy diet
siqua
sirrosis. See *cirrhosis.*
skirus. See *scirrhous.*
sludge
somatostatinoma
sorenterea. See *psorenteria.*
spasm
spastic
    s. colon
sphincter
    esophagogastric s.
    Oddi's s.
    pyloric s.
sphincteroplasty
sphincterotomy
splanchnic
splanchnicectomy
splanchnolith
splanchnologia
splanchnomegaly
splanchnomicria
splanchnopathy
splanchnopleure
splanchnoptosis
splanchnosclerosis
splanchnostaxis

splank-. See words beginning
    splanch-.
spleen
splenic flexure syndrome
splenomegaly
splenopancreatic
splenopathy
splenorrhagia
splenosis
spondylitis
sprue
    tropical s.
Ssabanejew-Frank gastrostomy
stagnant loop syndrome
Stamm's gastrostomy
Staphylococcus
    S. aureus
stasis
    ileal s.
    venous s.
status
    s. gastricus
steatorrhea
steatosis
stenosis
    pyloric s.
steroid
stoma
stomach
    cup-and-spill s.
    leather bottle s.
stomatitis
stool
    s. culture
    s. guaiac
    lienteric s.
strangulation
stratum
    s. longitudinale tunicae
        muscularis coli
    s. longitudinale tunicae
        muscularis intestini
        tenuis
Streptococcus
stricture
subdiaphragmatic
submucosa

subserosal
succus
    s. entericus
    s. gastricus
    s. pancreaticus
succussion
    s. splash
sudo-. See words beginning
    pseudo-.
sulcus
    s. intermedius
suppository
    glycerin s.
swallow
    barium s.
syndrome
    acquired immuno-
        deficiency s.
    afferent loop s.
    Banti's s.
    Barrett's s.
    Behçet's s.
    blind loop s.
    Boerhaave's s.
    Courvoisier-Terrier s.
    Dubin-Johnson s.
    dumping s.
    Ehlers-Danlos s.
    functional bowel s.
    Gardner's s.
    gastrocardiac s.
    Glénard's s.
    glioma-polyposis s.
    Hanot-Rössle s.
    irritable bowel s.
    Maffucci's s.
    malabsorption s.
    Mallory-Weiss s.
    Meigs' s.
    Ogilvie's s.
    Oldfield's s.
    Osler's s.
    Paterson-Brown-Kelly s.
    Peutz-Jeghers s.
    Plummer-Vinson s.
    sump s.
    Turcot s.

syndrome (continued)
    wasting s.
    Wermer's s.
    Zellweger s.
    Zollinger-Ellison s.
system
    portal s.
Szabo's test
tabes
    t. mesenterica
tachygastria
tampon
    Corner's t.
tamponade
    esophageal t.
Tangier disease
tapeworm
telangiectasia
    hemorrhagic t.
telephium
tenesmus
tenia
    t. mesocolica
    t. omentalis
teratoma
test
    acid clearance t.
    acid reflux t.
    alkaline phosphatase t.
    Althausen's t.
    bentiromide t.
    Bernstein's t.
    Carnot's t.
    Congo red t.
    Diagnex blue t.
    D-xylose absorption t.
    fecal fat t.
    glucose absorption t.
    Gmelin's t.
    histamine t.
    hydrogen breath t.
    lactose tolerance t.
    liver function t.
    Lundh t.
    Moynihan's t.
    qualitative fecal fat t.
    radioallergosorbent t.

test (continued)
    Sahli's t.
    Salomon's t.
    Schilling t.
    secretin t.
    secretin-pancreozymin t.
    serum bilirubin t.
    stool guaiac t.
    string t.
    Szabo's t.
    Topfer's t.
    Udránszky's t.
    vitamin A absorption t.
    xylose tolerance t.
test meal
    Boas' t. m.
    Boyden's t. m.
    Dock's t. m.
    Ehrmann's alcohol t. m.
    Ewald's t. m.
    Fischer's t. m.
    Leube's t. m.
    motor t. m.
    Riegel's t. m.
    Salzer's t. m.
Theile's glands
thromboembolic
thrombosis
thymus
tif-. See words beginning
    typh-.
tomography
    computed t.
    computerized axial t.
    positron emission t.
    ultrasonic t.
Topfer's test
torsion
tracheoesophageal
tract
    alimentary t.
    biliary t.
    gastrointestinal t.
transhepatic
treatment
    Murphy's t.
    Ochsner's t.

Treitz's
    arch
    fossa
    hernia
    ligament
    muscle
trichobezoar
Trichuris
    T. trichiura
triplication
Troisier's node
Trousseau's sign
trunci
    t. intestinales
truncus
    t. celiacus
Trypanosoma
    T. cruzi
tube
    Argyle's t.
    Baker's t.
    Blakemore's t.
    Cantor's t.
    duodenal t.
    Levin t.
    Miller-Abbott t.
    nasogastric t.
    Rubin's t.
    Sengstaken's t.
    Wangensteen's t.
tuberculosis
    esophageal t.
    intestinal t.
tumor
    desmoid t.
    islet cell t.
tunica
    t. fibrosa hepatis
    t. fibrosa lienis
    t. mucosa ventriculi
    t. mucosa vesicae felleae
    t. muscularis coli
    t. muscularis intestini
      tenuis
    t. muscularis recti
    t. muscularis ventriculi
    t. serosa

tunica (continued)
    t. serosa coli
    t. serosa hepatis
    t. serosa intestini tenuis
    t. serosa lienis
    t. serosa peritonei
    t. serosa ventriculi
    t. serosa vesicae felleae
Turcot syndrome
typhlenteritis
typhlitis
typhlocholecystitis
typhlocolitis
Udránszky's test
UGI – upper gastrointestinal
ukilea. See *euchylia.*
uklorhidrea. See *euchlorhydria.*
ukolea. See *eucholia.*
ulcer
    Cushing's u.
    duodenal u.
    esophageal u.
    gastric u.
    jejunal u.
    peptic u.
    postbulbar u.
    stercoral u.
    stomal u.
    stress u.
ulceration
ulcerative
ultrasonography
umbilicus
United Ostomy Association
unrest
    peristaltic u.
upepsea. See *eupepsia.*
urease
uremia
uremic
vagal
vagotomy
vagus
varices
    esophageal v.
vasospasm
Vater's ampulla

vermiform
Vibrio cholerae
villi
      colonic v.
      jejunal v.
villus
Virchow's node
viscus
vitamin A absorption test
volvulus
vomit
vomitus
      v. cruentus
      v. matutinus
Wangensteen's tube
wart
      venereal w.
wasting syndrome
web
      esophageal w's
Wermer's syndrome

Whipple's disease
whipworm
Winslow's foramen
Wirsung's duct
Wolf-Schindler gastroscope
Wolman's disease
Wood's lamp
xiphoid
xylose tolerance test
Yersinia
      Y. enteritis
Zellweger syndrome
Zenker's diverticulum
zifoid. See *xiphoid.*
Zollinger-Ellison syndrome
Zugsmith's sign
zymogen
      z. granules
      lab z.
zymosis
      z. gastrica

Immunology

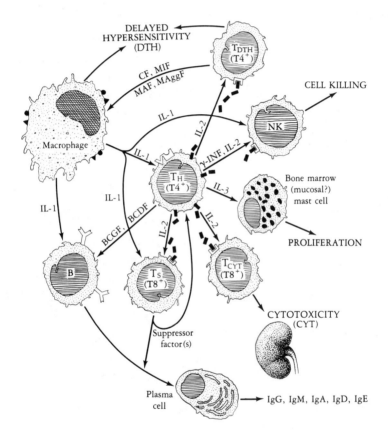

Immunology
With Special Reference to AIDS*

AA – arachidonic acid
AAAF – albumin
    autoagglutinating factor
ABC – antigen-binding capacity
Abelson's murine leukemia
    virus
ABMA – anti-basement
    membrane antibody
ABO blood group
absorption
ABV – Adriamycin, bleomycin,
    and vinblastine
Achilles
acid-fast bacilli
acid-labile alpha interferon
acquired immunodeficiency
    syndrome
acromegaly
ACTH stimulation test
Actinomyces
    A. israelii
actinomycin
acuity
acycloguanosine
acyclovir
ADA – adenosine deaminase
ADCC – antibody dependent
    cytotoxicity
Addison's disease
adenine arabinoside
adenopathy
adenosine deaminase
    deficiency
adenosine monophosphate
adenovirus
adherence

adjuvant
    Freund's a.
adjuvanticity
adrenal
    a. gland
    a. hyperplasia
    a. insufficiency
adrenalitis
Adriamycin
Adson's maneuver
adsorption
AEF – allogeneic effect factor
aerosolized pentamidine
affinity
    a. chromatography
    functional a.
    a. labeling
African green monkey
Ag – antigen
agammaglobulinemia
    Bruton's a.
agar
agarose
agglutin
agglutination
    passive a.
agglutinin
    cold a.
agglutinogen
agranulocytosis
agretope
AHF – antihemophilic factor
AIDS – acquired immuno-
    deficiency syndrome
AIDS related complex
AIDS related virus

---

*Medications and investigational drugs pertinent to AIDS are included in this section.

albinism
albumin
albuminuria
alcaptonuria-ochronosis
alexin
alimentation
alkaline phosphatase
alkalosis
allele
allelic
    a. exclusion
allelomorph
allergen
allergic
    a. bronchopulmonary
      aspergillosis
    a. granulomatosis
    a. orchitis
    a. rhinitis
allergy
allesthesia
alloagglutinin
alloantibody
alloantigen
allogeneic
allograft
allogroup
alloimmune
alloimmunization
allotype
    Am a.
    Gm a.
    Km a.
    latent a.
    nominal a.
    simple a.
    a. suppression
allotypic
    a. determinant
allotypy
alopecia
alpha
    a.-difluoromethyl-
      ornithine
    a.-fetoprotein
    a. heavy chain disease
    a.-helix

alpha (continued)
    a.-interferon
    a.-methyldopa
    a. 1-thymosin
ALS–antilymphocyte serum
ALT–alanine aminotransferase
alveolar
alveolitis
alveolus
AL-721
amebiasis
American Rheumatism
    Association
AmFAR–American
    Foundations for AIDS
    Research
amikacin
amine
amino acid
aminoglycoside
amoxicillin
amphetamine
amphotericin B
ampicillin
amyl nitrite
amyloid
amyloidosis
ANA–antinuclear antibody
anal intercourse
analogue
anamnesis
anamnestic
    a. response
ANA–negative lupus
anaphylatoxin
    a. inactivator
anaphylaxis
anaplastic
anatoxic
anatoxin
Ancobon
androgen
anemia
    autoimmune hemolytic a.
    hemolytic a.
    pernicious a.

anergy
    cutaneous a.
angiitis
    necrotizing a.
angioedema
angiogram
    fluorescein a.
angiomatous
angiosarcoma
anilingus
ankylosing
    a. hyperostosis
    a. spondylitis
anorectal
anorectum
anorexia
anoscopic
ansamycin
antibiotic
antibody
    anti-basement mem-
      brane a.
    anticytoplasmic a.
    antinuclear a.
    anti-peptide a.
    antireceptor a.
    anti–T-cell a.
    autoimmune a.
    autologous a.
    blocking a.
    combining-site a.
    complement-fixing a.
    cross-reacting a.
    cytophilic a.
    a. deficiency syndrome
    a.-dependent cell-
      mediated cytotoxicity
    Donath-Landsteiner a.
    enhancing a.
    a. excess
    heteroclitic a.
    heterogenetic a.
    heterophile a.
    homocytotropic a.
    humoral a.
    hybrid a.
    hybridoma a.

antibody (continued)
    isophil a.
    maternal a.
    monoclonal a.
    neutralizing a.
    non-precipitation a.
    skin-sensitizing a.
    TSH-displacing a.
    warm-reactive a.
anticholinergic
anticoagulant
    circulating a.
anticodon
anti-complementary
anticytoplasmic
antigen
    allogeneic a.
    alum-precipitated a.
    a.-antibody complex
    autologous a.
    bacterial a.
    a.-binding capacity
    carcinoembryonic a.
    Chido-Rodgers a.
    cross-reacting a.
    cryptococcal a.
    differentiation a.
    Duffy's a.
    endogenous a.
    a. excess
    exogenous a.
    Forssman's a.
    H a.
    hepatitis a.
    hepatitis B core a.
    hepatitis B surface a.
    heterogeneic a.
    heterophile a.
    histocompatibility a.
    homologous a.
    human leukocyte a.
    human thymus
      lymphocyte a.
    Ia a.
    idiotypic a.
    isophile a.
    leukocyte common a.

antigen (continued)
    lymphocyte function
      associated a.-1, 2, 3
    Ly a.
    O a.
    oncofetal a.
    organ-specific a.
    Oz a.
    plasma cell a.
    a. presentation
    a. presenting cell
    proliferating cell nuclear a.
    QA a.
    skin-specific
      histocompatibility a.
    surface a.
    synthetic a.
    T-cell a.
    thymus-dependent a.
    thymus-independent a.
    transplantation a.
    tumor-associated a.
    tumor-specific a.
    viral capsid a.
antigenemia
antigenemic
antigenic
    a. antibody lattice
      formation
    a. binding receptor
    a. competition
    a. determinant
    a. drift
    a. modulation
    a. shift
    a. variation
antigenicity
antiglobulin
antiglomerular
antihistamine
anti-histone
anti-immunoglobulin
antilymphocyte serum
antimetabolite
antimicrobial
antimoniotungstate
antimycobacterial

antineoplastic
antiprotozoal
antiretroviral
antiserum
    monospecific a.
    monovalent a.
    multivalent a.
    polyvalent a.
antithymocyte serum
antitoxin
antivenom
antiviral
Antrypol
aorta
aortitis
apatite-associated large joint lysis
APC – antigen-presenting cell
apheresis
aphtha(ae)
apolipoprotein E
appendicular
APPG – aqueous procaine
    penicillin G
ARA – American Rheumatism
    Association
ara-A – adenine arabinoside
ara-C – cytosine arabinoside
arachidonate
arachidonic acid
arachnodactyly
    contractural a.
ARC – AIDS related complex
arcade
    vascular a.
ARS – AIDS related syndrome
arterial blood gases
arteritis
    coronary a.
    Takayasu's a.
    temporal a.
arthralgia
arthritis
    atypical mycobacterial a.
    bacterial a.
    candidal a.
    degenerative a.
    enteropathic a.

arthritis (continued)
    erosive a.
    fungal a.
    gonococcal a.
    gouty a.
    gram-negative bacilli a.
    hemochromatotic a.
    infectious a.
    inflammatory a.
    meningococcal a.
    monoarticular a.
    a. mutilans
    mycobacterial a.
    neuropathic a.
    nongonococcal bacterial a.
    psoriatic a.
    pyogenic a.
    reactive a.
    rheumatoid a.
    rubella a.
    sarcoid a.
    septic a.
    traumatic a.
    tuberculous a.
    viral a.
arthrocentesis
arthrochalasis multiplex
    congenita
arthrography
arthropathy
    Charcot's a.
arthroplasty
arthroscopic
arthroscopy
arthrotomy
Arthus' reaction
ARV–AIDS related virus
ascariasis
Aschoff's cell
ascites
ascorbate
aseptic meningitis
aspartate aminotransferase
aspergilloma
aspergillosis
    allergic bronchopul-
      monary a.

Aspergillus
    A. fumigatus
    A. niger
aspiration
aspirin
assay
    enzyme-linked
      immunosorbent a.
    hemolytic plaque a.
    immunofluorescent a.
    immunoradiometric a.
    Jerne plaque a.
    plaque-forming cell a.
    polyethylene glycol
      precipitation a.
    Raji cell a.
    staphylococcal protein A
      binding a.
association constant
AST–aspartate aminotransferase
asthma
Atabrine
ataxia
    a.-telangiectasia
ATLL–adult T-cell leukemia-
    lymphoma
atopic
atopy
atrophy
    optic a.
    Sudeck's a.
ATS–antithymocyte serum
attenuated
atypical
augmentation
aurotherapy
autoantibody
    anti-platelet a's
autoantigen
autobody
autograft
autoimmune
autoimmunity
autoinfection
autologous
autonomic
autoradiography

autosome
avascular
avidin
avidity
axial
axillary
axis
axoplasmic
azathioprine
azidothymidine
azotemia
AZT – azidothymidine
AZT – 3'-azido-3'-
    deoxythymidine
bacille Calmette-Guérin
bacillus
    Friedländer's b.
Bacillus
    B. amyloliquefaciens H.
bacteremia
bacteria
bacterial
bactericidin
bacterid
bacteriolysin
bacteriolysis
bacteriophage
    lambda b.
Bacterium
Bactrim
Balantidium
    B. coli
basophil
B cell
B cell function
B cell growth factor I, II
B cell mitogen
B cell stimulating factor 1, 2
B lymphocyte
BCG – bacille Calmette-Guérin
BCP – basic calcium phosphate
Behçet's disease
Belganyl
Bence Jones protein
benoxaprofen
beta
    b.-interferon

beta (continued)
    b.-2 microglobulin
    b.-pleated sheet
binding
    b. constant
    b. protein
BFP – biologic false-positive
biopsy
biosynthesis
biotin
Birbeck's granule
bisexual
bivalency
    monogamous b.
bivalent
blast
    b. transformation
blastogenesis
blastogenic
Blastomyces
    B. dermatitidis
blastomycosis
Blenoxane
bleomycin
blepharoconjunctivitis
blood groups
    ABO
    Duffy
    Kell-Cellano
    Kidd
    Lutheran
    MNSs
    Rh
blot test
blotting
    Northern b.
    Southern b.
    Western b.
body
    Cowdry type A
        intranuclear inclusion
        b's
    jugular's b's
    Russell's b's
Bombay phenotype
bone marrow suppression
bradykinin

breeding
    random b.
bronchial
bronchiolitis
bronchoalveolar
    b. lavage
bronchoscopy
bronchovascular
brucellosis
Bruton's agammaglobulinemia
bullous
Burkitt-like lymphoma
Burkitt's lymphoma
bursa
bursitis
    anserine b.
    iliopectineal b.
    ischiogluteal b.
    prepatellar b.
    septic b.
    traumatic b.
    trochanteric b.
Buschke-Löwenstein tumor
busulfan
butyl nitrite
C1 inhibitor
C1, 2, 3, 4, 5, 6, 6–7, 7, 8, 9
    deficiency
C3a, C5a receptor
cachectin
calcification
calcinosis
calcitonin
CALLA – common acute
    lymphocytic leukemia
    antigen
Calmette-Guérin bacille
Campylobacter
    C. cinaedi
    C. fennelliae
    C. fetus enteritis
campylobacteriosis
cancer
    testicular c.
Candida
    C. albicans
    C. proctitis

Candida (continued)
    C. stomatitis
candidal
candidemia
candidiasis
    bronchial c.
    cutaneous c.
    pulmonary c.
Caner-Decker syndrome
Caplan's syndrome
capping
capsule
    articular c.
capsulitis
    adhesive c.
carcinoid
carcinoma
    squamous cell c.
cardiomegaly
cardiomyopathy
cardiopulmonary
cardiovascular
carpometacarpal
cartilage
    articular c.
catabolic
catabolism
catheter
    indwelling c.
catheterization
CD – cluster of differentiation
CDC – Centers for Disease
    Control
CDR – complementarity-
    determining region
CEA – carcinoembryonic antigen
ceftriaxone
cell
    accessory c.
    adherent c.
    antigen-presenting c.
    Aschoff's c.
    B c.
    blast c.
    bone marrow c.
    c.-mediated immunity
    cytotoxic c.

cell (continued)
> dendritic epidermal c.
> enterochromaffin c.
> epithelioid c.
> follicular dendritic c.
> helper c.
> hematopoietic stem c.
> homozygous typing c.
> hybrid c.
> hyperchromatic c.
> immunologically
>> competent c.
> inclu-
>> sion c.
> inducer c.
> intracytoplasmic inclu-
>> sion c.
> K c.
> killer c.
> Kupffer's c.
> Langerhans' c.
> LE c.
> Lyl B c.
> lymphoreticular c.
> M c.
> mast c.
> maturation B c.
> mediator c.
> mononuclear c.
> myeloid c.
> natural killer c.
> non-adherent c.
> null c.
> phagocytic c.
> plaque-forming c.
> plasma c.
> pre-B c.
> Reed-Sternberg giant c.
> sinusoidal endothelial c.
> spindle-shaped c.
> stem c.
> suppressor c.
> T c.
> T4 c.
> T8 c.
> target c.

cell (continued)
> T-cytotoxic c.
> T-suppressor c.
> thymic epithelial c.
> thymus nurse c.
> veiled c.
> white c's

cell-mediated immune response
cellular
> c. immune deficiency
> c. immunity

cellularity
centimorgan
Cephalosporium
> *C. granulomatis*

cerebrospinal fluid
cervicitis
CFU-S – colony-forming unit –
> spleen

Chagas' disease
challenge
chancre
Charcot's arthropathy
Charcot-Leyden crystal
Charcot-like arthropathy
Chédiak-Higashi syndrome
chemiluminescence
chemotactic
chemotaxis
chemotherapeutic
chemotherapy
Chido-Rodgers antigen
chimera
chimerism
Chlamydia
> *C. psittaci*
> *C. trachomatis*

chlamydial
chlorambucil
chloramphenicol
chlorpromazine
cholangitis
> sclerosing c.

cholecystitis
cholesterol

chondritis
    auricular c.
chondrocalcinosis
chondrocyte
chondromalacia
chorea
    Sydenham's c.
chorioamnionitis
choriomeningitis
chorioretinitis
choroid
choroidal
chromosome
    c. walking
chrysotherapy
Churg-Strauss syndrome
chymotrypsin
ciliary
cimetidine
cineradiography
cirrhosis
    Laennec's c.
cisplatin
cisterna chyli
clathrin
Cleveland procedure
clindamycin
CLL-chronic lymphocytic
    leukemia
clofazimine
clonal
clone
clonotypic
clostridia
Clostridium
    C. difficile
clotrimazole
clotting factor
clubbing
cM – centimorgan
CMR – carpometacarpal ratio
CMV – cytomegalovirus
CNS – central nervous system
coagulation
coalesce
cocaine

co-capping
coccidian protozoan
Coccidioides
    C. immitis
coccidioidin
coccidioidomycosis
    primary extrapul-
    monary c.
coccyx
cocultivation
co-dominance
codon
cofactors
cognate
    c. interaction
    c. recognition
cohesive end
coitus
colchicine
colitis
    amebic c.
    ulcerative c.
collagen
    intimal c.
collagenase
collagenolysis
colon
colonization
    jejunal c.
colony-stimulating factor
colorectal
column
    Morgagni's c.
complement
    c. deficiency
    c. deviation
    c. fixation
    c. level
    c.-mediated anaphylaxis
    c. receptor 1,2,3,4
    c. sequence
    c. test
complementarity-determining
    region
complementation

complex
    Golgi's c.
complotype
Compound Q
Compound S
concanavalin A
concentrate
    lyophilized c.
concomitant
condyloma
    c. acuminatum
    c. latum
conformation
conformational
    c. determinant
congenic
congenital
conglutination
conglutinin
conjunctiva
    bulbar c.
    ocular c.
    palpebral c.
    tunica c.
conjunctival
conjunctivitis
contaminated
contamination
contrasuppression
Coombs' test
coproantibody
corneal
coronary
corpuscle
    Hassall's c.
corticosteroid
Corynebacterium
    C. infantisepticum
    C. parvulum
cosmid
costochondritis
costoclavicular
co-trimoxazole
cotton wool spots
Cowdry type A intranuclear
    inclusion bodies
CPK – creatine phosphokinase

CPPD – calcium pyrophosphate
    dihydrate
C-reactive protein
CREST – *c*alcinosis, *R*aynaud's
    phenomenon, *e*sophageal
    dysfunction, *s*clerodactyly,
    and *t*elangiectasia
CREST syndrome
criteria
    Jones c.
Crithidia
    C. lucilliae
Crohn's disease
cromolyn
CRP – C-reactive protein
cryoglobulin
cryoglobulinemia
cryoprecipitate
cryopreserved
cryotherapy
crypt
    anal c's
cryptococcal
    c. meningitis
    c. meningoencephalitis
cryptococcosis
Cryptococcus
    C. neoformans
cryptosporidial
cryptosporidiosis
    biliary c.
Cryptosporidium
    C. listeria
crystal
    Charcot-Leyden c.
crystalluria
CSF – cerebrospinal fluid
    colony stimulating factor
CT – computerized tomography
C-type retrovirus
cul-de-sac
cunnilingus
Cushing's syndrome
cutaneous anergy
cutis laxa
CVI – common variable
    immunodeficiency

cyclobenzaprine
cycloheximide
cyclophosphamide
cycloserine
cyclosporin A
cyclosporine
cysticercosis
cystitis
cytochalasin
    c. B
cytoid
cytokine
cytolysin
cytolytic
cytomegalic
cytomegalovirus
cytometry
    flow c.
cytopathic
cytopenia
cytosine arabinoside
cytoskeleton
cytotoxic
    c. T lymphocyte
    c. T lymphocyte precursor
cytotoxicity
cytotoxic-suppressor
cytotropic
DAF – decay antibody-
   accelerating factor
danazol
Danysz's phenomenon
dapsone
Daraprim
DDAVP – desamino-D-arginine
   vasopressin
DDCT – dideoxycytidine
debilitating
DEC – dendritic epidermal cell
decubitus
deficiency
    acquired C1 inhibitor d.
    adenosine deaminase d.
    C1, 2, 3, 4, 5, 6, 6 – 7, 7,
      8, 9 d.
    cytochrome b d.
    Factor D, H, I d.

deficiency (continued)
    kappa chain d.
    leukocyte adhesion d.
    tyrosine aminotrans-
      ferase d.
    X-linked hypogamma-
      globulinemia with
      growth hormone d.
deformity
    swan neck d.
degradation
degranulation
delta
    d. antigen
    d. hepatitis
demarcation
dementia complex
demyelinated
demyelinating
dendritic
dengue
dentinogenesis
    d. imperfecta
deoxy-D-glucose
deoxyribonuclease
deoxyribonucleic acid
depletion
de Quervain's
    syndrome
    tenosynovitis
dermatitis
    atopic d.
    d. herpetiformis
dermatomal herpes zoster
dermatomyositis
dermatophytosis
dermis
desensitization
desetope
detachment
determinant
    antigenic d.
    conformational d.
    hidden d.
    immunogenic d.
    isoallotypic d.
    isotypic d.

determinant (continued)
 Kern's isotypic d.
 Km allotypic d.
 Mcg isotypic d.
 Oz isotypic d.
 sequential d.
detoxification
dextran
DFMO – difluoro-
 methylornithine
DGI – disseminated gonococcal
 infection
DHPG – 9-[(1,3-dihydroxy-
 2-propoxy)methyl]guanine
diabetes
 d. mellitus
dialysis
diarrhea
diazotization
Dick test
dideoxycytidine
differentiated
differentiation
 thymus cell d.
difluoromethylornithine
DiGeorge's syndrome
digoxin
dihydroxypropoxymethylguanine
dilatation
 sinusoidal d.
dinitrochlorobenzene
dinitrophenol
diphtheroid
DIPJ – distal interphalangeal joint
diploid
diplopia
disease
 Addison's d.
 alpha chain d.
 autoimmune d.
 Behçet's d.
 celiac d.
 Chagas' d.
 connective tissue d.
 Crohn's d.
 cytomegalic inclusion d.
 dense-deposit d.

disease (continued)
 endocrine d.
 Forestier's d.
 gamma heavy chain d.
 Gaucher's d.
 graft-versus-host d.
 Graves' d.
 heavy chain d.
 Hodgkin's d.
 immunodeficiency d.
 inflammatory bowel d.
 Jakob-Creutzfeldt d.
 Kashin-Beck d.
 Kawasaki d.
 Kellgren's d.
 Legg-Calvé-Perthes d.
 Leiner's d.
 Lyme d.
 lysosomal storage d.
 mixed connective tissue d.
 mu heavy chain d.
 Osgood-Schlatter d.
 Paget's d.
 Parkinson's d.
 runt d.
 sickle cell d.
 Still's d.
 von Willebrand's d.
 wasting d.
 Whipple's d.
 Wilson's d.
disequilibrium
 linkage d.
DISH – diffuse idiopathic skeletal
 hyperostosis
diskitis
diskography
disseminated
 d. candidiasis
 d. cytomegalovirus
dissemination
dissociation
 d. constant
distribution
 Sips d.
DJD – degenerative joint disease
DNA – deoxyribonucleic acid

DNA chain terminator
DNA histone
DNA ligase
DNA nucleotidylexotransferase
DNA polymerase
DNA virus
DNCB—dinitrochlorobenzene
domain
Donath-Landsteiner antibody
doxorubicin
doxycycline
D-penicillamine
DPVNS–diffuse pigmented
    villonodular synovitis
DTH–delayed-type
    hypersensitivity
duct
        thoracic d.
Duffy
        antigen
        blood group
Duncan's syndrome
D-xylose absorption
dysfunction
        myocardial d.
        sensorineural d.
dysgammaglobulinemia
dysgenesis
        reticular d.
dysphagia
dyspnea
E, EA, EAC rosette
EAE–experimental allergic
    encephalomyelitis
eburnation
EBV–Epstein-Barr virus
ECF–eosinophil chemotactic
    factor
ECF-A–eosinophil chemotactic
    factor of anaphylaxis
Echinococcus
eczema
edathamil
edema
        hereditary angioneurotic e.
edematous

effect
        Lyon's e.
effusion
        pleural e.
Ehlers-Danlos syndrome
EIA–enzyme immunoassay
eicosanoid
ejaculation
electroimmunodiffusion
electromyography
electron-microscopic
electrophoresis
electroporation
electrotransfer test
ELISA–enzyme-linked
    immunosorbent assay
emperic
emperipolesis
empyema
en coup de sabre
encapsulated
encephalitis
encephalomyelitis
        disseminated e.
encephalopathy
encysted
endemic
endocarditis
        bacterial e.
        Libman-Sacks e.
endocrine
endocytosis
endogenous
Endolimax
        E. nana
endonuclease
endoscopic
endoscopy
endosome
endothelial
endotoxic
endotoxin
enhancement
enhancer
Entamoeba
        E. histolytica
enteric

enteritis
    regional e.
enterobiliary
Enterobius
    E. vermicularis
enterocolitis
enteropathy
    gluten-sensitive e.
entropion
Envacor test
enzyme
eosinophil
eosinophilia
eosinophilic
    e. exudates
epicondylitis
epidemiology
epidermis
epipodophyllotoxin
epinephrine
epiphysitis
epithelial
epithelialize
epitope
Epstein-Barr virus
equilibrium
    e. constant
    e. dialysis
equivalence
ER – endoplasmic reticulum
eruption
    Kaposi's varicelliform e.
erythema
    e. chronicum migrans
    e. marginatum
    e. multiforme
    e. nodosum
erythematous
erythroblastosis
    e. fetalis
erythrocyte
Escherichia
    E. coli
esophageal
esophagitis
    Candida e.
    herpetic e.
esophagogram

esophagram
esotoxin
ESR – erythrocyte sedimentation
    rate
estradiol
estrogen
ETAF – epithelial thymic-
    activating factor
ethambutol
ethionamide
etiology
etoposide
euglobulin
euthanasia
exanthem
exanthematous
excystation
exocytosis
exogenous
exon
exophytic
exotoxin
expectorate
extrahepatic
extrainguinal
extralymphatic
extranodal
extraocular
extrapulmonary
    e. tuberculosis
extrathoracic
extravasation
exudate
FACS – fluorescence-activated
    cell sorting
facteur thymique serique
factor
    albumin autoagglu-
      tinating f.
    allogeneic effect f.
    angiogenesis f.
    colony stimulating f.
    decay accelerating f.
    D, H, I deficiency f.
    eosinophil chemotactic f.
    epithelial thymic-
      activating f.

factor (continued)
    F. I, II, III, IV, V, VII,
       VIII, IX, X, XI, XII,
       XIII
    Hageman's f.
    hepatocyte stimulating f.
    leukocyte inhibitory f.
    lymphocyte-activating f.
    macrophage-activating f.
    migration inhibitory f.
    nephritic f.
    neutrophil chemotactic f.
    osteoclast-activating f.
    platelet-activating f.
    T-cell growth f.
    thymus-replacing f.
    tumor necrosis f.
FAIDS – feline AIDS
familial
fasciitis
fatigue
fecal fat quantitation
feces
fellatio
Felty's syndrome
FeLV – feline leukemia virus
ferritin
fever
    rheumatic f.
FIA – fluoroimmunoassay
fibroblast
fibroma
fibromyalgia
fibronectin
fibrosarcoma
fibrosis
fibrositis
Fiessinger-Leroy syndrome
FIGE – field inversion gel
    electrophoresis
filariform larvae
fingerprinting
Fisher-Race theory
Fisher's exact test
fissure
fisting
fistula

flocculation
flora
flucytosine
fluorescein
    f. isothiocyanate
fluorescence
    f.-activated cell sorter
    f. enhancement
    f. quenching
fluorescent
fluorocytosine
fluorography
fluoroimmunoassay
FMF – familial Mediterranean
    fever
foci
folinic acid
follicle
follicular
footprinting
Forestier's disease
"formes frustes"
formyl-methionyl-leucyl-
    phenylalanine
Forssman's antigen
foscarnet
Fourneau 309
fragellin
fragment
    Fab f.
    F (ab')$_2$ f.
    Fabc f.
    Facb f.
    Fb f.
    Fc f.
    Fv f.
    Klenow's f.
    restriction f.
    Spengler's f.
Frei test
Freund's adjuvant
friability
Friedländer's
    bacillus
    pneumonia
fulminant
funduscopic

fungal
fungemia
fungemic
Fungizone
fungus
  opportunistic f.
  pathogenic f.
  subcutaneous f.
  systemic f.
furazolidone
fusion
  protoplast f.
GAG – glycosaminoglycan
gait
  Trendelenburg's g.
gallium
  g. scanning
gametocyte
gamma
  g. globulin
  g. interferon
gammopathy
  monoclonal g.
  polyclonal g.
ganciclovir
ganglia
gastritis
  syphilitic g.
gastroenteritis
gastrointestinal
Gaucher's disease
gene
  g. bank
  g. code
  env g.
  gag g.
  g. mapping
  pol g.
  tat g.
genetic
  g. code
genome
genotype
Germanin
germ-line theory
Giardia
  G. lamblia

giardiasis
gingival
gingivitis
  gonococcal g.
gliotic
GLNS – gay lymph node
  syndrome
globulin
glomerular
glomerulonephritis
  acute post-streptococcal g.
glomerulosclerosis
glucocorticoid
glucosidase
gluten
glycoprotein
Gm allotype
GM-CSF – granulocyte-
  macrophage colony-
  stimulating factor
gold therapy
Golgi's complex
gonococcemia
gonorrhea
  Neisseria g.
  oropharyngeal g.
  pharyngeal g.
  rectal g.
Goodpasture's syndrome
Good's syndrome
Gottron's papule
gout
  tophaceous g.
gradient
graft
  g. rejection
  g.-versus-host disease
Gram-Weigert staining
granule
  Birbeck's g.
granulocyte
granulocytopenia
granuloma
granulomatosis
  allergic g.
  lymphomatoid g.
  Wegener's g.

granulomatous
Graves' disease
GRID – gay-related
    immunodeficiency disease
griseofulvin
group
        Kell-Cellano blood g.
        Kidd blood g.
        Lutheran blood g.
Guillain-Barré syndrome
GVH – graft-versus-host
H antigen
HA – hyaluronic acid
Haemate-P
Haemophilus
        H. aegyptius
        H. ducreyi
        H. gallinarum
        H. influenzae
Hageman's factor
hairpin loop
hairy leukoplakia
Haitian immigration
hallux valgus
Ham test
haploid
haplotype
hapten
Hashimoto's thyroiditis
Hassall's corpuscle
HAT medium
HBcAg – hepatitis B core antigen
HBsAg – hepatitis B surface
    antigen
Heaf test
Heberden's node
helminth
helminthic
helper cells
helper-suppressor cell ratio
hemagglutination
      passive h.
hemagglutinin
hemangioma
hemarthritis
hematochezia
hematologic

hematological
hematopoietic
hematoxylin-eosin staining
hemianopsia
hemiparesis
hemispheric
hemochromatosis
hemochromatotic
hemocystinuria
hemocytoblast
hemodialysis
hemodynamic
hemoglobinuria
      paroxysmal cold h.
      paroxysmal nocturnal h.
hemolysin
hemolysis
      passive h.
hemolytic
      h. anemia
hemophilia
hemophiliac
hemorrhage
hemorrhoid
hemosiderosis
Henoch-Schönlein purpura
heparin
hepatic
hepatitis
      h. B antigen
      delta h.
      infectious h.
      non-A h.
      non-B h.
      peliosis h.
      serum h.
      syphilitic h.
      type A, type B h.
      viral h.
hepatobiliary
hepatocyte
hepatomegaly
hepatosplenomegaly
heredity
heredofamilial
heritable
herniation

heroin
herpes
    anorectal h.
    h. genitalis
    pharyngeal h.
    h. simplex
    h. virus
    h. zoster
    h. zoster ophthalmicus
Herpesvirus
    H. hominis
    H. simiae
herpetic
    h. proctitis
    h. whitlow
herpetiformis
    dermatitis h.
heterocliticity
heterodimer
heteroduplex
heterogeneity
heterograft
heterokaryon
heterologous
heterophile
heterosexual
heterotopic
heterozygous
Hexamita
Heymann's nephritis
hidradenitis
    suppurative h.
high-zone tolerance
hinge region
histaminase
histamine
histiocyte
histiocytic
histochemical
histocompatibility
histogenesis
histologic
histone
histopathology
Histoplasma
    H. capsulatum

histoplasmin
histoplasmoma
histoplasmosis
    disseminated h.
    ocular h.
histotope
HIV – human immunodeficiency
    virus
HIVAGEN test
HLA – human leukocyte antigen
HOA – hypertrophic
    osteoarthroscopy
hoarseness
Hodgkin's disease
homocystinuria
homodimer
homograft
homologous
homology unit
homonymous
    h. hemianopsia
homosexual
homosexuality
homotransplantation
homozygous
hormone
    thymic h.
horror autotoxicus
HPA-23 (antimonium tungstate)
HSV – herpes simplex virus
HTC – homozygous typing cell
HTLA – human thymus
    lymphocyte antigen
HTLV – human T-cell leukemia
    virus
    human T-cell lympho-
    tropic virus
HTLV-MA – HTLV membrane
    antigen
HTLV provirus
HTLV I, II, III, IV
human immunodeficiency virus
humoral
    h. immune response
    h. immunity
hyaline

hybridization
    DNA h.
    in situ h.
hybridoma
    B lymphocyte h.
    T lymphocyte h.
hydralazine
hydrocortisone
hydroperoxyeicosatetraenoic acid
hydroxyapatite
hydroxychloroquine
5-hydroxytryptamine
hydroxyzine
Hymenolepis
    H. fraterna
    H. nana
hyperalimentation
hypercellularity
hypercholesterolemia
hyperemia
    conjunctival h.
hyperemic
hyperesthesia
hypergammaglobulinemia
hyperglobulinemia
hyperimmune
    h. globulin
hyperimmunization
hyperimmunoglobulinemia E
hyperkalemia
hyperlipoproteinemia
hypermobility
hyperostosis
hyperparathyroidism
hyperpigmentation
hyperplasia
    mesangial h.
hypersensitivity
hypertension
hypertriglyceridemia
hypertrophic
hyperuricemia
hypervariable
hypocellular
hypocellularity
hypocomplementemia

hypogammaglobulinemia
hypoglycemia
hypokalemia
hyponatremia
hypoparathyroidism
hypopigmentation
hypoplasia
hyposensitization
hyposplenism
hypotension
hypothesis
    unitarian h.
hypothyroidism
hypouricemia
hypoxanthine
hypoxemia
HZV – herpes zoster virus
I invariant
Ia antigen
IBD – inflammatory bowel
    disease
ibuprofen
IC – immune complex
IDDM – insulin-dependent
    diabetes mellitus
idiopathic
    i. thrombocytopenic
    purpura
idiotope
idiotype
idiotypic
idoxuridine
IDU – 2′-deoxy-5-iodouridine
IEP – immunoelectrophoresis
IF – immunofluorescence
IFA – immunofluorescent assay
IFN – interferon
IgA – gamma A immunoglobulin
IgD – gamma D immunoglobulin
IgE – gamma E immunoglobulin
IgG – gamma G immunoglobulin
IgM – gamma M
    immunoglobulin
IgM response
IgY – gamma Y immunoglobulin
ileitis

IL-1 – interleukin-1
IL-2 – interleukin-2
IL-3 – interleukin-3
immune
    i. deviation
    i. elimination
    i. hemolysis
    i. interferon
    i. neutropenia
    i. paralysis
    i. serum
    i. serum globulin
    i. suppression
    i. surveillance
immunity
    herd i.
    humoral i.
    passive i.
immunization
    passive i.
    prophylactic i.
immunoassay
    solid-phase i.
immunobiology
immunoblastic
immunoblotting
immunochemical
immunochemistry
immunocompetence
immunocompetency
immunocompetent
immunocompromised
immunoconglutination
immunocyte
immunodeficiency
    cellular i.
    human i.
    primary i.
    X-linked hyper-IgM i.
immunodeficient
immunodepression
immunodiffusion
    radial i.
immunodominant
immunoelectrophoresis
    rocket i.
immunofixation

immunofluorescence
immunofluorescent
immunogen
immunogenetics
immunogenic
immunogenicity
immunoglobulin
    i. A, D, E, G, M, Y
    i. alpha chain
    i. class
    i. class switching
    i. delta chain
    i. domain
    i. epsilon chain
    i. fold
    i. gamma chain
    i. gene rearrangement
    i. genes
    i. heavy chain
    i. kappa chain
    i. lambda chain
    i. light chain
    membrane i.
    monoclonal i.
    i. mu chain
    secreted i.
    i. subclass
    i. superfamily
immunohistochemical
immunohistologic
immunoincompetent
immunologic
    i. imbalance
    i. memory
    i. surveillance
immunological
immunology
immunomodulary
immunomodulating
immunomodulation
immunoparasitology
immunoperoxidase staining
immunophysiology
immunopotentiation
immunoprophylaxis
immunoradiometric
immunoregulation

immunoregulatory
immunostimulant
immunosuppressed
immunosuppression
immunosuppressive
immunotherapy
immunotoxicology
immunotoxin
immunovar
Imodium
impetigo
impotence
IMREG-1
inanition
inbred strain
inbreeding
inclusion
    nuclear i's
incubation
indium
indomethacin
induration
infarction
infection
    bacterial i.
    cryptosporidial i.
    "gay bowel i."
    hepatitis B virus i.
    herpes simplex i.
    herpes zoster i.
    metazoan i.
    nosocomial i.
    opportunistic i.
    parasitic i.
    perinatal i.
    protozoan i.
    pyogenic i.
    viral i.
infectious
    i. mononucleosis
inferotemporal
infiltrates
infiltration
    mesentery i.
    parenchymal i.
inflammation
inflammatory

influenza
INH – isonicotine hydrazine
inhibitor
    C1 i.
inoculation
inoculum
inosine pranobex
in situ
    i.s. hybridization
integrin family
intercellular
interferon
    acid-labile alpha i.
    i.-alpha
    i.-beta
    i.-gamma
interfollicular
interleukin 1, 2, 3, 4, 5, 6
interphalangeal
interstitial
intervening sequence
intervertebral
intestinal
intracranial
intracytoplasmic inclusion cell
intrahepatic
intranuclear
intraocular
intraorbital
intrauterine
intravascular
intravenous
intravenously
intrinsic
    i. affinity
    i. association constant
intron
Intron-A
intussusception
in utero
invariant
    i. chain
    I i.
invasive
inversion
in vitro
in vivo

iodoquinol
iproniazid
iridocyclitis
iritis
irradiation
ischemia
ischemic
iscom
ISG – immune serum globulin
isoagglutinin
isoallotypic determinant
isoantibody
isoantigen
isoelectric
 i. focusing
 i. point
isogeneic
isograft
isohemagglutinin
isohydric
isoimmunization
isoniazid
Isoprinosine
isoproterenol
isoschizomer
Isospora
 I. belli
isosporiasis
isotope
isotype
isotypic
Ixodes
 I. dammini
JA – juvenile arthritis
Jacob-Creutzfeldt disease
jaundice
Jerne plaque assay
joint
 cricoarytenoid j.
 manubriosternal j.
 metacarpophalangeal j.
 sacroiliac j.
 sternoclavicular j.
 temporomandibular j.
 uncovertebral j.
Jones' criteria
Jones-Mote reaction

JRA – juvenile rheumatoid
 arthritis
jugular
junctional
juvenile
 j. onset diabetes
 j. rheumatoid arthritis
kala-azar
kallikrein
Kaposi's
 K. sarcoma
 K. varicelliform eruption
karyotype
Kashin-Beck disease
Kauffmann-White scheme
Kawasaki disease
K cell
Kell-Cellano blood group
Kellgren's disease
keratitis
 dendritic k.
keratoconjunctivitis
 k. sicca
Kern's isotypic determinant
ketoconazole
Kidd blood group
killer cells
kilobase
kinin
kininogen
Klebsiella
 K. pneumoniae
Klenow's fragment
KLH – keyhole limpet
 hemocyanin
Klippel-Trenaunay syndrome
Km allotype
Km allotypic determinant
KS – Kaposi's sarcoma
Kupffer's cell
Kveim reaction
kwashiorkor
kyphoscoliosis
kyphosis
 Scheuermann's juvenile k.
LAD – leukocyte adhesion
 deficiency

Laennec's cirrhosis
LAF – lymphocyte-activating
    factor
lagophthalmos
lambda
        l. bacteriophage
lamina
Langerhans' cell
larva
        l. migrans
laryngeal
larynx
LAS – lymphadenopathy
    syndrome
LATS – long-acting thyroid
    stimulator
lattice theory
LAV – lymphadenopathy-
    associated virus
lavage
LCM – lymphocytic
    choriomeningitis
LDL – low-density lipoprotein
LE cell
lectin
Legg-Calvé-Perthes disease
Legionella pneumophila
    pneumonia
Leiner's disease
Leishmania
leishmaniasis
lepromatous leprosy
lepromin
leprosy
lesion
        cavitary pulmonary l.
Leu-2
Leu-3
Leu-7
Leu-11
leukemia
        acute lymphoblastic l.
        chronic lymphocytic l.
        hairy cell l.
        lymphocytic l.
        myelogenous l.
        myeloid l.

leukemia (continued)
        myelomonocytic l.
leukoagglutinin
leukocyte
        l. inhibitory factor
        passenger l's
        polymorphonuclear l's
leukocytoclastic
leukocytosis
leukoencephalopathy
leukopenia
leukoplakia
        hairy l.
leukotriene
levamisole
LGV – lymphogranuloma
    venereum
Libman-Sacks endocarditis
LIF – leukocyte inhibiting factor
ligand
LIP – lymphocytic interstitial
    pneumonitis
lipodystrophy
lipopolysaccharide
lipoprotein
liposome
lipoxygenase
Listeria
        L. monocytogenes
listeriosis
LM 427
locus
        minor histocompatibility l.
        T l.
Lomotil
low-zone tolerance
lumbar puncture
lumbosacral
lumen
luminal
lupus
        discoid l.
        l. erythematosus
        l. nephritis
Lutheran blood group
Ly antigen
Lyl B cell

Lyme disease
lymph
    l. node
    l. nodule
lymphadenitis
lymphadenopathy
lymphatic
lymphoblast
lymphocyte
    l.-activating factor
    l. recirculation
    suppressor T l.
    l. transformation
lymphocytic
lymphocytopenia
lymphocytosis
lymphocytotoxic
lymphocytotropic
lymphoepithelial
lymphogranuloma
    l. venereum
lymphoid
lymphokine
lymphoma
    adult T-cell leukemia l.
    Burkitt-like l.
    Burkitt's l.
    follicular l.
    histiocytic l.
    large-cell l.
    lymphoblastic l.
    nodular l.
    non-Hodgkin's l.
lymphomatosis
lymphopenia
lymphoproliferative
lymphoreticular
lymphotoxin
lymphotropic
Lyon's effect
lyophilized
lysin
lysis
    reactive l.
lysogen
lysosomal
lysosome

lysozyme
lysylbradykinin
MAC–membrane attack
    complex
macaques
macroglobulin
macroglobulinemia
    Waldenström's m.
macrophage
    activated m.
    alveolar m.
    suppressor m.
macula
macular
maculopapular
maculopathy
    ischemic m.
MAF–macrophage-activating
    factor
malabsorption
malaise
malakoplakia
malaria
malignancy
malignant
malnutrition
maneuver
    Adson's m.
Mantoux test
marasmus
marfanoid hypermobility
    syndrome
Marfan's syndrome
margination
marijuana
Mason Pfizer monkey virus
Masugi nephritis
Matuhasi-Ogata phenomenon
maturation
M cell
Mcg isotypic determinant
McLeod's phenotype
MCTD–mixed connective tissue
    disease
MDP–muramyl dipeptide
measles
mebendazole

mediastinal
medium
    HAT m.
megakaryocyte
melanoma
    multiple m.
melphalan
membrane
    basement m.
meninges
meningitides
meningitis
    cryptococcal m.
    lymphocytic m.
    mycobacterial m.
meningococcal
meningococci
meningococcus
meningoencephalitis
meniscectomy
meniscus
menstruation
6-mercaptopurine
mescaline
mesenteric
metabolic
metaproterenol
metastatic
metazoa
methaqualone
methenamine silver staining
method
    Ouchterlony m.
    Wintrobe's m.
methotrexate
methyltestosterone
metronidazole
MG – myasthenia gravis
MHC – major histocompatibility
    complex
mice
    New Zealand m.
miconazole
microaneurysm
microbicidal
microcephalic
microecology

microglia
microglobulin B$_2$
microimmunofluorescent test
microscopy
    electron m.
Microsulfon
microvascular
microvasculopathy
MIF – migration inhibitory factor
minocycline
mithramycin
mitogen
    pokeweed m.
    T-cell m's
mitogenic
mitogenicity
MLC – mixed lymphocyte culture
MLR – mixed lymphocyte
    reaction
MNSs blood group
modulation
molecular
    m. hybridization probe
    m. mimicry
molecule
    T-4 m.
molluscum
    m. bodies
    m. contagiosum
monarthritis
monoclonal
monocyte
monocyte-macrophage
monocytopenia
monocytosis
monokine
mononuclear
mononucleosis
    infectious m.
monovalent
Moranyl
Moraxella
    M. bovis
    M. liquefaciens
Morgagni's column
morphea
Morton's neuroma

motility
MPGN – membrano-
 proliferative
 glomerulonephritis
MPMV – Mason Pfizer monkey
 virus
MPO – myeloperoxidase
MRI – magnetic resonance
 imaging
mucicarmine staining
mucocutaneous
    m. candidiasis
    m. herpes simplex
mucopolysaccharides
mucopurulent
mucosal
mucous
multifactorial
multifocal
multinucleated
multivalent
multivesicular
mumps
murine
    m. T cell phenotype
musculoskeletal
mutant
mutation
    somatic m.
myalgia
myasthenia gravis
Mycelex
mycobacteria
mycobacterial
mycobacteriosis
Mycobacterium
    M. avium-intracellulare
    M. bovis
    M. chelonei
    M. fortuitum
    M. haemophilum
    M. kansasii
    M. scrofulaceum
    M. tuberculosis
    M. ulcerans

Mycoplasma
    M. hominis
mycoplasmal
Mycostatin
mycotic
myelocyte
myelography
myeloma
    multiple m.
myelomatosis
myeloneuropathy
myelopathy
myeloperoxidase
myocardial
myocarditis
myocyte
myopathy
myositis
    m. ossificans
Naganol
Naphuride
naproxen
nasopharyngeal
National Institutes of Allergy &
 Infectious Diseases
natural killer cells
NBT – nitroblue
 tetrazolium
NCF – neutrophil chemotactic
 factor
necleoside
necropsy
necrosis
necrotic
necrotizing
Neisseria
    N. gonorrhoeae
    N. lactamica
    N. meningitidis
    N. mucosa
neoantigen
neonatal
neoplasm
neoplastic
neopterin
nephelometry

nephritis
  Heymann's n.
  Masugi n.
nephropathy
nephrotic syndrome
network theory
neuritis
neuroanatomic
neuroarthropathy
neurologic
neurological
neuroma
  Morton's n.
neuromuscular
neuro-ophthalmic
neuro-ophthalmology
neuropathic
neuropathy
  optic n.
  peripheral n.
neurophysiologic
neuropsychiatric
neuroradiological
neurotrophic
neutralization
neutropenia
neutrophil
neutrophilic
New Zealand mice
Nezelof's syndrome
NIAID – National Institutes of
  Allergy & Infectious
  Diseases
nick translation
nifedipine
nightsweats
nitrofurantoin
Nizoral
NK – natural killer
Nocardia
  N. asteroides
  N. otitidis-caviarum
nocardiosis
node
  Heberden's n's
  mesenteric n's

nodosa
  periarteritis n.
nodular
nodule
  glial n's
nonaesthenic
non-B hepatitis
noncleaved
non-Hodgkin's lymphoma
nonoxynol-9
nonsecretor
nonspecific
nonvisceral
Northern blotting
Norwalk virus
nosocomial
NSAID – non-steroidal anti-
  inflammatory drugs
nucleic acid
nucleoside
  n. analogue
  n. phosphorylase
nystatin
O antigen
OA – osteoarthritis
OAF – osteoclast-activating factor
obesity
obscuration
obstipation
obstruction
obtunded
occult
ochronosis
odynophagia
OI – opportunistic infection
  osteogenesis imperfecta
OKT4
OKT8
oligoarthritis
oligoclonal
oligosaccharide
  asparagine-linked o.
oncogene
oncogenesis
oncogenic
oncologist

oncology
Oncovin
oocyst
opacification
opaque
ophthalmia
ophthalmic
ophthalmicus
ophthalmologist
ophthalmoscopy
opportunistic
opsonin
opsonization
optic
oral thrust
orbicularis oculi
orbit
orchitis
ORF – open reading frame
organelles
organism
     transgenic o.
organotropism
original antigenic sin
orogenital
oropharynx
Ortho-mune
orthotopic
Osgood-Schlatter disease
osteitis
     o. deformans
osteoarthritis
     erosive o.
osteochondritis
     o. dissecans
osteochondrosis
osteogenesis
     o. imperfecta
osteohypertrophic nevus
    flammeus
osteoid
osteoma
osteomalacia
osteomyelitis
osteonecrosis
osteophyte

osteoporosis
     juxta-articular o.
OT – old tuberculin
Ouchterlony method
outbreeding
oxygen
oxygenation
oxyphenbutazone
Oz
     O. antigen
     O. isotypic determinant
pachydermoperiostitis
PAF – platelet-activating factor
Paget's disease
PAHO – Pan American Health
    Organization
PAIDS – pediatric AIDS
palindrome
palindromic
pallor
palpebral
PAN – polyarteritis nodosa
Pan American Health
    Organization
pancreas
pancreatic
pancytopenia
panencephalitis
panlymphopenia
panniculitis
pannus
papain
paperadioimmunosorbent test
papilledema
papilloma
papillomavirus
papillotomy
papovavirus
papular
papule
    Gottron's p.
paramacular
parameter
paramyxovirus
paraprotein
parasite
parasitemia

parasitic
parasitism
parasitologic
parasympathetic
parathyroid
parathyroidectomy
paratope
parenchyma
    hepatic p.
parenteral
paresis
Parkinson's disease
paromomycin
parotitis
parovirus
parvovirus
pasteurized Factor VIII
    concentrate
patches
    Peyer's p's
patching
paternity
pathogen
pathogenesis
pathogenicity
pathophysiologic
pathway
    lipoxygenase p.
pauciarticular
Paul-Bunnell test
PCA – passive cutaneous
    anaphylaxis
PCNA – proliferating cell nuclear
    antigen
PCP – pneumocystis carinii
    pneumonia
PCR – polymerase chain
    reaction
PEG – polyethylene glycol
Pel-Ebstein fever
pemphigoid
    bullous p.
pemphigus
    p. vulgaris
penicillamine
penicillin
Pentam 300

pentamidine
    p. isethionate
pepsin
peptide
    chemotactic p.
    signal p.
perception
perforation
perforin
periarteritis
    p. nodosa
periarthritis
pericarditis
pericyte
perihepatitis
    gonococcal p.
perinatal
periodontal disease
peripapillary
peripheral
peripolesis
periportal
perirectal
perithelial
peritonitis
perivascular
permeability
pertussis
petechial
Peyer's patches
Pfeiffer's phenomenon
PFGE – pulsed field gradient gel
    electrophoresis
PFS – primary fibromyalgia
    syndrome
PGL – persistent generalized
    lymphadenopathy
PHA – phytohemagglutinin
phagocyte
    mononuclear p.
phagocytosis
phagolysosome
phagosome
pharyngeal
pharyngitis
    gonococcal p.
    streptococcal p.

phenomenon
  Danysz's p.
  Matuhasi-Ogata p.
  Pfeiffer's p.
  Raynaud's p.
  vacuum p.
phenotype
  Bombay p.
  dominant p.
  McLeod's p.
  murine T cell p.
phenotypic
phenylbutazone
phloxine-tartrazine stain
phorbol ester
phospholipase A, A$_2$, B, C, D
phosphonoformate
phosphoribosyl pyrophosphate
phosphorylase
photosensitivity
phylogenetic
phytohemagglutinin
pinocytosis
pinworm
pituitary
pityriasis
placenta
placentation
plaque-forming cell assay
plasma
plasmacytoid
plasmapheresis
plasmid
Plasmodium
platelet
plateletpheresis
pleocytosis
  mononuclear p.
pleomorphic
pleural
pleuropulmonary
plot
  Sips p.
  Wu-Kabat p.
PLT – primed lymphocyte typing
PMN – polymorphonuclear
  neutrophil

PMR – polymyalgia rheumatica
pneumococcal polysaccharide
pneumococcus
pneumocystic
Pneumocystis
  P. carinii
pneumocystosis
pneumonia
  eosinophilic p.
  Friedländer's p.
  giant cell p.
  *Legionella pneumo-
    phila* p.
  Pneumocystis carinii p.
  staphylococcal p.
pneumonitis
  hypersensitivity p.
  lymphoid interstitial p.
PNH – paroxysmal nocturnal
  hemoglobinuria
poliomyelitis
poliovirus
polyacrylamide gel
polyagglutination
polyarteritis
  p. nodosa
polyarthritis
polyarticular
polychondritis
  relapsing p.
polyclonal
  p. hypergamma-
    globulinemia
  p. hyperglobulinemia
polyethylene glycol
polyimmunoglobulin
polymerase chain reaction
polymicrobial
polymorphism
polymorphonuclear
polymyalgia
  p. rheumatica
polymyositis
polyneuritis
polynucleotide
polyomavirus
polypeptide

polyploid
polypoid
polysaccharide
polyvalent
postnatal
postneonatal
postpartum
poxvirus
PPD–purified protein derivative
PPNG–penicillinase-producing
    Neisseria gonorrhoeae
Prausnitz-Küstner reaction
precipitation
precipitin
        p. curve
        p. reaction
prednisone
pregnancy
PRIST–paperadio-
    immunosorbent test
privileged site
probenecid
procainamide
procedure
        Cleveland p.
procollagenase
proctalgia
proctitis
        p. obliterans
        pseudoinfectious p.
        traumatic p.
proctocolitis
prodromal
prodrome
progenitor
progeny
prognostic marker
proliferation
proliferative
promiscuity
promoter
properdin
prophylaxis
propranolol
proptosis
prostacyclin
prostaglandin

protease
protein
        A, G, S p.
        Bence Jones p.
proteinuria
proteoglycan
protocol 019
protoplast
protozoa
protozoal
protozoan
proviral
prozone
pruritus
pseudoallele
pseudocyst
pseudoencapsulated
pseudogene
pseudoglobulin
pseudogout
pseudohyphae
pseudolymphoma
Pseuaomonas
pseudomycelia
psoriasis
psychogenic
psychoneuroimmunology
pulmonary
        p. nodulosis
        p. sarcoidosis
purine
purpura
        Henoch-Schönlein p.
        hypergammaglobu-
            linemic p.
        thrombocytopenic p.
PWA–person with AIDS
pyoderma
        p. gangrenosum
        streptococcal p.
pyogenic
pyrantel pamoate
pyrazinamide
pyrimethamine
pyrogen
        endogenous p.
pyroglobulin

pyroglobulinemia
pyrophosphate
Qa antigen
quantitation
quantitative
quaternary
quiescent
Quin-2
RA – rheumatoid arthritis
rabies
radiation
radiculopathy
radioallergosorbent
radioimmunoassay
radioimmunoelectrophoresis
radioimmunoprecipitation
radioimmunosorbent
radioisotope
radiology – See *Radiology and Nuclear Medicine* section.
radionuclide
radiotherapy
ragweed
Raji cell assay
RAST – radioallergosorbent test
rate
    Westergren sedimentation r.
Raynaud's phenomenon
reaction
    acute phase r.
    Arthus' r.
    Jones-Mote r.
    Kveim r.
    Prausnitz-Küstner r.
    quantitative precipitin r.
    Schultz-Dale r.
    Shwartzman's r.
reactivation
reagin
Rebuck's skin window technique
receptor
    C3a, C5a r.
    homing r.
    polyimmunoglobulin r.
    transferrin r.
recombinant

Reed-Sternberg giant cell
region
    framework r.
Reiter's syndrome
renal
    r. calculi
    r. toxicity
    r. transplantation
replication
RES – reticuloendothelial system
resorbed
respiratory
response
    anamnestic r.
restitope
reticular
reticulin staining
reticuloendothelial
    r. blockade
    r. system
reticuloendotheliosis
    leukemic r.
reticulohistiocytosis
    multicentric r.
reticuloma
reticulosarcoma
reticulum
    r. cell carcinoma
    endoplasmic r.
retina
retinal
    r. detachment
retinitis
    cytomegalovirus r.
retinoblastoma
retinochoroidal
retinochoroiditis
retinopathy
retroperitoneal
Retrovir
retroviral
retrovirus
    lymphotropic r.
RFLP – restriction fragment length polymorphism
Rh
    R. blood group

Rh (continued)
  R. immunization
  R. incompatibility
  R. isoantigen
rhegmatogenous
rhesus macaque
rheumatic
  r. disease
  r. factor
rheumatism
  palindromic r.
rheumatoid
  r. arthritis
  r. factor
  r. nodule
  r. vasculitis
rheumatologic
rhinitis
  allergic r.
rhodamine
  r. isothiocyanate
RIA – radioimmunoassay
ribavirin
ribonucleic acid
ribonucleoprotein
ribose
ribosome
ricin
rifabutine
rifampin
rimming
RIP – radio-
  immunoprecipitation
RIST – radioimmunosor-
  bent test
R-loop
RNA – ribonucleic acid
RNA polymerase
RNA splicing
RNA virus
RNP – ribonucleoprotein
rosea-like
rosette
  E, EA, EAC r.
Roth's spots
rovamycin
rubella

rubeola
Russell's body
Sabin-Feldman dye test
Sabin's vaccine
SACE – serum angiotensin-
  converting enzyme
saccharide
  O-linked s.
sacral
sacroiliitis
  pyogenic s.
sacrum
SAIDS – Simian AIDS
salicylate
saliva
salivary
Salk's vaccine
Salmonella
  S. choleraesuis
  S. enteritidis
  S. proctitis
  S. serogroup D
salmonellosis
Sandimmune
sarcoid
sarcoidosis
sarcoma
  epithelioid s.
  immunoblastic s.
  Kaposi's s.
scan
  CT (computerized
  tomography) s.
scanning
  gallium s.
scheme
  Kauffmann-White s.
Scheuermann's juvenile kyphosis
schistosomiasis
schizont
schizophreniform
Schultz-Dale reaction
SCID – severe combined
  immunodeficiency
scintigraphy
scleredema
sclerodactyly

scleroderma
scleromalacia
sclerosing
sclerosis
    multiple s.
    progressive systemic s.
    systemic s.
scoliosis
secretor
secretory
    s. component deficiency
    s. compound
    s. IgA
seizure
semen
sensitization
sepsis
septicemia
    perinatal s.
sequence
    consensus s.
    Shine-Dalgarno s.
    signal s.
sequestered
sequestration
sera
seroconversion
serologic
serological
seronegative
seropositive
seropositivity
seroprevalence
serositis
serotherapy
serotonin
serotype
serous
serpin
Serratia
    S. liquefaciens
    S. marcescens
    S. proteamaculans
serum
    s. albumin
    s. amyloid A component
    s. amyloid P component

serum (continued)
    antilymphocyte s.
    antithymocyte s.
    convalescent s.
    s. sickness
    s. urate level
    s. uric acid
sexual transmission
Sézary's syndrome
Shigella
    S. flexneri
    S. sonnei
shigellosis
Shine-Dalgarno sequence
shingles
shock
    anaphylactoid s.
    endotoxic s.
Shwachman's syndrome
Shwartzman's reaction
sialophorin
sigmoidoscopy
sign
    Tinel's s.
    trolley-track s.
    Yergason's s.
simian AIDS
sinus
    marginal s.
sinusitis
sinusoid
sinusoidal endothelial cell
Sips
    distribution
    plot
Sjögren's syndrome
SLE–systemic lupus
    erythematosus
SLP–sex-limited protein
somatic
sonography
Southern blotting
specificity
spectinomycin
spectrotype
Spengler's fragment
sperm

spheroplast
sphincterotomy
spindle-shaped cells
spiramycin
spirochetes
    nontreponemal s.
spirochetosis
spleen
splenectomy
splenomegaly
spondylitis
    ankylosing s.
spondyloarthropathy
spondylolisthesis
spondylosis
    s. deformans
Sporothrix
    S. schenckii
sporotrichosis
sporozooid
sporozoite
sputum
SRS-A – slow reacting substance
    of anaphylaxis
stain/staining
    fluorescent auramine-
      rhodamine s.
    Gram-Weigert s.
    hematoxylin-eosin s.
    immunoperoxidase s.
    methenamine silver s.
    mucicarmine s.
    phloxine-tartrazine s.
    reticulin s.
    toluidine blue s.
    Ziehl-Neelsen s.
staphylococcal
Staphylococcus
    S. aureus
    S. epidermidis
    S. pyogenes
    S. simulans
stasis
steatosis
    macrovesicular s.
    microvesicular s.

stenosis
    papillary s.
steroid
steroidogenesis
Stewart-Treves syndrome
Still's disease
stomatitis
streptococcal
streptococcemia
Streptococcus
    S. bovis
    Group A *S.*
    S. pneumoniae
    S. pyogenes
streptomycin
Strongyloides
    S. stercoralis
strongyloidiasis
SUA – serum uric acid
subcutaneous
subluxation
submucosal
suboptimal
subset
Sudeck's atrophy
suicide
sulfadiazine
sulfadoxine-pyrimethamine
sulfamethoxazole
sulfinpyrazone
superonasal
superotemporal
suppression
suppressor T-cells
suramin sodium
Svedberg's unit
Sydenham's chorea
sympathomimetic
syncytial
syndesmophyte
syndrome
    acquired
      immunodeficiency s.
    antibody deficiency s.
    bare lymphocyte s.
    Caner-Decker s.
    Caplan's s.

syndrome (continued)
    carpal tunnel s.
    Chédiak-Higashi s.
    Churg-Strauss s.
    cold agglutinin s.
    CREST s.
    cubital tunnel s.
    Cushing's s.
    de Quervain's s.
    DiGeorge's s.
    Duncan's s.
    Ehlers-Danlos s.
    Felty's s.
    Fiessinger-Leroy s.
    Goodpasture's s.
    Good's s.
    Guillain-Barré s.
    hyper IgE s.
    hyper IgM s.
    Klippel-Trenaunay s.
    marfanoid hyper-
        mobility s.
    Marfan's s.
    mucocutaneous lymph
        node s.
    Nezelof's s.
    occipital horn s.
    overlap s.
    postcardiotomy s.
    primary fibromyalgia s.
    Reiter's s.
    Sézary's s.
    Shwachman's s.
    sicca s.
    Sjögren's s.
    Stewart-Treves s.
    tarsal tunnel s.
    thoracic outlet s.
    Tietze's s.
    ulnar tunnel s.
    wasting s.
    Wiskott-Aldrich s.
    X-linked
        lymphoproliferative s.
syngeneic
synovectomy

synovial
    s. biopsy
    s. chondrosarcoma
    s. histopathology
    s. osteochondromatosis
    s. sarcoma
    s. stromal cells
synoviography
synovitis
    villonodular s.
synovium
synthetic CD4
syphilis
    anorectal s.
syringomyelia
systemic
    s. lupus erythematosus
    s. sclerosis
    s. vasculitis
TA-AIDS – transfusion-associated
    AIDS
tachycardia
tachyphylaxis
tachypnea
tachyzoite
Taenia
    T. saginata
    T. solium
Takayasu's arteritis
tapeworm
TAT – transacting transcriptional
    regulation
T cell
T cell antigen
T cell function
T-cell growth factor
T cell proliferation
T4 cell
T8 cell
T-cytotoxic cell
TCGF – T-cell growth factor
technetium
    t. diphosphonate
    t. pertechnetate
technique
    Rebuck's skin window t.

telangiectasia
  ataxia-t.
  hereditary hemorrhagic t.
  t. lymphatica
tendinitis
tendon
  achilles t.
tenesmus
tenosynovitis
  de Quervain's t.
terminator
  DNA-chain t.
tertiary
  t. granule
  t. structure
test
  ACTH stimulation t.
  blot t.
  complement fixation t.
  Coombs' t.
  Dick t.
  electrotransfer t.
  Envacor t.
  Frei t.
  Ham t.
  Heaf t.
  HIVAGEN t.
  immunofluorescence t.
  interfacial t.
  Mantoux t.
  microimmunofluo-
    rescent t.
  mucin clot t.
  neutralization t.
  nitroblue tetrazolium
    dye t.
  paperadioimmuno-
    sorbent t.
  patch t.
  Paul-Bunnell t.
  pulmonary function t.
  radioallergosorbent t.
  radioimmunosorbent t.
  ring t.
  Sabin-Feldman dye t.
  scratch t.
  streptozyme t.

test (continued)
  transcriptase reverse t.
  tuberculin t.
  virus neutralization t.
  Vollmer t.
  Western blot t.
  Winn t.
testosterone
tetracycline
thalassemia
  sickle-cell t.
T helper cell
theophylline
theory
  Fisher-Race t.
  germ-line t.
  side-chain t.
  template t.
thermoascus crustaceus
thioguanine
thiokinase
thiol
thiolase
thiolester
thrombocyte
thrombocytopenia
  t. purpura
thrombocytopenic
thrombocytosis
thrombosis
thromboxane
thrush
thymectomy
thymic
  t. hypoplasia
  t. peptide
  t. transplantation
thymocyte
Thymolan
thymoma
thymosin
thymosin-alpha-1
thymulin
thymus
thyroid
thyroiditis
  Hashimoto's t.

thyroiditis (continued)
    lymphocytic t.
Tietze's syndrome
tinea
    t. capitis
    t. corporis
    t. versicolor
Tinel's sign
titer
titration
T lymphocyte
TNF–tumor necrosis
    factor
tolerance
tolerogen
tolerogenic
tolmetin
tomography
tonometer
tonsil
Torula
    T. capsulatus
    T. histolytica
torulosis
toxicity
toxin
    antitetanus t.
Toxocara
toxoid
Toxoplasma
    T. gondii
toxoplasmin
toxoplasmosis
trachomatis
TRAIDS–transfusion related
    AIDS
transaminase
transbronchial
transcobalamin
transcriptase
transcytosis
transduction
transfection
transfectoma
transfer
    passive t.
transformation

transfusion
    exchange t.
transglutaminase
transient
transmissible
transmission
transplacental
transplantation
    bone marrow t.
Trendelenburg's gait
Treponema
    T. pallidum
treponemal
TRF–thymus-replacing factor
trichiasis
trichinosis
Trichomonas
Trichophyton
trichosanthin
trimethoprim-sulfamethoxazole
trisodium phosphonoformate
trisulfapyrimidine
TRNG–tetracycline-resistant
    Neisseria gonorrhoea
troches
trolley-track sign
trophozoite
tropism
trypanocidal
Trypanosoma
trypanosomiasis
trypsin
tryptase
TSA–tumor-specific antigen
T-suppressor cell
tuberculin test
tuberculosis
tubular
tubulin
tubuloreticular particles
tumor
    Burkitt-like t.
    Burkitt's t.
    Buschke-Löwenstein t.
    t. immunity
    t.-specific antigen

tyrosine
    t. aminotransferase
      deficiency
tyrosinemia
ubiquitin
ulcer
    corneal u.
    decubitus u.
ulceration
ulcerative
    u. colitis
ulnar
    u. drift
    u. nerve
    u. tunnel syndrome
undifferentiated
unit
    Svedberg's u.
univalent
urate
urethritis
URF – unidentified reading frame
uric acid
uricosuric
urticaria
    u. pigmentosa
uveal
uveitis
vaccination
vaccinatum
    eczema v.
vaccine
    attenuated v.
    pertussis v.
    polyvalent v.
    Sabin's v.
    Salk's v.
    smallpox v.
    typhoid v.
    viral v.
vaccinia
    v. gangrenosa
    v. immune globulin
vacuolar
    v. myelopathy
vaginitis
valence

variability
variable
varicella
    v.-zoster virus
variolation
vascular
vasculitis
    hypersensitivity v.
vasoactive-spasmogenic mediator
vasodilator
vasopermeability
VCA – viral capsid antigen
vector
    expression v.
Velban
venom
ventricle
VePesid
vertebra
vertebral
    v. artery
    v. compression fracture
    v. osteomyelitis
vesicular
vidarabine
VIG – vaccinia immune globulin
villonodular
vilona
vinblastine
vincristine
violaceous
Vira-A
Virazole
viremia
virology
virostatic
virucidal
virulence
virus
    Abelson's murine
      leukemia v.
    Epstein-Barr v.
    herpes zoster v.
    human immuno-
      deficiency v.
    human T-cell
      lymphotropic v.

virus (continued)
    neurotrophic v.
    v. neutralization test
    Norwalk v.
    varicella-zoster v.
visceral
vitreous
VLA – *very late appearing* antigen
VNS – villonodular synovitis
Vollmer test
von Willebrand's disease
VP-16-epipodophyllotoxin
vulva
VZV – varicella-zoster virus
Waldenström's
    macroglobulinemia
wart
    venereal w's
WAS – Wiskott-Aldrich
    syndrome
wasting syndrome
Wegener's granulomatosis
Westergren sedimentation rate
Western
    blotting
    blot test
whiplash
Whipple's disease
white graft
whitlow
Wilson's disease
window
    skin w.
Winn test

Wintrobe's method
Wiskott-Aldrich syndrome
Wu-Kabat plot
xanthoma
xenograft
xerophthalmia
xerostomia
XLA – X-linked
    agammaglobulinemia
X-linked
    hypogammaglobulinemia
X-linked infantile
    agammaglobulinemia
X-linked lymphoproliferative
    syndrome
Yergason's sign
Yersinia
Z thumb
zeta
    z. potential
    z. sedimentation rate
zidovudine
Ziehl-Neelsen stain
ZIG – zoster immune globulin
zoster
    disseminated z.
    dermatomal z.
    herpes z.
    z. immune globulin
    varicella z.
Zovirax
ZSR – zeta sedimentation rate
zygomycosis
zymosan

Internal Medicine

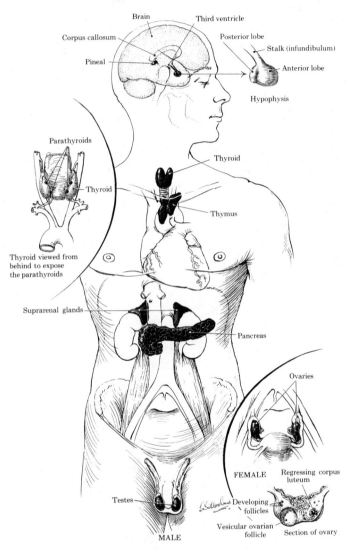

THE ENDOCRINE GLANDS

(Courtesy of Dorland's Illustrated Medical Dictionary, 26th ed. Plate XIX. Philadelphia, W. B. Saunders Company, 1981.)

Internal Medicine

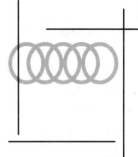

AAV – adeno-associated virus
Abderhalden-Fanconi syndrome
abdomen
abdominal
abdominalgia
Abercrombie's syndrome
abetalipoproteinemia
ABO blood groups
abortion
Abrami's disease
Abrikossoff's tumor
abscess
    caseocavernous a.
    eosinophilic a.
    epidural a.
    Pautrier's a.
    pyogenic a.
acalcerosis
Acanthocheilonema
    A. perstans
acanthocheilonemiasis
acanthocytosis
acantholysis
acanthosis
    a. nigricans
acapnia
acariasis
acatalasia
acaulinosis
achalasia
Achard-Thiers syndrome
achlorhydria
achondroplasia
achroacytosis
achylanemia
acidemia
acidosis
    diabetic a.

acidosis (continued)
    hypercapnic a.
    hyperchloremic a.
    metabolic a.
    nonrespiratory a.
    renal tubular a.
    respiratory a.
    starvation a.
    uremic a.
aciduria
Acinetobacter
acinus
acne
    a. pustulosa
    a. vulgaris
Acosta's disease
acoustic
acremoniosis
acrocentric
acrocephalopoly-
    syndactyly
acrocyanosis
acrodermatitis
    a. chronica atrophicans
    a. enterohepatica
acrodynia
acrokeratosis
    a. paraneoplastica
acromegaly
acropachyderma
ACTH – adrenocorticotropic
    hormone
Actinomyces
    A. muris
actinomycetoma
actinomycosis
adamantinoma
    pituitary a.

adamantinoma (continued)
    a. polycysticum
Adams-Stokes
    disease
    syndrome
ADCC – antibody-dependent
    cellular cytotoxicity
addisonian
Addison's disease
ADE – acute disseminated
    encephalomyelitis
adenalgia
adenia
    leukemic a.
adenine
adenitis
    acute epidemic infec-
       tious a.
    acute salivary a.
    cervical a.
    phlegmonous a.
adenoacanthoma
adenoangiosarcoma
adenocarcinoma
adenocystoma
    papillary a.
       lymphomatosum
adenofibroma
adenohypophysis
adenoids
adenoma
    acidophilic a.
    adamantinum a.
    chromophobe a.
    chromophobic a.
    langerhansian a.
    pituitary a.
    a. sebaceum
adenomata
    colloid a.
    follicular a.
adenomatosis
adenomatous
adenomeloblastoma
adenomyoepithelioma
adenomyofibroma
adenomyomatosis

adenopathy
adenosarcoma
adenosarcorhabdomyoma
adenosclerosis
adenosis
adenosylcobalamin
adenotyphus
adenovirus
ADH – antidiuretic hormone
adhesion
adipose
adiposis
    a. dolorosa
    a. hepatica
    a. tuberosa simplex
    a. universalis
adjuvant
ADP – adenosine
   diphosphate
adrenal
    a. cortex
    a. crisis
    a. gland
    a. hyperplasia
    a. hypoplasia
    Marchand's a's
    a. medulla
    a. steroids
    a. virilism
adrenalectomize
adrenalectomy
adrenaline
adrenalism
adrenalitis
adrenalopathy
adrenalotropic
adrenarche
adrenergic
adrenic
adrenin
adreninemia
adrenitis
adrenocortical
adrenocorticomimetic
adrenocorticotrophic
adrenocorticotropic
adrenogenital
adrenogenous

adrenogram
adrenokinetic
adrenoleukodystrophy
adrenolytic
adrenomedullotropic
adrenomegaly
adrenopathy
adrenopause
adrenoprival
adynamia
    a. episodica hereditaria
aerophagia
afazea. See *aphasia.*
afferent
afibrinogenemia
aftha. See *aphtha.*
agalactia
agalactous
agalorrhea
agammaglobulinemia
aganglionosis
ageusia
aglutition
agnosia
agoraphobia
agranulemia
agranulocytopenia
agranulocytosis
agranulosis
ague
    brass-founders' a.
    catenating a.
    dumb a.
    quartan a.
    quintan a.
    quotidian a.
    shaking a.
    tertian a.
Ahumada – Del Castillo
    syndrome
AIDS. See *AIDS* section.
akalazea. See *achalasia.*
akathisia
akawlinosis. See *acaulinosis.*
akilahnemea. See
    achylanemia.
akinesia

akondroplazea. See
    achondroplasia.
akroahsitosis. See *achroacytosis.*
akromikrie
alastrim
Albers-Schönberg's syndrome
albinism
Albright's syndrome
albuminemia
albuminuria
albumosuria
alcaptonuria
alcoholic
alcoholism
aldosterone
aldosteronism
Aldrich's syndrome
aleukemia
aleukia
    a. hemorrhagica
alexia
alkalemia
alkaloid
    plant a.
alkalosis
alkylating agent
alkylator
allantiasis
allele
allergen
allergic
allergy
alloantibody
alopecia
alpha-fetoprotein
alphavirus
ALS – amyotrophic lateral
    sclerosis
alveolar
alveolitis
alveolus(i)
alymphocytosis
alymphoplasia
Alzheimer's disease
amanitotoxin
amastigote
amaurosis
    albuminuric a.

amaurosis (continued)
    a. fugax
amebiasis
    hepatic a.
amebic
ameboma
ameloblastoma
amenorrhea
amine
    aromatic a.
amino acid
aminoaciduria
AML–acute monocytic
    leukemia
    acute myeloblastic
      leukemia
    acute myelocytic
      leukemia
AMML–acute myelomonocytic
    leukemia
amnesia
ampulla of Vater
amylase
amyloidosis
amylosuria
amyotrophy
    diabetic a.
anabolic
anabolism
anafil-. See words beginning
    anaphyl-.
analbuminemia
anaphase
anaphylactia
anaphylactic
anaphylactoid
anaphylaxis
anaplasia
anaplasmosis
anaplastic
anasarca
ancylostomiasis
Anders' disease
Andersen's disease
androblastoma
androgen

anemia
    achrestic a.
    aplastic a.
    Bagdad Spring a.
    Biermer-Ehrlich a.
    Chvostek's a.
    congenital nonspherocytic
      hemolytic a.
    Cooley's a.
    Dresbach's a.
    Edelmann's a.
    Fanconi's a.
    glucose-6-phosphate
      dehydrogenase
      deficiency a.
    hemolytic a.
    Herrick's a.
    hypochromic a.
    hypoplastic a.
    icterohemolytic a.
    Lederer's a.
    macrocytic a.
    Mediterranean a.
    megaloblastic a.
    microcytic a.
    myelophthisic a.
    normochromic a.
    normocytic a.
    pernicious a.
    sickle cell a.
    sideroblastic a.
    sideropenic a.
    spherocytic a.
    thrombopenic a.
anencephaly
anergy
aneurysm
angiitis
    visceral a.
angina
    a. cordis
    monocytic a.
    a. nervosa
    a. pectoris
    Plaut's a.
    Schultz's a.

angina (continued)
    vasomotor a.
angiocardiography
angiodysplasia
angioedema
angiography
angiohemophilia
angiokeratoma
    a. corporis diffusum
angiolupoid
angioma
angiomatosis
    hemorrhagic familial a.
angiomatous
angiomyosarcoma
angioneuralgia
angioneurosis
angioneurotic
angiopancreatitis
angioplasty
angiosarcoma
angiostrongyliasis
Angiostrongylus
    A. cantonensis
    A. costaricensis
angiotensin
anhidrosis
anhydremia
anion
aniridia
anisocytosis
anisuria
ankylosing
    a. spondylitis
ANLL – acute nonlymphocytic
    leukemia
anomaly
    Ebstein's a.
    Hegglin's a.
    May-Hegglin a.
    Pelger-Huët a.
    Undritz' a.
anorectal
anorexia
    a. nervosa
anorexic

anoscopy
anoxemia
anoxia
ansilostomiasis. See
    ancylostomiasis.
antagonist
    metabolic a.
anthracosis
    a. linguae
anthrax
anthrocosilicosis
antibiotic
anticholinergic
antidiuretic hormone (ADH)
antifolate
antigen
    carcinoembryonic a.
    Kell a.
    Kidd's a.
antihistamine
antimetabolite
antinuclear
antipurine
antipyrimidine
antral
antrectomy
antrum
anuria
aorta
aortic
aortitis
apancrea
apancreatic
aparathyrosis
aphasia
    Broca's a.
aphtha
aphthous
APL – acute promyelocytic
    leukemia
aplasia cutis
aplastic
apnea
    deglutition a.
    sleep a.
apneic

apocrine
apoplexy
appendicitis
apraxia
ARA-C–cytosine arabinoside
arachnodactyly
arachnoiditis
Arakawa-Higashi syndrome
arbovirus
ARC–AIDS-related complex
areflexia
areolitis
arginosuccinicaciduria
Arias' syndrome
ariboflavinosis
Armanni-Ehrlich's degeneration
Armstrong's disease
arrhythmia
arsenical
arteriography
arterioles
arteriosclerosis
arteriovenous
arteritis
arthralgia
    a. saturnina
arthritis
    degenerative a.
    gouty a.
    a. hiemalis
    hypertrophic a.
    Jaccoud's a.
    juvenile a.
    Lyme a.
    a. nodosa
    psoriatic a.
    rheumatoid a.
    tuberculous a.
arthrography
arthrogryposis
arthropathia
    a. ovaripriva
    a. psoriatica
arthrosis
Arthus response
asbestos
asbestosis

ascariasis
Ascaris
    A. lumbricoides
Ascher's syndrome
ascites
ascorbemia
Aseli's pancreas
asfiksea. See *asphyxia.*
Asiatic cholera
asiderosis
asinus. See *acinus.*
aspergilloma
aspergillosis
Aspergillus
    A. flavus
    A. fumigatus
    A. oryzae
asphyxia
aspiration
asplenia
assay
    estrogen receptor a.
astereognosis
asterixis
asthenia
    a. gravis hypophyseogenea
asthma
    Heberden's a.
asthmatic
astrocyte
astrocytoma
asystole
ataxia
    Friedreich's a.
atelectasis
atherosclerosis
atherothrombosis
athetosis
athyreosis
atresia
atrial
    a. fibrillation
    a. flutter
atrioventricular
atrium
atrophy
    Sudeck's a.

attack
    Stokes-Adams a.
Aufrecht's disease
auscultation
Australian X disease
autoimmune
autolysis
autonomic
autosomal
avitaminosis
Ayerza's
    disease
    syndrome
azmah. See *asthma.*
azoospermia
azotemia
AZT – azidothymidine
Baber's syndrome
babesiosis
Babinski's sign
bacillemia
bacilluria
Bacillus
    B. anthracis
    B. cereus
    B. stearothemophilus
    B. subtilis
bacteremia
bacteriocidal
bacteriuria
Bagdad Spring anemia
balantidiasis
Baló's disease
Balser's fatty necrosis
Banti's
    disease
    syndrome
Bard-Pic syndrome
Barlow's syndrome
Bar's syndrome
bartonellosis
Bartter's syndrome
basaloma
Basedow's disease
basilar
Bassen-Kornzweig
    syndrome

bath
    paraffin b.
BCNU –
    bischloroethylnitrosourea
Bearn-Kunkel syndrome
Beauvais' disease
Begbie's disease
Behçet's
    disease syndrome
Behr's disease
Bell's palsy
Bence Jones
    myeloma
    protein
    proteinuria
benign
Bennett's disease
benzpyrene
Berger's disease
beriberi
Bernard's syndrome
Bernard-Sergent syndrome
berylliosis
Besnier-Boeck disease
bezoar
Biermer-Ehrlich anemia
Biett's disease
bilharziasis
biliary
    b. atresia
    b. cirrhosis
bilirubinemia
bilirubinuria
biofeedback
biopsy
    bone marrow b.
    excisional b.
    incisional b.
    needle b.
bischloroethylnitrosourea
bisinosis. See *byssinosis.*
Blastomyces
    B. dermatitidis
blastomycosis
blennorrhea
Bloom's syndrome
Blumenthal's disease

Blumer's shelf
Blum's syndrome
BMR – basal metabolic rate
Boeck's
    disease
    sarcoid
Boerhaave's syndrome
Bohr's
    effect
    equation
Borrelia
    B. burgdorferi
botulism
Bouchard's nodes
Bouillaud's syndrome
Bowen's disease
BPV – benign positional vertigo
brachydactyly
brachymetacarpia
Bradley's disease
bradycardia
bradykinesia
"breakbone" fever
Brill-Symmers disease
Brill-Zinsser disease
Brinton's disease
Broca's aphasia
bromohyperhidrosis
bronchiectasis
bronchiolitis
bronchitis
bronchoalveolar
bronchoconstriction
bronchodilation
bronchogenic
bronchography
bronchopneumonia
bronchoscopy
bronchospasm
brucellosis
Bruhl's disease
bruising
bruit
    Verstraeten's b.
Brunsting's syndrome
brwe. See *bruit.*
bubonalgia

bubonulus
Budd-Chiari syndrome
Budd's cirrhosis
Buerger's disease
bulimia
bullous
Burkitt's
    lymphoma
    tumor
bursitis
Busse-Buschke disease
Butter's cancer
BX – biopsy
byssinosis
CA – cancer
cachectin
cachexia
café au lait spots
caisson disease
calcemia
calcification
calcinosis
    c. interstitialis
    c. universalis
calcitonin
calcium
calculus
California encephalitis
calor
    c. febrilis
    c. fervens
    c. innatus
    c. internus
Campylobacter
    C. fetus
    C. jejuni
cancellous
cancer
    acinous c.
    adenoid c.
    c. atrophicans
    Butter's c.
    cellular c.
    cerebriform c.
    colorectal c.
    dendritic c.
    dermoid c.

cancer (continued)
  endothelial c.
  epidermal c.
  epithelial c.
  fungous c.
  glandular c.
  hematoid c.
  c. in situ
  Lobstein's c.
  medullary c.
  melanotic c.
  retrograde c.
  scirrhous c.
  solanoid c.
  spider c.
  tubular c.
  villous duct c.
  withering c.
canceration
canceremia
cancericidal
cancerous
cancroid
Candida
  C. albicans
  C. parapsilosis
  C. tropicalis
candidiasis
candidosis
canker sore
Capillaria
  C. hepatica
  C. philippinensis
Caplan's syndrome
capsid
capsulitis
carbuncle
carcinoembryonic
carcinogen
carcinogenesis
carcinogenic
carcinoid
carcinolytic
carcinoma
  acinous c.
  adenocystic c.
  adenoid cystic c.

carcinoma (continued)
  c. adenomatosum
  adrenal c.
  alveolar c.
  ampullary c.
  anaplastic c.
  basal cell c.
  c. basocellulare
  basosquamous cell c.
  bronchioalveolar c.
  bronchiolar c.
  bronchogenic c.
  cavitated c.
  cerebriform c.
  chorionic c.
  colloid c.
  comedo c.
  corpus c.
  cribriform c.
  c. cutaneum
  cylindrical c.
  cylindrical cell c.
  ductal c.
  c. durum
  embryonal c.
  encephaloid c.
  c. en cuirasse
  epibulbar c.
  epidermoid c.
  epithelial c.
  c. epitheliale adenoides
  erectile c.
  c. erysipeloides
  exophytic c.
  c. exulcere
  c. fibrosum
  gelatiniform c.
  gelatinous c.
  giant cell c.
  c. gigantocellulare
  glandular c.
  granulosa cell c.
  hair-matrix c.
  hematoid c.
  hepatocellular c.
  Hürthle cell c.
  hyaline c.

carcinoma (continued)
    hypernephroid c.
    infiltrating ductal cell c.
    c. in situ
    intraepidermal c.
    intraepithelial c.
    Kulchitzky-cell c.
    lenticular c.
    c. lenticulare
    lipomatous c.
    lobular c.
    c. mastitoides
    medullary c.
    c. melanodes
    melanotic c.
    metastatic c.
    c. molle
    mucinous c.
    c. muciparum
    c. mucocellulare
    mucoepidermoid c.
    c. mucosum
    c. myxomatodes
    nasopharyngeal c.
    nevoid basal cell c.
    c. nigrum
    oat cell c.
    c. ossificans
    osteoid c.
    papillary c.
    periportal c.
    preinvasive c.
    prickle cell c.
    pultaceous c.
    radiogenic c.
    renal cell c.
    c. sarcomatodes
    schneiderian c.
    scirrhous c.
    c. scroti
    signet-ring cell c.
    c. simplex
    solanoid c.
    spheroidal cell c.
    spindle cell c.
    c. spongiosum
    squamous c.

carcinoma (continued)
    squamous cell c.
    string c.
    c. telangiectaticum
    c. telangiectodes
    transitional cell c.
    c. tuberosum
    tuberous c.
    verrucous c.
    c. villosum
carcinomata
carcinomatoid
carcinomatosis
carcinomatous
carcinosarcoma
carcinosis
cardiac
cardiogenic
cardiomegaly
cardiospasm
cardiothoracic
cardiothyrotoxicosis
cardiovascular
cardioversion
carditis
carnosinemia
carotenemia
carotid
carotidynia
carpal tunnel syndrome
Carrión's disease
cartilage
Castellani's disease
catabolism
cataplexy
catecholamine
catheter
    Swan-Ganz c.
cat scratch disease
cauda
    c. equina
causalgia
cavernous
cavitation
CEA – carcinoembryonic antigen
celiac
celialgia

celiopathy
cell
        bone marrow c's
        daughter c.
        germinal c's
        Kupffer's c's
        Leydig's c's
        parent c.
        somatic c's
        target c's
        transducer c's
        transitional c's
cellulitis
cephalalgia
cerebellar
cerebellopontine
cerebellum
cerebral
cerebrospinal
cerebrovascular
cerumen
cestodiasis
CGD – chronic granulomatous
    disease
chagoma
chancre
chancroid
Charcot's cirrhosis
Chédiak-Higashi syndrome
cheilitis
cheilosis
CHEM – chemotherapy
chemodectoma
chemoreceptor
chemotaxis
chemotherapeutic
chemotherapy
      combination c.
Cheyne-Stokes respiration
Chiari-Frommel syndrome
chickenpox
chiggers
chilblain(s)
Chinese restaurant syndrome
Chlamydia
      C. psittaci
      C. trachomatis

chloremia
chloridorrhea
chlorosis
chloruremia
cholangiocarcinoma
cholangiogram
cholangiography
cholangiohepatitis
cholangiohepatoma
cholangiole
cholangiolitis
cholangioma
cholangiopancreatography
cholangitis
    catarrhal c.
    c. lenta
cholecystectomy
cholecystitis
cholecystography
cholecystolithiasis
cholecystostomy
choledocholithiasis
cholelithiasis
cholemia
    familial c.
    Gilbert's c.
cholepathia
    c. spastica
choleperitoneum
cholera
    Asiatic c.
    bilious c.
    c. morbus
    c. nostras
cholestasis
cholestatic
cholesteatoma
cholesteremia
cholesterol
cholesteroleresis
cholesterolosis
cholesteroluria
cholesterosis
cholinergic
chondriosome
chondritis
chondrocalcinosis

chondromalacia
chondromatosis
chondrosarcoma
chordoma
chorea
    Sydenham's c.
choreoathetosis
choriocarcinoma
chorioepithelioma
    c. malignum
choriomeningitis
    lymphocytic c.
    pseudolymphocytic c.
chorionic
Christmas disease
chromatography
chromoblastomycosis
chromomycosis
chromosome
    Philadelphia c.
chubby puffer syndrome
Chvostek's anemia
Chvostek-Weiss sign
chylomicronemia
chylopericardium
chylothorax
cineangiography
cineradiography
cirrhosis
    alcoholic s.
    atrophic c.
    biliary c.
    Budd's c.
    Charcot's c.
    Cruveilhier-Baumgarten c.
    Glisson's c.
    Hanot's c.
    Laennec's c.
    Maixner's c.
    portal c.
    Todd's c.
Citrobacter
    C. freundii
cladosporiosis
Cladosporium
    C. bantianum
    C. trichoides

claudication
    intermittent c.
climacteric
climacterium
    c. praecox
CLL – chronic lymphocytic
    leukemia
clonorchiasis
clostridia
clostridial
    c. myonecrosis
Clostridium
    C. botulinum
    C. difficile
    C. perfringens
    C. tetani
    C. welchii
CMF – Cytoxan, methotrexate,
    5-fluorouracil
CML – chronic myelocytic
    leukemia
    chronic myelogenous
    leukemia
CMV – cytomegalovirus
coarctation
coccidioidomas
coccidioidomycosis
coccidiosis
coccygodynia
code
    genetic c.
    molecular c.
colibacillosis
colic
    renal c.
    stercoral c.
    ureteral c.
    uterine c.
colisepsis
colitis
collagen vascular disease
colonization
colonoscopy
Colorado tick fever virus
colorectal
colostomy
comedocarcinoma

communicable
complex
      Ghon c.
Concato's disease
concussion
condyloma
      c. acuminata
congenital
Conn's syndrome
constipation
contracture
      Dupuytren's c.
convulsion
Cooley's anemia
Cooper's disease
COP–Cytoxan, Oncovin,
   prednisone
COPD–chronic obstructive
   pulmonary disease
coproporphyria
cor
      c. pulmonale
      c. triatriatum
cordotomy
cornification
coronary–See *Cardiovascular
   System* section
corpus
      c. callosum
      c. luteum
      c. striatum
cortex
      adrenal c.
corticoid
corticoreticular
corticosteroid
cortisol
cortisone
corynebacteria
Corynebacterium
      C. diphtheriae
      C. parvum
      C. vaginale
coryza
Courvoisier's
    law
    sign

coxarthrosis
Coxiella
      C. burnetii
Coxsackie virus
cretinism
Crohn's disease
croup
CRS–Chinese restaurant
   syndrome
Cruveilhier-Baumgarten
      cirrhosis
      syndrome
cryoglobulinemia
cryoprecipitate
cryosurgery
cryptococcosis
cryptorchidism
culture
Curschmann's disease
curse
      Ondine's c.
cushingoid
Cushing's syndrome
CVA–cerebrovascular accident
CVP–Cytoxan, vincristine,
   prednisone
cyanosis
cycle
    growth c.
    Krebs-Henseleit urea c.
cyclothymic
cylindroma
cyst
cystadenocarcinoma
cystadenoma
cystadenosarcoma
cystathioninuria
cystic
cysticercosis
cystinemia
cystinosis
cystinuria
cystitis
cystoadenoma
cystocarcinoma
cystomyoma
cystomyxoadenoma

cystomyxoma
cystosarcoma
        c. phylloides
cytology
        exfoliative c.
cytomegalic
cytomegalovirus
cytomycosis
cytopenia
cytoplasm
cytoreduction
cytosine arabinoside
cytotoxic
cytotoxicity
dacryoadenitis
dacryocystitis
dactylitis
dactylolysis
        d. spontanea
dance
        St. Vitus' d.
Darier-Roussy sarcoid
Darling's disease
Dawson's inclusion
DCCT–Diabetes Control and
    Complications Trial
Debove's disease
decalcification
decompression sickness
decubitus
dedifferentiated
dedifferentiation
degeneration
        amyloid d.
        Armanni-Ehrlich d.
        hepatolenticular d.
        hyaline d.
degenerative
Degos'
        disease
        syndrome
dehydration
Déjérine-Sottas disease
delirium
        d. tremens
dementia
De Morgan's spots

demyelination
dengue
deoxyribonucleic acid
deoxyribose
depigmentation
depolarization
deradenitis
deradenoncus
dermalaxia
dermametropathism
dermamyiasis
dermataneuria
dermatitis
dermatoarthritis
dermatofibroma
dermatomucosomyositis
dermatomycosis
dermatomyositis
dermatophytid
dermatophytosis
dermatosis
dermis
dermographism
dermopathy
DES–diethylstilbestrol
desequestration
deshydremia
dethyroidism
detoxification
DHL–diffuse histocytic
    lymphoma
DI–diabetes insipidus
diabetes
        d. alternans
        brittle d.
        d. insipidus
        Lancereaux's d.
        latent d.
        d. mellitus
Diabetes Control and
    Complications Trial
diabetic
        d. ketoacidosis
dialysis
diapedesis
diaphoresis
diaphoretic

diaphragm
diaphragma
    d. sellae
diarrhea
diarrheogenic
diaspironecrobiosis
diaspironecrosis
diastematomyelia
diathermy
diathesis
dicroceliasis
diet
    Ebstein's d.
diethylstilbestrol
differentiated
differentiation
    cellular d.
diffuse
diffusion
difilobothriasis. See
    diphyllobothriasis.
difth-. See words beginning
    diphth-.
digestion
digitalization
DiGuglielmo's syndrome
diphtheria
diphtheroid
diphyllobothriasis
diplegia
diplococcemia
diplopia
dis-. See words beginning *dys-.*
discography
discoid
disease
    Abrami's d.
    Acosta's d.
    acute demyelinating d.
    Adams-Stokes d.
    Addison's d.
    Alzheimer's d.
    Anders' d.
    Andersen's d.
    angiopasmodic d.
    Armstrong's d.
    Aufrecht's d.

disease (continued)
    Australian X d.
    autoimmune d.
    Ayerza's d.
    Baló's d.
    Banti's d.
    Basedow's d.
    Beauvais' d.
    Begbie's d.
    Behçet's d.
    Behr's d.
    Bennett's d.
    Berger's d.
    Besnier-Boeck d.
    Biett's d.
    Blumenthal's d.
    Boeck's d.
    Bowen's d.
    Bradley's d.
    Brill-Symmer d.
    Brill-Zinsser d.
    Brinton's d.
    Bruhl's d.
    Buerger's d.
    Busse-Buschke d.
    caisson d.
    Carrión's d.
    Castellani's d.
    cat-scratch d.
    celiac d.
    Chagas' d.
    Christmas d.
    collagen d.
    combined
      immunodeficiency d.
    Concato's d.
    Cooper's d.
    Crohn's d.
    Curschmann's d.
    Darling's d.
    Debove's d.
    Degos' d.
    Déjérine-Sottas d.
    demyelinating d.
    Dressler's d.
    Durand's d.
    Ebstein's d.

disease (continued)
>   Economo's d.
>   Fabry's d.
>   Fenwick's d.
>   Filatov's d.
>   Flajani's d.
>   Friedländer's d.
>   Gamna's d.
>   Gandy-Nanta d.
>   Gaucher's d.
>   Gilbert's d.
>   Gilchrist's d.
>   glycogen storage d.
>   Graves' d.
>   Hand-Schüller-
>   Christian d.
>   Hanot's d.
>   Hansen's d.
>   Hartnup's d.
>   Hashimoto's d.
>   Heberden's d.
>   Heerfordt's d.
>   hemolytic d.
>   heredoconstitutional d.
>   Hers' d.
>   Hirschsprung's d.
>   Hodgkin's d.
>   Horton's d.
>   Huchard's d.
>   Huntington's d.
>   Hutinel's d.
>   Jodbasedow's d.
>   Kahler's d.
>   Kirkland's d.
>   Krabbe's d.
>   Landouzy's d.
>   legionnaires' d.
>   Letterer-Siwe d.
>   Lignac's d.
>   Luft's d.
>   Lyme d.
>   Marie's d.
>   mast cell d.
>   Mathieu's d.
>   Meleda d.
>   Meniere's d.
>   Mikulicz's d.

disease (continued)
>   Möbius' d.
>   Monge's d.
>   Morquio's d.
>   Nicolas-Favre d.
>   Niemann-Pick d.
>   Niemann's d.
>   Ollier's d.
>   Opitz's d.
>   Osler's d.
>   Osler-Vaquez d.
>   Paget's d.
>   parenchymatous d.
>   Parkinson's d.
>   Parrot's d.
>   Parry's d.
>   Parsons' d.
>   Pavy's d.
>   Pfeiffer's d.
>   Pick's d.
>   Plummer's d.
>   Pompe's d.
>   Poncet's d.
>   Pott's d.
>   pulseless d.
>   Raynaud's d.
>   Refsum's d.
>   Reiter's d.
>   rheumatic heart d.
>   Riedel's d.
>   Rokitansky's d.
>   Runeberg's d.
>   San Joaquin Valley d.
>   Schaumann's d.
>   Sheehan's d.
>   Simmonds' d.
>   Smith-Strang d.
>   Sternberg's d.
>   Still's d.
>   Stuart-Bras d.
>   Symmers' d.
>   Tangier d.
>   Tay-Sachs d.
>   tsutsugamushi d.
>   von Gierke's d.
>   von Recklinghausen's d.
>   von Willebrand's d.

disease (continued)
    Weil's d.
    Werner's d.
    Wernicke's d.
    Whipple's d.
    Widal-Abrami d.
    Willis' d.
    Wilson's d.
    zymotic d.
dissection
    block d.
disseminated
distomiasis
    hemic d.
    hepatic d.
diuresis
diverticulitis
diverticulosis
diverticulum
    Meckel's d.
    Zenker's d.
DKA – diabetic ketoacidosis
DM – diabetes mellitus
DMARDs – disease-modifying
    anti-rheumatic drugs
DNA – deoxyribonucleic acid
DNA virus
doll's eye test
Doppler ultrasound
dormant
dot
    Schüffner's d's
dowager's hump
dracunculiasis
Dresbach's
    anemia
    syndrome
Dressler's disease
dropsy
drugs. See *Drugs and Chemistry*
    section.
drusen
duct
    Wirsung's d.
    wolffian d's
dumping syndrome
duodenitis

duodenum
Dupuytren's contracture
Durand's disease
dwarf
    achondroplastic d.
    hypopituitary d.
dwarfism
    pituitary d.
dysarthria
dysautonomia
    Riley-Day d.
dysbetalipoproteinemia
dyschondroplasia
dyscrasia
    blood d.
    lymphatic d.
dyscrinism
dysdiemorrhysis
dysdipsia
dysendocrisiasis
dysentery
    amebic d.
dysesthesia
dysfibrinogenemia
dysgammaglobulinemia
dysgerminoma
dysglobulinemia
dyshepatia
dyshidrosis
dyskeratosis
dyskinesia
dysmenorrhea
dysmyelination
dysostosis
    d. multiplex
dyspancreatism
dysparathyroidism
dyspareunia
dyspepsia
dysphagia
dyspinealism
dyspituitarism
dysplasia
    olfactogenital d.
dyspnea
dysponderal
dyspragia

dysproteinemia
dyssebacia
dysthymic
dysthyroidism
dystonia
dysuria
eastern equine encephalomyelitis
Ebstein's
        anomaly
        diet
        disease
EBV – Epstein-Barr virus
ecchymosis
eccrine
eccyclomastoma
echinococcosis
Echinococcus
echinostomiasis
echocardiography
echovirus
eclampsia
Economo's disease
ecphyma
        e. globulus
ectasia
ecthyma
ectodermal
        e. dysplasia
ectodermosis
        e. erosiva pluriorificialis
ectopia
ectopic
ectopy
eczema
Edelmann's anemia
edema
        Milroy's e.
        nonpitting e.
        pedal e.
        Pirogoff's e.
        prehepatic e.
edematous
edentulous
effect
        Bohr e.
        Somogyi e.
efferent

effusion
Ehlers-Danlos syndrome
ejaculatory
ekfima. See *ecphyma.*
ekimosis. See *ecchymosis.*
ekino-. See words beginning
    echino-.
eksanthema. See *exanthema.*
eksiklomastoma. See
    eccyclomastoma.
ekthima. See *ecthyma.*
ekzema. See *eczema.*
elastofibroma
        e. dorsi
elastoma
elastorrhexis
elastosis
electrocardiography
electrocauterization
electrocautery
electrocoagulation
electroconvulsive
electroencephalography
electrolysis
electrolytes
electromyography
electronystagmography
electrophoresis
electropyrexia
elephantiasis
ellipsoid
        e. of spleen
elliptocytosis
emaciation
embolectomy
embolemia
embolism
embolomycotic
embolus
embryopathy
EMC – encephalomyocarditis
emesis
emetatrophia
emphysema
empyema
encapsulated

encephalitis
  acute disseminated e.
  acute necrotizing e.
  bulbar e.
  California e.
  demyelinating e.
  eastern equine e.
  hemorrhagic e.
  Japanese B e.
  Murray Valley e.
  Russian spring-summer e.
  St. Louis e.
  e. siderans
  Strümpell-Leichtenstern e.
  tick-borne e.
  viral e.
  von Economos e.
  western equine e.
  West Nile e.
encephalomeningitis
encephalomyelitis
  eastern equine e.
  Venezuelan equine e.
  western equine e.
encephalopathy
  hepatic e.
  Wernicke's e.
enchondromatosis
endarterectomy
endarteritis
endobronchial
endocarditis
  bacterial e.
endocardium
endocrine
endocrinosis
endocytosis
endometriosis
endometritis
endometrium
endomyocardium
endorphin(s)
endoscopy
endosonography
endothelial
endothelioangiitis
endothelioblastoma

endotheliocytosis
endotheliomatosis
endotheliomyoma
endotheliomyxoma
endotheliosis
endothelium
endotoxicosis
endotoxin(s)
endotracheal
enema
enkondromatosis. See
    enchondromatosis.
ensefal-. See words beginning
    encephal-.
entamebiasis
Entamoeba
    E. histolytica
enteritis
    e. necroticans
enterobiasis
enteroclysis
enterocolitis
enteropathy
enterovirus
enthesis
enuresis
enzyme
eosinopenia
eosinophilia
    Löffler's e.
eosinophilopoietin
ependymoma
epidemic
epidermal
epidermis
epidermodysplasia
epidermoid
epidermolysis
    e. bullosa
epidermophytosis
epididymis
epididymitis
epidura
epigastric
epiglottitis
epilepsy
    abdominal e.

epilepsy (continued)
    catamenial e.
    corticoreticular e.
    gelastic e.
    grand mal e.
    myoclonus e.
    petit mal e.
    photosensitive e.
    psychomotor e.
    rolandic e.
    sylvian e.
epiloia
epiphysis
epipodophyllotoxin
episcleritis
epispadias
epistaxis
    Gull's renal e.
epithelial
epithelioblastoma
epithelioma
epithelium
epituberculosis
Epstein-Barr virus
equation
    Bohr e.
equilibrium
ER – estrogen receptors
Erb's sign
erethism
ergotism
erisipela de la costa
eructation
erysipelas
erythema
    e. annulare
    e. chronicum migrans
    e. induratum
    e. marginatum
    e. multiforme
    e. nodosum
    e. toxicum
erythematous
erythermalgia
erythralgia
erythrasma
erythremia

erythroblastoma
erythroblastomatosis
erythroblastopenia
erythroblastosis
erythrocyanosis
erythrocyte
erythrocythemia
erythrocytosis
    leukemic e.
    e. megalosplenica
erythroderma
erythrodontia
erythrogenesis
    e. imperfecta
erythroid
erythroleukemia
erythroleukosis
erythromelalgia
erythromelia
erythroneocytosis
erythropenia
erythroplakia
erythropoiesis
erythropoietin
eschar
Escherichia
    E. coli
esophagitis
esophagography
esophagus
espundia
estriasis. See *oestriasis.*
estrogen
Eubacterium
eunuchism
    pituitary e.
eunuchoidism
eustachian
euthanasia
euthyroid
euthyroidism
Evans's syndrome
Ewing's sarcoma
exanthem
    e. subitum
Exc. – excision
exenteration

exfoliative
exhaustion
exogenous
exophthalmometry
exophthalmos
exostosis
expectoration
exsanguination
extracellular
extrapyramidal
Faber's syndrome
Fabry's disease
facies
    Parkinson's f.
facioscapulohumeral
    f. dystrophy
factitious
fagositosis. See *phagocytosis.*
Fallot's tetralogy
Falta's triad
familial
Fanconi's
    anemia
    syndrome
FAP–familial adenomatous
    polyposis
farinjitis. See *pharyngitis.*
Farre's tubercles
fasciculation
fasciitis
    eosinophilic f.
    necrotizing f.
fascioliasis
fasciolopsiasis
fasciotomy
fatigue
favism
FBS–fasting blood sugar
Felty's syndrome
fenetidinurea. See *phenetidinuria.*
fenilketonurea. See
    phenylketonuria.
feno-. See words beginning
    pheno-.
Fenwick's disease
feo-. See words beginning *pheo-.*
ferritin

ferrokinetics
festination
fetor
    f. hepaticus
fetoscopy
fever
    "breakbone" f.
    etiocholanolone f.
    Haverhill f.
    hay f.
    hemorrhagic f.
    Malta f.
    Oroya f.
    phlebotomus f.
    Q f.
    quartan f.
    quinine f.
    quintana f
    quotidian f.
    rat-bite f.
    rheumatic f.
    Rift Valley f.
    Rocky Mountain
      spotted f.
    saddleback f.
    San Joaquin f.
    scarlet f.
    South American
      hemorrhagic f.
    Southeast Asian
      mosquito-borne
      hemorrhagic f.
    streptobacillary f.
    typhoid f.
    undulant f.
    West Nile f.
    yellow f.
fiber
    Purkinje's f.
fibrillation
fibrinogen
fibrinogenemia
fibrinogenopenia
fibrinolysis
fibrinopenia
fibroadamantoblastoma
fibroadenia

fibroadenoma
fibroadenosis
fibroblastoma
fibrocyst
fibrocystic
fibrocystoma
fibroelastosis
fibrogenesis
fibrolymphoangioblastoma
fibroma
fibromatoid
fibromatosis
fibromyoma
fibromyositis
fibromyxosarcoma
fibrosarcoma
fibrosis
    cystic f.
fibrositis
fibrous
    f. dysplasia
    f. plaque
Fick method
fikomycosis. See *phycomycosis.*
filariasis
Filatov's disease
fire
    St. Anthony's f.
fissure
fistula
Fitz-Hugh-Curtis syndrome
Fitz's
    law
    syndrome
flagellosis
Flajani's disease
flatulence
flavivirus
Flavobacterium
flebitis. See *phlebitis.*
flebo-. See words beginning
  phlebo-.
fleckmilz
fluoroscopy
folate
follicle-stimulating hormone
follicular

folliculitis
folliculogenesis
food poisoning
    Bacillus cereus f. p.
    enterococcal f. p.
foot and mouth disease
Forbes-Albright syndrome
fovea
fractionation
fragilitas
    f. sanguinis
fragilocytosis
Francisella
    F. tularensis
Friedländer's disease
Friedmann's vasomotor
    syndrome
Friedreich's ataxia
frostbite
fructokinase
fructose
fructosemia
fructosuria
FSH – follicle-stimulating
    hormone
FU – fluorouracil
fucosidosis
fundus
fungating
FUO – fever of unknown origin
furuncle
furunculosis
Fusobacterium
G-1 period
G-2 period
Ga – gallium
Gaisböck's syndrome
galactokinase
galactorrhea
galactosemia
gallbladder
gallstones
gamma
    g. chain disease
    g. globulin
    g.-interferon
    g. rays

gamma (continued)
    g. streptococci
Gamna's disease
Gandy-Gamna
    nodules
    spleen
Gandy-Nanta disease
ganglia
gangliocytoma
ganglion
    Troisier's g.
ganglioneuroma
gangrene
    Raynaud's g.
Gardnerella
    G. vaginalis
Gardner's syndrome
gargoylism
gastrectasia
gastrectomy
gastric
gastrin
gastrinoma
gastritis
gastroenteritis
gastroesophageal
gastrointestinal
gastroma
gastroparesis
Gaucher's
    disease
    splenomegaly
gene
generation time
genetic code
genital
genitalia
genitourinary
genome
    mitochondrial g.
geotrichosis
geriatric
German measles
germinal
germinoma
Ghon complex

Giardia
    G. lamblia
giardiasis
gigantism
Gilbert's
    cholemia
    disease
Gilchrist's
    disease
    mycosis
gingivitis
gingivostomatitis
gland
    adrenal g.
    endocrine g.
    exocrine g.
    parathyroid g.
    pineal g.
    pituitary g.
    suprarenal g.
    thymus g.
    thyroid g.
glanders
Glanzmann's syndrome
glaucoma
glial
glioblastoma
    g. multiforme
glioma
Glisson's cirrhosis
globoid
globular
globulinemia
globus
    g. hystericus
    g. pallidus
glomangioma
glomerular
glomerulitis
glomerulocapillary
    g. sclerosis
glomerulonephritis
glomerulosclerosis
    intercapillary g.
glomerulus
glomus body
glossitis

glossodynia
glossopharyngeal
glucagon
glucagonoma
glucocorticoid
glucocorticosteroid
gluconeogenesis
glucose
glucosuria
glue sniffing
glutathionemia
glycemia
glycogen
glycogenolysis
glycoglycinuria
glycolysis
glycopenia
glycopolyuria
glycoprotein
glycoside
glycosphingolipidosis
glycosuria
goiter
    adenomatous g.
    colloid g.
    endemic g.
    exophthalmic g.
    fibrous g.
    follicular g.
    intrathoracic g.
    nodular g.
    papillomatous g.
    parenchymatous g.
    substernal g.
    toxic g.
gonad(s)
gonadoblastoma
gonadotropic hormone
gonadotropin
gongylonemiasis
gonococcal
gonococcemia
gonococcus(i)
gonorrhea
Goodpasture's syndrome
Gopalan's syndrome

gout
    abarticular g.
    articular g.
    calcium g.
    chalky g.
    latent g.
    lead g.
    misplaced g.
    oxalic g.
    polyarticular g.
    renal g.
    retrocedent g.
    rheumatic g.
    saturnine g.
    tophaceous g.
gouty
Gradenigo's syndrome
grading
Graefe's sign
granulation
granuloblastosis
granulocytopenia
granulocytosis
granuloma
    amebic g.
    eosinophilic g.
    Hodgkin's g.
    g. inguinale
    necrotic g.
    pyogenic g.
granulomatosis
    bronchocentric g.
    g. infantiseptica
    lymphomatoid g.
    g. siderotica
    Wegener's g.
granulomatous
granulopoiesis
granulosa
Graves' disease
Grawitz's tumor
grippe
groin
growth
    g. cycle
    g. fraction
    g. hormone

GTT – glucose tolerance test
guanine
Gubler's icterus
Guillain-Barré syndrome
Gull's renal epistaxis
gumma
Günther's syndrome
Gymnodinium
    G. breve
gynecologic
gynecology
gynecomastia
Haemophilus
    H. aphrophilus
    H. ducreyi
    H. influenzae
    H. parainfluenzae
    H. vaginalis
halitosis
hamartoma
hamartomatosis
Hamman-Rich syndrome
Hand-Schüller-Christian disease
Hanger-Rose skin test
Hanot's
    cirrhosis
    disease
Hansen's disease
Harris' syndrome
Hartnup's disease
Hashimoto's
    disease
    struma
    thyroiditis
hashitoxicosis
haustrum (haustra)
Haverhill fever
Hayem's icterus
Hayem-Widal syndrome
HD – Hodgkin's disease
headache
    cluster h.
    Horton's h.
    migraine h.
heartburn
Heberden's
    asthma

Heberden's (continued)
    disease
    nodes
    rheumatism
Heerfordt's
    disease
    syndrome
Hegglin's anomaly
Heidenhaim's syndrome
Heimlich maneuver
helical
helminthiasis
    cutaneous h.
    h. elastica
    h. wuchereri
hemagglutination
hemangioblastoma
hemangioma
hemangiomatosis
hemangiopericytoma
hemangiosarcoma
hemarthrosis
hematemesis
hematochezia
hematocrit
hematogenesis
hematologic
hematology
hematoma
    epidural h.
hematomycosis
hematomyelia
hematopenia
hematopoiesis
hematoporphyria
hematuria
heme
hemiachromatopsia
hemianopia
hemicrania
hemiparesis
hemiplegia
hemisporosis
hemobilinuria
hemoblastosis
Hemoccult test
hemochromatosis

hemoconcentration
hemocytoblastoma
hemodialysis
hemodynamic crisis
hemoglobin
hemoglobinemia
hemoglobinuria
hemolysis
hemolytic
hemoperfusion
hemophilia
    h. A
    h. B
    h. B, Leyden
    h. C
    h. neonatorum
    vascular h.
hemopneumothorax
hemoptysis
hemorrhage
hemorrhoids
hemosiderosis
hemostasis
hemothorax
hemuresis
Henle's loop
Henoch-Schönlein purpura
hepar
    h. adiposum
    h. lobatum
hepatalgia
hepatargia
hepatatrophia
hepatic
hepatism
hepatitis
    acute h.
    aggressive h.
    alcoholic a.
    anicteric h.
    autoimmune h.
    chronic h.
    infectious h.
    peliosis h.
    serum h.
    type D h.
    type non-A h.

hepatitis (continued)
    type non-B h.
    viral h.
hepatization
hepatocele
hepatocirrhosis
hepatocyte
hepatodynia
hepatodystrophy
hepatoglobinemia
hepatohemia
hepatolenticular
hepatolienal
hepatoma
hepatomalacia
hepatomegaly
hepatomphalos
hepatonephritis
hepatonephromegaly
hepatoperitonitis
hepatophyma
hepatoportal
hepatoptosis
hepatorenal
hepatorrhagia
hepatorrhexis
hepatosis
hepatosplenitis
hepatosplenomegaly
hepatotoxicity
heredity
heredopathia
    h. atactica
      polyneuritiformis
Hermansky-Pudlak syndrome
hermaphroditism
hernia
    hiatus h.
herniation
herpangina
herpes
    h. catarrhalis
    h. generalisatus
    h. genitalis
    h. gestationis
    h. labialis
    h. meningoencephalitis

herpes (continued)
    h. neonatalis
    h. simplex
    h. varicella-zoster virus
    h. virus
    h. zoster
herpesvirus
herpetiform
Herrick's anemia
Hers' disease
heteradenia
heterogeneity
heteropancreatism
heterophyiasis
HGF – hyperglycemic-
    glycogenolytic factor
HGH – human growth hormone
hibernoma
hiccup
Hickey-Hare test
Hickman's catheter
hidradenitis
    h. suppurativa
hidrorrhea
hidrosadenitis
    h. axillaris
    h. destruens suppurativa
hidrosis
hilar
Hines-Bannick syndrome
hippocampus
Hirschsprung's disease
hirsutism
histidinemia
histiocytomatosis
histiocytosis
    h. X
histocompatibility
Histoplasma
    H. capsulatum
histoplasmosis
HIV – human immunodeficiency
    virus
Hodgkin's
    disease
    granuloma
    lymphoma

Hoesch's test
Homans' sign
homeostasis
homocystinuria
homosexual
hookworm
hormone
Horner's syndrome
Horton's
    disease
    headache
    syndrome
host cell
Huchard's disease
human immunodeficiency virus
humidification
Hunter's syndrome
Huntington's disease
Hurler's syndrome
Hürthle cell carcinoma
Hutchinson's triad
Hutinel's disease
hyaline
hyaloserositis
hybridoma
hydatid
hydatidiform
hydatidoma
hydatidosis
hydrarthrosis
hydration
hydremia
hydrocarbon
    aromatic h.
hydrocephalus
hydrocytosis
hydrogen
hydromyelia
hydronephrosis
hydrophobia
hydrops
hydroxylysinemia
hydroxyprolinemia
hydroxyurea
hyloma
hymenolepiasis
hyperaeration

hyperaldosteronism
hyperaminoaciduria
hyperamylasemia
hyperargininemia
hyperbilirubinemia
hyperbradykininism
hypercalcemia
hypercalciuria
hypercapnia
hypercarbia
hyperceruloplasminemia
hyperchloremia
hypercholesterolemia
hypercholesterolia
hyperchromatic
hyperchromatism
    macrocytic h.
hyperchromia
hypercortisolism
hypercupremia
hypercystinuria
hyperemesis
    h. hiemis
hyperemia
hyperesthesia
hyperfibrinogenemia
hypergammaglobulinemia
hypergenesis
hypergeusia
hyperglobulinemia
hyperglycemia
hyperglycemic-glycogenolytic
    factor
hyperglyceridemia
hyperglycinemia
hyperglycinuria
hypergonadism
hyperhidrosis
    h. lateralis
hyperhistaminemia
hyperhistidinemia
hyperhistidinuria
hyperhydroxyprolinemia
hyperimmunoglobulinemia
hyperinsulinemia
hyperinsulinism
hyperkalemia

hyperkeratomycosis
hyperkeratosis
hyperketonemia
hyperketonuria
hyperkinemia
hyperkinesia
hyperkinetic
hyperlipemia
hyperlipidemia
hyperlipoproteinemia
hyperliposis
hyperlordosis
hyperlysinemia
hyperlysinuria
hypernatremia
hypernephroma
hypernitremia
hypernormocytosis
hyperostosis
hyperoxaluria
hyperoxemia
hyperparathyroidism
hyperpathia
hyperpepsinemia
hyperphagia
hyperphenylalaninemia
hyperphosphatemia
hyperphosphaturia
hyperphosphoremia
hyperpigmentation
hyperpituitarism
    basophilic h.
    eosinophilic h.
hyperplasia
hyperpnea
hyperpotassemia
hyperproinsulinemia
hyperprolactinemia
hyperprolinemia
hyperproteinemia
hyperpyrexia
hypersecretion
hypersensitivity
hypersomnia
hypersplenism
hypertension
hypertensive

hyperthermia
hyperthrombinemia
hyperthrombocytemia
hyperthyroidism
hyperthyroiditis
hypertrichiasis
hypertrichosis
  h. lanuginosa
hypertriglyceridemia
hypertrophy
    Marie's h.
hyperuricemia
hyperuricosuria
hypervalinemia
hyperventilation
hypervitaminosis
hypervolemia
hypoadrenalemia
hypoadrenalism
hypoaeration
hypoalbuminemia
hypoalbuminosis
hypoaldosteronemia
hypoaldosteronism
hypoaminoacidemia
hypocalcemia
hypocalcitoninemia
hypocapnia
hypocarbia
hypochloremia
hypochlorhydria
hypochondriasis
hypochromasia
hypochromemia
    idiopathic h.
hypochromia
hypochrosis
hypocitraturia
hypocomplementemia
hypocrinism
hypocupremia
hypocythemia
hypodermoclysis
hypodermolithiasis
hypoendocrinism
hypoesthesia
hypoestrogenemia

hypofibrinogenemia
hypogammaglobulinemia
hypogeusia
hypoglycemia
hypogonadism
hypogonadotropism
hypogranulocytosis
hypohepatia
hypohidrosis
hypoinsulinemia
hypoinsulinism
hypokalemia
hypolepidoma
hypoleukocytosis
hypolipidemia
hypomagnesemia
hyponatremia
hyponeocytosis
hyponitremia
hypoparathyroidism
hypoperfusion
hypophosphatasia
hypophosphatemia
hypophyseal
hypophysectomy
hypophysis
hypopiesia
hypopiesis
hypopituitarism
hypoplasia
hypoproteinemia
hypoprothrombinemia
hypopyon
hyporeflexia
hyposecretion
hyposialadenitis
hypospadias
hyposplenism
hyposthenuria
hypotension
    orthostatic h.
hypothalamic
hypothalamus
hypothermia
    endogenous h.
hypothrombinemia
hypothyroidism

hypotonia
hypotonic
hypotonicity
hypoventilation
hypovitaminosis
hypovolemia
hypoxemia
hypoxia
HZ – herpes zoster
IADH – inappropriate
    antidiuretic hormone
IASP – International Association
   for the Study of Pain
ichthyosarcotoxism
ichthyosis
ictal
icteric
icteroanemia
icterohepatitis
icterus
      acholuric hemolytic i.
        with splenomegaly
      bilirubin i.
      i. castrensis gravis
      i. castrensis levis
      i. catarrhalis
      cythemolytic i.
      i. gravis
      Gubler's i.
      Hayem's i.
      i. hemolyticus
      i. infectiosus
      i. praecox
      i. simplex
      spirochetal i.
      i. typhoides
      urobilin i.
      i. viridans
ictus
idiopathic
IGF-1 – insulin-like growth
   factor-1
iksodiasis. See *ixodiasis.*
ikterik. See *icteric.*
iktero-. See words beginning
   ictero-.

ikterus. See *icterus.*
iktheosarkotoksizm. See
    ichthyosarcotoxism.
iktheosis. See *ichthyosis.*
iktus. See *ictus.*
ileitis
ileocolitis
ileostomy
ileum
ileus
imaging. See *Radiology and*
    Nuclear Medicine section.
immotile cilia syndrome
immune response
immunity
immunization
immunocompromised
immunodeficiency
immunoelectrophoresis
immunoglobulin
immunologic
immunosuppression
impedance
      i. plethysmography
imperforate
impetigo
impotence
inanition
inappropriate antidiuretic
   hormone
incarnatio
      i. unguis
inclusion
      Dawson's i.
incontinence
incontinentia
      i. pigmenti
incubation
Indian tick typhus
indoluria
inebriation
inert
infarction
      myocardial i.
infection
infectious

infective
infertility
infestation
infiltrative
inflammation
inflammatory
influenza
infundibuloma
inguinal
inguinodynia
inhalation
inhibition
    contact i.
inoculation
inocystoma
inotropic
in situ
insomnia
insulin
insulinemia
insulinogenesis
insulinoma
insuloma
interleukin-1, -2, -3, -4
intermittent
    i. claudication
    i. porphyria
International Association for the
    Study of Pain
intersexuality
interstitial
interstitialoma
interstitium
intertrigo
intestine
intimal
intravenous
intubation
intussusception
invasive
in vitro
in vivo
iodine
ionic
ionizing

iritis
    diabetic i.
    gouty i.
irradiation
irritable bowel syndrome
ischemia
islet
    i's of Langerhans
isonormocytosis
isopathy
Isospora
    I. hominis
isosthenuria
isotope
isthmus
Ixodes
    I. dammini
    I. persulcatus
    I. ricinus
ixodiasis
Jaccoud's arthritis
Janeway's spots
Japanese B encephalitis
jargonaphasia
jaundice
    hemolytic j.
    obstructive j.
JCA – juvenile chronic arthritis
JCAH – Joint Commission on
    Accreditation of Hospitals
jejunoileitis
Job's syndrome
jodbasedow
juvenile
juxtaglomerular
K – potassium
kahkeksea. See *cachexia.*
Kahler's disease
kala-azar
kalemia
kaliopenia
kaliuresis
kallikrein-kinin system
Kallmann's syndrome
Kaposi's sarcoma
Karnofsky's scale

Kartagener's syndrome
karyotype
katzenjammer
Kawasaki syndrome
Kayser-Fleischer ring
Kell antigen
kemotherape. See *chemotherapy.*
keratin
keratinocyte
keratitis
keratoderma
    k. blennorrhagica
keratoma
keratomalacia
keratosis
Kerley's B lines
kernicterus
Kernig's sign
ketoacidosis
ketonemia
ketonuria
ketosis
Kidd antigen
kifosis. See *kyphosis.*
kilosis. See *cheilosis.*
Kimmelstiel-Wilson syndrome
kinetics
    cell population k.
kinetosis
Kirkland's disease
Klebsiella
Kleine-Levin syndrome
Klinefelter's syndrome
klor-. See words beginning *chlor-.*
Kocher's syndrome
koilonychia
koksake. See *Coxsackie.*
kolange-. See words beginning
    cholangi-.
kole-. See words beginning *chole-.*
kolera. See *cholera.*
koles-. See words beginning
    choles-.
kondritis. See *chondritis.*
kondro-. See words beginning
    chondro-.
König's syndrome

kopf-tetanus
Koplik's spots
kordoma. See *chordoma.*
korea. See *chorea.*
koreo-. See words beginning
    chorio-.
Korotkoff's sounds
Krabbe's disease
Krebs-Henseleit urea cycle
kromoblastomikosis. See
    chromoblastomycosis.
Kulchitzky-cell carcinoma
Kundrat's lymphosarcoma
Kupffer's cells
Kussmaul's respiration
Kveim-Siltzbach test
kwashiorkor
kyphoscoliosis
kyphosis
labyrinthitis
lactacidemia
lactase
lactation
lactic
    l. acidosis
Lactobacillus
    L. acidophilus
    L. casei
lactogenic hormone
lactoperoxidase
lactose
lactosuria
Laennec's cirrhosis
la grippe
Lancereaux's diabetes
Landouzy's
    disease
    purpura
Langerhans
    islets of L.
laparoscopy
laparotomy
    staging l.
laryngitis
laryngotracheobronchitis
larynx
latent

Laurence-Moon-Biedl syndrome
law
    Courvoisier's l.
    Fitz's l.
Läwen-Roth syndrome
LE–lupus erythematosus
LED–lupus erythematosus
    disseminatus
Lederer's anemia
Legionella
legionnaires' disease
leiomyoma
leiomyosarcoma
Leishmania
    L. donovani
leishmaniasis
lentigo
    l. maligna melanoma
    l. simplex
leopard syndrome
leprosy
leptomeninges
leptomeningitis
leptoprosopia
Leptospira
    L. interrogans
leptospirosis
    l. icterohemorrhagica
Leriche's syndrome
Lesch-Nyhan syndrome
Leser-Trélat sign
lethal
lethargy
Letterer-Siwe disease
leukapheresis
leukemia
    acute nonlymphocytic l.
    acute promyelocytic l.
    aleukemic l.
    aleukocythemic l.
    basophilic l.
    blast cell l.
    blastic l.
    l. cutis
    embryonal l.
    eosinophilic l.
    granulocytic l.

leukemia (continued)
    hairy cell l.
    hemocystoblastic l.
    histiocytic l.
    leukopenic l.
    lymphatic l.
    lymphoblastic l.
    lymphocytic l.
    lymphogenous l.
    lymphoid l.
    lymphoidocytic l.
    lymphosarcoma cell l.
    mast cell l.
    megakaryocytic l.
    micromyeloblastic l.
    monocytic l.
    myeloblastic l.
    myelocytic l.
    myelogenous l.
    myeloid granulocytic l.
    nonlymphocytic l.
    plasma cell l.
    plasmacytic l.
    prolymphocytic l.
    promyelocytic l.
    Rieder cell l.
    Schilling's l.
    smoldering l.
    splenomedullary l.
    splenomyelogenous l.
    stem cell l.
    subleukemic l.
    undifferentiated cell l.
leukoagglutinin(s)
leukocyte
leukocytoclasis
leukocytosis
leukocyturia
leukodystrophy
leukoencephalitis
leukoerythroblastosis
leukolymphosarcoma
leukopenia
leukoplakia
Leydig's cells
LH–luteinizing hormone
libido

lichen
Lignac-Fanconi syndrome
Lignac's disease
line
    Kerley's B l's
    Sergent's white l.
linitis
    l. plastica
liomioma. See *leiomyoma.*
liomiosarkoma. See
    leiomyosarcoma.
lipemia
lipid(s)
lipiduria
lipoatrophy
lipoblastosis
lipochondrodystrophy
lipodystrophia
    l. progressiva
lipodystrophy
lipogenesis
lipoma
lipomatosis
lipoprotein
    l. lipase
    l. metabolism
    l. X
lipoproteinemia
liposarcoma
lipoxygenase
Listeria
    L. monocytogenes
lithotripsy
livedo
    l. reticularis
liver
    amyloid l.
    brimstone l.
    cirrhotic l.
    lardaceous l.
Loa
    L. loa
loaiasis
Lobstein's cancer
locus
    l. ceruleus

Löffler's
    eosinophilia
    syndrome
loiasis
loop
    l. of Henle
lordosis
Lowe syndrome
LTH – luteotropic hormone
Lucio's phenomenon
lues
    l. hepatis
Luft's
    disease
    syndrome
lumbago
    ischemic l.
lupus
    discoid l.
    l. erythematosus
    l. nephritis
    l. pernio
    l. profundus
luteinizing hormone
Lyme
    arthritis
    disease
lymphadenectasis
lymphadenhypertrophy
lymphadenia
    l. ossea
lymphadenitis
    caseous l.
    paratuberculous l.
lymphadenocyst
lymphadenogram
lymphadenography
lymphadenoid
lymphadenoleukopoiesis
lymphadenoma
lymphadenopathy
    giant follicular l.
lymphadenosis
lymphoadenovarix
lymphangiectasia
lymphangiectasis
lymphangioendothelioblastoma

lymphangioendothelioma
lymphangiofibroma
lymphangiogram
lymphangiography
lymphangioleiomyomatosis
lymphangiosarcoma
lymphangitis
lymphatic
lymphatism
lymphedema
    l. praecox
lymphemia
lymphoadenopathy
lymphoblastic
lymphoblastoma
    giant follicular l.
lymphoblastomatosis
lymphocystosis
lymphocyte
lymphocythemia
lymphocytic
lymphocytoma
lymphocytopenia
lymphocytosis
lymphodermia
lymphoepithelioma
lymphogranuloma
    l. venereum
lymphogranulomatosis
lymphoidotoxemia
lymphokine
lymphoma
    Burkitt's l.
    clasmocytic l.
    giant follicular l.
    granulomatous l.
    Hodgkin's l.
    lymphoblastic l.
    lymphocytic l.
    non-Hodgkin's l.
    stem-cell l.
lymphomatosis
lymphopathia
    l. venereum
lymphopenia
lymphoproliferative
lymphoreticular

lymphosarcoleukemia
lymphosarcoma
    Kundrat's l.
    lymphocytic l.
lymphosarcomatosis
lymphotoxemia
lysemia
lysosomal
lysozyme(s)
lyssavirus
M period
MacLeod's capsular rheumatism
macroadenoma
macrocytosis
macrodystrophia
    m. lipomatosa progressiva
macrogenitosomia
    m. praecox
macroglobulinemia
    Waldenström's m.
macrophage
macropsia
macrosomatia
    m. adiposa congenita
maculation
    pernicious m.
maculopapular
maduromycosis
magnetic resonance imaging
Maixner's cirrhosis
mal
    m. de mer
malabsorption
maladie (Fr.)
malaise
malakoplakia
malaria
malformation
malignancy
malignant
mali-mali
malnutrition
Malta fever
mamillary
mamillitis
mamma
mammary

mammogram
mammography
mammoplasia
maneuver
    Heimlich m.
mannosidosis
maple syrup urine disease
marasmus
Marchand's adrenals
marche à petits pas
Marchiafava-Micheli syndrome
Marfan's syndrome
Marie's
    disease
    hypertrophy
    sign
    syndrome
marijuana
Maroteaux-Lamy syndrome
masculinization
mastadenoma
mastalgia
mastatrophy
mastauxe
mastectomy
masthelcosis
mastitis
mastocarcinoma
mastochondroma
mastocytosis
mastoid
mastoiditis
mastoncus
mastopathia
    m. cystica
mastopathy
mastoplastia
mastoptosis
Mathieu's disease
May-Hegglin anomaly
measles
    German m.
Meckel's diverticulum
meconium
mediastinitis
mediastinum
Medicaid

Medicare
medications. See *Drugs and Chemistry* section.
Mediterranean anemia
medulla
    adrenal m.
medullary
medulloblastoma
megacolon
megakaryoblastoma
megakaryocytosis
megalerythema
megalgia
megaloblastic
megaloblastosis
meibomian gland
meiosis
melanocyte
melanoma
melanosis
    m. coli
melanuria
melasma
    m. addisonii
    m. suprarenale
melatonin
Meleda disease
melena
melenemesis
melioidosis
membrane
    nuclear m.
menarche
Meniere's
    disease
    syndrome
meninges
meningioma
meningismus
meningitis
meningoblastoma
meningococcal
meningococcemia
meningoencephalitis
meningomyelitis
meningomyelocele
meningopneumonitis

meningotyphoid
meniscocytosis
menometrorrhagia
menopause
menorrhagia
menstrual
menstruation
meralgia
     m. paresthetica
6-mercaptopurine
Merseburg triad
mesangiocapillary
mesenteric
     m. adenitis
mesenteritis
mesentery
mesocardia
mesothelioma
metabolic
metabolism
metagonimiasis
metamorphosis
     fatty m.
metaphase
metaplasia
     myeloid m.
     pseudopyloric m.
     squamous m.
metastasis(es)
metastasize
metastatic
metatarsal
methemalbuminemia
methemoglobinemia
methionine
method
     Fick m.
mets – metastases
microaneurysm
microangiopathy
microcephaly
microcythemia
microcytosis
microlithiasis
microorganism
micturition

mielo-. See words beginning
     myelo-.
migraine
miks-. See words beginning *myx-.*
mikso-. See words beginning
     myxo-.
Mikulicz's
     disease
     syndrome
miliaria
Milroy's edema
mineralization
mineralocorticoid(s)
Minkowski-Chauffard syndrome
miosis
mirinjitis. See *myringitis.*
mitochondria
mitochondrial DNA
mitochondrion
mitosis
mitral
     m. insufficiency
     m. regurgitation
     m. stenosis
     m. valve
mittelschmerz
Möbius'
     disease
     sign
modality
molecule
molluscum
     m. contagiosum
Monge's disease
mongolism
monilethrix
moniliasis
monocytopenia
monocytosis
mononeuritis
mononuclear
mononucleosis
     infectious m.
MOPP – nitrogen mustard,
     Oncovin, prednisone,
     procarbazine
morbidity
morbilliform

Morquio's
    disease
    syndrome
mosaicism XO/XY
MP – mercaptopurine
mRNA – messenger RNA
MS – multiple sclerosis
MTX – methotrexate
mucinous
mucocele
mucolipidosis
mucopolysaccharidosis
mucopolysacchariduria
mucopurulent
mucormycosis
mucosa
mucosanguineous
mucositis
    m. necroticans
        agranulocytica
mucous
mucoviscidosis
mucus
müllerian
mumps
Münchausen's syndrome
murmur
    heart m.
Murray Valley encephalitis
muscarinic
musculoskeletal
mutagen
mutagenesis
mutagenic
mutation
    spontaneous genetic m.
mutism
myalgia
myasthenia
    m. gravis
myasthenic
myatonia
    m. congenita
myatrophy
mycethemia
mycetismus
mycetoma

mycobacteria
mycobacteriosis
Mycobacterium
    M. avium-intracellulare
    M. bovis
    M. fortuitum-chelonae
    M. kansasii
    M. leprae
    M. marinum
    M. scrofulaceum
    M. szulgai
    M. tuberculosis
    M. xenopi
mycoplasma
mycosis
    m. fungoides
    Gilchrist's m.
    splenic m.
mycotoxicosis
mydriasis
myelemia
myelin
myelinolysis
myelinopathy
myelitis
myeloblastemia
myeloblastoma
myeloblastomatosis
myeloblastosis
myelocythemia
myelocytoma
myelocytomatosis
myelodysplastic
myelofibrosis
myelogenous
myelography
myeloid
    m. metaplasia
myeloma
    Bence Jones m.
    giant cell m.
    multiple m.
myelomatosis
myelomeningocele
myelopathy
myeloproliferative
myelosarcoma

myelosarcomatosis
myelosclerosis
myelosis
myelosuppression
myelotoxicosis
myiasis
myoblastoma
myocardia
myocardiac
myocardial
      m. contractions
      m. infarction
      m. ischemia
myocarditis
      acute bacterial m.
myocardium
myocardosis
myoclonus
myoedema
myofascial
myoglobinuria
myoglobulinuria
myokymia
myolysis
      m. cardiotoxica
myoma
myonecrosis
myositis
      m. ossificans
myotonia
      m. congenita
      m. dystrophica
myringitis
myxadenitis
myxadenoma
myxangitis
myxasthenia
myxedema
myxoblastoma
myxochondrofibrosarcoma
myxochondroma
myxochondrosarcoma
myxodermia
myxofibrosarcoma
myxoidedema
myxoma
myxomatosis

myxosarcoma
myxovirus
Na – sodium
nanism
      Paltauf's n.
narcolepsy
nasal
nasogastric
National Academy of Sciences
National Cancer Institute
National Clearinghouse of
      Poison Control
National Diabetes Data Group
National Dialysis Registry
National Heart, Lung and Blood
      Institute
National Institutes of Health
natremia
natriuresis
nausea
Necator
      N. americanus
necrobiosis
      n. lipoidica
      n. lipoidica diabeticorum
necrosis
      Balser's fatty n.
      decubital n.
      icteric n.
necrotic
NED – no evidence of disease
nefritis. See *nephritis.*
nefro-. See words beginning
      nephro-.
Neisseria
      N. gonorrhoeae
      N. lactamica
      N. meningitidis
nemathelminthiasis
nematodiasis
neoplasia
neoplasm
neospinothalamic
nephritic
nephritis
nephroblastoma
nephrocalcinosis

nephrocarcinoma
nephrocirrhosis
nephrocystitis
nephrocystosis
nephrogram
nephrolithiasis
nephroma
nephron
nephronophthisis
nephroptosis
nephropyelitis
nephrosclerosis
nephrosis
nephrostomy
nephrotic
NER – no evidence of recurrence
NERD – no evidence of
   recurrent disease
neuralgia
neurasthenia
neuritis
neuroacanthocytosis
neuroamebiasis
neuroblastoma
neurodermatitis
neuroendocrinology
neurofibroma
neurofibromatosis
neurogenic
neurohypophysis
neurolabyrinthitis
neuroleptic
neurologic
neuroma
     acoustic n.
neuromyasthenia
neuromyopathic
neuromyositis
neuromyotonia
neuron
neuronopathy
neurosyphilis
neurotensin
neurotransmitter
neutropenia
neutrophilia
Nicolas-Favre disease

nidus
Niemann-Pick disease
Niemann's
     disease
     splenomegaly
Nikolsky's sign
Nocardia
     N. asteroides
     N. intracellularis
nocardiosis
noctalbuminuria
nocturia
node
     Bouchard's n's
     Heberden's n's
     lymph n's
     Osler's n's
     Parrot's n.
     Schmorl's n's
nodular
nodule
     cold n.
     Gandy-Gamna n's
non-Hodgkin's lymphoma
nonsteroidal
Noonan's syndrome
noradrenaline
norepinephrine
nosocomial
NPDL – nodular, poorly
   differentiated lymphocytes
NSAIDs – non-steroidal anti-
   inflammatory drugs
nucleic acid
nucleolus
nucleoprotein
nucleosomes
nucleotide
nucleus
numo-. See words beginning
   pneumo-.
nystagmus
obesity
     endogenous o.
     exogenous o.
obstipation
obtundation

occlusion
ochrodermatosis
ochrodermia
ochronosis
oculogyric crisis
odon-eki
odoriferous
odynophagia
oestriasis
ofthal-. See words beginning
    ophthal-.
17-OHS – 17-
    hydroxycorticosteroid
okro-. See words beginning
    ochro-.
oksalosis. See *oxalosis.*
okseuriasis. See *oxyuriasis.*
oligemia
oligoanuria
oligochromemia
oligocythemia
oligodendrocyte
oligodendroglioma
oligomenorrhea
oligophrenia
    phenylpyruvic o.
oligoplasmia
oligoptyalism
oligospermia
oligotrophia
oliguria
Ollier's disease
omentum
onchocerciasis
oncocytoma
oncogene
oncogenesis
oncogenic
oncology
oncotaxis
Ondine's curse
onyalai
onycholysis
onychomycosis
oophoritis
    o. parotidea
ophthalmia

ophthalmoplegia
opisthorchiasis
opisthotonos
Opitz's disease
opsoclonus
orchiectomy
orchitis
    o. parotidea
    o. variolosa
orf
ornithosis
orofaciodigital syndrome
Oroya fever
orthopnea
orthostatic
oscillopsia
Osler's
    disease
    nodes
    sign
    syndrome
Osler-Vaquez disease
osmolality
osmotic
osteitis
    o. deformans
    o. fibrosa cystica
osteoarthritis
osteoarthropathy
osteoarthrosis
osteodystrophy
osteoectasia
osteogenesis
    o. imperfecta
osteolysis
osteoma
osteomalacia
osteomyelitis
osteonecrosis
osteopenia
osteopetrosis
osteoporosis
osteosarcoma
osteosarcomatous
osteosclerosis
ostium
    o. primum

ostium (continued)
    o. secundum
otorrhea
ovary(ies)
overhydration
oxalate
oxalosis
oxygenation
oxytocin
oxyuriasis
Oxyuris
    O. vermicularis
pachydermoperiostosis
pachymeningitis
Paget's disease
pagophagia
pake-. See words beginning
    pachy-.
paleospinothalamic
    p. tract
pallor
palpation
palpitation
palsy
    Bell's p.
Paltauf's nanism
pancarditis
pancolitis
pancreas
    Aseli's p.
    p. divisum
    Willis' p.
    Winslow's p.
pancreatalgia
pancreatemphraxis
pancreathelcosis
pancreatic
pancreatitis
pancytopenia
pandysautonomia
panencephalitis
panhypopituitarism
panneuritis
    p. epidemica
panniculitis
panniculus
pannus

pansitopenea. See *pancytopenia*.
pantatrophia
pantatrophy
Papanicolaou smear
papilla
papillary
papilledema
papillitis
papilloadenocystoma
papillocarcinoma
papilloma
papillomatosis
papillomatous
papillomavirus
papillosarcoma
Pap smear
papular
papule
papuloerythematous
papulosquamous
paracentesis
paracoccidioidomycosis
parafollicular
paragonimiasis
Paragonimus
    P. westermani
paragranuloma
parahemophilia
parakeratosis
paralysis
paralytic
parameningeal
paramyotonia
    p. congenita
paramyxovirus
paraplegia
pararotavirus
parascarlatina
parasite
parasitemia
parasitic
parasitosis
paraspinal
parasympathetic
parasystole
parathormone
parathyroid

parathyroidoma
parathyroprival
parathyroprivia
parathyrotoxicosis
paraventricular
paravertebral
parenchymal
paresis
paresthesia
parkinsonian
parkinsonism
 postencephalitis p.
Parkinson's
 disease
 facies
 syndrome
paroksizm. See *paroxysm.*
paroksizmal. See *paroxysmal.*
paronychia
parotid
parotidoscirrhus
parotidosclerosis
parotitis
 p. phlegmonosa
paroxysm
paroxysmal
Parrot's
 disease
 node
 ulcer
Parry's disease
pars
 p. anterior
 p. distalis
 p. intermedia
 p. recta
 p. tuberalis
Parsons' disease
parvovirus
pasteurellosis
patch test
Paterson-Brown-Kelly syndrome
pathoglycemia
Paul's treatment
Pautrier's abscess
Pavy's disease
PBI – protein-bound iodine

peadra. See *piedra.*
pectenosis
pectoralgia
pectus
 p. excavatum
pediculosis
pedunculated
Pel-Ebstein pyrexia
Pelger-Huët anomaly
pellagra
pelohemia
Pemberton's sign
pemfigoid. See *pemphigoid.*
pemfigus. See *pemphigus.*
pemphigoid
pemphigus
 p. erythematosus
 p. foliaceus
 p. neonatorum
 p. vegetans
 p. vulgaris
penicilliosis
pentastomiasis
pentatrichomoniasis
pentosemia
pentosuria
pepsin
peptide
peptococci
peptostreptococci
percussion
percutaneous
perforation
perfusion
perianal
periarteritis
 p. nodosa
pericardial
pericarditis
pericardium
pericolic
periostitis
peripheral
peritoneal
peritoneoscopy
peritoneum
peritonitis

perityphlitis
perlèche
perlingual
pertussis
pestilence
pestis
      p. ambulans
      p. bubonica
      p. siderans
petechia(ae)
petechiasis
Pfeiffer's disease
Pfuhl's sign
phagocytosis
phantom limb
pharmacokinetics
pharmacology
pharyngitis
pharynx
phenetidinuria
phenolemia
phenoluria
phenomenon
      Lucio's p.
      Raynaud's p.
      Rumpel-Leede p.
      Somogyi p.
phenylketonuria
pheochromoblastoma
pheochromocytoma
Philadelphia chromosome
phlebitis
phleboclysis
phlebothrombosis
phobia
phonation
phosphate
phosphaturia
photocoagulation
photodermatitis
photon
photophobia
photoscan
phototherapy
phycomycosis
pian
      p. bois

piarhemia
pica
Pick's disease
pickwickian syndrome
PID – pelvic inflammatory disease
piedra
pineal
pinocytosis
pinworm
Pirogoff's edema
pituitarism
pituitary
pityriasis
      p. alba
      p. lichenoides et
         varioliformis
      p. rosea
      p. rubra pilaris
placebo
plague
planum
      p. temporale
plasmacytoma
plasmacytosis
plasmapheresis
Plasmodium
      P. falciparum
platelet
plateletpheresis
platybasia
platypnea
Plaut's angina
pleocytosis
pleomastia
pleomorphic
plethysmography
pleura
pleuralgia
pleurisy
pleuritic
pleuritis
pleurocholecystitis
pleurodynia
pleuropneumonia-like
plombage
Plummer's disease

Plummer-Vinson syndrome
PMS – premenstrual
    syndrome
PND – paroxysmal nocturnal
    dyspnea
pneumaturia
pneumococcal
pneumococcemia
pneumococcosis
pneumococcus
pneumoconiosis
Pneumocystis
        P. carinii
pneumocystosis
pneumomediastinum
pneumonia
        pneumococcal p.
        Pneumocystis carinii p.
pneumonitis
pneumoperitoneum
pneumothorax
Pneumovax
Pneumovirus
podagra
podalgia
poikilocytosis
poikiloderma
poikilodermatomyositis
poisoning
        mushroom p.
polioencephalitis
poliomyelencephalitis
poliomyelitis
        bulbar p.
poliothrix
poliovirus
pollinosis
polyadenitis
polyadenosis
polyamine(s)
polyangiitis
polyarteritis
        p. nodosa
polyarthritis
polychondritis
polychromatophilia
polycyclic

polycystic
polycythemia
        myelopathic p.
        p. rubra vera
        splenomegalic p.
        p. vera
polycytosis
polydactyly
polydipsia
polydysplasia
polyemia
polygenic
polymorphism
polymorphonuclear
polymyalgia
        p. rheumatica
polymyositis
polyneuritis
polyneuropathy
        erythredema p.
polyopsia
polyostotic
polyp
polypectomy
polypeptide(s)
polyphagia
polypoid
polyposis
        p. coli syndrome
polypus
polyradiculitis
polyradiculoneuritis
polyrrhea
polysarcia
polyserositis
polysplenia
polyuria
POMP – prednisone, Oncovin,
    methotrexate, 6-mercap-
    topurine
Pompe's disease
Poncet's
        disease
        rheumatism
popliteal
porphobilinogen
porphyria

Pott's disease
pouch
    Rathke's p.
poxvirus
Prader-Willi syndrome
precordium
preeclampsia
prematurity
premenstrual
priapism
PRL – prolactin
proctalgia
    p. fugax
proctencleisis
proctitis
    epidemic gangrenous p.
proctocolitis
proctodynia
proctorrhagia
proctorrhea
proctoscopy
proctosigmoiditis
proctosigmoidoscopy
progeria
progesterone
progestin
projectile
prolactin
prolactinoma
proopiomelanocortin
proptosis
prostaglandin(s)
    D_2
    $E_{1,2}$
    $F_{1,2}$
prostate
prostatism
prostatitis
prostatodynia
prosthesis
prostration
protein
    Bence Jones p.
proteinemia
proteinosis
proteinuria
    Bence Jones p.

proteinuria (continued)
    orthostatic p.
proteolysis
Proteus
    P. mirabilis
    P. morganii
prothrombin
prothrombinopenia
protocol
protocoproporphyria
protoporphyria
protozoa
provirus
"prune-belly" syndrome
prurigo
pruritus
    p. ani
psammocarcinoma
psammoma
psammosarcoma
pseudoacanthosis
    p. nigricans
pseudoaldosteronism
pseudocyst
pseudohemophilia
    p. hepatica
pseudohermaphrodism
pseudohyperkalemia
pseudohyponatremia
pseudohypoparathyroidism
pseudoleukemia
    p. lymphatica
pseudolymphoma
Pseudomonas
    P. aeruginosa
    P. cepacia
    P. mallei
    P. pseudomallei
pseudoproteinuria
pseudo-pseudohypo-
    parathyroidism
pseudoxanthoma
    p. elasticum
psilosis
psittacosis
psoriasis
psychogenic

psychosis
pterygium
PTH – parathormone
    parathyroid hormone
ptosis
puberty
pulmonary
pulmonic
pulpa
    p. lienis
pulpitis
pulsus
    p. alternans
    p. paradoxus
PUO – pyrexia of unknown origin
purging
purine
Purkinje's fiber
purpura
    actinic p.
    allergic p.
    p. cachectica
    cocktail p.
    dependent nonthrombo-
        cytopenic p.
    p. fulminans
    p. hemorrhagica
    Henoch-Schönlein p.
    hyperglobulinemic p.
    idiopathic p.
    Landouzy's p.
    nonpalpable p.
    orthostatic p.
    p. rheumatica
    senile p.
    p. simplex
    thrombocytopenic p.
    p. variolosa
    vascular p.
pustule
pyarthrosis
pyelitis
pyelography
pylonephritis
pyelonephrosis
pyemia
    cryptogenic p.

pyknodysostosis
pyloric stenosis
pyoderma
pyomyositis
pyrexia
    Pel-Ebstein p.
pyrimidine
pyrogen
pyrogenic
pyroglobulinemia
pyropoikilocytosis
pyrosis
pyruvemia
pyuria
Q fever
quadriplegia
quarantine
Queensland tick typhus
quinsy
RA – rheumatoid arthritis
rabdomioma. See *rhabdomyoma.*
rabdomyosarcoma. See
    rhabdomyosarcoma.
rabies
rachitis
radiation
    ionizing r.
    non-ionizing r.
radicular
radiculopathy
radioactive
radioactivity
radiocurable
radiography
radioimmunoassay
radioiodine
radioisotope
radioligand
radiology. See *Radiology and*
    Nuclear Medicine section.
radioneuritis
radionuclide
radioreceptor
radioresistant
radiosensitive
radiotherapy
radium

RAI – radioactive iodine
RAIU – radioactive iodine uptake
rakitis. See *rachitis.*
ranula
    pancreatic r.
RAST – radioallergosorbent test
Rathke's pouch
RAtx – radiation therapy
Raynaud's
    disease
    gangrene
    phenomenon
reaction
    Weil-Felix r.
receptor
    estrogen r.
recessive
recrudescence
rectosigmoid
rectovaginal
rectum
reflux
Refsum's disease
regimen
regurgitation
    aortic r.
Reifenstein's syndrome
Reiter's
    disease
    syndrome
REM – rapid eye movement
remission
Rénon-Delille syndrome
renovascular
replication
resection
    block r.
respiration
    Cheyne-Stokes r.
    Kussmaul's r.
respiratory
response
    Arthus r.
resuscitation
retching
reticular
reticulocytopenia

reticulocytosis
reticuloendothelioma
reticuloendotheliosis
    leukemic r.
reticulohistiocytosis
reticuloid
reticulonodularity
reticulosarcoma
reticulosis
reticulum
    endoplasmic r.
    sarcoplasmic r.
retinitis
retinoblastoma
retinochoroiditis
retinopathy
retroperitoneal
retropulsion
retrovirus
Reye's syndrome
rhabdomyolysis
rhabdomyoma
rhabdomyosarcoma
rheumapyra
rheumarthritis
rheumatalgia
rheumatic
rheumatism
    Heberden's r.
    MacLeod's capsular r.
    Poncet's r.
rheumatoid
    r. arthritis
rhinitis
rhinophyma
rhinorrhea
rhinoscleroma
rhinosporidiosis
rhinovirus
rhonchi
RIA – radioimmunoassay
ribonucleic acid
ribose
ribosome
Richter's syndrome
rickets

Rickettsia
 R. akari
 R. australis
 R. canada
 R. conorii
 R. prowazekii
 R. rickettsii
 R. siberica
 R. tsutsugamushi
 R. typhi
rickettsial
rickettsialpox
rickettsiosis
Riedel's
 disease
 struma
Rieder cell leukemia
Rift Valley fever
rigidity
Riley-Day
 dysautonomia
 syndrome
ring
 Kayser-Fleischer r.
 Schatzki's r.
rinitis. See rhinitis.
rino-. See words beginning rhino-.
RNA – ribonucleic acid
RNA-dependent DNA
 polymerase
RNA reverse transcriptase
RNA virus
robertsonian translocation
Rocky Mountain spotted fever
Rokitansky's disease
Romaña's sign
Romberg-Paessler syndrome
Romberg's sign
rongki. See rhonchi.
rooma-. See words beginning
 rheuma-.
rosacea
Rosenbach's syndrome
roseola
roseoliform
 r. exanthem
roseolus

rotavirus
Roth's spot
Rotor's syndrome
roundworm
rubella
 r. scarlatinosa
rubeola
 r. scarlatinosa
rubor
rubra
Rumpel-Leede phenomenon
Runeberg's
 disease
 type
rupia
Russian spring-summer
 encephalitis
Sabin-Feldman dye test
sacroiliitis
sacrum
saddleback fever
St. Anthony's fire
St. Louis encephalitis
St. Vitus' dance
salicylate
salicylism
Salmonella
 S. typhi
 S. typhosa
salmonellosis
salpingitis
samokarsinoma. See
 psammocarcinoma.
samoma. See psammoma.
samosarkoma. See
 psammosarcoma.
Sanfilippo's syndrome
San Joaquin fever
San Joaquin Valley disease
sarcocarcinoma
sarcoid
 s. of Boeck
 Darier-Roussy s.
 Schaumann's s.
 Spiegler-Fendt s.
sarcoidosis
sarcolemma

sarcoma
    Ewing's s.
    Kaposi's s.
    meningeal s.
    osteogenic s.
    reticulum cell s.
sarcomphalocele
sarcoplasmic
sarcosepsis
sarcosinemia
sarcosis
sarcosporidiosis
SBE – subacute bacterial
    endocarditis
scabies
scale
    Karnofsky's s.
scalenus anticus syndrome
scan
    brain s.
    CT (computed
      tomography) s.
    thyroid s.
scapuloperoneal
scarlatina
scarlet fever
Schatzki's ring
Schaumann's
    disease
    sarcoid
    syndrome
Scheie's syndrome
Schilling's leukemia
Schirmer's test
schistosomiasis
    cutaneous s.
    hepatic s.
Schmidt's syndrome
Schmorl's node
Schoffner's dot
Schultz's angina
schwannoma
scintigraphy
scirrhoma
scirrhous
scleral
scleredema

scleritis
sclerodactylia
    s. annularis ainhumoides
sclerodactyly
scleroderma
scleromalacia
sclerosis
    amyotrophic lateral s.
    multiple s.
scoleciasis
scoliosis
scopulariopsosis
scotodinia
scotoma
scrofula
scrofuloderma
scurvy
sebaceous
seborrheic
    s. dermatitis
    s. keratosis
sefalaljeah. See cephalalgia.
seizure
self-replication
sella turcica
seminoma
Senear-Usher syndrome
senile
    s. dementia
sensory
sepsis
    s. lenta
    puerperal s.
septicemia
septicophlebitis
septicopyemia
septic shock
Sergent's white line
serositis
serotonin
serous
serpiginous
serum sickness
sessile
Sézary's syndrome
sferositosis. See spherocytosis.
shangker. See chancre.

shangkroid. See *chancroid.*
Sheehan's disease
shelf
    Blumer's s.
Shigella
shigellosis
shingles
shock
    insulin s.
sialadenitis
sialidoses
sialoadenitis
sialoangiitis
sialometaplasia
sialorrhea
    s. pancreatica
sickle cell anemia
sick sinus syndrome
sideroblastic
siderocyte
siderosis
sigmoidoscopy
sign
    Babinski's s.
    Chvostek-Weiss s.
    Courvoisier's s.
    Erbs's s.
    Graefe's s.
    Homans' s.
    Kernig's s.
    Leser-Trélat s.
    Marie's s.
    Möbius' s.
    Nikolsky's s.
    Osler's s.
    Pemberton's s.
    Pfuhl's s.
    Romaña's s.
    Romberg's s.
    Stellwag's s.
    Troisier's s.
    Trousseau's s.
    Unschuld's s.
silicatosis
silicosis
silicotuberculosis
silosis. See *psilosis.*

Simmonds' disease
simultanagnosia
singultus
sinusitis
sirrosis. See *cirrhosis.*
sitakosis. See *psittacosis.*
sitophobia
Sjögren's syndrome
skistosomiasis. See
    schistosomiasis.
SLE – systemic lupus
    erythematosus
sleep apnea
smallpox
smear
    Papanicolaou (Pap) s.
    Tzanck s.
Smith-Strang disease
somatization
somatostatin
somatostatinoma
somatotropin
somnambulism
Somogyi
    effect
    phenomenon
sonofluoroscopy
sonography
sootsoogamooshe. See
    tsutsugamushi.
soriasis. See *psoriasis.*
sound
    Korotkoff's s.
South African tick typhus
South American hemorrhagic
    fever
Southeast Asian mosquito-borne
    hemorrhagic fever
spasticity
S period
spermatogenesis
spherocytosis
sphincter
sphingolipidoses
Spiegler-Fendt sarcoid
spina bifida
spinocerebellar

spirochetosis
spleen
    accessory s.
    Gandy-Gamna s.
    lardaceous s.
splenadenoma
splenalgia
splenatrophy
splenauxe
splenculus
splenectasis
splenectomy
splenectopia
splenelcosis
splenemia
splenemphraxis
spleneolus
splenepatitis
splenetic
splenic
    s. flexure syndrome
splenicterus
splenitis
    spodogenous s.
splenocele
splenocleisis
splenocolic
splenocyte
splenodynia
splenogenous
splenogram
splenogranulomatosis
    s. siderotica
splenography
splenohepatomegaly
splenokeratosis
splenolymphatic
splenolysin
splenolysis
splenoma
splenomalacia
splenomedullary
splenomegaly
    Gaucher's s.
    hemolytic s.
    hypercholesterolemic s.
    myelophthisic s.

splenomegaly (continued)
    Niemann's s.
    siderotic s.
    spodogenous s.
splenometry
splenomyelogenous
splenomyelomalacia
splenoncus
splenonephric
splenonephroptosis
splenopancreatic
splenoparectasis
splenopathy
splenopexy
splenophrenic
splenoptosis
splenorrhagia
splenosis
splenotoxin
splenotyphoid
splenulus
spondylarthritis
spondylitis
    von Bechterew-Strümpell
        s.
spondylolisthesis
spondylosis
spongiosis
sporotrichosis
spot
    café au lait s's
    De Morgan's s's
    Janeway's s's
    Koplik's s's
    Roth's s's
squamous
st – stage (of disease)
stage
    Tanner s.
staging
staphylococcal scalded skin
    syndrome
staphylococcus
Staphylococcus
    S. aureus
    S. epidermidis
    S. faecalis

Staphylococcus (continued)
 S. saprophyticus
 S. viridans
stasis syndrome
status
 s. asthmaticus
 s. choleraicus
 s. degenerativus
 s. epilepticus
 s. lymphaticus
 s. parathyreoprivus
 s. praesens
 s. thymicolymphaticus
STD – sexually transmitted
 disease
steal syndrome
steatorrhea
Stein-Leventhal syndrome
Stellwag's sign
stenosis
 aortic s.
 hypertrophic pyloric s.
 meatal s.
 mitral s.
 papillary s.
 pulmonic s.
 pyloric s.
 subaortic s.
 tracheal s.
 tricuspid s.
stereoanesthesia
sterility
Sternberg's disease
sternutatio
 s. convulsiva
steroid
Stevens-Johnson syndrome
Still's disease
Stokes-Adams attack
stomatitis
stomatocytosis
strabismus
Strachan-Scott syndrome
stratum
 s. corneum
 s. germinativum
 s. spinosum cells

streptocerciasis
streptococcus
Streptococcus
 S. bovis
 S. faecalis
 S. milleri
 S. mutans
 S. pneumoniae
 S. pyogenes
 S. viridans
streptolysin
 s. O
streptozyme test
striation
striatonigral
stricture
stridor
stroke
strongyloidiasis
struma
 s. basedowificata
 Hashimoto's s.
 s. lymphomatosa
 s. ovarii
 Riedel's s.
Strümpell-Leichtenstern
 encephalitis
Stuart-Bras disease
stupor
stuporous
subaortic
subarachnoid
subcutaneous
subdural
subphrenic
substrate
sucrosemia
Sudeck's atrophy
sudo-. See words beginning
 pseudo-.
sulfhemoglobinemia
sunstroke
superoxide
supraventricular
Sutton-Rendu-Osler-Weber
 syndrome
Swan-Ganz catheter

Sydenham's chorea
Symmers' disease
sympathectomy
sympathoadrenal
sympathochromaffin
sympathomimetic
synapsis
syncope
    carotid sinus s.
syndrome
    Abderhalden-Fanconi s.
    Abercrombie's s.
    Achard-Thiers s.
    Adams-Stokes s.
    addisonian s.
    adrenogenital s.
    Ahumada-Del Castillo s.
    Albers-Schönberg s.
    Albright's s.
    Aldrich's s.
    aortic arch s.
    Arakawa-Higashi s.
    argentaffinoma s.
    Arias' s.
    Ascher's s.
    Ayerza's s.
    Baber's s.
    Banti's s.
    Bard-Pic s.
    Barlow's s.
    Bar's s.
    Bartter's s.
    basal cell nevus s.
    Bassen-Kornzweig s.
    Bearn-Kunkel s.
    Behçet's s.
    Bernard's s.
    Bernard-Sergent s.
    Bloom's s.
    Blum's s.
    Boerhaave's s.
    Bouillaud's s.
    Brunsting's s.
    Budd-Chiari s.
    Caplan's s.
    carcinoid s.
    carpal tunnel s.

syndrome (continued)
    cervical rib s.
    Chédiak-Higashi s.
    Chiari-Frommel s.
    Chinese restaurant s.
    chubby puffer s.
    Conn's s.
    Cruveilhier-Baumgarten s.
    Cushing's s.
    defibrination s.
    Degos' s.
    DiGuglielmo's s.
    Dresbach's s.
    dysglandular s.
    ectopic ACTH s.
    Ehlers-Danlos s.
    Evans' s.
    Faber's s.
    Fanconi's s.
    Felty's s.
    Fitz-Hugh-Curtis s.
    Fitz's s.
    Forbes-Albright s.
    Friedmann's vasomotor s.
    Gaisböck's s.
    Gardner's s.
    Glanzmann's s.
    Goodpasture's s.
    Gopalan's s.
    Gradenigo's s.
    Guillain-Barré s.
    Günther's s.
    Hamman-Rich s.
    Harris' s.
    Hayem-Widal s.
    Heerfordt's s.
    Heidenhain's s.
    hemopleuropneumonic s.
    hepatorenal s.
    Hermansky-Pudlak s.
    Hines-Bannick s.
    Horner's s.
    Horton's s.
    Hunter's s.
    Hurler's s.
    hydralazine lupus s.
    hyperventilation s.

syndrome (continued)
    hyperviscosity s.
    Job's s.
    Kallmann's s.
    Kartagener's s.
    Kawasaki s.
    Kimmelstiel-Wilson s.
    Kleine-Levin s.
    Klinefelter's s.
    Kocher's s.
    König's s.
    Laurence-Moon-Biedl s.
    Läwen-Roth s.
    leopard s.
    Leriche's s.
    Lesch-Nyhan s.
    Lignac-Fanconi s.
    Löffler's s.
    Lowe's s.
    Luft's s.
    lymphoproliferative s.
    malabsorption s.
    Marchiafava-Micheli s.
    Marfan's s.
    Marie's s.
    Maroteaux-Lamy s.
    Meniere's s.
    Mikulicz's s.
    Minkowski-Chauffard s.
    Morquio's s.
    Münchausen's s.
    neurocutaneous s.
    nevoid basaloma s.
    Noonan's s.
    Osler's s.
    pancreaticohepatic s.
    parkinsonian s.
    Parkinson's s.
    Paterson-Brown-Kelly s.
    pickwickian s.
    Plummer-Vinson s.
    polyglandular s.
    polyposis coli s.
    Prader-Willi s.
    "prune-belly" s.
    Reifenstein's s.
    Reiter's s.

syndrome (continued)
    Rénon-Delille s.
    Reye's s.
    Richter's s.
    Riley-Day s.
    Romberg-Paessler s.
    Rosenbach's s.
    Rotor's s.
    rubella s.
    Sanfilippo's s.
    scalenus anticus s.
    Schaumann's s.
    Scheie's s.
    Schmidt's s.
    Senear-Usher s.
    Sézary's s.
    Sjögren's s.
    statis s.
    steal s.
    Stein-Leventhal s.
    Stevens-Johnson s.
    Strachan-Scott s.
    Sutton-Rendu-Osler-
        Weber s.
    Takayasu's s.
    Tietze's s.
    toxic shock s.
    Troisier-Hanot-Chauffard
        s.
    Troisier's s.
    Turner's s.
    von Hippel-Lindau s.
    Wallenberg's s.
    Waterhouse-Friderichsen
        s.
    Weil's s.
    Weinstein's s.
    Wermer's s.
    Werner's s.
    Willebrand's s.
    Wiskott-Aldrich s.
synechiae
synovial
synoviography
synovioma
synovitis
synovium

synthesis
    DNA s.
    protein s.
syphilis
syringomyelia
system
    kallikrein-kinin s.
    TNM staging s.
systemic
systolic
T_3-triiodothyronine
T_4-thyroxine
tabes
    diabetic t.
    t. dorsalis
taboparesis
tachyarrhythmias
tachycardia
tachyphylaxis
tachypnea
Takayasu's syndrome
tamponade
Tangier disease
Tanner stage
tapeworm
tardive
    t. akathisia
    t. dyskinesia
    t. dystonia
target cell(s)
Tay-Sachs disease
Tc-technetium
telalgia
telangiectasia
telangiectasis
template
tendinitis
tenesmus
tenosynovitis
teratoma
test
    alpha-fetoprotein t.
    beta-HCG t.
    CEA (carcinoembryonic
        antigen) t.
    cellophane tape t.
    doll's eye t.

test (continued)
    estrogen receptor assay t.
    Hanger-Rose skin t.
    Hemoccult t.
    Hickey-Hare t.
    Hoesch's t.
    indirect hemagglutination
        t.
    Kveim-Siltzbach t.
    latex agglutination t.
    patch t.
    radioallergosorbent t.
    Sabin-Feldman dye t.
    Schirmer's t.
    streptozyme t.
    Wassermann's t.
    Widal's t.
testicular
testis (testes)
tetanus
tetany
    hyperventilation t.
    parathyroid t.
    parathyroprival t.
    rheumatic t.
    thyroprival t.
tetralogy
    t. of Fallot
thalassemia
thelarche
thermography
thoracentesis
thoracic
thorax
thrombasthenia
thromboangiitis
    t. obliterans
thromboarteriosclerosis
    t. obliterans
thrombocytasthenia
thrombocythemia
thrombocytopenia
thrombocytopenic purpura
thrombocytopoiesis
thrombocytosis
thromboembolism
thrombolysis

thrombopenia
thrombophlebitis
thromboplastin
thrombosis
thrombus
thrush
thymectomy
thymine
thymolipoma
thymoma
thymus
thyrocalcitonin
thyroid
thyroidism
thyroiditis
    ligneous t.
thyroid-stimulating hormone
thyromegaly
thyrophyma
thyroprival
thyrotoxicosis
    t. factitia
thyroxine
tic
    t. douloureux (*doo-loo-roo*)
tick paralysis
Tietze's syndrome
time
    generation t.
tinnitus
TNM–tumor, nodes, metastases
TNM staging system
Todd's cirrhosis
tomography
tonsillitis
tophus
    t. syphiliticus
torticollis
torulosis
tosis. See *ptosis.*
Toxemia
toxic
toxicity
toxicology
toxicosis
toxocariasis

Toxoplasma
    T. gondii
toxoplasmosis
trachea
tracheitis
trachelagra
tracheobronchitis
tracheostomy
trachoma
translocation
    robertsonian t.
transplantation
    allogeneic marrow t.
treatment
    Paul's t.
    Yeo's t.
trematode(s)
trematodiasis
tremor
Treponema
    T. carateum
    T. pallidum
    T. pertenue
treponemal
treponematosis
treponemiasis
triad
    Falta's t.
    Hutchinson's t.
    Merseburg t.
    Whipple's t.
trichinosis
trichocephaliasis
trichoglossia
Trichomonas
    T. vaginalis
trichomoniasis
trichophytosis
trichorrhexis
    t. nodosa
trichostrongylosis
trichuriasis
tricyclic
trigeminal
    t. neuralgia
triglyceride(s)
triiodothyronine

trikinosis. See *trichinosis.*
triko-. See words beginning
   tricho-.
trikuriasis. See *trichuriasis.*
trismus
trisomy 13, 18, 21, 22, X
tRNA – transfer RNA
trofedema. See *trophedema.*
Troisier-Hanot-Chauffard
   syndrome
Troisier's
     ganglion
     sign
     syndrome
trophedema
Trousseau's sign
truncal
truncus
     t. arteriosus
Trypanosoma
     T. brucei
     T. cruzi
     T. gambiense
     T. rhodesiense
trypanosomiasis
TSH – thyroid-stimulating
   hormone
TSS – toxic shock syndrome
tsutsugamushi disease
tubercle
     Farre's t's
tuberculin
tuberculosis
tuberous
tubulointestinal
tularemia
tumor
     Abrikossoff's t.
     Burkitt's t.
     fungating t.
     Grawitz' t.
     islet cell t.
     mixed-tissue t.
     mucinous t.
     nonresponsive t.
     radiocurable t.
     radioresistant t.

tumor (continued)
     radiosensitive t.
     responsive t.
     serous t.
     solid t.
     Wilms' t.
Turner's syndrome
tylosis
type
     Runeberg's t.
typhoid
typhoidette
typhus
     Indian tick t.
     Queensland tick t.
     South African tick t.
tyrosinemia
tyrosinosis
Tzanck smear
UCTS – undifferentiated
   connective tissue syndrome
ulcer
     aphthous u.
     cutaneous u.
     decubitus u.
     duodenal u.
     Parrot's u.
     peptic u.
     serpiginous u.
ulcerating
ulceration
ulcerative
     u. colitis
ultrasonography
ultrasound
     Doppler u.
uncinariasis
undifferentiated
Undritz' anomaly
undulant fever
Unschuld's sign
unsinariasis. See *uncinariasis.*
unukizm. See *eunuchism.*
uptake
     radioactive iodine u.
uracil
urate

urea
uremia
uremic
ureter
ureterocele
urethra
urethritis
URI – upper respiratory infection
uricosuria
urinary
urine
urobilinemia
urobilinuria
urogram
urography
urokinase
urolithiasis
urticaria
uterus
uthanazea. See *euthanasia.*
uthiroid. See *euthyroid.*
uthiroidism. See *euthyroidism*
utricle
uveitis
uveomeningitis
uvula
vaccination
    smallpox v.
vaccine
vaccinia
    v. gangrenosa
vagina
vaginitis
vaginosis
vagotomy
vagovagal
valine
varicella
varices
variola
varix
vascular
vasculitis
vasomotor
vasopressin
Vater's ampulla
venereal

Venezuelan equine
    encephalomyelitis
venography
VEP – visual evoked potential
vermiculous
verruca
    v. peruana
    v. vulgaris
verrucous
Verstraeten's bruit
vertigo
vestibular system
vinyl chloride
viremia
viricidal
virilism
    adrenal v.
    prosopopilary v.
virion
virology
virus
    Colorado tick fever v.
    Coxsackie v.
    DNA v.
    Epstein-Barr v.
    herpes v.
    HIV v.
    oncogenic v.
    RNA v.
visceral
viscus
vitiligo
vitium
    v. conformationis
    v. primae formationis
voiding
vomiting
vomitus
von Bechterew-Strümpell
    spondylitis
von Economo's encephalitis
von Gierke's disease
von Hippel-Lindau syndrome
von Recklinghausen's disease
von Willebrand's disease
vookereriasis. See *wuchereriasis.*
vulvovaginitis

Waldenström's
    macroglobulinemia
Wallenberg's syndrome
Wasserman's test
Waterhouse-Friderichsen
    syndrome
WEE – western equine
    encephalitis
Wegener's granulomatosis
Weil-Felix reaction
Weil's
    disease
    syndrome
Weinstein's syndrome
Wermer's syndrome
Werner's
    disease
    syndrome
Wernicke's
    aphasia
    disease
    encephalopathy
West Nile
    encephalitis
    fever
western equine enceph-
    alitis
wheezing
Whipple's
    disease
    triad
whitlow
whooping cough
Widal-Abrami disease
Widal's test
Willebrand's syndrome
Willis'
    disease
    pancreas
Wilms' tumor
Wilson's disease
Winslow's pancreas
Wirsung's duct
Wiskott-Aldrich syndrome

wolffian duct
World Health Organization
Wuchereria
    W. bancrofti
wuchereriasis
xanthelasma
xanthinuria
xanthogranuloma
xanthoma
    x. diabeticorum
xanthomatosis
xanthosis
    x. diabetica
X chromosome
xenogeneic
xerocytosis
xeroderma pigmentosum
xerophthalmia
xerosis
xerostomia
yaws
Y chromosome
yellow fever
yellow nail syndrome
Yeo's treatment
Yersinia
    Y. enterocolitica
    Y. pseudotuberculosis
zan.- See words beginning *xan-.*
zantho-. See words beginning
    xantho-.
Zenker's diverticulum
zerofthalmea. See *xerophthalmia.*
zerosis. See *xerosis.*
zerostomia
zona
    z. fasciculata
    z. glomerulosa
    z. reticularis
zosteriform
zoster sine herpete
zygomycosis
zymolysis

Obstetrics and Gynecology

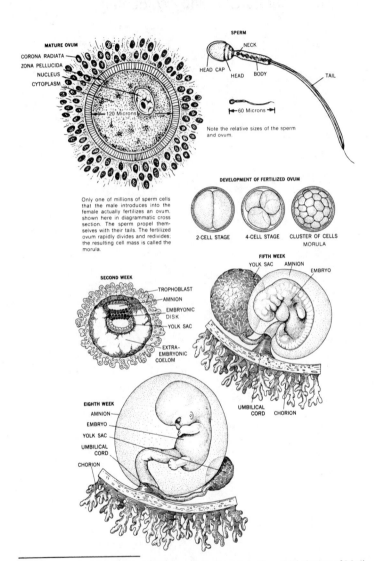

MATURE OVUM

CORONA RADIATA
ZONA PELLUCIDA
NUCLEUS
CYTOPLASM

120 Microns

SPERM

NECK
HEAD CAP
HEAD   BODY
TAIL

60 Microns

Note the relative sizes of the sperm and ovum.

Only one of millions of sperm cells that the male introduces into the female actually fertilizes an ovum, shown here in diagrammatic cross section. The sperm propel themselves with their tails. The fertilized ovum rapidly divides and redivides; the resulting cell mass is called the morula.

DEVELOPMENT OF FERTILIZED OVUM

2-CELL STAGE   4-CELL STAGE   CLUSTER OF CELLS
MORULA

SECOND WEEK

TROPHOBLAST
AMNION
EMBRYONIC DISK
YOLK SAC
EXTRA-EMBRYONIC COELOM

FIFTH WEEK

YOLK SAC   AMNION
EMBRYO

UMBILICAL CORD   CHORION

EIGHTH WEEK

AMNION
EMBRYO
YOLK SAC
UMBILICAL CORD
CHORION

(Courtesy of Miller, B. F., and Keane, C. B.: Encyclopedia and Dictionary of Medicine, Nursing and Allied Health, 2nd ed. Philadelphia, W. B. Saunders Company, 1978.)

Obstetrics and Gynecology

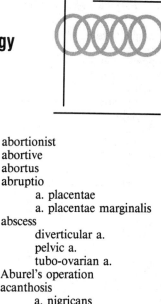

AB – abortion
abactio
abactus venter
abdomen
abdominal
abdominohysterectomy
abdominohysterotomy
Abell's operation
ablatio
    a. placentae
ABO compatible
ABO incompatibility
ABO incompatible
abort
aborticide
abortifacient
abortion
    afebrile a.
    ampullar a.
    cervical a.
    complete a.
    contagious a.
    criminal a.
    epizootic a.
    habitual a.
    imminent a.
    incomplete a.
    induced a.
    inevitable a.
    infectious a.
    justifiable a.
    missed a.
    saline a.
    septic a.
    spontaneous a.
    therapeutic a.
    threatened a.
    tubal a.
    vibrio a.

abortionist
abortive
abortus
abruptio
    a. placentae
    a. placentae marginalis
abscess
    diverticular a.
    pelvic a.
    tubo-ovarian a.
Aburel's operation
acanthosis
    a. nigricans
accouchement
    a. force
accoucheur
acephalocystis racemosa
Achard-Thiers syndrome
acidosis
acquired immunodeficiency
    syndrome
acrocyanosis
acrohysterosalpingectomy
acrosomal
Adair's tenaculum
adenitis
    vestibular a.
adenoacanthoma
adenocarcinoma
    clear cell a.
adenofibroma
adenohypophysis
adenoma
    a. endometrioides
        ovarii
    a. ovarii testiculare
    a. tubulare testiculare
        ovarii

467

adenomyofibroma
adenomyoma
adenomyomatosis
adenomyometritis
adenomyosis
adenomyositis
adenopathy
adenosis
    vaginal a.
adhesion
    filamentous a.
    periadnexal a.
adnexa
    a. uteri
adnexal
adnexectomy
adnexitis
adnexogenesis
adnexopexy
adnexorganogenic
adrenal
adrenarche
adrenocorticoid
adrenocorticotropic
adrenopause
aerocolpos
afibrinogenemia
afterbirth
after-coming head
afterpains
agenesis
    müllerian a.
    renal a.
    vaginal a.
agenitalism
agonist
    beta-adrenergic a.
Ahlfeld's sign
Ahumada-Del Castillo
   syndrome
AID – artificial insemination
   donor
aidoiitis
AIDS – acquired
   immunodeficiency
   syndrome. See *Immunology*
   section.

albuginea
    a. ovarii
albumin
Aldrich's operation
Alexander-Adams operation
Alexander's operation
algomenorrhea
algorithm
Allen-Masters syndrome
All-Flex diaphragm
Allis'
    clamp
    forceps
alopecia
    postpartum a.
amenia
amenorrhea
    absolute a.
    dysponderal a.
    hypothalamic a.
    lactation a.
    ovarian a.
    pathologic a.
    physiologic a.
    pituitary a.
    "postpill" a.
    premenopausal a.
    primary a.
    relative a.
    secondary a.
amenorrheal
ametria
aminoglycoside(s)
amniocentesis
amniochorial
amniogenesis
amniogram
amniography
amnioma
amnion
amnionic
amnionitis
amniorrhea
amniorrhexis
amnioscopy
amniotic
    a. fluid

amniotin
amniotome
        Baylor's a.
        Beacham's a.
amniotomy
ampule
ampulla
ampullary
analgesia
anastomosis
        ureterotubal a.
androgen
android
androstenedione
anemia
anencephaly
anesthesia. See *General Surgical Terms.*
angiokeratoma
        vulvar a.
angioma
angiomata
        cherry a.
angiotensin
angle
        costovertebral a.
anisocytosis
ankylocolpos
anorexia
        a. nervosa
anovaginal
anovaria
anovarism
anovular
anovulation
anovulatory
anovulia
anovulomenorrhea
anoxia
        a. neonatorum
anteflexed
anteflexio
        a. uteri
anteflexion
antenatal
antepartal
antepartum

anteversion
anteverted
anthropoid
antiandrogenic
antigen
antigravity suit
antihypertensive
antineoplastic
antrum
anus
Apgar
        rating
        score
A & P repair – anterior and
        posterior repair
aplasia
apoplexia
        a. uteri
apoplexy
        uterine a.
        uteroplacental a.
appendicitis
appendix
applicator
        Ernst's a.
arachidonic acid
arcuate
areno-. See words beginning
        arrheno-.
areola
areolar
Arey's rule
Arias-Stella's phenomenon
Arnoux's sign
arrhenoblastoma
arrhenogenic
arrhenoma
arrhenomimetic
artery
        hypogastric a.
        hypophyseal a.
        iliac a.
        ilioinguinal a.
        ovarian a.
        peroneal a.
        pudendal a.
        umbilical a.

artery (continued)
    uterine a.
arthritis
    rheumatoid a.
ascensus
    a. uteri
Aschheim-Zondek test
ascites
Asherman's syndrome
asphyxia
aspiration
    vacuum a.
aspirator
    blue tip a.
    red tip a.
    vacuum a.
    yellow tip a.
assimilation
asynclitism
atelectasis
athenospermia
Atlee's dilator
atony
    uterine a.
atopomenorrhea
ATP–adenosine triphosphate
atresia
atrium
    a. vaginae
atrophy
atypical
Auerbach's plexus
augmentation
ausculatory
autoimmune disease
autosomal
Auvard-Remine speculum
Auvard's
    cranioclast
    weighted speculum
avascular
axillary
Ayerst's knife
AZ test–Aschheim-Zondek test
Babcock's clamp
bacilli
    Döderlein's b.

Backhaus towel clamp
bacteriuria
Bacteroides
    B. fragilis
Baer's vesicle
bag
    Champetier de Ribes' b.
    Voorhees' b.
Bailey-Williamson forceps
balanic
Baldwin's operation
Baldy's operation
Baldy-Webster operation
Balfour's retractor
Ballantine's clamp
ballotable
ballottement
Ball's operation
Bandl's ring
Bard-Parker blade
Barkow
    colliculus of B.
barren
Barrett-Allen forceps
Barrett's
    forceps
    tenaculum
bartholinitis
Bartholin's
    cyst
    gland
Barton's
    forceps
    traction handle
basalis
Basedow's disease
basiotripsy (fetal)
Basset's operation
Baudeloque's operation
Baylor's amniotome
BBT–basal body temperature
Beacham's amniotome
Beatson's operation
Beccaria's sign
Beck. See *Boeck.*
Beclard's sign
Behçet's disease

Bellow's pack
Bel-O-Pak
Benaron's forceps
benign
Berlind-Auvard speculum
Berry's forceps
beta-blocker
Beuttner's method
bicornuate
bifid
bilirubin
Billroth's forceps
Bill's traction handle
bimanual
Biocept-G test
biophysical
biopsy(ies)
    bite b.
    cervical b.
    cold knife conization b.
    cone b.
    endometrial b.
    excisional b.
    four point b.
    multiple b.
    needle b.
    punch b.
    sponge b.
    wedge b.
biparietal diameter
biphasic
Birnberg's bow
Bischoff's operation
Bishop's score
Bissell's operation
bivalve
Black-Wylie dilator
bladder
    b. blade
    dome of b.
    b. flap
    hypotonic b.
blade
    Bard-Parker b.
    bistoury b.
    bladder b.
blennorrhea

block
    paracervical b.
    pudendal b.
blood
    cord b.
Blot's perforator
body
    Call-Exner b's
    Donovan's b's
    psammoma b's
Boeck's sarcoidosis
boggy
Bolt's sign
Bond's forceps
Bonnaire's method
Bonney's
    hysterectomy
    test
bosselated
Bouilly's operation
Bovie unit
bow
    Birnberg's b.
Bowen's disease
box
    Stockholm b.
Bozeman's
    forceps
    operation
BPD – biparietal diameter
Braasch's forceps
Bracht's maneuver
Brandt-Andrews maneuver
Brandt's
    brassiere
    technique
    treatment
Brantley-Turner retractor
brassiere
    Brandt's b.
Braune's canal
Braun-Fernwald sign
Braun-Jardine-DeLee hook
Braun's
    cranioclast
    hook
    scissors

Braun's (continued)
    tenaculum
Braxton-Hicks
    contraction
    sign
    version
breech. See also presentation.
    b. delivery
    b. extraction
    b. presentation
Breisky's
    disease
    pelvimeter
Brenner's tumor
Brentano's syndrome
Breu's mole
Brewer's speculum
Bricker's operation
Broder's classification
Brouha's test
bruit
Brunschwig's operation
brwe. See *bruit.*
Buie clamp
bulbus
    b. vestibuli vaginae
Bumm's curet
Burch's operation
BUS glands–Bartholin's,
    urethral, and Skene's glands
Buxton clamp
cachectic
cachexia
    c. ovariopriva
calculation
    Johnson's c.
Call-Exner body
Camper's fascia
canal
    Braune's c.
    cervical c.
    endocervical c.
    c. of Nuck
canalis
    c. cervicis uteri
Candida
    C. albicans

Candida (continued)
    C. vulvovaginitis
cannula
    Holman-Mathieu c.
    Hudgins' c.
    Jarcho's c.
    Kahn's c.
    Neal's c.
    Rubin's c.
cannulation
capacitation
caput
    c. medusae
    c. succedaneum
carcinoma
    clear cell c.
    comedo c.
    cylindromatous c.
    ductal c.
    embryonal c.
    epidermoid c.
    granulosa cell c.
    gyriform c.
    infiltrating c.
    c. in situ
    intraepithelial c.
    invasive c.
    macrofolliculoid c.
    microfolliculoid c.
    parenchymatous c.
    squamous cell c.
carcinomatosis
carcinophilic
carcinosarcoma
cardiac
cardiomyopathy
cardiorespiratory
cardiovascular
carina
    c. fornicis
    c. urethralis vaginae
caruncle
    hymenal c's
    urethral c.
carunculae hymenales
catamenia
catamenial

catamenogenic
catecholamine
catheter
    Foley c.
    French c.
    Fritsch's c.
    indwelling c.
    Wurd's c.
catheterization
cauterization
cauterized
cautery
    Percy's c.
cavity
    endometrial c.
cavum
    c. uteri
CDC—calculated date of
    confinement
celiocolpotomy
celiohysterectomy
celiohysterotomy
celiosalpingectomy
celiosalpingotomy
celiotomy
    vaginal c.
cell
    atypical c.
    bank c.
    basket c.
    ciliated c.
    clue c.
    cornified c.
    c. cycle
    decidual c.
    endocervical c.
    endometrial c.
    epithelial c.
    epithelioid c.
    granulosa c.
    hilar c.
    intercalary c.
    keratinized c.
    Langhan's c.
    Leydig's c.
    luteum c.
    mesothelial c.

cell (continued)
    navicular c.
    Paget's c.
    parabasal c.
    precornified c.
    squamous c.
    superficial c.
    syncytial c.
    "tadpole" c.
    target c.
    tart c.
    theca lutein c.
    Walthard's c.
cephalad
cephalic
cephalometry
cephalopelvic disproportion
cerclage
cervical
    c. biopsy
    c. canal
    c. caps
    c. collar
    c. conization
    c. fascia
    c. os
cervicectomy
cervicitis
    granulomatous c.
    traumatic c.
cervicocolpitis
    c. emphysematosa
cervicovaginal
cervicovaginitis
cervicovesical
cervimeter
cervitome
    Milex c.
cervix
    conglutination of c.
    incompetent c.
    c. uteri
cesarean. See under *section.*
CGT—chorionic gonadotropin
Chadwick's sign
Chamberlen's forceps
Champetier de Ribes's bag

chancre
chancroid
chart
 Liley's c.
chemotherapy
Chiari-Frommel syndrome
Chlamydia
chloasma
 c. gravidarum
 c. uterinum
chlorosis
 c. vulvae
cholestasis
cholesterol
chondromalacia
 c. fetalis
chorioadenoma
 c. destruens
chorioamnionitis
choriocarcinoma
chorioepithelioma
chorion
 c. frondosum
chorionic
 c. gonadotropin
 c. villi
chorioplacental
chromohydrotubation
chromosomal
cicatrix
circumcision
circumoral
clamp
 Allis' c.
 Babcock's c.
 Backhaus towel c.
 Ballantine's c.
 Buie c.
 Buxton c.
 Heaney's c.
 Kane's c.
 Kelly's c.
 Kocher's c.
 Lahey's c.
 Ochsner's c.
 Pennington's c.
 Reich's c.

clamp (continued)
 Willett's c.
 Yellen c.
classification
 Broder's c.
 White's c.
Claudius' fossa
clean catch urine
cleavage
cleidotomy (fetal)
cleidotripsy
climacteric
climacterium
 c. praecox
clip
 Hulka's c.
clitoral
clitoridauxe
clitoridean
clitoridectomy
clitoriditis
clitoridotomy
clitoris
 bifid c.
 crura of c.
 prepuce of c.
clitorism
clitoritis
clitoromania
clitoromegaly
clitorotomy
cloaca
Cloquet's node
closure
 Latzko's c.
coagulation
coagulopathy
 disseminated intravas-
  cular c.
coccyx
Coffey's operation
coil
 Margulles' c.
coitophobia
coitus
 c. á la vache
 c. incompletus

coitus (continued)
  c. interruptus
  c. reservatus
coleocele
coleocystitis
coleoptosis
coleospastia
coleotomy
Colles' fascia
colliculus
  c. of Barkow
  cervical c. of female
   urethra
Collin's
  forceps
  pelvimeter
  speculum
  test
Collyer's pelvimeter
colon
  sigmoid c.
colostrum
  c. gravidarum
  c. puerperarum
colovaginal
colpalgia
colpatresia
colpectasia
colpectasis
colpectomy
colpeurysis
colpismus
colpitic
colpitis
  c. emphysematosa
  emphysematous c.
  c. granulosa
  c. mycotica
colpocele
colpoceliocentesis
colpoceliotomy
colpocleisis
colpocystitis
colpocystocele
colpocystoplasty
colpocystotomy
colpocystoureterocystotomy

colpocytogram
colpocytology
colpodynia
colpoepisiorrhaphy
colpohyperplasia
colpohysterectomy
colpohysteropexy
colpohysterorrhaphy
colpohysterotomy
colpolaparotomy
colpomicroscope
colpomicroscopic
colpomicroscopy
colpomycosis
colpomyomectomy
colpoperineoplasty
colpoperineorrhaphy
colpopexy
colpoplasty
colpopoiesis
colpopolypus
colpoptosis
colporectopexy
colporrhagia
colporrhaphy
colporrhexis
colposcope
colposcopy
colpospasm
colpostat
colpostenosis
colpostenotomy
colpotherm
colpotomy
colpoureterocystotomy
colpoureterotomy
colpoxerosis
columnar
comedocarcinoma
comedomastitis
commissura
  c. labiorum anterior
  c. labiorum posterior
  c. labiorum pudendi
commissure
  anterior c. of labia
  posterior c. of labia

compatible
conception
conceptus
condom
conduplicato
    c. corpore
condyloma
    c. acuminatum
    c. latum
    c. subcutaneum
condylomata
condylomatoid
condylomatosis
condylomatous
condylotomy
configuration
    arcuate c.
confinement
congenital
conglutinatio
    c. orificii externi
conglutination
conization
    cold knife c.
conjugata
    c. vera obstetrica
conjugate
    diagonal c.
    obstetric c.
contraception
contraceptive
contraction
    Braxton-Hicks c.
    premonitory c's
Coombs' test
copious
copulation
cord
    c. blood
    clamping c.
    c. compression
    medullary c's
    ovigerous c's
    umbilical c.
Corey's forceps
Corner-Allen test
cornu

cornua
cornual
coronal
corpora atretica
corpus
    c. albicans
    c. cavernosum clitoridis
    c. clitoridis
    c. glandulosum
    c. hemorrhagicum
    c. luteum
    c. spongiosum urethrae muliebris
    c. uteri
    uterine c.
cortex
corticosteroid
costovertebral
cotyledon
Couvelaire uterus
CPD – cephalopelvic disproportion
crab louse
cranioclasis (fetal)
cranioclast
    Auvard's c.
    Braun's c.
    Zweifel-DeLee c.
craniotome
craniotomy (fetal)
Credé's method
cretin
cretinism
CRF – corticotropin-releasing factor
cribriform
crista
    c. urethralis femininae
    c. urethralis muliebris
Crohn's disease
crowning
crura
crus
    c. clitoridis
    c. of clitoris
    c. glandis clitoridis
cryostat

cryosurgery
cryotherapy
cryptomenorrhea
crystalline
CS – cesarean section
C-section – cesarean section
cuboidal
cul-de-sac
    Douglas' c.d.s.
culdocentesis
culdoscope
    Decker's c.
culdoscopy
Cullen's sign
cumulus
    c. oophorus
    ovarian c.
    c. ovaricus
cuneihysterectomy
cup
    Silastic c.
curet
    banjo c.
    Bumm's c.
    Greene's c.
    Gusberg's c.
    Hannon's c.
    Heaney's c.
    Holden's c.
    Holtz's c.
    Hunter's c.
    Kelly-Gray c.
    Kelly's c.
    Kevorkian's c.
    Kushner-Tandatnick c.
    Lounsbury's c.
    Novak's c.
    Randall's c.
    Récamier's c.
    Reich-Nechtow c.
    serrated c.
    Sims' c.
    Skene's c.
    Thomas' c.
curettage
    fractional c.
    suction c.

curette. See *curet.*
curettement
Curtius' syndrome
curve
    oxygen dissociation c.
Cusco's speculum
Cushing's syndrome
CVA – costovertebral angle
CWP – childbirth without pain
cyanotic
cycle
    aberrant c.
    anovulatory c.
    endometrial c.
    genesial c.
    gonadotropic c.
    menstrual c.
    myometrial c.
    oogenetic c.
    ovarian c.
    reproductive c.
    sexual c.
cyclic
cyema
cyesedema
cyesiognosis
cyesiology
cyesis
cyestein
cyogenic
cyonin
cyophoria
cyophoric
cyotrophy
cyst
    adnexal c.
    atheromatous c.
    Bartholin's c.
    blue dome c.
    chocolate c.
    chorionic c.
    corpus luteum c.
    dermoid c.
    embryonal c.
    endometrial c.
    epoophoron c.
    follicular c.

cyst (continued)

    gartnerian c.

    granulosa lutein c.

    hemorrhagic c.

    hymenal c.

    inclusion c.

    inflammatory c.

    lutein c.

    c. of Morgagni

    morgagnian c.

    nabothian c.

    Naboth's c's

    oophoritic c.

    ovarian c.

    paroophoritic c.

    parovarian c.

    pedicled c.

    polycystic c.

    retention c.

    Sampson's c.

    sebaceous c.

    theca-lutein c.

    tubo-ovarian c.

    vaginal inclusion c.

    wolffian c.

cystadenocarcinoma

cystadenofibroma

cystadenoma

    mucinous c.

    pseudomucinous c.

    serous c.

cystectomy

cystic

    c. fibrosis

    c. mastitis

cystitis

cystocele

cystoelytroplasty

cystography

cystolutein

cystoma

    myxoid c.

    c. serosum simplex

cystomatitis

cystomatous

cystometrogram

cystosarcoma

    c. phylloides

cystoscopy

cystourethrocele

cystourethrogram

    bead-chain c.

cystourethroscopy

cytogenic

cytogenetic

cytomegalovirus

cytoplasm

cytotoxic

cytotrophoblast

Dacron shield

Dalkon shield

Danforth's

    method

    sign

David's disease

Davis' operation

D & C–dilatation and curettage

    diagnostic D & C

    suction D & C

De Alvarez's forceps

Deaver's retractor

deceleration

decidua

    basal d.

    d. basalis

    capsular d.

    d. capsularis

    menstrual d.

    d. menstrualis

    parietal d.

    d. parietalis

    reflex d.

    d. reflexa

    d. serotina

    d. vera

decidual

decidualitis

deciduate

deciduation

deciduitis

deciduoma

deciduomatosis

decipara
Decker's
    culdoscope
    operation
defervesced
deficiency
    21-hydroxylase enzyme d.
deflection
    vesicouterine d.
defundation
defundectomy
DeLee's
    forceps
    maneuver
    pelvimeter
    retractor
    tenaculum
delivery
    breech d.
    low forceps d.
    mid forceps d.
    spontaneous d.
denidation
depression
    postpartum d.
    reactive d.
dermatosis
    vulvar d.
dermoid
Dermoplast spray
DES – diethylstilbestrol
descensus
    d. uteri
    uterine d.
desensin
Desjardin's forceps
desultory
detachment
    annular d.
detrusor
Deventer's
    diameter
    pelvis
device
    Fletcher-Suit after-
      loading d.

Devilbiss' speculum
Devilbiss-Stacey speculum
Dewees' sign
Dewey's forceps
dextroposition
dextrorotation
Dextrostix
dextroverted
diabetes
    d. mellitus
diagnostic D & C
diameter
    Deventer's d.
    Löhlein's d.
diaphanography
diaphragm
    All-Flex d.
    Ramses' d.
    urogenital d.
    vaginal d.
diastasis
    d. recti abdominis
DIC – disseminated intravascular
    coagulopathy
Diday's law
didelphia
didelphic
Dienst's test
dihysteria
dilatation
    d. and curettage
    d. and evacuation
dilated
dilation
dilation and curettage
dilator
    Atlee's d.
    Black-Wylie d.
    Goodell's d.
    Hank-Bradley d.
    Hank's d.
    Hegar's d.
    Hurtig's d.
    Jolly's d.
    Kelly's d.
    Palmer's d.

dilator (continued)
    Pratt's d.
    Reich-Nechtow d.
    Starlinger's d.
    Wylie's d.
diovulatory
diphasia
dis-. See also words beginning
   dys-.
disc
    embryonic d.
discission
discrete
disease
    autoimmune d.
    Basedow's d.
    Behçet's d.
    Bowen's d.
    Breisky's d.
    Crohn's d.
    David's d.
    fibrocystic d.
    Fox-Fordyce d.
    Graves' d.
    Halban's d.
    Lignac-Fanconi d.
    Maher's d.
    Niemann-Pick d.
    Paget's d.
    pelvic inflammatory d.
    Schroeder's d.
    Tay-Sachs d.
    Valsuani's d.
    von Willebrand's d.
disproportion
    cephalopelvic d.
dissection
diverticulum
    urethral d.
DNA – deoxyribonucleic
   acid
Döderlein's
    bacilli
    operation
Doleris' operation
Donald-Fothergill operation
Donald's operation

Donovania
    D. granulomatis
Donovan's body
doptone
douche
Douglas'
    cul-de-sac
    fold
    line
    method
    pouch
douglascele
douglasitis
Dow-Corning implant
Down's syndrome
Doyen's
    operation
    retractor
    scissors
    vaginal hysterectomy
drain
    Penrose d.
drip
    pitocin d.
drugs. See *Drugs and Chemistry*
   section.
DUB – dysfunctional uterine
   bleeding
Dubovitz's syndrome
duct
    Gartner's d.
    mesonephric d.
    müllerian d.
    omphalomesenteric d.
    ovarian d.
    paramesonephric d's
    Reichel's cloacal d.
    Skene's d.
    vitelline d.
    wolffian d.
ductuli transversi epoophori
ductus
    d. arteriosus
    d. epoophori
      longitudinalis
    d. venosus

Dudley's
    hook
    operation
Dührssen's
    operation
    tampon
duipara
Duncan's mechanism
Duplay's
    hook
    tenaculum
D 5 & W – 5% dextrose and water
dye
    indigo carmine d.
dyschezia
dysfunction
dysfunctional
    d. uterine bleeding
dysgenesis
    gonadal d.
    mosaic gonadal d.
dysgerminoma
dyskaryosis
dyskinesia
    uterine d.
dysmaturity
dysmenorrhea
    d. intermenstrualis
    plethoric d.
    psychogenic d.
dyspareunia
dysplasia
dyspnea
dysponderal
dystocia
dystrophy
    hyperplastic d.
    myotonic d.
Eastman's retractor
easy-pulls
EBL – estimated blood loss
eclampsia
ectasia
    mammary duct e.
ectocervix
ectoderm
    dorsal e.

ectopic
EDC – estimated date of
        confinement
     expected date of
        confinement
edema
Eder's forceps
effaced
effacement
effect
    Poseiro's e.
EGA – estimated gestational age
electrocauterization
electrocoagulation
electrometrogram
elephantiasis
    e. of vulva
elevator
    Soonawalla uterine e.
Elliott's
    forceps
    treatment
Ellis-van Creveld syndrome
emansio mensium
embolus
embryo
embryoctony
embryogenesis
embryogenetic
embryogenic
embryology
embryonal
embryonate
embryonic
embryoniform
embryonism
embryonization
embryonoid
embryopathia
    e. rubeolaris
embryopathology
embryopathy
embryotocia
embryotome
embryotomy
emesis
    e. gravidarum

emmenagogic
emmenagogue
emmenia
emmenic
emmeniopathy
emmenology
Emmert-Gellhorn pessary
Emmet's
    hook
    operation
    retractor
    scissors
Emmet-Studdiford
    perineorrhaphy
en bloc
encephalopathy
    bilirubin e.
endocervical
    e. canal
    e. mucosa
    e. polyp
endocervicitis
endocervix
endocolpitis
endocrine
endoderm
    ventral e.
endodermal
endolymphatic
endometrectomy
endometria
endometrial
endometrioid
endometrioma
endometriosis
    e. externa
    e. interna
    ovarian e.
    e. ovarii
    e. uterina
    e. vesicae
endometriotic
endometritis
    bacteriotoxic e.
    decidual e.
    e. dissecans
    exfoliative e.

endometritis (continued)
    glandular e.
    membranous e.
    postpartum e.
    puerperal e.
    syncytial e.
endometrium
    hyperplastic e.
    secretory e.
    Swiss-cheese e.
endomyoparametritis
endorphin(s)
endosalpingitis
endosalpingoma
endosalpingosis
endosalpinx
endotoxic
endouterine
engorge
engorgement
entad
ental
enteritis
enterocele
enteropathy
enucleated
epichorion
epimenorrhagia
epimenorrhea
episioclisia
episioelytrorrhaphy
episioperineoplasty
episioperineorrhaphy
episioplasty
episiorrhaphy
episiostenosis
episiotomy
    Matsner e.
epithelial
epithelialized
epithelioid
epithelioma
    e. of Malherbe
epithelium
    dysplastic e.
epoophorectomy
epoöphoron

Ernst's applicator
eroded
erosion
erythroblastosis
     e. fetalis
     e. neonatorum
Escherichia
     E. coli
escutcheon
esophagitis
     reflux e.
Estes' operation
esthiomene
estradiol
estrogen
etrohysterectomy
EUA – examination under
    anesthesia
eunuchoid
eutocia
evacuation
eversion
evert
examination
     bimanual e.
     gynecologic e.
     hanging drop e.
     postpartal e.
     speculum e.
     vaginorectal e.
exenteration
exercise
     Kegel's e.
exfetation
exometritis
exophytic
expulsion
external os
extraction
     breech e.
     vacuum e.
extraembryonic
     e. celom
extragenital
extraperitoneal
extrauterine
extravaginal

falciform
Falk-Shukuris operation
Falk's operation
fallectomy
fallopian tube
fallostomy
fallotomy
Falope's ring
Farre's line
Farris' test
fascia
     Camper's f.
     cervical f.
     Colles' f.
     endopelvic f.
     pubovesicocervical f.
     Scarpa's f.
     subvesical f.
     transversalis f.
fecalith
femur length
fenestrated
fenestration
Ferguson's
     reflex
     scissors
Fergusson's speculum
ferning
Ferris' forceps
fertile
fertility
fertilization
fetal
     f. alcohol syndrome
     f. allograft
     f. asphyxia
     f. breathing
     f. circulation
     f. distress
     f. head
     f. heart sound
     f. heart tone
     f. hemolysis
     f. hydantoin syndrome
     f. hydrops
     f. monitor
     f. oophoritis

fetal (continued)
    f. oxygenation
    f. postmaturity syndrome
    f. skull
    f. structure
    f. tachycardia
    f.-to-maternal ratio
    f. warfarin syndrome
    f. weight
    f. well-being
fetal position
    LFA – left frontoanterior
    LFP – left frontoposterior
    LFT – left frontotransverse
    LMA – left mentoanterior
    LMP – left mentoposterior
    LMT – left
      mentotransverse
    LOA – left occipitoanterior
    LOP – left
      occipitoposterior
    LOT – left
      occipitotransverse
    LSA – left sacroanterior
    L. Sc. A. – left
      scapuloanterior
    L. Sc. P. – left
      scapuloposterior
    LSP – left sacroposterior
    LST – left sacrotransverse
    RFA – right frontoanterior
    RFP – right frontoposterior
    RFT – right
      frontotransverse
    RMA – right
      mentoanterior
    RMP – right
      mentoposterior
    RMT – right
      mentotransverse
    ROA – right
      occipitoanterior
    ROP – right
      occipitoposterior
    ROT – right
      occipitotransverse
    RSA – right sacroanterior

fetal position (continued)
    R. Sc. A. – right
      scapuloanterior
    R. Sc. P. – right
      scapuloposterior
    RSP – right sacroposterior
    RST – right
      sacrotransverse
fetation
feticide
feticulture
fetogram
fetography
fetomaternal
fetometry
fetoplacental
fetoscopy
fetus
    f. acardiacus
    f. amorphus
    calcified f.
    f. compressus
    harlequin f.
    f. in fetu
    macerated f.
    mummified f.
    paper-doll f.
    papyraceous f.
    f. papyraceus
    parasitic f.
    f. sanguinolentis
    sireniform f.
Feulgen stain
FHR – fetal heart rate
FHS – fetal heart sound
FHT – fetal heart tone
Fibrindex test
fibrinogen
fibroadenoma
fibrocystadenoma
fibrocystic
fibroid
fibroidectomy
fibroma
fibromyoma
fibromyomata
fibromyomectomy

fibrothecoma
FIGO – International Federation
    of Gynecology and
    Obstetrics
filamentous
fimbria
    ovarian f.
    f. ovarica
fimbriae of uterine tube
fimbriae tubae uterinae
fimbrial
fimbriated
fimbriectomy
fimbriocele
fistula
    rectolabial f.
    rectovaginal f.
    ureterovaginal f.
    urinary f.
    vaginoperineal f.
    vesicocervical f.
    vesicovaginal f.
    vulvorectal f.
Fitz-Hugh's syndrome
flebitis. See *phlebitis.*
Fleming's
    knife
    operation
Fletcher-Suit afterloading
    device
Fletcher-Van Doren forceps
flexion
flora
fluffs
fluid
    amniotic f.
    crystalline f.
fluor
    f. albus
FMR – fetal-to-maternal ratio
Foerster's forceps
fold
    Douglas' f.
    Pawlik's f.
    rectouterine f.
    vesicouterine f.
Foley catheter

follicle
    graafian f's
    nabothian f's
    Naboth's f's
    ovarian f.
    primordial f.
    secondary f.
follicle-stimulating hormone
follicular
folliculoma
fontanelle
forceps
    Allis' f.
    Bailey-Williamson f.
    Barrett-Allen f.
    Barrett's f.
    Barton's f.
    Benaron's f.
    Berry's f.
    Billroth's f.
    Bond's f.
    Bozeman's f.
    Braasch's f.
    Chamberlen's f.
    Collin's f.
    Corey's f.
    De Alvarez's f.
    DeLee's f.
    Desjardin's f.
    Dewey's f.
    Eder's f.
    Elliott's f.
    Ferris' f.
    Fletcher-Van Doren f.
    Foerster's f.
    Garrigue's f.
    Gaylor's f.
    Gellhorn's f.
    Gelpi-Lowrie f.
    Glenner's f.
    Gordon's f.
    Gutglass' f.
    Hale's f.
    Hartman's f.
    Hawkins' f.
    Hawks-Dennen f.
    Heaney-Ballantine f.

forceps (continued)
Heaney-Kanter f.
Heaney-Rezek f.
Heaney's f.
Heise's f.
Henrotin's f.
Hirst-Emmett f.
Hodge's f.
Iowa f.
Jacobs' f.
Jarcho's f.
Kelly's f.
Kennedy's f.
Kielland-Luikart f.
Kielland's f. (Kjelland's f.)
Kittner's f.
Krause's f.
Laufe-Barton-Kielland f.
Laufe-Piper f.
Laufe's f.
Levret's f.
Long Island f.
Long's f.
Luikart's f.
Luikart-Simpson f.
Maier's f.
Mann's f.
Maryan's f.
McLane's f.
McLane-Tucker f.
McLane-Tucker-Luikart f.
Mitchell-Diamond f.
mouse-tooth f.
Mundie's f.
Newman's f.
obstetric f.
O'Hanlon's f.
Overstreet's f.
ovum f.
Palmer's f.
Pean's f.
Phaneuf's f.
Piper's f.
placental f.
polyp f.
Randall's stone f.
ring f.

forceps (continued)
Rochester-Carmalt f.
Rochester-Ochsner f.
Rochester-Pean f.
Russell's f.
Schroeder's f.
Schubert's f.
Schwartz's f.
Schweizer's f.
Segond's f.
Senn f.
Simpson-Luikart f.
Simpson's f.
Skene's f.
Smith's f.
Somers' f.
sponge f.
Staude-Moore f.
Staude's f.
stone f.
Tarnier's f.
Teale's f.
Thoms' f.
Thoms-Allis f.
Thoms-Gaylor f.
Tischler's f.
tissue f.
Tucker-McLean f.
Van Doren f.
vulsellum f.
Walton's f.
Walton-Schubert f.
Weisman's f.
Wertheim-Cullen f.
Wertheim's f.
Willett's f.
Wittner's f.
Yeoman's f.
forewaters
fornices
fornix
fossa
Claudius' f.
navicular f.
f. navicularis
obturator f.
f. of vestibule of vagina

fossa (continued)
    f. of Waldeyer
    ovarian f.
    f. ovarica
    f. vestibuli vaginae
Fothergill's operation
fourchette
Fox-Fordyce disease
fractional
Frangenheim-Goebell-Stoeckel
  operation
frenal
French catheter
frenulum
    f. labiorum pudendi
    f. of clitoris
frenum
    f. of labia
Freund's
    law
    operation
Friedman-Lapham test
Friedman's
    retractor
    test
frigid
frigidity
Fritsch-Asherman syndrome
Fritsch's
    catheter
    operation
Frommel's operation
"frozen pelvis"
FSH – follicle-stimulating
  hormone
FTLB – full-term living birth
FTND – full-term normal
  delivery
fulcrum
fulguration
functionalis
fundal
fundectomy
fundus
    f. of uterus
    f. of vagina
    f. uteri

fundus (continued)
    f. vaginae
fungating
funis
Gabastou's hydraulic method
galactocele
galactorrhea
galactosemia
galacturia
Galli-Mainini test
gamete
Gardnerella
    G. vaginalis
Gariel's pessary
Garrigue's
    forceps
    speculum
Gartner's duct
gastrocolpotomy
gastrointestinal
    g. bypass
Gauss' sign
Gaylor's forceps
GC – gonococcus
    gonorrhea
Gehrung pessary
Gellhorn's
    forceps
    pessary
Gelpi-Lowrie forceps
Gelpi's retractor
genesial
genetic
genital
    g. ridge
    g. tract
genitalia
genitourinary
Genupak tampon
gestation
gestational
    g. age
    g. sac
    g. trophoblastic neoplasia
gestosis
Gigli's operation
Gilliam-Doleris operation

Gilliam's operation
Giordano's operation
gland
    adrenal g.
    Bartholin's g.
    BUS g's
    Littre's g's
    Naboth's g's
    Skene's g.
    thyroid g.
    urethral g.
    vestibular g.
glans
    g. clitoridis
    g. of clitoris
Glenner's
    forceps
    retractor
glomerular
    g. filtration rate
glucocorticoid
glucose
glycoprotein
GnRH – gonadotropin-releasing
   hormone
Goebel-Stoeckel operation
Goffe's operation
goiter
Golden's sign
gonad
gonadal
    g. dysgenesis
gonadoblastoma
gonadogenesis
gonadotropic
gonadotropin
gonococcus
gonorrhea
Goodall-Power operation
Goodell's
    dilator
    law
    sign
Gordan-Overstreet
   syndrome
Gordon's forceps
Gottschalk's operation

graafian
    g. follicle
    g. ovule
"grandmother" theory
Grant-Ward operation
granuloma
    g. inguinale
    pyogenic g.
granulosa
    g. lutein
    g. theca cell
Graves'
    disease
    speculum
gravid
gravida I, II, III, etc.
gravidic
gravidism
graviditas
    g. examnialis
    g. exochorialis
gravidity
gravidocardiac
gravidopuerperal
Gravindex test
Grawitz's tumor
Green-Armytage operation
Greene's curet
grip
    Pawlik's g.
GTN – gestational trophoblastic
   neoplasia
gumma
Gusberg's curet
Gutglass' forceps
Guttmann's
    retractor
    speculum
GYN – gynecology
gynandrism
gynandroblastoma
gynatresia
gynecogen
gynecography
gynecoid
gynecoil
gynecologic

gynecological
gynecologist
gynecology
gynecopathy
gynecotokology
gyneduct
gynogamon
gynomerogon
gynomerogony
gynopathic
gynopathy
gynoplastics
gynoplasty
Haase's rule
Haemophilus
    H. ducreyi
    H. vaginalis
Halban's
    disease
    sign
Hale's forceps
Halsted's radical
    mastectomy
Hamilton's method
Hank-Bradley dilator
Hank's dilator
Hannon's curet
Hardy-Duddy speculum
Harrison's method
Hartman's forceps
Haultaim's operation
Hawkins' forceps
Hawks-Dennen forceps
hCG – human chorionic
    gonadotropin
Heaney-Ballantine forceps
Heaney-Kanter forceps
Heaney-Rezek forceps
Heaney's
    clamp
    curet
    forceps
    needle holder
    retractor
    vaginal hysterectomy
Heaney-Simon retractor
heartburn

Hegar's
    dilator
    operation
    sign
Heise's forceps
hemangioma
hematocele
    parametric h.
    pudendal h.
    retrouterine h.
    vaginal h.
hematochlorine
hematocolpometra
hematocolpos
hematogenous
hematologic
hematoma
hematome
hematometra
hematosalpinx
hematuria
hemelytrometra lateralis
hemoglobin
hemoglobinopathy
hemolytic
hemoperitoneum
hemorrhage
hemorrhoids
hemostasis
Henrotin's
    forceps
    speculum
hepatic
hepatitis B
hermaphroditism
herpes
    h. genitalis
    h. gestationis
    h. menstrualis
    h. progenitalis
    h. simplex
heterosexual
heterozygous
Hicks'
    sign
    version

hidradenitis
  h. suppurativa
hidradenoma
hilar
hilus
  h. of ovary
  h. ovarii
Hirst-Emmett forceps
Hirst's operation
hirsutism
His' rule
histocompatibility
Hodge's
  forceps
  maneuver
  pessary
Hoehne's sign
Hogben's test
Holden's curet
Holman-Mathieu cannula
Holtz's curet
homeostasis
hood
  Rock-Mulligan h.
hook
  Braun-Jardine-DeLee h.
  Braun's h.
  Dudley's h.
  Duplay's h.
  Emmet's h.
  Kelly's h.
  Mayo's h.
  Newman's h.
  Schwartz's h.
hormonal
hormone
  luteinizing h.
  thyrotropin-releasing h.
hormonotherapy
horn
  h. of clitoris
  h. of uterus
Horrocks' maieutic
hPL – human placental lactogen
HSG – hysterosalpingogram
Hudgins' cannula
Huffman-Graves speculum

Huhner's test
Hulka's clip
human chorionic gonadotropin
Hunter's
  curet
  ligament
Huntington's operation
Hurtig's dilator
hyaline
Hyam's operation
hydatid
  h. of Morgagni
hydatidiform
hydramnios
hydrocele
  h. feminae
  h. muliebris
  Nuck's h.
hydrocephalus
hydrocolpos
hydroparasalpinx
hydrops
  h. fetalis
  h. folliculi
hydrorrhea
  h. gravidarum
hydrosalpinx
  h. follicularis
  intermittent h.
  h. simplex
hydrotubation
hydroureter
hydrovarium
hydroxylase
  17α-h.
  11β-h.
  21-h.
hydroxysteroid
  3β-h.
hymen
  annular h.
  h. bifenestratus
  h. biforis
  circular h.
  cribriform h.
  denticular h.
  falciform h.

hymen (continued)
    fenestrated h.
    imperforate h.
    infundibuliform h.
    lunar h.
    septate h.
    h. septus
    h. subseptus
hymenal
    h. band
    h. ring
hymenectomy
hymenitis
hymenorrhaphy
hymenotome
hymenotomy
hyperbilirubinemia
hyperemesis
    h. gravidarum
hyperestrogenism
hyperflexion
hypermenorrhea
hypernephroma
hyperovaria
hyperovarianism
hyperovarism
hyperplasia
    adenomatous h.
    adrenal h.
    endometrial h.
    hilus cell h.
    postmenopausal h.
    proliferative h.
    stromal h.
hyperplastic
hyperprolactinemia
hyperstimulation
hypertension
hyperthecosis
hyperthyroidism
hypertonic
hypertrophy
hypofibrinogenemia
hypofunction
hypogalactia
hypoglycemia
hypomastia

hypomenorrhea
hypo-ovaria
hypoplasia
hypospadias
    female h.
hypothalamic
hypothalamus
hypothermia
hypothyroidism
hypotonic
hypovaria
hypovarianism
hypoxia
hysteralgia
hysteratresia
hysterectomy
    abdominal h.
    Bonney's h.
    cesarean h.
    chemical h.
    complete h.
    Doyen's vaginal h.
    extrafascial h.
    Heaney's vaginal h.
    intrafascial h.
    Latzko's radical h.
    Mayo-Ward vaginal h.
    paravaginal h.
    partial h.
    Porro's h.
    radical h.
    Ries-Wertheim h.
    Schauta-Amreich vaginal
      h.
    Schauta's radical vaginal
      h.
    Spalding-Richardson h.
    subtotal h.
    supracervical h.
    supravaginal h.
    total h.
    total abdominal h.
    vaginal h.
    Ward-Mayo vaginal h.
    Wertheim's radical h.
hystereurynter
hystereurysis

hysterobubonocele
hysterocarcinoma
hysterocele
hysterocervicotomy
hysterocleisis
hysterocolpectomy
hysterocolposcope
hysterocystic
hysterocystopexy
hysterocytocleisis
hysterodynia
hysterogastrorrhaphy
hysterogram
hysterograph
hysterography
hysterolaparotomy
hysterolith
hysterology
hysterolysis
hysterometer
hysterometry
hysteromyoma
hysteromyomectomy
hysteromyotomy
hystero-oophorectomy
hystero-ovariotomy
hysteropathy
hysteropexia
hysteropexy
hysteroptosia
hysteroptosis
hysterorrhaphy
hysterorrhexis
hysterosalpingectomy
hysterosalpingogram
hysterosalpingography
hysterosalpingo-oophorectomy
hysterosalpingostomy
hysteroscope
      Storz's h.
hysteroscopic
hysteroscopy
hysterospasm
hysterostat
hysterostomatocleisis
hysterostomatome
hysterostomatomy

hysterothermometry
hysterotome
hysterotomotokia
hysterotomy
hysterotrachelectasia
hysterotrachelectomy
hysterotracheloplasty
hysterotrachelorrhaphy
hysterotrachelotomy
hysterotubography
hysterovaginoenterocele
idiometritis
ileus
I.M. cocktail – intramuscular
      cocktail
immune
immunoglobulin
immunologic
immunology
imperforate
implant
      Dow-Corning i.
implantation
incision. See *General Surgical
      Terms.*
incompatibility
incontinence
      overflow i.
      stress i.
      urge i.
      urinary i.
index
      Mengert's i.
indices
indigo carmine dye
induced
induction
inertia
      uterine i.
infarction
Infectious Disease Society for
      Obstetrics and Gynecology
infertilitas
      i. feminis
infertility
infundibula
infundibular

infundibuliform
infundibulum
    i. of fallopian tube
    i. of uterine tube
    i. tubae uterinae
inguinolabial
inlet
    pelvic i.
insemination
    artificial i. donor
    heterologous i.
    homologous i.
in situ
insufficiency
    uteroplacental i.
insufflation
    methylene blue i.
    tubal i.
insufflator
    Kidde's tubal i.
intercalary
intercourse
intermenstrual
intermural
internal os
interphase
intersexual
interstitial
intertrigo
intracavitary
intracervical
intracranial
intraepithelial
intrafetation
intraligamentous
intramural
intranatal
intraovarian
intrapartum
intraperitoneal
intraplacental
intratubal
intrauterine
    i. fetal death
    i. growth retardation
intrauterine device (IUD)
    bow IUD

intrauterine device (IUD) (continued)
    coil IUD
    copper-7 IUD
    Lippes' loop IUD
    Mazlin spring IUD
    Progestasert IUD
    Tatum-T IUD
intravaginal
intravenous
introitus
    marital i.
    parous i.
    i. vaginae
in utero
inversion
    i. of uterus
in vitro
in vivo
involution
Iowa forceps
IPD – inflammatory pelvic disease
Irving's operation
Isaac's differential distortion
    divergent method
ischemia
ischial
ischiopubic
ischiopubiotomy
ischiorectal
ischiovaginal
isoimmunization
    rhesus i.
isthmica nodosa
isthmic-cornual
isthmus
    i. of fallopian tube
    i. of uterus
    i. tubae uterinae
    tubal i.
    i. uteri
IU – international unit
IUD – intrauterine device
IUGR – intrauterine growth
    retardation
IV cocktail – intravenous cocktail
Jackson's retractor

Jacobs'
forceps
tenaculum
Jacquemier's sign
Jarcho's
cannula
forceps
Johnson's calculation
Jolly's dilator
Jonas-Graves speculum
Jones' operation
Jungbluth
vasa propria of J.
Kahn-Graves speculum
Kahn's
cannula
tenaculum
kakektic. See *cachectic*.
kakexia. See *cachexia*.
Kallmann's syndrome
Kane's clamp
Kanter's sign
Kapeller-Adler test
karyotype
Kegel's exercise
Keith's needle
Kelly-Gray curet
Kelly's
clamp
curet
dilator
forceps
hook
operation
scissors
Kennedy's
forceps
operation
keratinized
Kergaradec's sign
kernicterus
Kerr's cesarean section
Kevorkian's curet
Keyes' biopsy punch
Kidde's tubal insufflator
Kielland-Luikart forceps

Kielland's forceps (Kjelland's
forceps)
Kittner's forceps
Kleihauer-Betke test
Klinefelter's syndrome
Kline's flocculation test
kloasma. See *cloasma*.
Klotz's syndrome
Kluge's method
knife
Ayerst's k.
Fleming's k.
Pace's k.
kocherization
kocherized
Kocher's clamp
Kocks' operation
koleo-. See words beginning
coleo-.
kolostrum. See *colostrum*.
kolp-, kolpo-. See words
beginning *colp-, colpo-*.
kondilo-. See words beginning
condylo-.
kondro-. See words beginning
chondro-.
korio-. See words beginning
chorio-.
kotiledon. See *cotyledon*.
kraurosis
k. vulva
Krause's forceps
Kristeller's method
Kroener's operation
Kronig's cesarean section
Krukenberg's tumor
krura. See *crura*.
kryo-. See words beginning *cryo-*.
Kuldo-. See words beginning
culdo-.
Kupperman's test
Kushner-Tandatnick curet
Küstner's
law
operation
sign

kyphosis
    dorsal k.
kyphotic
labia
    l. majora
    l. majus
    l. minora
labial
labium
    l. majus
    l. minus
labor
    atonic l.
    desultory l.
    dyskinetic l.
    habitual l.
    induced l.
    instrumental l.
    mimetic l.
    obstructed l.
    postponed l.
    precipitate l.
    prodromal l.
    protracted l.
    spontaneous l.
laceration
    fishmouth l.
    perianal l.
lactation
lacteal
lactic
lactobacilli
lactogen
    human placental l.
lactogenic
lacuna
    intervillous l.
Ladin's sign
Lahey's clamp
Laminaria tent
lamination
Landou's sign
Langhan's
    cell
    stria
laparocolpohysterotomy

laparocystotomy
laparohysterectomy
laparohystero-oophorectomy
laparohysterosalpingo-
    oophorectomy
laparohysterotomy
laparokelyphotomy
laparomonodidymus
laparomyomectomy
laparosalpingectomy
laparosalpingo-oophorectomy
laparosalpingotomy
laparoscope
    Wolf's l.
laparoscopic
laparoscopy
laparotomy
    exploratory l.
laparotrachelotomy
laparouterotomy
laser
Lash's operation
latent phase
Latzko's
    cesarean section
    closure
    operation
    radical hysterectomy
Laufe-Barton-Kielland forceps
Laufe-Piper forceps
Laufe's forceps
law
    Diday's l.
    Freund's l.
    Goodell's l.
    Küstner's l.
    Leopold's l.
    Levret's l.
    Pajot's l.
layer
    Nitabuch's l.
LeFort's operation
leiomyoma
    l. uteri
leiomyomata
    l. uteri

leiomyosarcoma
Leopold's
 law
 maneuver
 operation
Lerous' method
leukocytosis
leukokraurosis
leukophlegmasia
leukoplakia
 l. vulvae
leukorrhea
levator ani
level
 pregnanediol l.
Levret's
 forceps
 law
Leydig's cell
LFA–left frontoanterior
LFP–left frontoposterior
LFT–left frontotransverse
LH–luteinizing hormone
libido
lichen
 l. sclerosis
ligament
 anterior l.
 broad l.
 cardinal l.
 Hunter's l.
 infundibulopelvic l.
 keystone l.
 lacunar l.
 lateral l.
 Mackenrodt's l.
 ovarian l.
 posterior l.
 pubocervical l.
 rectouterine l.
 round l.
 sacrogenital l.
 sacrouterine l.
 suspensory l.
 uterosacral l.
 vesicouterine l.

ligamenta
 l. ovarii proprium
 l. teres uteri
ligation
 tubal l.
Lignac-Fanconi disease
Liley's chart
line
 Douglas' l.
 Farre's l.
linea
 l. alba
 l. nigra
lio-. See words beginning *leio-*.
lipoid
Lippes' loop IUD
liquor
 l. amnii
 l. chorii
 l. folliculi
Listeria
 L. monocytogenes
lithopedion
Littre's glands
littritis
Litzmann's obliquity
LMA–left mentoanterior
LMP–last menstrual period
 left mentoposterior
LMT–left mentotransverse
LNMP–last normal menstrual
 period
LOA–left occipitoanterior
lochia
 l. alba
 l. cruenta
 l. purulenta
 l. rubra
 l. sanguinolenta
lochial
lochiocolpos
lochiocyte
lochiometra
lochiometritis
lochiopyra
lochiorrhagia
lochiorrhea

lochioschesis
lochiostasis
lochometritis
lochoperitonitis
Löhlein's diameter
Long Island forceps
Long's forceps
loop
    Lippes' l.
LOP – left occipitoposterior
LOT – left occipitotransverse
Lounsbury's curet
Løvset's maneuver
LSA – left sacroanterior
L. Sc. A. – left scapuloanterior
L. Sc. P. – left scapuloposterior
LSP – left sacroposterior
LS ratio – lecithin-sphingomyelin
    ratio
LST – left sacrotransverse
Lugol's stain
Luikart-Bill traction handle
Luikart's forceps
Luikart-Simpson forceps
lumen
    uterine l.
    vaginal l.
lumpectomy
luteal
luteectomy
lutein
luteinic
luteinization
luteoid
luteoma
luteum
lying-in
lymphadenectomy
lymphatic
lymphogranuloma
    l. benignum
    Schaumann's benign l.
    venereal l.
    l. venereum
lyo-. See words beginning *leio*
lyra
    l. uteri

lyra (continued)
    l. uterina
    l. vaginae
lyre
    l. of uterus
    l. of vagina
maceration
Mackenrodt's
    ligament
    operation
macroadenoma
macroscopic
macrosomia
macula
    m. gonorrhoeica
    Saenger's m.
Madlener operation
Maher's disease
Maier's forceps
maieusiomania
maieusiophobia
maieutic
    Horrocks' m.
Malherbe
    epithelioma of M.
malposition
malpresentation
mammary
mammectomy
mammogram
mammography
mammoplasty
Manchester
    operation
    ovoid
maneuver. See also *method.*
    Bracht's m.
    Brandt-Andrews m.
    DeLee's m.
    Hodge's m.
    Leopold's m.
    Løvset's m.
    Massini's m.
    Mauriceau's m.
    Mauriceau-Smellie m.
    Mauriceau-Smellie-
        Veit m.

maneuver (continued)
    McDonald's m.
    Müller-Hillis m.
    Munro-Kerr m.
    Phaneuf's m.
    Pinard's m.
    Prague m.
    Ritgen's m.
    Saxtorph's m.
    Scanzoni's m.
    Schatz's m.
    Van Hoorn's m.
    Wigand's m.
Mann's forceps
Marchetti test
Marckwald's operation
Margulles' coil
Marlex atraumatic tenaculum
Marshall-Marchetti-Krantz
    operation
Marshall-Marchetti
    operation
    test
marsupialization
Martin's
    operation
    pelvimeter
Martius' operation
Maryan's forceps
masculinovoblastoma
Mason-Auvard speculum
Massini's maneuver
mastectomy
    Halsted's radical m.
    modified m.
    radical m.
    segmental m.
    Willy Meyer radical m.
mastitis
    cystic m.
    plasma cell m.
mastodynia
mastogram
mastography
matrix
    intercellular m.
Matsner episiotomy

maturation
    ovarian follicular m.
Mauriceau's maneuver
Mauriceau-Smellie maneuver
Mauriceau-Smellie-Veit
    maneuver
Mayer-Rokitansky-Küster
    syndrome
Mayer's speculum
Mayo-Fueth operation
Mayo-Harrington scissors
Mayor's sign
Mayo's
    hook
    needle
    scissors
Mayo-Sims scissors
Mayo-Ward vaginal
    hysterectomy
maza
mazic
Mazlin spring IUD
McCall-Schuman operation
McCall's operation
McCune-Albright syndrome
McDonald's
    maneuver
    operation
McDowell's operation
McIndoe operation
McLane's forceps
McLane-Tucker forceps
McLane-Tucker-Luikart forceps
meatus
    urinary m.
mechanism
    Duncan's m.
    Schultze's m.
meconium
medications. See *Drugs and
    Chemistry* section.
megaloclitoris
megavoltage
Meigs-Cass syndrome
Meigs' syndrome
meiosis
melanoma

melasma
    m. gravidarum
membrane
    hyaline m.
    mucous m.
menalgia
menarche
menarchial
Mendelson's syndrome
Mengert's index
Menge's
    operation
    pessary
menhidrosis
meningocele
menolipsis
menometrorrhagia
menopausal
menopause
menophania
menoplania
menorrhagia
menorrhalgia
menorrhea
menorrheal
menoschesis
menosepsis
menostasis
menostaxis
menotoxic
menotoxin
menoxenia
menses
menstrual
menstruant
menstruate
menstruation
    anovular m.
    anovulatory m.
    nonovulational m.
    ovulatory m.
    regurgitant m.
    retrograde m.
    scanty m.
    supplementary m.
    suppressed m.
    vicarious m.

menstruous
menstruum
mesenchymal
mesenteric
mesoderm
mesometritis
mesometrium
mesonephric
mesonephroma
mesonephros
mesosalpinx
mesothelial
mesothelioma
mesovarium
metabolism
metacyesis
metaplasia
    squamous m.
method. See also *maneuver*.
    Beuttner's m.
    Bonnaire's m.
    Credé's m.
    Danforth's m.
    Douglas' m.
    Gabastou's hydraulic m.
    Hamilton's m.
    Harrison's m.
    Isaac's differential
        distortion divergent m.
    Kluge's m.
    Kristeller's m.
    Lerous's m.
    Pajot's m.
    Pomeroy's m.
    Puzo's m.
    rhythm m.
    Schultze's m.
    Schuman's m.
    Smellie's m.
    Watson's m.
methylene blue insufflation
metra
metralgia
metranoikter
metratonia
metratrophia
metrechoscopy

metrectasia
metrectomy
metrectopia
metreurynter
metreurysis
metria
metritis
 m. dissecans
 dissecting m.
 puerperal m.
metrocampsis
metrocarcinoma
metrocele
metrocolpocele
metrocystosis
metrocyte
metrodynia
metroendometritis
metrofibroma
metrogenous
metrogonorrhea
metrography
metroleukorrhea
metromalacia
metromalacoma
metromenorrhagia
metroparalysis
metropathia
 m. haemorrhagica
metropathic
metropathy
metroperitoneal
metroperitonitis
metrophlebitis
metroplasty
metroptosis
metrorrhagia
 m. myopathica
metrorrhea
metrorrhexis
metrosalpingitis
metrosalpingogram
metrosalpingography
metroscope
metrostaxis
metrostenosis

metrotome
metrotomy
metrotoxin
metrotubography
Metzenbaum scissors
MH – marital history
microinvasive
microtransducer
micturition
midsegment
Milex cervitome
Miller's
 operation
 speculum
Millin-Read operation
Mitchell-Diamond forceps
mitochondria
mitosis
mitotic
mittelschmerz
mole
 Breu's m.
 hydatidiform m.
molimen
molimina
molluscum
 m. contagiosum
mongoloid
monilial
monitoring
 fetal m.
monocyesis
mons
 m. pubis
 m. ureteris
 m. veneris
Montgomery strap
morcellated
morcellation
morcellement
Morgagni
 cyst of M.
 hydatid of M.
morula
mosaicism
Moschcowitz's operation

motile
MRI – magnetic resonance
    imaging
mucinous
mucocolpos
mucosa
        endocervical m.
mucus
Mueller's needle
Müller-Hillis maneuver
müllerian
müllerianoma
müllerianosis
mülleriosis
Müller's
        operation
        tubercle
multigravida
multiloculated
multipara
multiparity
multiparous
multiphasic
Mundie's forceps
Munnell's operation
Munro-Kerr maneuver
muscle
        bulbocavernosus m.
        external oblique m.
        gluteus maximus m.
        internal oblique m.
        ischiocavernosus m.
        levator ani m.
        obturator internus m.
        pubovaginal m.
        pyramidalis m.
        recti m.
        rectouterine m.
        sphincter ani m.
        transverse abdominus m.
        transverse perineal m.
myasthenia
        m. gravis
Mycoplasma
        M. genitalis
myelocele

myoma
myomagenesis
myomata
        m. uteri
myomatectomy
myomatosis
myomatous
myomectomy
myometrial
myometritis
myometrium
myomohysterectomy
myomotomy
myosalpingitis
myosalpinx
myosarcoma
myosis
mytotic. See *mitotic.*
nabothian
Naboth's
        cysts
        follicles
        glands
        ovules
        vesicles
Nägele's
        obliquity
        pelvis
        rule
nausea
navicular
NB — newborn
Neal's cannula
necrosis
necrotic
needle
        Keith's n.
        Mayo's n.
        Mueller's n.
        Pereyra n.
        Shirodkar n.
        Touhey's n.
        Verres' n.
        Vim-Silverman n.
        Voorhees' n.

needle holder
    Heaney's n.h.
Neisseria
    N. gonorrhoeae
Nelson's scissors
neonatal
neonate
neonatologist
neonatology
neoplasia
    gestational tropho-
        blastic n.
    intraepithelial n.
neoplasm
    adrenal n.
    stromal cell n.
neosalpingostomy
nerve
    ilioinguinal n.
    pudendal n.
    uterine n.
neumo-. See words beginning
    pneumo-.
neural
neurectomy
    presacral n.
neuropeptide
nevus
    vulvar n.
Newman's
    forceps
    hook
Nickerson's medium smear
Niemann-Pick disease
Nitabuch's layer
node
    Cloquet's n.
    iliac n.
    obturator n.
    para-aortic lymph n.
nodule
    discrete n.
noma
    n. pudendi
    n. vulvae
norethindrone test
norethynodrel test

Nott's speculum
Novak's curet
Nuck
    canal of N.
    hydrocele of N.
nucleus
nulligravida
nullipara
nulliparity
nulliparous
numo-. See words beginning
    pneumo-.
nympha
nymphae
nymphectomy
nymphitis
nymphocaruncular
nymphohymeneal
nymphomania
nymphomaniac
nymphoncus
nymphotomy
OB—obstetrics
OB-GYN—obstetrics and
    gynecology
obliquity
    Litzmann's o.
    Nägele's o.
    Roederer's o.
obliteration
obstetrical
obstetrician
obstetrics
obstruction
occipital
occipitoanterior
occipitoposterior
occlusion
    fimbrial o.
    isthmic cornual o.
    midsegment o.
    tubal o.
Ochsner's clamp
octigravida
octipara
O'Hanlon's forceps
oligohydramnios

oligohypermenorrhea
oligohypomenorrhea
oligomenorrhea
oligo-ovulation
oligospermia
Olshausen's
    operation
    sign
omphalocele
oncology
oocyesis
oocyte
oocytin
oogenesis
oogenetic
oogonia
oophoralgia
oophorectomize
oophorectomy
oophoritis
oophorocystectomy
oophorocystosis
oophorogenous
oophorohysterectomy
oophoroma
oophoron
oophoropathy
oophoropeliopexy
oophoropexy
oophoroplasty
oophororrhaphy
oophorosalpingectomy
oophorosalpingitis
oophorostomy
oophorotomy
oophorrhagia
operation
    Abell's o.
    Aburel's o.
    Aldrich's o.
    Alexander-Adams o.
    Alexander's O.
    Baldwin's o.
    Baldy's o.
    Baldy-Webster o.
    Ball's o.
    Basset's o.

operation (continued)
    Baudeloque's o.
    Beatson's o.
    Bischoff's o.
    Bissell's o.
    Bouilly's o.
    Bozeman's o.
    Bricker's o.
    Brunschwig's o.
    Burch's o.
    Coffey's o.
    Davis' o.
    Decker's o.
    Döderlein's o.
    Doleris' o.
    Donald-Fothergill o.
    Donald's o.
    Doyen's o.
    Dudley's o.
    Dührssen's o.
    Emmet's o.
    Estes' o.
    Falk's o.
    Falk-Shukuris o.
    Fleming's o.
    Fothergill's o.
    Frangenheim-Goebell-
      Stoeckel o.
    Freund's o.
    Fritsch's o.
    Frommel's o.
    Gigli's o.
    Gilliam-Doleris o.
    Gilliam's o.
    Giordano's o.
    Goebel-Stoeckel o.
    Goffe's o.
    Goodall-Power o.
    Gottschalk's o.
    Grant-Ward o.
    Green-Armytage o.
    Haultaim's o.
    Hegar's o.
    Hirst's o.
    Huntington's o.
    Hyam's o.
    interposition o.

operation (continued)
  Irving's o.
  Jones' o.
  Kelly's o.
  Kennedy's o.
  Kocks' o.
  Kroener's o.
  Küstner's o.
  Lash's o.
  Latzko's o.
  LeFort's o.
  Leopold's o.
  Mackenrodt's o.
  Madlener o.
  Manchester o.
  Marckwald's o.
  Marshall-Marchetti o.
  Marshall-Marchetti-
    Krantz o.
  Martin's o.
  Martius' o.
  Mayo-Fueth o.
  McCall's o.
  McCall-Schuman o.
  McDonald's o.
  McDowell's o.
  McIndoe o.
  Menge's o.
  Miller's o.
  Millin-Read o.
  Moschcowitz's o.
  Müller's o.
  Munnell's o.
  Olshausen's o.
  O'Sullivan's o.
  Oxford's o.
  Pean's o.
  Peterson's o.
  Pomeroy's o.
  Porro's o.
  Porro-Veit o.
  Pozzi's o.
  Récamier's o.
  Ries-Wertheim o.
  Rizzoli's o.
  Rubin's o.
  Saenger's o.

operation (continued)
  Scanzoni's o.
  Schauffler's o.
  Schauta's o.
  Schauta-Wertheim o.
  Schröder's o.
  Schuchardt's o.
  Shirodkar o.
  Simon's o.
  Spalding-Richardson o.
  Spinelli's o.
  Strassman-Jones o.
  Sturmdorf's o.
  Taussig-Morton o.
  Taussig's o.
  Te Linde o.
  Thomas's o.
  Torpin's o.
  Tuffier's o.
  Twombly's o.
  Twombly-Ulfelder o.
  Uchida's o.
  Vernon-David o.
  Warren's o.
  Water's o.
  Watkins' o.
  Watkins-Wertheim o.
  Webster's o.
  Wertheim's o.
  Wertheim-Schauta o.
  Wharton's o.
  Whitacre's o.
  Williams' o.
  Williams-Richardson o.
  Wylie's o.
orifice
  abdominal o. of uterine
    tube
  external urethral o.
  hymenal o.
  o. of uterus
  vaginal o.
orificium
  o. externum uteri
  o. hymenis
  o. internum uteri
  o. vaginae

os
Osiander's sign
osteoporosis
ostium
    o. abdominale tubae
       uterinae
    o. uteri
    o. uterinum tubae uterinae
    o. vaginae
O'Sullivan-O'Connor
    retractor
    speculum
O'Sullivan's operation
outlet
    marital o.
ova
ovarian
ovariectomy
ovaries
ovarin
ovariocele
ovariocentesis
ovariocyesis
ovariodysneuria
ovariogenic
ovariohysterectomy
ovarioncus
ovariopathy
ovariopexy
ovariorrhexis
ovariosalpingectomy
ovariosteresis
ovariostomy
ovariotestis
ovariotherapy
ovariotomist
ovariotomy
ovariotubal
ovariprival
ovaritis
ovarium
ovarotherapy
ovary
Overstreet's forceps
oviduct
ovoid
    Manchester o.

ovotestis
ovotherapy
ovula
ovulate
ovulation
ovulatory
ovule
    graafian o's
    Naboth's o's
    primitive o.
    primordial o.
ovulogenous
ovulum
ovum
    blighted o.
Oxford's operation
oxygen
oxygenation
oxytocic
oxytocin
oxyuriasis
Pace's knife
pack
    Bellow's p.
packing
    iodoform gauze p.
Pagano-Levin medium smear
Paget's
    cell
    disease
Pajot's
    law
    method
Palmer's
    dilator
    forceps
palpation
pampiniform
pancreatitis
panhysterectomy
panhystero-oophorectomy
panhysterosalpingectomy
panhysterosalpingo-
    oophorectomy
Papanicolaou's
    smear
    stain

papilla
papilloma
    intraductal p.
Pap test
papulosis
    bowenoid p.
papyraceous
para – primipara
para 0, I, II, III, etc.
paracentesis
paracervical
paracolic
paracolpitis
paracolpium
paracyesis
paragomphosis
parametria
parametrial
parametric
parametritic
parametritis
parametrium
paraovarian
pararectal
parasalpingeal
parasalpingitis
parasitic
parathyroid
paratubal
parauterine
paravaginal
paravaginitis
paravesical
parenchymatous
paries
      p. anterior vaginae
parietal
parity
paroophoric
paroophoritis
paroöphoron
parous
parovarian
parovariotomy
parovaritis
parovarium

pars
    p. fetalis placentae
    p. uterina placentae
    p. uterina tubae uterinae
partes genitales externae
    muliebres
partes genitales femininae
    externae
parturient
parturifacient
parturiometer
parturition
partus
    p. agrippinus
    p. caesareus
    p. immaturus
    p. maturus
    p. precipitatus
    p. prematurus
    p. serotinus
    p. siccus
patent
path – pathology
patulous
pavilion
    p. of the oviduct
Pawlik's
    fold
    grip
    triangle
Pean's
    forceps
    operation
peau d'orange
Pederson's speculum
pedicle
pediculosis
pedunculated
pelvic
    p. congestion syndrome
    p. exenteration
    p. inflammatory disease
    p. inlet
    p. outlet
    p. plane diameter
    p. thrombophlebitis

pelvicellulitis
pelvicephalography
pelvicephalometry
pelvicliseometer
pelvifixation
pelvigraph
pelvilithotomy
pelvimeter
    Breisky's p.
    Collin's p.
    Collyer's p.
    DeLee's p.
    Martin's p.
    Thoms' p.
    William's p.
pelvimetry
pelvis
    p. aequabiliter justo major
    p. aequabiliter justo minor
    android p.
    p. angusta
    anthropoid p.
    beaked p.
    brachypellic p.
    contracted p.
    Deventer's p.
    dolichopellic p.
    "frozen" p.
    funnel-shaped p.
    gynecoid p.
    mesatipellic p.
    Nägele's p.
    pithecoid p.
    p. plana
    platypellic p.
    platypelloid p.
    Robert's p.
    rostrate p.
pendulous
Pennington's clamp
Penrose drain
Peptococcus
Peptostreptococcus
Percy's cautery
Pereyra
    needle

Pereyra (continued)
    procedure
perforator
    Blot's p.
    Smellie's p.
periadnexal
pericolpitis
perimetric
perimetrium
perimetrosalpingitis
perinatal
perineal
perineauxesis
perineocele
perineocolporectomyomectomy
perineometer
perineoplasty
perineorrhaphy
    Emmet-Studdiford p.
perineosynthesis
perineotomy
perineovaginal
perineovaginorectal
perineovulvar
perineum
perioophoritis
perioophorosalpingitis
perioothecitis
perioothecosalpingitis
perisalpingitis
perisalpingo-ovaritis
perisalpinx
peritoneal
peritonealize
peritoneopexy
peritoneum
    parietal p.
peritonitis
periuterine
perivaginal
perivaginitis
per primam
pessary
    cup p.
    diaphragm p.
    doughnut p.

pessary (continued)
- Emmert-Gellhorn p.
- Gariel's p.
- Gehrung p.
- Gellhorn's p.
- gynefold p.
- Hodge's p.
- lever p.
- Menge's p.
- ring p.
- Smith-Hodge p.
- Smith's p.
- stem p.
- Thomas' p.
- Wylie's p.
- Zwanck's p.

petechia
Peterson's operation
Phaneuf's
- forceps
- maneuver

phase
- luteal p.
- menstrual p.
- proliferative p.
- secretory p.

phenomenon
- Arias-Stella p.
- fern p.
- Strassmann's p.

phenotypic
phenylketonuria
Phenylstix
phimosis
- p. vaginalis

phlebitis
phlegmasia
- p. alba dolens
- p. alba dolens
  - puerperarum
- cellulitic p.

phototherapy
Phthirus
- *P. pubis*

Picot's speculum
PID – pelvic inflammatory disease

pielo-. See words beginning
- *pyelo-*.

PIF – prolactin-inhibiting factor
Pinard's
- maneuver
- sign

pio-. See words beginning *pyo-*.
Piper's forceps
Piskacek's sign
pithecoid
pitocin drip
pituitary
- p. disease
- p. gland
- p.-hypothalamus

placenta
- accessory p.
- p. accreta
- adherent p.
- annular p.
- battledore p.
- bidiscoidal p.
- bilobate p.
- bilobed p.
- p. bipartita
- bipartite p.
- chorioallantoic p.
- choriovitelline p.
- p. circumvallata
- circumvallate p.
- cirsoid p.
- p. cirsoides
- deciduous p.
- p. diffusa
- p. dimidiata
- dimidiate p.
- discoid p.
- p. discoidea
- duplex p.
- endotheliochorial p.
- epitheliochorial p.
- p. febrilis
- p. fenestrata
- fetal p.
- p. foetalis
- fundal p.

placenta (continued)
> furcate p.
> hemochorial p.
> hemoendothelial p.
> horseshoe p.
> incarcerated p.
> p. increta
> labyrinthine p.
> lobed p.
> p. marginalis
> p. marginata
> maternal p.
> p. membranacea
> multilobate p.
> multilobed p.
> p. multipartita
> p. nappiformis
> nondeciduous p.
> p. obsoleta
> panduriform p.
> p. panduriformis
> p. percreta
> p. praevia
> p. praevia centralis
> p. praevia marginalis
> p. praevia partialis
> p. previa
> p. reflexa
> p. reniformis
> retained p.
> Schultze's p.
> p. spuria
> stone p.
> p. succenturiata
> succenturiate p.
> syndesmochorial p.
> p. triloba
> trilobate p.
> p. tripartita
> tripartite p.
> p. triplex
> p. truffée
> p. uterina
> uterine p.
> velamentous p.
> villous p.

placenta (continued)
> yolk-sac p.
> zonary p.
> zonular p.

placentae
> ablatio p.
> abruptio p.
> marginalis p.

placental
> p. abruption
> p. "barrier"
> p. tissue
> p. vascular anastomosis

placentation
placentitis
placentocytotoxin
placentogenesis
placentogram
placentography
placentoid
placentologist
placentology
placentoma
placentopathy
placentotherapy
plaque
plasmapheresis
platypellic
platypelloid
plethoric
plexus
> Auerbach's p.
> p. cavernosus clitoridis
> cavernous p. of clitoris
> ovarian p.
> p. ovaricus
> pampiniform p.
> p. pampiniformis
> uterine p.
> uterovaginal p.
> p. uterovaginalis
> vaginal p.
> p. venosus vaginalis
> venous p.

plica
> p. rectouterina

plicae
p. ampullares tubae
uterinae
p. isthmicae tubae
uterinae
p. palmatae
p. tubariae tubae uterinae
p. vaginae
plication
PMP–previous menstrual period
pneumoamnios
pneumogynecogram
pneumonia
neonatal p.
pneumoperitoneum
pneumothorax
polycyesis
polycystic
polycystoma
polyhydramnios
polyhypermenorrhea
polyhypomenorrhea
polymenorrhea
polyostotic
polyp
cervical p.
endocervical p.
endometrial p.
leiomyomatous p.
sessile p.
polypectomy
polypoid
Pomeroy's
method
operation
Porro's
cesarean section
hysterectomy
operation
Porro-Veit operation
portio
p. supravaginalis cervicis
p. vaginalis cervicis
Poseiro's effect
position. See *fetal position* and
General Surgical Terms.
postabortal

postacrosomal
postcoital
post coitum
postmenopausal
postmenstrua
postpartum
p. blues
p. hemorrhage
Potter's version
pouch
p. of Douglas
vesicouterine p.
Pozzi's operation
PPA–phenylpyruvic acid
Prague maneuver
Pratt's dilator
precocity
preeclampsia
pregnancy
abdominal p.
afetal p.
bigeminal p.
cornual p.
ectopic p.
entopic p.
exochorial p.
extrauterine p.
gemellary p.
heterotopic p.
hydatid p.
hysteric p.
interstitial p.
intraligamentary p.
intramural p.
intraperitoneal p.
intrauterine p.
mesenteric p.
molar p.
mural p.
ovarioabdominal p.
oviducal p.
parietal p.
post-term p.
sacrofetal p.
sacrohysteric p.
spurious p.
stump p.

pregnancy (continued)
    term p.
    tubal p.
    tuboabdominal p.
    tuboligamentary p.
    tubo-ovarian p.
    tubouterine p.
    uteroabdominal p.
    utero-ovarian p.
    uterotubal p.
pregnanediol level
pregnant
Pregnosticon test
premature
prematurity
premenarchal
premenopausal
premenstrua
premenstrual
premenstruum
prenatal
prepuce
preputial
preputium
    p. clitoridis
presacral
presentation. See also *fetal*
    position.
    breech p.
    brow p.
    cephalic p.
    compound p.
    face p.
    footling p.
    footling breech p.
    frank breech p.
    full breech p.
    funis p.
    knee breech p.
    longitudinal p.
    mentoanterior face p.
    oblique p.
    parietal p.
    pelvic p.
    placental p.
    polar p.
    shoulder p.

presentation (continued)
    torso p.
    transverse p.
    trunk p.
    vertex p.
    vertex-vertex p.
previable
primigravid
primigravida
primipara
primiparity
primiparous
primitiae
primordial
    p. follicle
    p. germ cells
primordium
    uterovaginal p.
procedure
    Pereyra p.
    Shirodkar p.
    Stamey's p.
    Strap p.
    Temple p.
procidentia
progenital
Progestasert IUD
progestational
progesteroid
progesterone
progestin
progestogen
progestomimetic
progravid
prolactin
prolapse
    uterine p.
    vaginal p.
prolapsus
    p. uteri
proliferative
prostaglandin(s)
proteinuria
pruritus
Pryor-Pean retractor
psammoma bodies
pseudocorpus luteum

pseudocyesis
pseudoendometritis
pseudoerosion
pseudohermaphroditism
pseudomamma
pseudomenopause
pseudomenstruation
pseudomucin
pseudomucinous
pseudomyxoma
    p. peritonei
pseudopregnancy
psoas
psoriasis
psychosis
PU – pregnancy urine
pubarche
puberty
    precocious p.
    pseudoprecocious p.
pubic
pubocervical
pubovesicocervical
pudendal
pudendum
    p. femininum
    p. muliebre
puerpera
puerperal
puerperalism
puerperant
puerperium
pulmonary
    p. embolism
    p. maturity
punch
    Keyes' biopsy p.
punctation
punctiform
Puzo's method
pyelitis
    p. gravidarum
pyelocystitis
pyelonephritis
pylorospasm
pyocolpocele
pyocolpos

pyogenic
pyometra
pyometritis
pyometrium
pyo-ovarium
pyosalpingitis
pyosalpingo-oophoritis
pysalpingo-oothecitis
pyosalpinx
pyuria
Q-tip test
quadripara
quadruplets
quintipara
rachitic
radiation. See *Radiology and Nuclear Medicine* section.
radioimmunoassay
radioreceptor assay
radium
rakitic. See *rachitic.*
Ramses' diaphragm
ramus
    ischiopubic r.
Randall's
    curet
    sign
    stone forceps
Rasch's sign
rating
    Apgar r.
reaction
    acrosome r.
    depressive r.
Récamier's
    curet
    operation
recombinant
    r. DNA
rectocele
rectolabial
rectouterine
rectovaginal
rectum
reflex
    Ferguson's r.

regime
  Smith & Smith r.
Reichel's cloacal duct
Reich-Nechtow
  curet
  dilator
Reich's clamp
renal
  r. agenesis
  r. failure
  r. function
  r. transplant
renin
  r. angiotensin system
reproductive
respiration
respiratory
resuscitation
rete
  r. ovarii
retention
retractor
  Balfour's r.
  Brantley-Turner r.
  Deaver's r.
  DeLee's r.
  Doyen's r.
  Eastman's r.
  Emmet's r.
  Friedman's r.
  Gelpi's r.
  Glenner's r.
  Guttmann's r.
  Heaney's r.
  Heaney-Simon r.
  Jackson's r.
  O'Sullivan-O'Connor r.
  Pryor-Pean r.
  Rigby's r.
  Sims' r.
  Sims-Kelly r.
  Wesson's r.
retrocervical
retrocessed
retrocession
retrodisplacement
retroflexion

retroplacental
retroposition
retrouterine
retroversion
retroverted
Retzius' space
Reusner's sign
RFA – right frontoanterior
RFP – right frontoposterior
RFT – right frontotransverse
Rh blood type
rhesus
  r. factor
  r. isoimmunization
Rh factor – Rhesus factor
Rh neg. – Rhesus factor negative
Rho-Gam test
Rh pos. – Rhesus factor positive
Rh sensitization
Richardson's technique
Ries-Wertheim
  hysterectomy
  operation
Rigby's retractor
ring
  Bandl's r.
  Falope's r.
  hymenal r.
Ringer's lactate
Rinman's sign
Ritgen's maneuver
Rizzoli's operation
RMA – right mentoanterior
RMP – right mentoposterior
RMT – right mentotransverse
ROA – right occipitoanterior
Robert's pelvis
Rochester-Carmalt forceps
Rochester-Ochsner forceps
Rochester-Pean forceps
Rock-Mulligan hood
Roederer's obliquity
Rohr's stria
Rokitansky-Küster-Hauser
  syndrome
rooming-in
ROP – right occipitoposterior

ROT – right occipitotransverse
  rotation
    internal r.
Rotunda treatment
RRA – radioreceptor
  assay
RSA – right sacroanterior
R. Sc. A. – right scapuloanterior
R. Sc. P. – right scapuloposterior
RSP – right sacroposterior
RST – right sacrotransverse
rubella
Rubin's
    cannula
    operation
    test
ruga
rugae
    r. of vagina
    r. vaginales
rule
    Arey's r.
    Haase's r.
    His' r.
    Nägele's r.
Russell's forceps
Sabin-Feldman test
sacrouterine
sactosalpinx
Saenger's
    macula
    operation
Saf-t-coil
saline
Salmon's sign
salpingectomy
salpingemphraxis
salpingian
salpingitic
salpingitis
    chronic interstitial s.
    chronic vegetating s.
    hemorrhagic s.
    hypertrophic s.
    s. isthmica nodosa
    mural s.
    nodular s.

salpingitis (continued)
    parenchymatous s.
    s. profluens
    pseudofollicular s.
    purulent s.
    tuberculous s.
salpingocele
salpingocyesis
salpingogram
salpingography
salpingolithiasis
salpingolysis
salpingo-oophorectomy
salpingo-oophoritis
salpingo-oophorocele
salpingo-oothecitis
salpingo-oothecocele
salpingo-ovariectomy
salpingo-ovariotomy
salpingoperitonitis
salpingopexy
salpingoplasty
salpingorrhaphy
salpingostomatomy
salpingostomatoplasty
salpingostomy
salpingotomy
salpinx
Sampson's cyst
sanguineous
sarcoidosis
    Boeck's s.
sarcoma
    s. botryoides
Sarcoptes
    S. scabiei
Saxtorph's maneuver
Scanzoni's
    maneuver
    operation
scarification
    chemical s.
Scarpa's fascia
Schatz's maneuver
Schauffler's operation
Schaumann's benign
    lymphogranuloma

Schauta-Amreich vaginal
   hysterectomy
Schauta's
   operation
   radical vaginal
     hysterectomy
Schauta-Wertheim operation
Schiller's test
Schröder's operation
Schroeder's
   disease
   forceps
   scissors
   syndrome
   tenaculum
Schubert's forceps
Schuchardt's operation
Schuller's stain
Schultze's
   mechanism
   method
   placenta
Schuman's method
Schwartz's
   forceps
   hook
Schweizer's forceps
scissors
   Braun's s.
   Doyen's s.
   Emmet's s.
   Ferguson's s.
   Kelly's s.
   Mayo-Harrington s.
   Mayo's s.
   Mayo-Sims s.
   Metzenbaum s.
   Nelson's s.
   Schroeder's s.
   Sims' s.
   umbilical s.
   Waldmann's s.
sclerocystic
sclero-oophoritis
sclero-oothecitis
score
   Apgar s.

score (continued)
   Bishop's s.
   Silverman's s.
Scully's tumor
sebaceous
secretion
secretory
section
   cesarean s.
   cesarean s., cervical
   cesarean s., classic
   cesarean s., corporeal
   cesarean s., extraperitoneal
   cesarean s., Kerr's
   cesarean s., Kronig's
   cesarean s., Latzko's
   cesarean s., low
   cesarean s., Porro's
   cesarean s., transperitoneal
   cesarean s., transverse
   cesarean s., Water's
   frozen s.
secundigravida
secundina
secundinae
secundine
secundipara
secundiparity
secundiparous
sefalo-. See words beginning
   cephalo-.
segment
   equatorial s.
Segond's
   forceps
   spatula
seizures
semen
seminoma
   ovarian s.
Senn forceps
sepsis
   puerperal s.
septate
septicemia
septigravida
septimetritis

septipara
septum
    s. corporum
      cavernosorum clitoridis
    longitudinal s.
    placental s.
    rectovaginal s.
    s. rectovesicale
    transverse vaginal s.
    urogenital s.
serocystoma
serosa
serosal
serosanguineous
serous
Sertoli-Leydig cell tumor
serum alpha-fetoprotein
serviko-. See words beginning
    cervico-.
sessile
sex cords
sextigravida
sextipara
sexual
sexuality
Sheehan's syndrome
shield
    Dacron s.
    Dalkon s.
Shirodkar
    needle
    operation
    procedure
shock
    obstetric s.
    toxic s.
Shorr's stain
sign
    Ahlfeld's s.
    Arnoux's s.
    Beccaria's s.
    Beclard's s.
    Bolt's s.
    Braun-Fernwald s.
    Braxton-Hicks s.
    Chadwick's s.
    Cullen's s.

sign (continued)
    Danforth's s.
    Dewees' s.
    Gauss's s.
    Golden's s.
    Goodell's s.
    Halban's s.
    Hegar's s.
    Hicks' s.
    Hoehne's s.
    Jacquemier's s.
    Kanter's s.
    Kergaradec's s.
    Küstner's s.
    Ladin's s.
    Landou's s.
    Mayor's s.
    Olshausen's s.
    Osiander's s.
    Pinard's s.
    Piskacek's s.
    Randall's s.
    Rasch's s.
    Reusner's s.
    Rinman's s.
    Salmon's s.
    Spalding's s.
    Tarnier's s.
    Von Fernwald's s.
Silastic cup
Silverman's score
Simmonds' speculum
Simon's operation
Simpson-Luikart forceps
Simpson's
    forceps
    sound
Sims'
    curet
    retractor
    scissors
    sound
    speculum
Sims-Huhner test
Sims-Kelly retractor
Sinografin

sinus
    urogenital s.
skeletonized
Skene's
    curet
    duct
    forceps
    gland
SLE – systemic lupus
    erythematosus
smear
    buccal s.
    Nickerson's medium s.
    Pagano-Levin medium s.
    Papanicolaou's s.
smegma
    s. clitoridis
    s. embryonum
Smellie's
    method
    perforator
Smith & Smith regime
Smith-Hodge pessary
Smith's
    forceps
    pessary
sois. See *psoas.*
somatostatin
somatotropin release-inhibiting
    factor
Somers' forceps
sonogram
Soonawalla uterine
    elevator
sound
    Simpson's s.
    Sims' s.
    uterine s.
space
    pararectal s.
    paravesical s.
    presacral s.
    s. of Retzius
Spalding-Richardson
    hysterectomy
    operation
Spalding's sign

spatula
    Segond's s.
    Tauber's s.
spectrophotometry
speculum
    Auvard-Remine s.
    Auvard's weighted s.
    Berlind-Auvard s.
    Brewer's s.
    Collin's s.
    Cusco's s.
    Devilbiss' s.
    Devilbiss-Stacey s.
    duck-billed s.
    Fergusson's s.
    Garrigue's s.
    Graves' s.
    Guttmann's s.
    Hardy-Duddy s.
    Henrotin's s.
    Huffman-Graves s.
    Jonas-Graves s.
    Kahn-Graves s.
    Mason-Auvard s.
    Mayer's s.
    Miller's s.
    Nott's s.
    O'Sullivan-O'Connor s.
    Pederson's s.
    pediatric s.
    Picto's s.
    Simmonds' s.
    Sims' s.
    weighted s.
    Weisman-Graves s.
    wire bivalve s.
sperm
spermatogenesis
spermicidal
sphincter
    anal s.
    s. vaginae
Spinelli's operation
spinnbarkeit
spirochete
spray
    Dermoplast s.

squamocolumnar
SRIF – somatotropin release-
    inhibiting factor
stage
        Tanners's s's
stain
        Feulgen s.
        Lugol's s.
        Papanicolaou's s.
        Schuller's s.
        Shorr's s.
Stamey's procedure
staphylococci
Starlinger's dilator
Staude-Moore forceps
Staude's forceps
Stein-Leventhal syndrome
stellate
stenosis
stent
        foam rubber vaginal s.
sterility
sterilization
Steri-strips
steroid(s)
stick
        sponge s.
stillbirth
stillborn
Stockholm box
Storz' hysteroscope
strap
        Montgomery s.
Strap procedure
Strassman-Jones operation
Strassmann's phenomenon
streptococci
        group A, B, C (etc.) s.
stress
        s. incontinence
stria
        Langhans' s.
        Rohr's s.
striae
        s. gravidarum
stricture

Stroganoff's (Stroganov's)
    treatment
stroma
        s. of ovary
        ovarian s.
        s. ovarii
stromal
stromatosis
        endometrial s.
study
        air s.
        cytogenetic s.
Sturmdorf's operation
stylet
subinvolution
submucous
subperitoneal
subserous
subumbilical
subvesical
suction
        s. curettage
sudo-. See words beginning
        pseudo-.
sulcus
Sulkowich's test
superfecundation
supernumerary
suprapubic
supravaginal
surfactant
surgical procedures. See
        operation.
suspension
suture. See General Surgical
        Terms.
Swiss-cheese
        endometrium
Swyer's syndrome
Syed-Nesbit template
symphysis
        s. pubica
        s. pubis
symptothermal
synchondrosis
synclitism

syncopal
syncytial
syncytioma
syncytiotoxin
syndrome
    Achard-Thiers s.
    acid aspiration s.
    acquired
      immunodeficiency s.
    Ahumada-Del Castillo s.
    Allen-Masters s.
    androgen insensitivity s.
    Asherman's s.
    Brentano's s.
    Chiari-Frommel s.
    Curtius' s.
    Cushing's s.
    Down's s.
    Dubovitz's s.
    Ellis-van Creveld s.
    fetal alcohol s.
    fetal hydantoin s.
    fetal postmaturity s.
    fetal warfarin s.
    Fitz-Hugh's s.
    Fritsch-Asherman s.
    Gordon-Overstreet s.
    Kallmann's s.
    Klinefelter's s.
    Klotz's s.
    Mayer-Rokitansky-Küster
      s.
    McCune-Albright s.
    Meigs' s.
    Meigs-Cass s.
    Mendelson's s.
    pelvic congestion s.
    polycystic ovarian s.
    Rokitansky-Küster-
      Hauser s.
    Schroeder's s.
    Sheehan's s.
    Stein-Leventhal s.
    Swyer's s.
    testicular feminization s.
    Turner's s.

syndrome (continued)
    Young's s.
    Youssef's s.
synechia
    s. vulvae
synechiae
syo-. See words beginning
    cyo-.
syphilis
systemic lupus erythematosus
tachycardia
    fetal t.
tampon
    Dührssen's t.
    Genupak t.
tandem
Tanner's stages
Tarnier's
    forceps
    sign
Tatum-T IUD
Tauber's spatula
Taussig-Morton operation
Taussig's operation
Tay-Sachs disease
Teale's forceps
technique
    Brandt's t.
    Richardson's t.
telangiectatic
telangiecteric
Te Linde operation
template
    Syed-Nesbit t.
Temple procedure
tenaculum
    Adair's t.
    Barrett's t.
    Braun's t.
    DeLee's t.
    Duplay's t.
    Jacobs' t.
    Kahn's t.
    Marlex atraumatic t.
    Schroeder's t.
    sharp toothed t.

tent
    Laminaria t.
teratogen
teratogenicity
teratology
teratoma
teratome
tertigravida
tertipara
test
    agglutination inhibition t.
    Aschheim-Zondek t.
    AZ t.
    benzidine t.
    Biocept-G t.
    Bonney's t.
    Brouha's t.
    chorionic gonadotropin t.
    Collin's t.
    contraction stress t.
    Coombs' t.
    Corner-Allen t.
    cotton-tip applicator t.
    cross-matching t.
    dexamethasone
      suppression t.
    Dienst's t.
    Farris' t.
    fern t.
    fetal electrocardiogram t.
    Fibrindex t.
    foam stability t.
    Friedman-Lapham t.
    Friedman's t.
    frog t.
    Galli-Mainini t.
    Gravindex t.
    Hogben's t.
    Huhner's t.
    immunologic t.
    Kapeller-Adler t.
    Kleihauer-Betke t.
    Kline's flocculation t.
    Kupperman's t.
    Marchetti t.
    Marshall-Marchetti t.
    nitrazine t.

test (continued)
    nonstress t.
    norethindrone t.
    norethynodrel t.
    Pap t.
    Pregnosticon t.
    progesterone withdrawal t.
    Q-tip t.
    Rho-Gam t.
    Rubin's t.
    Sabin-Feldman t.
    Schiller's t.
    Sims-Huhner t.
    stimulation t.
    stress t.
    Sulkowich's t.
    Thorn t.
    thymol turbidity t.
    toad t.
    ultrasound t.
    Visscher-Bowman t.
    von Poehl's t.
    Wampole's t.
    Wilson's t.
    Xenopus laevis t.
testiculoma
    t. ovarii
thalassemia
theca
    t. cell
    t. externa
    t. folliculi
    t. interna
    t. lutein
thecoma
thecomatosin
thecosis
thelarche
theleplasty
thelerethism
thelitis
thelorrhagia
thermogram
thermography
Thomas'
    curet
    operation

Thomas' (continued)
    pessary
Thoms'
    forceps
    pelvimeter
Thoms-Allis forceps
Thoms-Gaylor forceps
Thorn test
thrombocytopenia
    thrombotic t.
thrombocytopenic
    t. purpura
thromboembolic
thrombolytic
thrombophlebitis
thrombosis
    venous t.
thyroid
    t. gland
    t.-stimulating hormone
    t. storm
thyrotoxicosis
Tischler's forceps
tissue
    endometrial t.
    interstitial t.
titer
    rubella t.
tocograph
tocography
tocology
tocolysis
tocolytic
toluidine blue
topography
TORCH – toxoplasmosis, other
    (syphilis), rubella,
    cytomegalovirus, herpes
    simplex
Torpin's operation
torsion
tortuosity
Touhey's needle
towel clamp
    Backhaus t.c.
toxemia
toxic shock

toxoplasmosis
trachelectomy
trachelitis
tracheloplasty
trachelorrhaphy
trachelosyringorrhaphy
trachelotomy
traction handle
    Barton's t.h.
    Bill's t.h.
    Luikart-Bill t.h.
transplacental
transvaginal
treatment
    Brandt's t.
    Elliott's t.
    Rotunda t.
    Stroganoff's (Stroganov's)
        t.
Treponema
    T. pallidum
TRH – thyrotropin-releasing
    hormone
triangle
    Pawlik's t.
Trichomonas vaginalis
trimester
triphasic
trisomy
trocar
trophoblast
T-strain mycoplasma
tubal
    t. ligation
    t. occlusion
    t. pregnancy
    t. sterilization
tube
    fallopian t.
    uterine t.
tubercle
    müllerian t.
    Müller's t.
tuberculosis
tuberosity
    ischial t.
tuboabdominal

tuboadnexopexy
tuboligamentous
tubo-ovarian
tubo-ovariotomy
tubo-ovaritis
tuboperitoneal
tuboplasty
tubouterine
tubovaginal
Tucker-McLean forceps
Tuffier's operation
tumor
    Brenner's t.
    corticoadrenal t.
    endodermal sinus t.
    germ-cell t.
    gonadal-stromal t.
    Grawitz's t.
    hilus cell t.
    hypernephroid t.
    Krukenberg's t.
    lipid-cell t.
    lipoid cell t.
    mesenchymal t.
    Scully's t.
    Sertoli-Leydig cell t.
    theca-cell t.
    Wilms' t.
tunica
    t. albuginea
    t. mucosa tubae uterinae
    t. mucosa urethrae
      femininae
    t. mucosa urethrae
      muliebris
    t. mucosa uteri
    t. mucosa vaginae
    t. muscularis cervicis uteri
    t. muscularis tubae
      uterinae
    t. muscularis urethrae
      femininae
    t. muscularis urethrae
      muliebris
    t. muscularis uteri
    t. muscularis vaginae
    t. serosa tubae uterinae

tunica (continued)
    t. serosa uteri
Turner's syndrome
twin(s)
    conjoined t's
    dizygotic t's
    fraternal t's
    identical t's
    monozygotic t's
Twombly's operation
Twombly-Ulfelder operation
UAP – uterine arterial pressure
UBF – uterine blood flow
UC – uterine contractions
Uchida's operation
ulcus
    u. phagedaenicum
      corrodens
    u. vulvae acutum
ultrasonography
ultrasound
umbilical cord
umbilicus
    amniotic u.
    decidual u.
unengaged
unicollis
unicornate
unicornis
unit
    Bovie u.
UPP – uterine perfusion pressure
Ureaplasma
    U. urealyticum
uremia
    puerperal u.
ureter
ureteroneocystostomy
ureterouterine
ureterovaginal
urethra
    u. feminina
    u. muliebris
urethral
    u. caruncle
    u. diverticulum
    u. syndrome

urethrocele
urethrocystography
urethrocystometry
urethrocystoscopy
urethropexy
urethroscopy
urethrovaginal
urethrovesical
urinalysis
urinary
    u. diversion
    u. fistula
    u. frequency
    u. incontinence
    u. sodium
    u. tract
uroflowmetry
urogenital
    u. diaphragm
    u. ridge
    u. sinus
urologic
uteralgia
uterectomy
uteri
    fibromyomata u.
uterine
uterismus
uteritis
uteroabdominal
uterocentesis
uterocervical
uterodynia
uterofixation
uterogestation
uterography
uterolith
uteromania
uterometer
uterometry
utero-ovarian
uteropexy
uteroplacental
    u. insufficiency
    u. ischemia
uteroplasty
uterorectal

uterosacral
uterosalpingography
uteroscope
uterothermometry
uterotomy
uterotonic
uterotropic
uterotubal
uterotubography
uterovaginal
uteroventral
uterovesical
uterus
    u. acollis
    arcuate u.
    u. arcuatus
    u. bicornis
    bicornuate u.
    u. biforis
    u. bilocularis
    u. bipartitus
    bosselated u.
    cochleate u.
    u. cordiformis
    Couvelaire u.
    u. didelphys
    duplex u.
    u. duplex
    fetal u.
    gravid u.
    u. incudiformis
    u. masculinus
    u. parvicollis
    pubescent u.
    u. septus
    u. simplex
    subseptate u.
    u. unicornis
    unicornuate u.
utriculoplasty
UVP—uterine venous pressure
vacuum
vagina
vaginae
vaginal
    v. plate
    v. septum

vaginal (continued)
    v. vault
vaginalectomy
vaginalis
    processus v.
    Trichomonas v.
vaginalitis
vaginapexy
vaginate
vaginectomy
vaginicoline
vaginiperineotomy
vaginismus
vaginitis
    v. adhaesiva
    atrophic v.
    catarrhal v.
    diphtheritic v.
    emphysematous v.
    glandular v.
    granular v.
    monilial v.
    papulous v.
    senile v.
    Trichomonas v.
vaginoabdominal
vaginocele
vaginocutaneous
vaginodynia
vaginofixation
vaginogenic
vaginogram
vaginography
vaginolabial
vaginometer
vaginomycosis
vaginopathy
vaginoperineal
vaginoperineorrhaphy
vaginoperineotomy
vaginoperitoneal
vaginopexy
vaginoplasty
vaginoscope
vaginoscopy
vaginotome
vaginotomy

vaginovesical
vaginovulvar
vagitus
    v. uterinus
    v. vaginalis
Valsuani's disease
Van Doren forceps
Van Hoorn's maneuver
varicella
varicocele
    ovarian v.
    utero-ovarian v.
vasa
    v. praevia
    v. propria of Jungbluth
vasectomy
vault
    vaginal v.
vectis
vein
    ovarian v.
velamentous
velamentum
venereal
ventrofixation
ventrohysteropexy
ventrosuspension
ventrovesicofixation
vernix
Vernon-David operation
Verres' needle
verruca
    v. acuminata
verrucous
version
    bipolar v.
    Braxton-Hicks v.
    cephalic v.
    Hicks' v.
    podalic v.
    Potter's v.
    Wigand's v.
    Wright's v.
vertex
vesicle
    Baer's v.
    chorionic v.

vesicle (continued)
    graafian v's
    Naboth's v's
vesicocervical
vesicouterine
vesicouterovaginal
vesicovaginal
vesicovaginorectal
vesiculae graafianae
vesiculae nabothi
vestibular
    v. bulb
vestibule
    v. of vagina
    urogenital v.
vestibuli vaginae
vestibulourethral
vestibulum
    v. vaginae
viability
viable
vibrio
vibrodilator
villi
villus
Vim-Silverman needle
virilism
visceral
Visscher-Bowman test
vitiligo
vomiting
Von Fernwald's sign
von Poehl's test
von Willebrand's disease
Voorhees'
    bag
    needle
vulva
    v. clausa
    v. conivens
    fused v.
    v. hians
vulvae
    kraurosis v.
    noma v.
vulval
vulvar

vulvectomy
vulvismus
vulvitis
    v. blenorrhagica
    creamy v.
    diabetic v.
    diphtheric v.
    diphtheritic v.
    eczematiform v.
    follicular v.
    irritative
    leukoplakic v.
    monilial v.
    phlegmonous v.
    plasma cell v.
    pseudoleukoplakic v.
    ulcerative v.
vulvocrural
vulvopathy
vulvorectal
vulvouterine
vulvovaginal
vulvovaginitis
Waldeyer's fossa
Waldmann's scissors
Walthard's cell
Walton-Schubert forceps
Walton's forceps
Wampole's test
Ward-Mayo vaginal
    hysterectomy
Warren's operation
wart
    venereal w's
Water's
    cesarean section
    operation
Watkins' operation
Watkins-Wertheim operation
Watson's method
Webster's operation
Weisman-Graves speculum
Weisman's forceps
Wertheim-Cullen forceps
Wertheim's
    forceps
    operation

Wertheim's (continued)
    radical hysterectomy
Wertheim-Schauta operation
Wesson's retractor
WF – white female
Wharton's operation
Whitacre's operation
White's classification
Wigand's
    maneuver
    version
Willett's
    clamp
    forceps
William's
    operation
    pelvimeter
Williams-Richardson operation
Willy Meyer radical mastectomy
Wilms' tumor
Wilson's test
Wittner's forceps
wolffian
    w. cyst
    w. duct
Wolf's laparoscope

Wright's version
Wurd's catheter
Wylie's
    dilator
    operation
    pessary
Xenopus laevis test
xerogram
xerography
xeromammogram
xeromammography
xeromenia
xeroradiography
Yellen clamp
Yeoman's forceps
yolk sac
Young's syndrome
Youssef's syndrome
zeromeneah. See *xeromenia.*
zona
    z. pellucida
Zwanck's pessary
Zweifel-DeLee cranioclast
zygosity
zygote

Ophthalmology

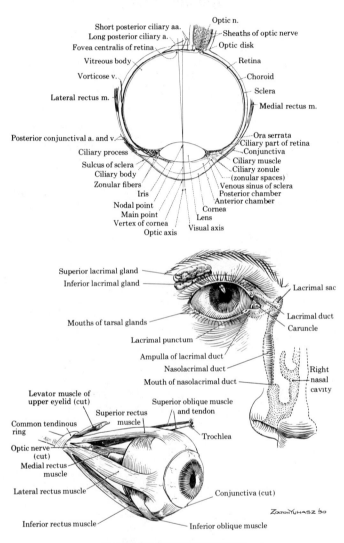

THE EYE AND RELATED STRUCTURES

(Courtesy of Dorland's Illustrated Medical Dictionary, 27th ed. Plate 16. Philadelphia, W. B. Saunders Company, 1988).

Ophthalmology

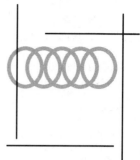

AA – amplitude of
    accommodation
AACG – acute angle closure
    glaucoma
Abadie's sign
abducens
    a. nerve
    a. palsy
abduction
aberrant regeneration
aberration
ab externus
abiotrophy
    retinal a.
ablatio
    a. retinae
ablation
ablepharia
ablepharon
ablepharous
ablephary
ablepsia
ablepsy
abrader
    Howard's a.
abrasio
    a. corneae
abrasion
abscess
abscessus
    a. siccus corneae
abscission
    corneal a.
absolute
    a. glaucoma
    a. hyperopia
    a. scotoma
absorptive lenses

AC – anterior chamber
AC/A ratio – accommodative
    convergence/accommo-
    dation ratio
Acc. – accommodation
accommodation
    absolute a.
    binocular a.
    excessive a.
    negative a.
    positive a.
    relative a.
    subnormal a.
accommodative
    a. convergence
    a. convergence/accom-
        modation ratio
    a. effort syndrome
    a. esotropia
    a. palsy
    a. spasm
    a. target
accommodometer
ACG – angle closure glaucoma
achlys
achroacytosis
achromatic
    a. lens
    a. perimetry
achromatopia
achromatopic
achromatopsia
achromatosis
acne
    a. ciliaris
acorea
acrocephalosyndactylia of Apert
acuity

acute angle closure glaucoma
adaptation
  retinal a.
adaptometer
adduction
adenocarcinoma
adenologaditis
adenoma
  acidophilic a.
  basophilic a.
  chromophobe a.
adenopathy
adenophthalmia
adherence syndrome
adhesions
adhesive syndrome
Adie's
  pupil
  syndrome
aditus
  a. orbitae
adnexa
  a. oculi
adrenergic
ADV – adenovirus
Aebli's scissors
aerial haze
affakia. See *aphakia.*
afferent
  a. defect
  a. nerve
afterimage
Agamodistomum
  A. ophthalmobium
Agnew's
  keratome
  operation
agnosia
  visual a.
agonist
Agrikola's retractor
AHM – anterior hyaloid
  membrane
akinesia
  O'Brien a.
  Van Lint a.
akinesis

akinetic
aklis. See *achlys.*
aknephascopia
akro-. See words beginning
  achro-.
alacrima
albedo
  a. retinae
albinism
Albright's disease
albuginea
  a. oculi
albugo
Alcon's cryophake
Alexander's law
alexia
  optical a.
Alezzandrini's syndrome
alignment
alkoptonuria
Allen's implant
alopecia
  a. orbicularis
Alpar's implant
alpha-hemolytic
Alport syndrome
Alström-Olsen syndrome
alternating
  a. esotropia
  a. strabismus
  a. sursumduction
amacrine cells
amaurosis
  albuminuric a.
  Burns' a.
  cat's eye a.
  central a.
  a. centralis
  cerebral a.
  congenital a.
  diabetic a.
  a. fugax
  hysteric a.
  intoxication a.
  Leber's a.
  saburral a.
  uremic a.

amaurotic
a. family idiocy
a. nystagmus
a. pupil
ambiopia
amblyopia
a. alcoholica
ametropic a.
arsenic a.
astigmatic a.
a. crapulosa
a. cruciata
deprivation a.
a. ex anopsia
nocturnal a.
postmarital a.
quinine a.
reflex a.
strabismic a.
tobacco a.
toxic a.
traumatic a.
uremic a.
amblyopiatrics
amblyoscope
American Hydron
ametrometer
ametropia
axial a.
curvature a.
index a.
position a.
refractive a.
ametropic
Amh. – mixed astigmatism with
myopia predominating
Ammon's operation
Amoils'
cryoextractor
cryoprobe
retractor
amotio
a. retinae
amphamphoterodiplopia
amplitude
a. of accommodation
a. of convergence

AMPPE – acute multifocal
placoid pigment
epitheliopathy
ampulla
a. canaliculi lacrimalis
a. ductus lacrimalis
ampullae
Amsler's
grid
needle
amyloidosis
anaglyph
Anagnostakis' operation
anaphoria
anatomic equator
Andogsky's syndrome
Anel's operation
anencephaly
anesthesia. See *General Surgical Terms* section.
aneurysm
Angelucci's syndrome
angiodiathermy
angiography
fluorescein a.
angioid streaks
angiokeratoma corporis diffusum
universale
angioma
angiomatosis
a. of retina
angiopathia retinae juvenilis
angiophakomatosis
angioscotoma
angle
a. alpha
anterior chamber a.
a. closure glaucoma
a. gamma
a. kappa
a. lambda
a. of anomaly
a. of deviation
a. of incidence
a. of refraction
a. of the anterior chamber
angular blepharitis

angulus
    a. iridocornealis
    a. oculi lateralis
    a. oculi medialis
anhidrosis
anicteric
aniridia
aniseikonia
aniseikonic
anisoaccommodation
anisocoria
anisometrope
anisometropia
anisometropic
anisophoria
anisopia
ankyloblepharon
    a. filiforme adnatum
ankylosing spondylitis
annular
    a. plexus
    a. scotomo
annulus. See also *anulus.*
    a. ciliaris
    a. of Zinn
    a. zinnii
anomalopia
anomaloscope
    Nagel's a.
anomalous
    a. retinal correspondence
    a. trichromatism
anomaly
    Peter's a.
anoopsia
anophoria
anophthalmia
anophthalmos
anophthalmus
anopia
anopsia
anorthopia
anotropia
antagonist
    contralateral a.
    ipsilateral a.

anterior
    a. chamber
    a. chamber angle
    a. chamber cleavage
    a. chamber top
    a. ciliary arteries
    a. corneal staphyloma
    a. focal point
    a. hyaloid membrane
    a. megalophthalmos
    a. pole
    a. segment
    a. synechia
    a. uveitis
Anthony's compressor
anthrax
antimetropia
anti-
    a-. mongoloid slant
    a-. reflective coating
    a-. suppression exercise
Anton-Babinski syndrome
Anton's symptom
anulus. See also *annulus.*
    a. conjunctivae
    a. iridis major
    a. iridis minor
    a. of conjunctiva
    a. tendineus communis
AO soft lens
A pattern
Apert's
    acrocephalosyndactylia
aperture
apex
aphake
aphakia
aphakic
aphasia
    visual a.
apical
    a. clearance
    a. radius
    a. zone
aplasia
    retinal a.
aponeurosis

apparatus
    Howard-Dolman a.
applanation
applanometer
applicator
    Gifford's a.
Aquaflex lens
aqueous
    a. flare
    a. humor
    a. outflow
aquocapsulitis
arachnodactyly
arachnoiditis
    optochiasmatic a.
ARC – abnormal retinal
      correspondence
    anomalous retinal
      correspondence
arch
    Salus' a.
areuate
    a. scotoma
arcus
    corneal a.
    a. juvenilis
    a. lipoides corneae
    a. palpebralis inferior
    a. palpebralis superior
    a. parieto-occipitalis
    a. senilis
    a. superciliaris.
area
    Broadmann's a's
argamblyopia
argema
argon laser trabeculoplasty
Argyll-Robertson pupil
argyria
argyrosis
Arlt-Jaesche operation
Arlt's
    disease
    line
    operation
    scoop
    sinus

Arlt's (continued)
    trachoma
Arroyo's sign
Arruga's
    expressor
    forceps
    implant
    operation
    protector
    trephine
arteriola
    a. macularis inferior
    a. macularis superior
    a. medialis retinae
    a. nasalis retinae inferior
    a. nasalis retinae superior
    a. temporalis retinae
      inferior
    a. temporalis retinae
      superior
arteriole
    medial a. of retina
    nasal a. of retina
    temporal a. of retina
arteritis
artery
    cilioretinal a.
    hyaloid a.
    long posterior ciliary a.
    posterior conjunctival a.
    retinal a.
    short posterior ciliary a.
arthritis
A-scan
Aseptron II
As. H. – hypermetropic
    astigmatism
As. M. – myopic astigmatism
Aspergillus
aspheric lens
aspheric lenticular spectacles
assay
Ast. – astigmatism
asteroid hyalosis
asthenocoria
asthenometer
asthenope

asthenopia
  accommodative a.
  muscular a.
  nervous a.
  retinal a.
  tarsal a.
asthenopic
astigmagraph
astigmatic
  a. axis
  a. clock
  a. dial
astigmatism
  a. against the rule
  compound a.
  corneal a.
  hypermetropic a.
  hyperopic a.
  lenticular a.
  mixed a.
  myopic a.
  oblique a.
  simple a.
  a. with the rule
astigmatometer
astigmatoscope
astigmatoscopy
astigmia
astigmic
astigmometer
astigmometry
astigmoscope
asymmetric
asymmetry
Atkinson's technique
atopic
atresia
  a. iridis
atrophia
  a. choroideae et retinae
  a. dolorosa
  a. gyrata of choroid
atrophy
  Behr's a.
  Fuchs' a.
  Schnabel's a.
  senile a.

atropinism
atropinization
atypical
  a. monochromacy
  a. monochromat
autokeratoplasty
autonomic
Auto-Plot
axanthopsia
Axenfeld's
  loop
  syndrome
axial
  a. hyperopia
  a. length
  a. myopia
axis
  a. of Fick
  optic a.
  visual a.
bacillus
  Koch-Weeks b.
Bacillus
  B. subtilis
Badal's operation
Baer's nystagmus
Bagolini lenses
Bahn's spud
Ballet's disease
Bamatter's syndrome
band
  b. keratopathy
  silicone b.
Barany's sign
Bardelli's operation
Bard-Parker
  blade
  knife
Barkan's
  knife
  operation
Barraquer-Colibri speculum
Barraquer-DeWecker scissors
Barraquer's
  brush
  erysiphake
  forceps

Barraquer's (continued)
    knife
    needle holder
    operation
    scissors
    speculum
    trephine
bar reader
barrel distortion
Barrio's operation
basal lamina
baseball lens
Basedow's disease
basophil
basophilic
Bassen-Kornzweig syndrome
Basterra's operation
Batten-Mayou disease
Bausch & Lomb
    cleaner
    lubricant
    solution
Beal's
    conjunctivitis
    syndrome
"bear tracks"
Beaupre's forceps
Beaver's
    blade
    handle
    keratome
    knife
bedewing
Beer's
    collyrium
    operation
Behçet's syndrome
Behr's
    atrophy
    disease
    pupil
    syndrome
Bekhterev's nystagmus
Bellows' cryoextractor
Bell's
    erysiphake
    palsy

Bell's (continued)
    phenomenon
Benedikt's syndrome
Bennett's forceps
Benson's disease
Berens'
    dilator
    forceps
    implant
    keratome
    operation
    punch
    retractor
    scissors
    spatula
    speculum
Berens-Rosa implant
Bergemeister's papilla
beriberi
Berke's
    clamp
    forceps
    operation
Berlin's
    disease
    edema
Berman's locator
Berneheimer's fibers
Best's disease
Biber-Haab-Dimmer
    degeneration
Bielschowsky-Jansky
    disease
Bielschowsky-Lutz-Cogan
    syndrome
Bielschowsky's
    disease
    operation
    test
Bietti's
    dystrophy
    syndrome
bifixation
bifocals
bifoveal
binasal
Binkhorst-Fyodorov lens

Binkhorst's
    implant
    lens
binocular
binocularity
binoculus
binophthalmoscope
binoscope
biomicroscope
biomicroscopy
    slit lamp b.
biopsy
bipolar
biprism
Birch-Hirschfeld lamp
Bishop-Harmon
    cannula
    forceps
bitemporal
bitoric contact lens
Bitot's spots
Bjerrum's
    scotoma
    scotometer
    screen
black sunburst
blade
    Bard-Parker b.
    Beaver's b.
    McPherson-Wheeler b.
Blair's operation
Blasius' operation
Blaskovics' operation
blastomycosis
Blatt's operation
bleb
    filtering b.
blef-. See words beginning *bleph-.*
blennorrhea
    b. adultorum
    inclusion b.
    b. neonatorum
blepharadenitis
blepharal
blepharectomy
blepharelosis
blepharism

blepharitis
    b. angularis
    b. ciliaris
    b. marginalis
    nonulcerative b.
    seborrheic b.
    b. squamosa
    b. ulcerosa
blepharoadenitis
blepharoadenoma
blepharoatheroma
blepharochalasis
blepharochromidrosis
blepharoclonus
blepharoconjunctivitis
blepharodiastasis
blepharoncus
blepharopachynsis
blepharophimosis
blepharophryplasty
blepharoplast
blepharoplasty
blepharoplegia
blepharoptosis
blepharopyorrhea
blepharorrhaphy
blepharospasm
blepharosphincterectomy
blepharostat
blepharostenosis
blepharosynechia
blepharotomy
blepharoxysis
Blessig-Iwanoff cysts
Blessig's cysts
blind
    color b.
blindness
    amnesic color b.
    Bright's b.
    color b.
    cortical psychic b.
    eclipse b.
    flash b.
    letter b.
    night b.
    snow b.

blindness (continued)
    twilight b.
blink reflex
Bloch-Stauffer syndrome
Bloch-Sulzberger syndrome
block
    O'Brien b.
    retrobulbar b.
    Van Lint b.
"blown pupil"
blow-out fracture
blue sclera
bobbing
body
    ciliary b.
    cytoid b.
    geniculate b.
    Landolt's b's
    Prowazek-Greeff b's
Boeck's sarcoid
Böhm's operation
Bonaccolto-Flieringa operation
Bonaccolto's
    forceps
    scleral ring
Bonnet-Dechaume-Blanc
    syndrome
Bonzel's operation
boosh de tah-per. See *bouche de
    tapir.*
Borthen's operation
Bossalino's operation
bouche
    b. de tapir
Bourneville's disease
Bovie unit
Bowen's disease
Bowman's
    membrane
    needle
    operation
    probe
boxcarring
Boyd's implant
Boynton's needle holder
Bracken's forceps
Braid's strabismus

Brailey's operation
branch vein occlusion
Brawley's retractor
Briggs' operation
Bright's
    blindness
    eye
Brodmann's areas
Bronson-Turz retractor
Brown-Dohlman implant
Brown's syndrome
Bruchner's test
Bruch's membrane
Brücke's
    fibers
    lens
    muscle
Bruecke
    tunica nervea of B
bruit
brush
    Barraquer's b.
    Haidinger's b's
Brushfield's spot
B scan ultrasonogram
BSV—binocular single vision
buckle
    scleral b.
Budinger's operation
bufilcon A
bulbar
bulbus
    b. oculi
Buller's shield
bullous
Bumke's pupil
bundle
    b. of Drualt
    papillomacular b.
Bunge's spoon
Bunker's implant
buphthalmia
buphthalmos
buphthalmus
bur
    Burwell's b.
Burch-Greenwood tucker

Burch's
    caliper
    operation
    pick
Burns' amaurosis
Burow's operation
Burwell's bur
Busacca nodule
BUT—breakup time
Buzzi's operation
BVA—best corrected visual
    acuity
b-wave
byerrum. See *Bjerrum.*
CAB—cellulose acetate butyrate
Cairns' operation
calcarine fissure
calculus
Calhoun-Merz needle
Calhoun's needle
caliculus
    c. ophthalmicus
caligo
    c. corneae
    c. lentis
    c. pupillae
caliper
    Burch's c.
    Castroviejo's c.
    Green's c.
    Jameson's c.
    Thorpe's c.
Callahan's operation
Calmette's ophthalmoreaction
caloric
    c. nystagmus
    c. testing
Campbell's retractor
campimeter
campimetry
canal
    Cloquet's c.
    Ferrein's c.
    hyaloid c.
    c. of Schlemm
    Petit's c.
    Sondermann's c's

canaliculi
canaliculitis
canaliculodacryocystostomy
canaliculorhinostomy
canaliculus
    c. lacrimalis
candela
Candida albicans
candle power
"candlewax drippings"
cannula
    Bishop-Harmon c.
    Castroviejo's c.
    Goldstein's c.
    Moncrieff's c.
    Randolph's c.
    Roper's c.
    Tenner's c.
Cantelli's sign
canthectomy
canthi
canthitis
cantholysis
canthoplasty
canthorrhaphy
canthotomy
canthus
    inner c.
    lateral c.
    medial c.
    outer c.
capillary
    c. hemangioma
capsitis
capsula
    c. lentis
capsule
    c. of Tenon
capsulectomy
capsulitis
capsulolenticular
capsulotome
    Darling's c.
capsulotomy
CAR—cancer-associated
    retinopathy

carcinoma
    epidermoid c.
cardinal
    c. movements
    c. points
carotid
    c. artery
    c. cavernous fistula
Carter's
    introducer
    operation
caruncle
    c. epicanthus
    lacrimal c.
caruncula
    c. lacrimalis
Casanellas' operation
Caspar's ring opacity
Castallo's retractor
Castroviejo-Arruga forceps
Castroviejo-Kalt needle holder
Castroviejo's
    caliper
    cannula
    dilator
    forceps
    keratome
    knife
    needle holder
    operation
    punch
    retractor
    scissors
    spatula
    speculum
    trephine
cataphoria
cataract
    adherent c.
    adolescent c.
    after c.
    arborescent c.
    aridosiliculose c.
    aridosiliquate c.
    axial c.
    black c.
    blood c.

cataract (continued)
    blue dot c.
    bony c.
    bottlemakers' c.
    brunescent c.
    calcareous c.
    capsular c.
    capsulolenticular c.
    caseous c.
    cerulean c.
    cheesy c.
    choroidal c.
    congenital c.
    contusion c.
    coralliform c.
    coronary c.
    cortical c.
    cupuliform c.
    cystic c.
    diabetic c.
    discission c.
    dry-shelled c.
    embryonal nuclear c.
    extracapsular c.
    fibroid c.
    floriform c.
    fusiform c.
    glassblowers' c.
    glaucomatous c.
    heat-ray c.
    hedger's c.
    heterochromic c.
    hypermature c.
    immature c.
    incipient c.
    infantile c.
    intracapsular c.
    intumescent c.
    irradiation c.
    juvenile c.
    Koby's c.
    lacteal c.
    lamellar c.
    lenticular c.
    lightning c.
    mature c.
    membranous c.

cataract (continued)
    morgagnian c.
    myotonic c.
    naphthalinic c.
    nuclear c.
    O'Brien's c.
    overripe c.
    perinuclear c.
    peripheral c.
    polar c.
    primary c.
    progressive c.
    puddler's c.
    punctate c.
    pyramidal c.
    reduplication c.
    ripe c.
    sanguineous c.
    secondary c.
    sedimentary c.
    senile c.
    siliculose c.
    siliquose c.
    snowflake c.
    snowstorm c.
    spindle c.
    stationary c.
    stellate c.
    subcapsular c.
    subtotal c.
    "sunflower" c.
    sutural c.
    syphilitic c.
    total c.
    toxic c.
    traumatic c.
    tremulous c.
    unripe c.
    Vogt's c.
    zonular c.
cataracta
    c. accreta
    c. brunescens
    c. cerulea
    c. complicata
    c. congenita
      membranacea
    c. coronaria

cataracta (continued)
    c. electrica
    c. membranacea accreta
    c. neurodermatica
    c. nigra
    c. ossea
    c. syndermotica
cataractous
catarrh
    vernal c.
cat cry syndrome
catheterization
cat's eye reflex
cautery
    Hildreth's c.
    Mueller's c.
    Rommel-Hildreth c.
    Rommel's c.
    Scheie's c.
    von Graefe's c.
    Wadsworth-Todd c.
    wetfield c.
    Ziegler's c.
cavernous
    c. hemangioma
    c. sinus
CCF – carotid cavernous fistula
cecal
cecocentral
"cell and flare"
cellophane
    c. retinopathy
cellulose acetate butyrate
Celsus' operation
center of rotation
centrad
central
    c. fixation
    c. fusion
    c. nervous system
    c. retinal artery
    c. retinal artery
      occlusion
    c. retinal vein
    c. retinal vein occlusion
    c. scotoma
    c. serous
      chorioretinopathy

central (continued)
    c. suppression
    c. visual acuity
centrocecal
cerclage
cerebellopontine angle tumor
cerebral
    c. dyschromatopsia
cerebro-ocular
CF – count fingers
c. gl. – correction with glasses
chalazia
chalazion
chalcosis
    c. lentis
chamber
    anterior c.
    aqueous c.
    posterior c.
    vitreous c.
Chandler's
    forceps
    syndrome
chart
    Donder's c.
    Duane's accommo-
       dative c.
    Landolt's c.
    Lebensohn's c.
    pseudoisochromatic c.
    Reuss' color c's
    Snellen's c.
cheiroscope
chemosis
Cheyne's nystagmus
chiasm
    optic c.
chiasma
    c. opticum
    c. syndrome
chiasmal
    c. arachnoiditis
Chlamydia trachomatis
chlamydial
chlorolabe
chloropsia
choriocapillaris
choriocele

chorioid
chorioidea
choked disk
chorioretinal
chorioretinitis
chorioretinopathy
choroid
choroidal
    c. detachment
    c. flush
    c. hemorrhage
    c. hyperfluorescence
    c. nevus
choroidea
choroideremia
choroiditis
    areolar c.
    Doyne's c.
    Förster's c.
    c. guttata senilis
    juxtapapillitic c.
    c. myopica
    c. serosa
    syphilitic c.
    Tay's c.
    toxoplasmic c.
choroidocyclitis
choroidoiritis
choroidopathy
choroidoretinitis
Choyce's implant
Choyce Mark VIII
    implant
chromatic
    c. aberration
    c. dispersion
    c. perimetry
chromatopsia
chromatoptometer
chromophobe
chromostereopsis
Cibasoft
cibisotome
cicatricial
cicatrix
cilia
ciliariscope
ciliarotomy

ciliary
    c. arteries
    c. body
    c. flush
    c. ganglion
    c. hyperemia
    c. muscle
    c. nerve
    c. process
    c. spasm
    c. vein
    c. zonule
ciliectomy
cilioretinal
    c. artery
    c. vein
cilioscleral
cilium
cillosis
cinching
circadian
    c. heterotropia
circinate
    c. exudate
    c. retinopathy
circle
    Willis' c.
circlet
    Zinn's c.
circumduction
clamp
    Berke's c.
    serrefine c.
Claude's syndrome
cleft
    corneal c.
Clens
Clerz
clinometer
clinoscope
clip
    Halberg c.
    tantalum c.
clock dial
Cloquet's canal
CME – cystoid macular
   edema

CMI – cytomegalic inclusion
CMV – cytomegalovirus
CNS – central nervous
   system
COAG – chronic open angle
   glaucoma
Coats'
    disease
    retinitis
    ring
"cobblestones"
co-contraction syndrome
Cogan's
    dystrophy
    syndrome
"cogwheeling"
Colibri's forceps
collarette
Collier's sign
collimator
Collin-Beard operation
collyria
collyrium
    Beer's c.
coloboma
    Fuchs' c.
    c. iridis
    c. lentis
    c. lobuli
    c. of choroid
    c. of iris
    c. of optic nerve
    c. of vitreous
    c. palpebrale
    c. retinae
Comberg lens
commissura
    c. palpebrarum lateralis
    c. palpebrarum medialis
    c. superior Meynerti
commissurae supraopticae
commissure
    arcuate c.
    Gudden's c.
    interthalamic c.
    Meynert's c.
    optic c.

commissure (continued)
    palpebral c.
    posterior c., chiasmatic
    supraoptic c's
commotio
    c. retinae
complementary
    c. afterimage
    c. chromaticities
    c. colors
compressor
    Anthony's c.
computed tomography
computerized
    tomography
conclination
concomitant
cone
    c. dystrophy
    c. monochromacy
    c. monchromat
    ocular c.
    retinal c.
    twin c's
    visual c.
conformer
    Fox's c.
confrontation fields
congenital
conical
conjugate
conjunctiva
conjunctival
conjunctiviplasty
conjunctivitis
    acne rosacea c.
    actinic c.
    allergic c.
    anaphylactic c.
    arc-flash c.
    atopic c.
    atropine c.
    bacterial c.
    Beal's c.
    blennorrheal c.
    calcareous c.
    catarrhal c.

conjunctivitis (continued)
    chemical c.
    chronic c.
    contact c.
    croupous c.
    diphtheritic c.
    diplobacillary c.
    eczematous c.
    Egyptian c.
    Elschnig's c.
    follicular c.
    gonococcal c.
    gonorrheal c.
    granular c.
    inclusion c.
    larval c.
    c. medicamentosa
    membranous c.
    meningococcus c.
    molluscum c.
    Morax-Axenfeld c.
    c. necroticans
        infectiosus
    neonatal c.
    parasitic c.
    Parinaud's c.
    Pascheff's c.
    c. petrificans
    phlyctenular c.
    prairie c.
    pseudomembranous c.
    purulent c.
    Samoan c.
    Sanyal's c.
    scrofular c.
    squirrel plague c.
    trachomatous c.
    c. tularensis
    uratic c.
    vernal c.
    viral c.
    welder's c.
    Widmark's c.
    Wucherer's c.
conjunctivodacryocystostomy
conjunctivoma
conjunctivoplasty

conjunctivorhinostomy
conoid
    Sturm's c.
conophthalmus
consensual
constricted
contacto gauge
contactoscope
Contino's
    epithelioma
    glaucoma
Contique
contralateral
    c. antagonist
    c. synergist
conus
convergence
    accommodative c.
    c. amplitudes
    fusional c.
    c. insufficiency
    proximal c.
    relative c.
    c. spasm
    voluntary c.
convergent
convergiometer
convex lens
convexoconcave lens
Copeland's
    implant
    retinoscope
copiopia
"copper wiring"
Coquille plano lens
Corbett's spud
coreclisis
corectasis
corectome
corectomedialysis
corectomy
corectopia
coredialysis
corediastasis
corelysis
coremorphosis
corenclisis

coreometer
coreometry
coreoplasty
corestenoma
coretomedialysis
coretomy
cornea
    conical c.
    c. farinata
    c. globosa
    c. guttata
    c. opaca
    c. plana
    sugar-loaf c.
    Vogt's c.
corneal
    c. abrasion
    c. apex
    c. astigmatism
    c. bedewing
    c. "button"
    c. cap
    c. dellen
    c. dystrophy
    c. erosion
    c. lens
    c. reflex
    c. scraping
    c. transplant
    c. ulcer
corneal graft
    lamellar c.g.
    mushroom c.g.
    penetrating c.g.
corneitis
corneoblepharon
corneoiritis
corneosclera
corneoscleral
corona
    c. ciliaris
    Zinn's c.
coroparelcysis
coroplasty
coroscopy
corotomy

corpus
c. adiposum orbitae
c. ciliaris
c. vitreum
correspondence
anomalous retinal c.
harmonious retinal c.
retinal c.
cortex
cerebellar c.
c. lentis
cortical
corticosteroid
Corynebacterium xerosis
"cotton wool" spots
couching
CPC – central posterior curve
CPEO – chronic progressive
external ophthalmoplegia
CRA – central retinal artery
cranial
craniofacial
craniophyaryngioma
craniosynostosis
CRAO – central retinal artery
occlusion
Credé's prophylaxis
crescent
cribriform
c. ligament
c. plate
crises
Pel's c's
Critchett's operation
crocodile tears
Crookes' lens
Crouzon's disease
CRV – central retinal vein
CRVO – central retinal vein
occlusion
cryodestruction
cryoextraction
cryoextractor
Amoils' c.
Bellows' c.
cryogenic
cryopexy

cryophake
Alcon's c.
Keeler's c.
cryoprobe
Amoils' c.
cryoptor
Thomas' c.
cryostat
cryosurgery
cryotherapy
crypt
c's of Fuchs
Cryptococcus neoformans
cryptoglioma
cryptophthalmia
cryptophthalmos
cryptophthalmus
crystalline
Csapody's operation
CT – cover test
CT scan
cuff
Honan's c.
cul-de-sac
conjunctival c.
cupped disc
cupping
cup-to-disc ratio
cupuliform
Curdy's sclerotome
curet
Gifford's c.
Green's c.
Heath's c.
Meyhoeffer's c.
Skeele's c.
Custodis' operation
cutaneous
Cutler-Beard operation
Cutler's implant
cyanolabe
cyanosis
c. bulbi
c. retinae
cyclectomy
cyclic
cyclicotomy

cyclitic
cyclitis
      heterochromic c.
      purulent c.
      serous c.
cycloanemization
cycloceratitis
cyclochoroiditis
cyclocryopexy
cyclocryotherapy
cyclodamia
cyclodialysis
cyclodiathermy
cycloduction
cycloelectrolysis
cyclogram
cyclokeratitis
cyclopentolate
cyclophoria
cyclophorometer
cyclopia
cycloplegia
cycloplegic
cyclops
cycloscope
cyclotome
cyclotomy
cyclotropia
cycloversion
cyl.–cylindrical lens
cylindrical
cyst
      Blessig-Iwanoff c's
      Blessig's c's
      meibomian c.
cystic microphthalmia
cystinosis
cystitome
cystitomy
cystoid macular edema
cystotome
      von Graefe's c.
      Wheeler's c.
cytomegalic inclusion disease
cytomegalovirus
cytotoxic
Czermak's operation

D.–diopter
dacryadenalgia
dacryadenitis
dacryadenoscirrhus
dacryagogatresia
dacryagogic
dacryagogue
dacrycystalgia
dacrycystitis
dacryelcosis
dacryoadenalgia
dacryoadenectomy
dacryoadenitis
dacryoblennorrhea
dacryocanaliculitis
dacryocele
dacryocyst
dacryocystalgia
dacryocystectasia
dacryocystectomy
dacryocystis
      phlegmonous d.
      syphilitic d.
      trachomatous d.
      tuberculous d.
dacryocystitis
dacryocystitome
dacryocystoblennorrhea
dacryocystocele
dacryocystogram
dacryocystography
dacryocystoptosis
dacryocystorhinostenosis
dacryocystorhinostomy
dacryocystorhinotomy
dacryocystostenosis
dacryocystostomy
dacryocystosyringotomy
dacryocystotome
dacryocystotomy
dacryogenic
dacryohelcosis
dacryohemorrhea
dacryolin
dacryolith
      Desmarres' d.
dacryolithiasis

dacryoma
dacryon
dacryops
dacryopyorrhea
dacryopyosis
dacryorhinocystotomy
dacryorrhea
dacryosinusitis
dacryosolenitis
dacryostenosis
dacryostomy
dacryosyrinx
Dalen-Fuchs nodule
Dalrymple's
    disease
    sign
D & N – distance and near
Darling's capsulotome
Daviel's
    operation
    scoop
    spoon
Davis'
    forceps
    knife needle
    spud
DDH – dissociated double
  hypertropia
debrider
    Sauer's d.
decentration
declination
decompression
degeneration
    Biber-Haab-Dimmer d.
    hyaline d.
    Kozlowski's d.
    lattice d.
    macular d.
    retinal lattice d.
    Vogt's d.
degenerative
de Grandmont's operation
dehiscence
    iris d.
Dejean's syndrome
delacrimation

dellen
deltafilcon A.
Del Toro's operation
Demours' membrane
demyelinate
demyelinization
dendrite
dendritic keratitis
denervation
deorsumduction
deorsumvergence
deorsumversion
depression
deprivation
depth of perception
Derf's needle holder
dermatochalasis
dermatoconjunctivitis
dermatomyositis
dermoid cyst
dermolipoma
Descartes' law
descemetitis
Descemet's membrane
descemetocele
Desmarres'
    dacryolith
    forceps
    knife
    law
    lid elevator
    retractor
    scarifier
detachment
    d. of retina
    d. of vitreous
    retinal d.
    rhegmatogenous d.
deterioration
deutan
deuteranomalopia
deuteranomaly
deuteranopia
deviation
    primary d.
    secondary d.
    skew d.

Devic's disease
DeVilbiss' irrigator
DeWecker-Pritikin scissors
DeWecker's
        operation
        scissors
dextroclination
dextrocular
dextrocularity
dextrocycloduction
dextrocycloversion
dextroduction
dextrotorsion
dextroversion
D-film
diabetes mellitus
diabetic retinopathy
dial
        clock d.
        fan d.
        Lancaster Regan d.
        "sunburst" d.
dialysis
        d. retinae
diastasis
        iris d.
diathermy
dichromatism
dichromatopsia
diffraction
diktyoma
dilator
        Berens' d.
        Castroviejo's d.
        Heath's d.
        Jones' d.
        Muldoon's d.
        d. muscle
        Nettleship-Wilder d.
        d. pupillae
diminution
Dimitry-Bell erysiphake
Dimitry's erysiphake
Dimitry-Thomas erysiphake
Dimmer's keratitis
dimple
        Fuchs' d's

diopsimeter
diopter
        prism d.
dioptometer
dioptometry
dioptoscopy
dioptre
dioptric
dioptrics
dioptrometer
dioptrometry
dioptroscopy
dioptry
diphtheroid
diplopia
        binocular d.
        crossed d.
        heteronymous d.
        homonymous d.
        monocular d.
        paradoxical d.
        pathologic d.
        physiologic d.
        torsional d.
diplopiometer
diploscope
disc
        anangioid d.
        ciliary d.
        d. diameter
        d. drusen
        optic d.
        Placido's d.
        Rekoss' d.
        stroboscopic d.
disciform
discission
disclination
disease
        Albright's d.
        Arlt's d.
        Ballet's d.
        Basedow's d.
        Batten-Mayou d.
        Behr's d.
        Benson's d.
        Berlin's d.

disease (continued)
    Best's d.
    Bielschowsky-Jansky d.
    Bielschowsky's d.
    Bourneville's d.
    Bowen's d.
    Coats' d.
    Crouzon's d.
    Dalrymple's d.
    Devic's d.
    Eales' d.
    Favre's d.
    Franceschetti's d.
    Gaucher's d.
    Graefe's d.
    Graves' d.
    Hand-Schüller-Christian
        d.
    Harada's d.
    Heerfordt's d.
    Hippel's d.
    Jensen's d.
    Kimmelstiel-Wilson d.
    Koeppe's d.
    Kuhnt-Junius d.
    Lauber's d.
    Leber's d.
    Lindau-von Hippel d.
    Masuda-Kitahara d.
    Mikulicz's d.
    Möbius' d.
    Niemann-Pick d.
    Norrie's d.
    Paget's d.
    Purtscher's d.
    Recklinghausen's d.
    Reis-Bücklers d.
    Reiter's d.
    Schilder's d.
    Sichel's d.
    Sjögren's d.
    Vogt's d.
    Vogt-Spielmeyer d.
    von Hippel-Lindau d.
    von Recklinghausen's d.
    Wagner's d.
    Weil's d.

disease (continued)
    Westphal-Strumpell d.
    Wilson's d.
disinsertion
disjugate
disk. See *disc.*
disparate
dissector
    Green's d.
dissociated
    d. nystagmus
    d. position
    d. vertical deviation
distichia
distichiasis
distometer
distortion
diurnal
divergence
    d. amplitudes
    d. excess
    d. insufficiency
divergent
Dix's spud
Doherty's implant
doll's head phenomenon
Donders'
    chart
    glaucoma
    law
    line
dot
    Gunn's d's
    Mittendorf's d.
    Trantas' d's
Dougherty's irrigator
Douvas' rotoextractor
downbeat nystagmus
down-gaze
Doyne's
    choroiditis
    iritis
Draeger tonometer
dropper
    Undine's d.
Drualt
    bundle of D.

drugs. See *Drugs and Chemistry* section.
drusen
dry eye syndrome
Duane's
    accommodative chart
    syndrome
duct
    lacrimal d.
    lacrimonasal d.
    nasolacrimal d.
    tear d.
duction
ductus
    d. lacrimales
Duke-Elder lamp
duochrome test
Dupuy-Dutemps operation
Durr's operation
DUSN–diffuse unilateral subacute neuroretinitis
Duverger and Velter's operation
DVA–distance visual acuity
DVD–dissociated vertical deviation
dyschromatopsia
dyscoria
dysmegalopsia
dysmetria
dysopia
    d. algera
dysopsia
dysplasia
dysplastic coloboma
dystrophy
    Bietti's d.
    Cogan's d.
    corneal d.
    Fehr's d.
    Fleischer's d.
    Franceschetti's d.
    Francois' d.
    Fuchs' d.
    Groenouw's d.
    Maeder-Danis d.
    Meesmann's d.
    Pillat's d.

dystrophy (continued)
    Salzmann's d.
    Schlichting's d.
    Schnyder's d.
E–esophoria
Eales' disease
Eber's forceps
ECCE–extracapsular cataract extraction
eccentric fixation
ecchymosis
echinophthalmia
echography
echo-ophthalmography
ectasia
    e. iridis
ectiris
ectochoroidea
ectocornea
ectopia
    e. lentis
    e. pupillae congenita
ectopic
ectropion
    e. cicatriceum
    cicatricial e.
    flaccid e.
    e. luxurians
    e. paralyticum
    e. sarcomatosum
    e. senilis
    e. spasticum
    e. uveae
ectropium
edema
    Berlin's e.
    Iwanoff's retinal e.
    Stellwag's brawny e.
Edinger-Westphal nucleus
edipism
efferent
egilops
Egyptian
    conjunctivitis
    ophthalmia
Ehrhardt's forceps
eightball hyphema

eikonometer
EKC – epidemic
    keratoconjunctivitis
elastosis
    e. dystrophica
Eldridge-Green lamp
electrode
        Gradle's e.
        Kronfeld's e.
        Pischel's e.
        Weve's e.
electrocoagulation
electromagnetic
    e. spectrum
electronystagmograph
electro-oculogram
electroparacentesis
electroperimetry
electroretinogram
electroretinography
elevator
        Desmarres' lid e.
ELISA – enzyme-linked
    immunosorbent assay
Elliot's
        operation
        trephine
Ellis' needle holder
Elschnig-O'Brien forceps
Elschnig's
        conjunctivitis
        forceps
        knife
        operation
        retractor
        spatula
        spoon
        spots
        syndrome
Ely's operation
Em. – emmetropia
embolism
        retinal e.
embolus
embryotoxon
emergent ray
emmetrope

emmetropia
emmetropic
endocrine
endogenous
endophthalmitis
        e. phakoanaphylactica
endothelial
endothelioma
        Sidler-Huguenin's e.
endothelium
        e. camerae anterioris oculi
        corneal e.
endpoint nystagmus
ENG – electronystagmograph
enophthalmos
enophthalmus
enstrophe
entophthalmia
entoptic
entoptoscope
entoptoscopy
entoretina
entropion
        e. cicatriceum
        cicatricial e.
        e. spasticum
        e. uveae
entropium
enucleate
enucleation
enzymatic
EOG – electro-oculogram
EOM – extraocular movement
epiblepharon
epibulbar
epicanthal
epicanthus
epicapsular
epicauma
epiphora
episclera
episcleral
episcleritis
        gouty e.
        e. partialis fugax
episclerotitis
epitarsus

epithelial
    e. downgrowth
epithelioma
    Contino's e.
epitheliosis
    e. desquamativa
      conjunctivae
epithelium
    e. anterius corneae
    e. corneae
    corneal e.
    e. of lens
    e. lentis
equator
    e. bulbi oculi
    e. lentis
    e. of crystalline lens
    e. of eyeball
    e. of lens
equatorial
    e. degeneration
    e. meridian
ERG – electroretinogram
erosion
erysipelas
erysiphake
    Barraquer's e.
    Bell's e.
    Dimitry-Bell e.
    Dimitry's e.
    Dimitry-Thomas e.
    Harrington's e.
    Kara's e.
    L'Esperance's e.
    Maumenee's e.
    Nugent-Green-Dimitry e.
    Post-Harrington e.
    Sakler's e.
    Searcy's e.
    Viers' e.
erythema
erythrolabe
erythropia
erythropsia
esodeviation
esophoria
esophoric

esotropia
esotropic
ET – esotropia
"E" test
ethmoid bone
E trisomy
euchromatopsy
euryopia
euthyphoria
euthyscope
Eversbusch's operation
eversion
evisceration
evulsio
    e. nervi optici
Ewald's law
exanthematous
excycloduction
excyclophoria
excyclotropia
excyclovergence
exenteration
exfoliation
exodeviation
exophoria
exophoric
exophthalmic
exophthalmogenic
exophthalmometer
    Hertel's e.
    Luedde's e.
exophthalmometric
exophthalmometry
exophthalmos
    endocrine e.
    pulsating e.
exophthalmus
exorbitism
exotropia
exotropic
expressor
    Arruga's e.
    Heath's e.
    Smith's e.
expulsive
externus
extinction

extorsion
extracapsular
extraction
    roto e.
extraocular
extrinsic
exudate
exudative
    e. retinitis
eye
    blear e.
    Bright's e.
    cinema e.
    dark-adapted e.
    epiphyseal e.
    exciting e.
    hare's e.
    Klieg e.
    lazy e.
    light-adapted e.
    monochromatic e.
    Nairobi e.
    parietal e.
    pineal e.
    pink e.
    schematic e.
    Snellen's reform e.
    squinting e.
    sympathizing e.
eyeball
eyebrow
eyecup
eyeground
eyelash
eyelid
eyestrain
facies
    Hutchinson's f.
facultative
    f. hyperopia
    f. suppression
Faden's procedure
fako-. See words beginning
    phaco-.
falciform fold
Farnsworth
    D-15 test

Farnsworth (continued)
    D-100 test
farsighted
farsightedness
Fasanella-Servat operation
fascia
    f. bulbi
    Tenon's f.
Favre's disease
FB – foreign body
f.c. – foot candles
Federov's implant
Fehr's dystrophy
FER – familial exudative
    retinopathy
Ferree-Rand perimeter
Ferrein's canal
Ferris-Smith retractor
Ferris-Smith-Sewall retractor
FFF fields – flicker, fusion,
    frequency fields
fiber
    Berneheimer's f's
    Brücke's f's
    Müller's f's
    optic nerve f.
    Sappey's f's
    von Monakow's f's
fiberoptic
fiberoptics
fiberscope
fibroma
fibroplasia
    retrolental f.
fibrosarcoma
fibrosis
Fick's
    axis
    halo
filamentary
Filatov-Marzinkowsky
    operation
Filatov's operation
Fink's retractor
Finnoff's transilluminator
Fisher's spud
"fishmouth" tear

fissure
    corneal f.
    palpebral f.
fistula
fixation
    f. axis
    binocular f.
    f. reflex
Flajani's operation
flare
Fleischer's
    dystrophy
    ring
Flexlens
Flieringa's ring
flikten-. See words beginning
    phlycten-.
floaters
Florentine iris
Flouren's law
fluorescein
    f. angiography
    f. dye disappearance
        test
    f. sodium
fluorescent
fluorophotometry
focus
Foerster's forceps
fogging
Foix's syndrome
fold
    epicanthal f.
    falciform f.
    semilunar f. of
        conjunctiva
follicle
follicular
folliculosis
Foltz's valve
Fontana's space
foot-candle
foramen
    optic f. of sclera
forceps
    Arruga's f.
    Barraquer's f.

forceps (continued)
    Beaupre's f.
    Bennett's f.
    Berens' f.
    Berke's f.
    Bishop-Harmon f.
    Bonaccolto's f.
    Bonn's f.
    Bracken's f.
    capsule f.
    Castroviejo-Arruga f.
    Castroviejo's f.
    chalazion f.
    Chandler's f.
    Colibri's f.
    Davis' f.
    Desmarres' f.
    Eber's f.
    Ehrhardt's f.
    Elschnig-O'Brien f.
    Elschnig's f.
    fixation f.
    Foerster's f.
    Fuchs' f.
    Gifford's f.
    Green's f.
    Hartman's f.
    Heath's f.
    Hess' f.
    Hess-Barraquer f.
    Hess-Horwitz f.
    Holth's f.
    Hunt's f.
    Jameson's f.
    Judd's f.
    Kalt's f.
    Katzin-Barraquer f.
    Kelman's f.
    Kerrison's f.
    Kirby's f.
    Knapp's f.
    Kronfeld's f.
    Kuhnt's f.
    Kulvin-Kalt f.
    Lambert's f.
    Lister's f.
    Littauer's f.

forceps (continued)
    McCullough's f.
    McPherson's f.
    mosquito f.
    Noble's f.
    Noyes' f.
    Nugent's f.
    O'Brien's f.
    Perritt's f.
    Pley's f.
    Prince's f.
    Quevedo's f.
    Reese's f.
    Rolf's f.
    Sauer's f.
    Schweigger's f.
    Shaaf's f.
    Smart's f.
    Spero's f.
    Stevens' f.
    Thorpe's f.
    Verhoeff's f.
    von Graefe's f.
    von Mondak's f.
    Waldeau's f.
    Ziegler's f.
fornices
fornix
    f. approach
    f.-based flap
    inferior f.
foro-. See words beginning
    phoro-.
Forster-Fuchs black spot
Förster's
    choroiditis
    operation
    uveitis
Foster-Kennedy syndrome
four-prism-diopter test
fovea
    f. centralis
    f. trochlearis
foveal
foveola
Foville's syndrome
Foville-Wilson syndrome

Fox's
    conformer
    implant
    irrigator
    operation
    shield
fpa – far point of accommodation
fracture
    blow-out f.
framing
Franceschetti's
    disease
    dystrophy
    operation
    syndrome
Francis' spud
François' dystrophy
Franklin glasses
Fresnel lens
Frey's implant
Fricke's operation
Friedenwald's
    operation
    ophthalmoscope
    syndrome
Friede's operation
Frost-Lang operation
Fuchs'
    atrophy
    coloboma
    crypts
    dimples
    dystrophy
    forceps
    heterochromia
    heterochromic cyclitis
    keratitis
    operation
    spot
    syndrome
Fuchs-Kraupa syndrome
Fukala's operation
fundus
    albinotic f.
    f. albipunctatus
    f. camera
    f. flavimaculatus

fundus (continued)
    f. oculi
    tessellated f.
    f. tigroid
funduscope
funduscopic
funduscopy
fungal
Fusarium
fusion
galactosemia
ganglion cell layer
gargoylism
gas-permeable lens
Gaucher's disease
Gaule's spots
Gayet's operation
gaze
    conjugate g.
    g. movement
    g. palsy
    g. paretic nystagmus
Gel Flex lens
geniculate body
geniculo-calcarine tract
geometric
    g. axis
    g. equator
    g. perspective
Georgariou's operation
gerontotoxon, gerontoxon
    g. lentis
Gerstmann's syndrome
Gibson's irrigator
Giemsa stain
Gifford-Galassi reflex
Gifford's
    applicator
    curet
    forceps
    operation
    reflex
    sign
Gillies' operation
Gill's knife
Girard procedure

Girard's operation
Giraud-Teulon law
glabella
gland
    inferior lacrimal g.
    Krause's g.
    lacrimal g.
    Manz's g's
    meibomian g.
    Moll's g.
    Rosenmüller's g.
    superior lacrimal g.
    tarsal g.
    Wolfring's g.
    zeisian g.
glanders
glands of Zeis
glasses
    Franklin g.
    Hallauer's g's
glaucoma
    g. absolutum
    acute angle closure g.
    air block g.
    angle-recession g.
    aphakic g.
    apoplectic g.
    auricular g.
    capsular g.
    chronic narrow angle g.
    chronic open angle g.
    closed angle g.
    g. consummatum
    Contino's g.
    Donders' g.
    enzyme g.
    fulminant g.
    hemorrhagic g.
    g. imminens
    infantile g.
    inflammatory g.
    juvenile g.
    lenticular g.
    malignant g.
    narrow angle g.
    neovascular g.

glaucoma (continued)
    noncongestive g.
    obstructive g.
    open angle g.
    phakogenic g.
    phakolytic g.
    pigmentary g.
    primary open angle g.
    g. simplex
    traumatic g.
    vitreous-block g.
    wide-angle g.
glaucomato-cyclitic crisis
glaucomatous
glaucosis
glioma
    g. endophytum
    g. exophytum
    g. retinae
globe
goblet cells
Goldmann's applanation
    tonometer
Goldstein's
    cannula
    retractor
Gomez-Marquez's operation
Gonin's operation
goniolens
goniophotocoagulation
goniophotography
goniopuncture
gonioscope
gonioscopy
goniosynechia
goniotomy
Gonnin-Amsler marker
gonoblennorrhea
gouge
    Todd's g.
Gowers' sign
GPC – giant papillary
    conjunctivitis
Gradenigo's syndrome
Gradle's
    electrode

Gradle's (continued)
    operation
    retractor
Graefe's
    disease
    knife
    operation
    sign
    syndrome
graft
    corneal g.
granuloma
    g. iridis
granulomatous
    g. uveitis
Graves' disease
gray line
Green's
    caliper
    curet
    dissector
    forceps
    hook
    knife
    needle holder
    replacer
Gregg's syndrome
Greig's syndrome
grid
    Amsler's g.
Grieshaber's
    keratome
    needle
    needle holder
    trephine
Groenholm's retractor
Groenouw's dystrophy
Grossmann's operation
Gruning's magnet
Gudden's commissure
Guillain-Barré syndrome
Guist's implant
Gullstrand's
    law
    slit lamp
gumma

gummatous
  g. meningitis
Gunn's
  dots
  syndrome
guttata
Gutzeit's operation
Guyton-Maumenee speculum
Guyton-Park speculum
Guyton's operation
gyrate atrophy
H. – hypermetropia
H – hyperphoria
Haab's
  magnet
  striae
Haag-Streit slit lamp
Haidinger's brushes
Haik's implant
Halberg clip
Hallauer's glasses
Hallermann-Streiff syndrome
Haller's layer
halo
  Fick's h.
  h. glaucomatosus
  glaucomatous h.
  h. saturninus
Halpin's operation
Halsey's needle holder
handle
  Beaver's h.
Hand-Schüller-Christian disease
haploscope
haptic
Harada's
  disease
  syndrome
Hardy-Rand-Ritter plates
Harrington's erysiphake
Harrison's scissors
Hartman's forceps
Hartstein's retractor
Hasner's
  operation
  valve
Hassall-Henle warts

HCL – hard contact lenses
head-tilt test
Heath's
  curet
  dilator
  expressor
  forceps
Heerfordt's disease
Heine's operation
HEMA – hydroxyethyl
  methacrylate
hemangioma
hemangiomatosis
hematoma
hemeralopia
hemianopia
  absolute h.
  altitudinal h.
  binasal h.
  bitemporal h.
  h. bitemporalis fugax
  congruous h.
  equilateral h.
  heteronymous h.
  homonymous h.
  incongruous h.
  nasal h.
  quadrantic h.
  temporal h.
  unilateral h.
  uniocular h.
hemianopic
hemianopsia
hemianoptic
hemianosmia
hemifacial microsomia
hemiopalgia
hemiopia
hemiopic
hemorrhage
  blot h.
  dot h.
hemorrhagic
Hemovac
Henle fiber layer
hepatolenticular degeneration
Herbert's operation

Hering's
    law
    test
    theory
herpes
    h. corneae
    h. iridis
    ocular h.
    h. ophthalmicus
    h. simplex
    h. zoster
herpetic
Hertel's exophthalmometer
Hertwig-Magendie syndrome
Hess'
    forceps
    operation
    spoon
Hess-Barraquer forceps
Hess-Horwitz forceps
Hess-Lees screen
heterochromia
    Fuchs' h.
    h. iridis
heterochromic
heteronymous
heterophoralgia
heterophoria
heterophoric
heterophthalmia
heterophthalmos
heteropsia
heteroptics
heteroscopy
heterotropia
hexachromic
high hyperopia
Hildreth's cautery
Hillis' retractor
Hippel-Lindau syndrome
Hippel's
    disease
    operation
hippus
Hirschberg's
    magnet
    method

histoplasmosis
histo spots
Hm. – manifest hyperopia
HM – hand motion
Hogan's operation
Hollenhorst's plaque
Holmgren's test
Holth's
    forceps
    operation
    punch
homokeratoplasty
homonymous
    h. diplopia
    h. hemianopia
    h. hemianopsia
Honan's cuff
hook
    fixation h.
    Green's h.
    Jameson's h.
    Kirby's h.
    Nugent's h.
    O'Connor's h.
    Smith's h.
    Stevens' h.
    Tyrell's h.
    von Graefe's h.
    Wiener's h.
Horay's operation
hordeolum
horizontal
    h. gaze
    h. meridian
    h. nystagmus
    h. raphe
Horner-Bernard syndrome
Horner's
    law
    muscle
    ptosis
    pupil
    syndrome
Horner-Trantas spots
horopter
    Vieth-Muller h.

horror
    h. fusionis
Horvath's operation
Hosford's spud
Hotz's operation
Howard-Dolman apparatus
Howard's abrader
HRR plates – Hardy-Rand-Ritter
    plates
Hruby lens
HSV – herpes simplex virus
Ht. – total hyperopia
Hudson's line
Hudson-Stähli line
Huey's scissors
Hughes'
    implant
    operation
Hummelsheim procedure
humor
    aqueous h.
    h. aquosus
    h. cristallinus
    crystalline h.
    ocular h.
    vitreous h.
    h. vitreus
Hunt's forceps
Hutchinson's
    facies
    pupil
    syndrome
hyaline
hyalinization
hyalitis
    asteroid h.
    h. punctata
    h. suppurativa
hyaloid
    h. canal
    h. membrane
hyalomucoid
hyalonyxis
hydrophilic lens
hydrophthalmia
hydrophthalmos
hydrophthalmus

hydrops
hyperemia
hyperfluorescence
hyperhidrosis
hyperkeratosis
hyperlipoproteinemia
hypermature
hypermetropia
hyperopia
    facultative h.
    manifest h.
hyperopic
hyperphoria
hypertelorism
    ocular h.
    orbital h.
hyptertensive
    h. retinopathy
hypertonia
    h. oculi
hypertonic
    h. saline
hypertropia
hyphema
hypofluorescence
hypophoria
hypoplasia
hypoplastic
hypopyon
hypotonia
    h. oculi
hypotonus
hypotony
hypotropia
hysterical
    h. amblyopia
    h. field
ianthinopsia
ICCE – intracapsular cataract
    extraction
ichthyosis
icteric
icterus
Iliff's operation
illusion
    Kuhnt's i.

image
    i. displacement
    i. jump
    i. point
    Purkinje's i.
    Purkinje-Sanson's i's
immature cataract
implant
    acorn-shaped i.
    acrylic i.
    Allen's i.
    Alpar's i.
    Arruga's i.
    Berens' i.
    Berens-Rosa i.
    Binkhorst's i.
    Boyd's i.
    Brown-Dohlman i.
    build-up i.
    Bunker's i.
    Choyce Mark VIII i.
    Choyce's i.
    conical i.
    Copeland's i.
    corneal i.
    Cutler's i.
    Doherty's i.
    Federov's i.
    Fox's i.
    Frey's i.
    glass sphere i.
    gold sphere i.
    Guist's i.
    Haik's i.
    hemisphere i.
    Hughes' i.
    Ivalon's i.
    Levitt's i.
    Lincoff's i.
    lucite i.
    magnetic i.
    McGhan's i.
    Mules' i.
    plastic sphere i.
    Plexiglas i.
    polyethylene i.
    Rayner-Choyce i.

implant (continued)
    reverse-shape i.
    scleral i.
    scleral buckler i.
    semishell i.
    shelf-type i.
    shell i.
    Silastic i.
    silicone i.
    Snellen's i.
    sphere i.
    spherical i.
    sponge i.
    Stone's i.
    surface i.
    tantalum i.
    Teflon i.
    tire i.
    Troutman's i.
    tunneled i.
    Vitallium i.
    Wheeler's i.
    wire mesh i.
implantation
Imre's
    operation
    treatment
incarceration
incipient
incision. See *General Surgical Terms* section.
inclusion bodies
incomitant strabismus
incongruous
incycloduction
incyclophoria
incyclotropia
incyclovergence
indentation tonometry
induration
infarct
infarction
infiltrates
infraduction
infranuclear
infraorbital
infraversion

insufficiency
    vascular i.
intercanthal
intercilium
internuclear
interpalpebral
interpupillary
interstitial
intorsion
intracapsular
intracranial
intraepithelial
intramarginal
    i. sulcus
intraocular
intraorbital
intraretinal
intrascleral
intrasheath
    i. tenotomy
intrinsic
introducer
    Carter's i.
intumescent
IOL-intraocular lens
IOP-intraocular pressure
ipsilateral
iridal
iridalgia
iridauxesis
iridectasis
iridectome
iridectomesodialysis
iridectomize
iridectomy
    basal i.
    optic i.
    peripheral i.
    preparatory i.
    sector i.
    stenopeic i.
    therapeutic i.
iridectopia
iridectropium
iridemia
iridencleisis
iridentropium

irideremia
irides
iridesis
iridiagnosis
iridial
iridian
iridic
iridization
iridoavulsion
iridocapsulitis
iridocapsulotomy
iridocele
iridochoroiditis
iridocoloboma
iridoconstrictor
iridocorneosclerectomy
iridocyclectomy
iridocyclitis
iridocyclochoroiditis
iridocystectomy
iridodesis
iridodiagnosis
iridodialysis
iridodiastasis
iridodilator
iridodonesis
iridokeratitis
iridokinesia
iridokinesis
iridokinetic
iridoleptynsis
iridology
iridolysis
iridomalacia
iridomesodialysis
iridomotor
iridoncus
iridoparalysis
iridopathy
iridoperiphakitis
iridoplegia
iridoptosis
iridopupillary
iridorhexis
iridoschisis
iridosclerotomy
iridosteresis

iridotasis
iridotomy
iris
    bombé i.
    i. coloboma
    i. crypts
    Florentine i.
    i. pigment dispersion
    i. prolapse
    i. sphincter
    i. stroma
    tremulous i.
    umbrella i.
irisopsia
iritic
iritis
    i. blenorrhagique á
      rechutes
    i. catamenialis
    diabetic i.
    Doyne's i.
    follicular i.
    gouty i.
    i. papulosa
    plastic i.
    purulent i.
    i. recidivans
      staphylococco-allergica
    serous i.
    spongy i.
    sympathetic i.
    tuberculous i.
    uratic i.
iritoectomy
iritomy
IRMA – intraretinal micro-
    vascular abnormalities
irradiance
irrigator
    DeVilbiss' i.
    Dougherty's i.
    Fox's i.
    Gibson's i.
    Rollet's i.
    Sylva's i.
Irvine-Gass syndrome
Irvine's scissors

ischemia
    i. retinae
ischemic
iseikonic lens
Ishihara's
    plate
    test
isochromatic
isocoria
isophoria
isopia
isopter
isoscope
Ivalon's implant
Iwanoff's retinal edema
Jacob's membrane
Jacobson's retinitis
Jaeger's
    keratome
    lid plate
    test
Jaesche-Arlt operation
Jameson's
    caliper
    forceps
    hook
    operation
jaundice
Javal's ophthalmometer
jaw-winking
Jendrassik's sign
Jensen procedure
Jensen's
    disease
    retinitis
jerk nystagmus
Johnson's syndrome
Jones'
    dilator
    test
Judd's forceps
junction
    sclerocorneal j.
    j. scotoma
juvenile
    j. gangliosidosis
    j. retinoschisis

juvenile (continued)
  j. xanthogranuloma
JXG-juvenile xanthogranuloma
kahla-. See words beginning
  chala-.
kalko-. See words beginning
  chalco-.
Kalt's
  forceps
  needle holder
Kaposi's sarcoma
kappa angle
Kara's erysiphake
Katzin-Barraquer forceps
Katzin's scissors
Kaufman's vitrector
Kayser-Fleischer ring
Keeler's cryophake
Keith-Wagener retinopathy
Kelman's
  forceps
  lens
  operation
kemosis. See *chemosis.*
Kennedy's syndrome
keratalgia
keratectasia
keratectomy
keratic
keratitis
  acne rosacea k.
  actinic k.
  aerosol k.
  alphabet k.
  anaphylactic k.
  arborescens k.
  artificial silk k.
  band k.
  k. bandelette
  k. bullosa
  dendriform k.
  dendritic k.
  Dimmer's k.
  k. disciformis
  epithelial k.
  exfoliative k.
  fascicular k.

keratitis (continued)
  k. filamentosa
  Fuchs' k.
  herpetic k.
  hypopyon k.
  interstitial k.
  lagophthalmic k.
  lattice k.
  marginal k.
  metaherpetic k.
  mycotic k.
  neuroparalytic k.
  neurotrophic k.
  k. nummularis
  oyster shuckers' k.
  parenchymatous k.
  k. petrificans
  phlyctenular k.
  k. profunda
  k. punctata
  k. punctata
    subepithelialis
  purulent k.
  k. pustuliformis profunda
  k. ramificata superficialis
  reaper's k.
  reticular k.
  ribbon-like k.
  rosacea k.
  Schmidt's k.
  sclerosing k.
  scrofulus k.
  serpiginous k.
  k. sicca
  striate k.
  stromal k.
  suppurative k.
  syphilitic k.
  Thygeson's k.
  trachomatous k.
  trophic k.
  vascular k.
  vasculonebulous k.
  vesicular k.
  xerotic k.
keratocele
keratocentesis

keratoconjunctivitis
    epidemic k.
    epizootic k.
    flash k.
    limbic k.
    phlyctenular k.
    k. sicca
    viral k.
    welder's k.
keratoconus
keratocyte
keratoderma
keratoectasia
keratoglobus
keratohelcosis
keratohemia
keratoid
keratoiridocyclitis
keratoiridoscope
keratoiritis
keratoleptynsis
keratoleukoma
keratoma
keratomalacia
keratomata
keratome
    Agnew's k.
    Beaver's k.
    Berens' k.
    Castroviejo's k.
    Grieshaber's k.
    Jaeger's k.
    Kirby's k.
keratometer
keratometric
keratometry
keratomileusis
keratomycosis
keratonosus
keratonyxis
keratopathy
    band k.
keratophakia
keratoplasty
    lamellar k.
    optic k.
    penetrating k.

keratoplasty (continued)
    tectonic k.
keratoprosthesis
keratorhexis
keratoscleritis
keratoscope
keratoscopy
keratotomy
    delimiting k.
keratotorus
keratouveitis
kerectasis
kerectomy
keroid
Kerrison's forceps
Kestenbaum's
    procedure
    rule
Key's operation
kias-. See words beginning *chias-*.
Kiloh-Nevin syndrome
Kimmelstiel-Wilson
    disease
    syndrome
kinescope
kinetic perimetry
Kirby's
    forceps
    hook
    keratome
    knife
    operation
    retractor
    scissors
    spoon
"kissing choroidals"
Klieg eye
Knapp-Imre operation
Knapp's
    forceps
    knife
    knife needle
    operation
    procedure
    retractor
    rule
    scissors

Knapp's (continued)
  scoop
  spatula
  speculum
  spoon
  streaks
  striae
knife
  Bard-Parker k.
  Barkan's k.
  Barraquer's k.
  Beaver's k.
  Castroviejo's k.
  Desmarres' k.
  Elschnig's k.
  Gill's k.
  Graefe's k.
  Green's k.
  Kirby's k.
  Knapp's k.
  Lancaster's k.
  Lundsgaard's k.
  McPherson-Wheeler k.
  McPherson-Ziegler k.
  McReynolds' k.
  Parker's k.
  Scheie's k.
  Smith-Green k.
  Tooke's k.
  von Graefe's k.
  Weber's k.
  Wheeler's k.
  Ziegler's k.
knife needle
  Davis' k.n.
  Knapp's k.n.
  von Graefe's k.n.
Koby's cataract
Koch-Weeks bacillus
Koeppe's
  disease
  nodule
Koerber-Salus-Elschnig
  syndrome
Kofler's operation
KOH – potassium hydroxide
kor-. See words beginning *chor-.*

korio-. See words beginning
  chorio-.
Kozlowski's degeneration
KP – keratitic precipitates
Kratz's lens
Kraupa's operation
Krause's
  gland
  syndrome
Kreiker's operation
Kriebig's operation
Krimsky's method
Kronfeld's
  electrode
  forceps
  retractor
Krönlein-Berke operation
Krönlein's operation
Krukenberg's spindle
Krupin's valve
Kuhnt-Junius disease
Kuhnt's
  forceps
  illusion
  operation
➥Kuhnt-Szymanowski operation
Kulvin-Kalt forceps
Kurz's syndrome
L & A – light and accommodation
labyrinthine
  l. nystagmus
Lacarrere's operation
lacquer cracks
lacrima
lacrimal
  l. apparatus
  l. artery
  l. bone
  l. canaliculi
  l. duct
  l. gland
  l. lake
  l. nerve
  l. papilla
  l. probe
  l. sac
lacrimalin

lacrimase
lacrimation
lacrimator
lacrimatory
lacrimonasal
lacrimotome
lacrimotomy
lacus
    l. lacrimalis
LaForce's spud
Lagleyze's operation
lagophthalmos
lagophthalmus
Lagrange's
    operation
    scissors
lake
    lacrimal l.
Lambert's forceps
lamella
lamellar
lamina
    l. basalis
    l. basalis choroideae
    l. basalis corporis ciliaris
    l. choriocapillaris
    l. cribrosa sclerae
    l. dots
    l. elastica anterior
    l. elastica posterior
    episcleral l.
    l. episcleralis
    l. fusca sclerae
    l. limitans anterior corneae
    l. limitans posterior
      corneae
    orbital l.
    l. orbitalis ossis
      ethmoidalis
    l. papyracea
    l. superficialis musculi
      levatoris palpebrae
      superioris
    l. suprachorioidea
    suprachoroid l.
    l. suprachoroidea
    l. vasculosa chorioideae

lamina (continued)
    l. vasculosa choroideae
    l. vitrea
lamp
    Birch-Hirschfeld l.
    Duke-Elder l.
    Eldridge-Green l.
    Gullstrand's slit l.
    Haag-Streit slit l.
    slit l.
Lancaster red-green test
Lancaster Regan dial
Lancaster's
    knife
    magnet
    speculum
lance
    Rolf's l.
Landolt's
    bodies
    chart
    operation
Langenbeck's operation
Lange's speculum
Larcher's sign
laser
    argon l.
    l. iridectomy
    l. photocoagulation
    ruby l.
    xenon arc l.
lattice degeneration
Lauber's disease
Laurence-Moon-Biedl syndrome
law
    Alexander's l.
    Descartes' l.
    Desmarres' l.
    Donders' l.
    Ewald's l.
    Flouren's l.
    Giraud-Teulon l.
    Gullstrand's l.
    Hering's l.
    Horner's l.
    Listing's l.
    Sherrington's l.

law (continued)
    Snell's l.
layer
    Haller's l.
    Henle fiber l.
lazy eye
LE–left eye
Lebensohn's chart
Leber's
    amaurosis
    disease
leiomyoma
leiomyosarcoma
lens(es)
    absorptive l.
    achromatic l.
    acrylic l.
    adherent l.
    AO soft l.
    aplanatic l.
    apochromatic l.
    Aquaflex l.
    aspheric l.
    Bagolini l.
    baseball l.
    biconcave l.
    biconvex l.
    bicylindrical l.
    bifocal l.
    Binkhorst-Fyodorov l.
    Binkhorst's l.
    bispherical l.
    bitoric contact l.
    Brücke's l.
    cataract l.
    Comberg l.
    concave l.
    concavoconcave l.
    concavoconvex l.
    contact l.
    converging l.
    convex l.
    convexoconcave l.
    Coquille plano l.
    Crookes' l.
    crystalline l.
    cylindrical l.

lens(es) (continued)
    decentered l.
    dispersing l.
    Fresnel l.
    gas permeable l.
    Gel Flex l.
    Hruby l.
    hydrophilic l.
    immersion l.
    iseikonic l.
    meniscus l.
    meter l.
    minus l.
    omnifocal l.
    orthoscopic l.
    periscopic l.
    planoconcave l.
    planoconvex l.
    prosthetic l.
    punktal l.
    retinal laser l.
    retroscopic l.
    Shearing's l.
    Sheets' l.
    silicone l.
    Simcoe l.
    Sinskey l.
    spherical l.
    Stokes' l.
    toric l.
    trifocal l.
lensometer
Lensrins
lentectomize
lentectomy
lenticonus
lenticular
lenticulo-optic
lenticulostriate
lenticulothalamic
lentiform
lentiglobus
leptotrichosis
    l. conjunctivae
L'Esperance's erysiphake
leukokoria

leukoma
 l. adhaerens
levator muscle
Levitt's implant
levoclination
levocycloduction
levocycloversion
levoduction
levotorsion
levoversion
Lewis' scoop
LGB-lateral geniculate body
lid everter
 Walker's l.e.
lid lag
lid plate
 Jaeger's l.p.
lid retraction
Liebreich's symptom
ligament
 canthal l.
 ciliary l.
 l. of Lockwood
 pectinate l.
 suspensory l. of lens
 Zinn's l.
limbal
 l. groove
 l. vasculitis
limbi palpebrales anteriores
limbi palpebrales posteriores
limbus
 l. conjunctivae
 l. corneae
 l. luteus retinae
 l. of cornea
limulus lysate test
Lincoff's
 implant
 operation
 sponge
Lindau-von Hippel disease
Lindner's
 operation
 spatula
line
 Arlt's l.

line (continued)
 Donders' l.
 Hudson's l.
 Hudson-Stähli l.
 Schwalbe's l.
 Stahli's l.
linea
 l. corneae senilis
linear
lipemia
 l. retinalis
lipoma
liposarcoma
liquor
 l. corneae
 Morgagni's l.
Lister-Burch speculum
Lister's forceps
Listing's law
lithiasis
 l. conjunctivae
Littauer's forceps
LKP-lamellar keratoplasty
locator
 Berman l.
Lockwood's
 ligament
 tendon
Löhlein's operation
Londermann's operation
loop
 Axenfeld's l.
 Meyer's l.
Lopez-Enriquez operation
Loring's ophthalmoscope
louchettes
Louis-Bar syndrome
loupe
 corneal l.
Löwenstein's operation
Lowe's
 ring
 syndrome
Luedde's exophthalmometer
luminance
Lundsgaard-Burch sclerotome
Lundsgaard's knife

lupus erythematosus
luxation
Lyle's syndrome
lymphangiectasis
lymphangioma
lymphoma
lymphosarcoma
lysozyme
Machek-Blaskovics operation
Machek-Gifford operation
Machek's operation
Mackay-Marg tonometer
macrophthalmia
macrophthalmous
macropsia
macula
    m. corneae
    m. lutea retinae
    m. retinae
macular
    m. degeneration
    m. displacement
    m. pucker
    m. sparing
    m. splitting
    m. star
maculocerebral
maculopapular
maculopathy
Maddox
    prism
    rod
    wing
Maeder-Danis dystrophy
Magitot's operation
magnet
    Gruning's m.
    Haab's m.
    Hirschberg's m.
    Lancaster's m.
    Storz's m.
magnification
Maier
    sinus of M.
Majewsky's operation
malaise

malignant
manifest
    m. hyperopia
    m. refraction
manner
    McLean's m.
Manz's gland
Marcus-Gunn phenomenon
Marfan's syndrome
Mariotte's spot
marker
    Gonnin-Amsler m.
Marlex mesh
Marlow's test
maser
Masselon's spectacles
Masuda-Kitahara disease
Mauksch's operation
Maumenee-Park speculum
Maumenee's erysiphake
Mauthner's test
maxilla
maxillary
Maxwell's
    ring
    spot
May's sign
McClure's scissors
McCullough's forceps
McGannon's retractor
McGavic's operation
McGhan's implant
McGuire's
    operation
    scissors
McIntire aspiration-irrigation
    system
McLaughlin's operation
McLean's
    manner
    scissors
    tonometer
McPherson-Castroviejo scissors
McPherson's
    forceps
    needle holder

McPherson's (continued)
  scissors
  spatula
  speculum
McPherson-Vannas scissors
McPherson-Wheeler
  blade
  knife
McPherson-Ziegler knife
McReynolds'
  knife
  operation
medial
medications. See *Drugs and Chemistry* section.
Meesmann's dystrophy
megalocornea
megalophthalmos
megalophthalmus
megophthalmos
meibomian
  cyst
  gland
meibomianitis
meibomitis
melanocyte
melanocytoma
melanoma
melanosis
  m. sclerae
Meller's
  operation
  retractor
Mellinger's speculum
membrana
  m. capsularis lentis
    posterior
  m. epipapillaris
membrane
  Bowman's m.
  Bruch's m.
  cyclitic m.
  Demours' m.
  Descemet's m.
  hyaloid m.
  Jacob's m.

membranectomy
meningioma
meniscus lens
meridian
meridiani bulbi oculi
meridional
mesh
  Marlex m.
  tantalum m.
meshwork
mesiris
mesodermal
mesoretina
metaherpetic
metamorphopsia
  m. varians
method
  Hirschberg's m.
metronoscope
Meyer's loop
Meyhoeffer's curet
Meynerti
  commissura superior of m.
Meynert's commissure
microaneurysm
microblepharia
microblepharon
microcoria
microcornea
microgonioscope
microimmunofluorescent
micronystagmus
microphakia
microphthalmia
microphthalmoscope
microphthalmus
micropsia
microptic
microsaccades
microscope
  Zeiss' m.
microvasculopathy
migraine
Mikulicz's
  disease
  syndrome

milium (milia)
Millard-Gubler syndrome
Miller's syndrome
miner's nystagmus
Minsky's operation
miosis
    irritative m.
    paralytic m.
    spastic m.
miotic
Mira
    photocoagulator
    unit
Mittendorf's dot
MLF – medial longitudinal
    fasciculus
Möbius'
    disease
    sign
    syndrome
Moll's gland
Moncrieff's
    cannula
    operation
monochromacy
monochromatism
monocular
monoculus
monofixation syndrome
Mooren's ulcer
Morax-Axenfeld conjunctivitis
Morax's operation
Morgagni's liquor
Mosher-Toti's operation
Motais' operation
motility
movement
    conjugate m.
Mueller's
    cautery
    retractor
    speculum
Muldoon's dilator
Mules'
    implant
    operation
    scoop

Müller's
    fibers
    muscle
    trigone
multiple sclerosis
Murdock-Wiener speculum
muscae volitantes
muscle
    abductor m's
    Brücke's m.
    ciliaris m.
    ciliary m.
    Horner's m.
    inferior oblique m.
    inferior rectus m.
    lateral rectus m.
    levator m.
    levator palpebrae
      superioris m.
    medial rectus m.
    Müller's m.
    obliquus inferior m.
    obliquus superior m.
    orbicular m. of eye
    orbital m.
    rectus inferior m.
    rectus lateralis m.
    rectus medialis m.
    rectus superior m.
    Riolan's m.
    superior oblique m.
    superior rectus m.
My. – myopia
mydriasis
mydriatic
myectomy
myelin
myelinated
myiocephalon
myiodesopsia
myodiopter
myope
myopia
    axial m.
    indicial m.
    pernicious m.
    prodromal m.

myopic
    m. crescent
    m. degeneration
myotomy
Naffziger's operation
Nagel's anomaloscope
Nairobi eye
nanophthalmos
nasociliary
nasolacrimal
near-sight
nearsighted
nearsightedness
nebula
needle
    Amsler's n.
    Bowman's n.
    Calhoun-Merz n.
    Calhoun's n.
    Grieshaber's n.
    Stocker's n.
    Weeks' n.
needle holder
    Barraquer's n.h.
    Boynton's n.h.
    Castroviejo-Kalt n.h.
    Castroviejo's n.h.
    Derf's n.h.
    Ellis' n.h.
    Green's n.h.
    Grieshaber's n.h.
    Halsey's n.h.
    Kalt's n.h.
    McPherson's n.h.
    Paton's n.h.
neodymium
neoplasm
neovascularization
nerve
    abducens n.
    infratrochlear n.
    optic n.
    trigeminal n.
    trochlear n.
    zygomatic n.
Nettleship-Wilder
  dilator

neurapraxia
neurectomy
    opticociliary n.
neurochorioretinitis
neurochoroiditis
neurodeatrophia
neuroepithelioma
neurofibroma
neurological
neuromyelitis
neuro-ophthalmic
neuroretinal
neuroretinitis
neuroretinopathy
    hypertensive n.
neurotomy
    opticociliary n.
neurotrophic
    n. keratitis
nevus
    Ota's n.
nicking
Nida's operation
Niemann-Pick disease
Nizetic's operation
Noble's forceps
nodal
nodularity
nodule
    Busacca's n.
    Dalen-Fuchs n.
    Koeppe's n.
Norrie's disease
Noyes' forceps
NPA – near point of
    accommodation
NPC – near point of convergence
NRC – normal retinal
    correspondence
nuclear
    n. sclerosis
nucleus
    Edinger-Westphal n.
    Perlia's n.
Nugent-Gradle scissors
Nugent-Green-Dimitry
    erysiphake

Nugent's
>forceps
>hook
Nv.–naked vision
NVA–near visual acuity
nyctalopia
nystagmic
nystagmiform
nystagmograph
nystagmoid
nystagmus
>aural n.
>Baer's n.
>Bekhterev's n.
>Cheyne's n.
>disjunctive n.
>end position n.
>gaze paretic n.
>labyrinthine n.
>miner's n.
>n.-myoclonus
>optokinetic n.
>oscillating n.
>paretic n.
>pendular n.
>"railroad" n.
>rotary n.
>"see-saw" n.
>undulatory n.
>vestibular n.
>vibratory n.
nystaxis
O'Brien's
>akinesia
>block
>cataract
>forceps
occipital cortex
occludable
occluder
occlusion
>branch retinal vein o.
O'Connor-Peter operation
O'Connor's
>hook
>operation

ocular
>o. adnexa
>o. albinism
>o. bobbing
>o. dysmetria
>o. flutter
>o. histoplasmosis
>o. hypertensive
>o. motility
>o. myoclonus
>o. pemphigus
>o. torticollis
oculentum
oculi
oculist
oculistics
oculocardiac reflex
oculocephalogyric
oculofacial
oculogyration
oculogyria
oculogyric
oculometroscope
oculomotor
oculomotorius
oculomycosis
oculonasal
oculopathy
>pituitarigenic o.
oculopupillary
oculoreaction
oculorespiratory reflex
oculospinal
oculozygomatic
oculus
ocutome
OD–oculus dexter–right eye
ODN–ophthalmodynamometry
ofthal-. See words beginning
>*ophthal-.*
opacification
opacity
>Caspar's ring o.
opaque
open angle glaucoma
"open sky" vitrectomy

operation
- Agnew's o.
- Ammon's o.
- Anagnostakis' o.
- Anel's o.
- Arlt-Jaesche o.
- Arlt's o.
- Arruga's o.
- Badal's o.
- Bardelli's o.
- Barkan's o.
- Barraquer's o.
- Barrio's o.
- Basterra's o.
- Beer's o.
- Berens' o.
- Berke's o.
- Bielschowsky's o.
- Blair's o.
- Blasius' o.
- Blaskovics' o.
- Blatt's o.
- Böhm's o.
- Bonaccolto-Flieringa o.
- Bonnett's o.
- Bonzel's o.
- Borthen's o.
- Bossalino's o.
- Bowman's o.
- Brailey's o.
- Briggs' o.
- Budinger's o.
- Burch's o.
- Burow's o.
- Buzzi's o.
- Cairns' o.
- Callahan's o.
- Carter's o.
- Casanellas' o.
- Castroviejo's o.
- Celsus' o.
- Collin-Beard o.
- Critchett's o.
- Csapody's o.
- Custodis' o.
- Cutler-Beard o.
- Czermak's o.

operation (continued)
- Daviel's o.
- de Grandmont's o.
- Del Toro's o.
- de Wecker's o.
- Dupuy-Dutemps o.
- Durr's o.
- Duverger and Velter's o.
- Elliot's o.
- Elschnig's o.
- Ely's o.
- equilibrating o.
- Eversbusch's o.
- Fasanella-Servat o.
- Filatov-Marzinkowsky o.
- Filatov's o.
- Flajani's o.
- Förster's o.
- Fox's o.
- Franceschetti's o.
- Fricke's o.
- Friedenwald's o.
- Friede's o.
- Frost-Lang o.
- Fuchs' o.
- Fukala's o.
- Gayet's o.
- Georgariou's o.
- Gifford's o.
- Gillies' o.
- Girard's o.
- Gomez-Marquez' o.
- Gonin's o.
- Gradle's o.
- Graefe's o.
- Grossmann's o.
- Gutzeit's o.
- Guyton's o.
- Halpin's o.
- Hasner's o.
- Heine's o.
- Herbert's o.
- Hess' o.
- Hippel's o.
- Hogan's o.
- Holth's o.
- Horay's o.

operation (continued)
: Horvath's o.
Hotz's o.
Hughes' o.
Iliff's o.
Imre's o.
Jaesche-Arlt o.
Jameson's o.
Kelman's o.
Key's o.
Kirby's o.
Knapp-Imre o.
Knapp's o.
Kofler's o.
Kraupa's o.
Kreiker's o.
Kriebig's o.
Krönlein-Berke o.
Krönlein's o.
Kuhnt's o.
Kuhnt-Szymanowski o.
Lacarrere's o.
Lagleyze's o.
Lagrange's o.
Landolt's o.
Langenbeck's o.
Lincoff's o.
Lindner's o.
Löhlein's o.
Londermann's o.
Lopez-Enriquez o.
Löwenstein's o.
Machek-Blaskovics o.
Machek-Gifford o.
Machek's o.
Magitot's o.
magnet o.
Majewsky's o.
Mauksch's o.
McGavic's o.
McGuire's o.
McLaughlin's o.
McReynolds' o.
Meller's o.
Minsky's o.
Moncrieff's o.
Morax's o.

operation (continued)
: Mosher-Toti's o.
Motais's o.
Mules' o.
Naffziger's o.
Nida's o.
Nizetic's o.
O'Connor-Peter o.
O'Connor's o.
Panas' o.
Paufique's o.
Peter's o.
Physick's o.
Polyak's o.
Poulard's o.
Power's o.
Quaglino's o.
Raverdino's o.
Richet's o.
Rowinski's o.
Rubbrecht's o.
Saemisch's o.
Scheie's o.
Schmalz's o.
Silva-Costa o.
Smith-Kuhnt-
Szymanowski o.
Smith's o.
Snellen's o.
Soria's o.
Sourdille's o.
Spaeth's o.
Speas' o.
Spencer-Watson o.
Stallard's o.
Stock's o.
Suarez-Villafranca o.
Szymanowski-Kuhnt o.
Szymanowski's o.
Tansley's o.
Terson's o.
Thomas' o.
Toti-Mosher o.
Toti's o.
Trantas' o.
Troutman's o.
Verhoeff's o.

operation (continued)
    Verwey's o.
    von Graefe's o.
    Waldhauer's o.
    Weekers' o.
    Weeks' o.
    West's o.
    Weve's o.
    Wheeler's o.
    Wicherkiewicz's o.
    Wiener's o.
    Wilmer's o.
    Wolfe's o.
    Worth's o.
    Ziegler's o.
operculum
Ophth. – ophthalmology
ophthalmagra
ophthalmalgia
ophthalmatrophia
ophthalmectomy
ophthalmencephalon
ophthalmia
    actinic ray o.
    catarrhal o.
    caterpillar o.
    o. eczematosa
    Egyptian o.
    electric o.
    o. electrica
    flash o.
    gonorrheal o.
    granular o.
    o. hivialis
    jequirity o.
    metastatic o.
    migratory o.
    mucous o.
    o. neonatorum
    neuroparalytic o.
    o. nodosa
    phlyctenular o.
    purulent o.
    scrofulous o.
    strumous o.
    sympathetic o.
    ultraviolet ray o.

ophthalmia (continued)
    varicose o.
ophthalmiatrics
ophthalmic
ophthalmin
ophthalmitic
ophthalmitis
ophthalmoblennorrhea
ophthalmocarcinoma
ophthalmocele
ophthalmocopia
ophthalmodesmitis
ophthalmodiagnosis
ophthalmodiaphanoscope
ophthalmodiastimeter
ophthalmodonesis
ophthalmodynamometer
ophthalmodynamometry
ophthalmodynia
ophthalmoeikonometer
ophthalmofunduscope
ophthalmograph
ophthalmography
ophthalmogyric
ophthalmoleukoscope
ophthalmolith
ophthalmologic
ophthalmologist
ophthalmology
ophthalmomalacia
ophthalmometer
    Javal's o.
ophthalmometroscope
ophthalmometry
ophthalmomycosis
ophthalmomyiasis
ophthalmomyitis
ophthalmomyositis
ophthalmomyotomy
ophthalmoneuritis
ophthalmoneuromyelitis
ophthalmopathy
ophthalmophacometer
ophthalmophantom
ophthalmophlebotomy
ophthalmophthisis
ophthalmoplasty

ophthalmoplegia
    basal o.
    exophthalmic o.
    o. externa
    fascicular o.
    o. interna
    internuclear o.
    nuclear o.
    orbital o.
    Parinaud's o.
    o. partialis
    o. progressiva
    Sauvineau's o.
    o. totalis
ophthalmoplegic
ophthalmoptosis
ophthalmoreaction
    Calmette's o.
ophthalmorrhagia
ophthalmorrhea
ophthalmorrhexis
ophthalmoscope
    Friedenwald's o.
    ghost o.
    Loring's o.
ophthalmoscopic
ophthalmoscopy
    binocular indirect o.
    direct o.
    medical o.
    metric o.
ophthalmostasis
ophthalmostat
ophthalmostatometer
ophthalmosteresis
ophthalmosynchysis
ophthalmothermometer
ophthalmotomy
ophthalmotonometer
ophthalmotonometry
ophthalmotoxin
ophthalmotrope
ophthalmotropometer
ophthalmovascular
ophthalmoxerosis
ophthalmoxyster
opportunistic
    o. infection

opsoclonia
opsoclonus
optesthesia
optic
    o. atrophy
    o. axis
    o. chiasm
    o. cup
    o. disc
    o. foramen
    o. nerve
    o. neuritis
    o. tract
    o. vesicle
optical
optician
opticianry
opticist
opticociliary
opticocinerea
opticokinetic
opticonasion
opticopupillary
optics
optist
optoblast
optogram
optomeninx
optometer
optometrist
optometry
optomyometer
optophone
optostriate
optotype
ora
    o. serrata
    o. serrata retinae
orbicularis
    o. ciliaris
    o. oculi
orbiculus
    o. ciliaris
orbit
orbita
orbitae
orbital
    o. apex

orbital (continued)
    o. cellulitis
    o. decompression
    o. fascia
    o. fat pads
    o. fissure
    o. floor fracture
    o. periosteum
    o. pseudotumor
    o. septum
orbitale
orbitalis
orbitonasal
orbitonometer
orbitonometry
orbitostat
orbitotemporal
orbitotomy
orthokeratology
orthometer
orthophoria
    asthenic o.
orthophoric
orthoptic
orthoptics
orthoptist
orthoptoscope
orthorater
orthoscope
orthoscopy
OS–oculus sinister–left eye
ossification
osteoma
Ota's nevus
otolith apparatus
OU–oculus unitas–both eyes
    oculus uterque–
      each eye
outflow channels
OWS–overwear
    syndrome
pachometer
pachyblepharon
pachyblepharosis
Paget's disease
palatine bone
palinopsia
pallor

palpebra
    tertius p.
palpebrae
palpebral
palpebralis
palpebrate
palpebration
palpebritis
palsy
    Bell's p.
PAN–periarteritis
    nodosa
Panas' operation
pannus
    p. carnosus
    p. crassus
    p. degenerativus
    p. eczematosus
    phlyctenular p.
    p. siccus
    p. tenuis
    p. trachomatosus
panophthalmia
panophthalmitis
panoptic
panretinal photocoagulation
pantankyloblepharon
panuveitis
papilla(ae)
    Bergemeister's p.
    lacrimal p.
    optic p.
papillary
papilledema
papillitis
papilloma
papillomacular
    p. bundle
papillomavirus
papilloretinitis
paracentesis
paracentral
parafovea
parallax
paralysis
paramacular
paramedian
parasympathetic

parenchyma
    p. of lens
paresis
paretic
Parinaud's
    conjunctivitis
    ophthalmoplegia
    syndrome
Parker's knife
Park's speculum
parophthalmia
parophthalmoncus
paropsis
pars
    p. caeca retinae
    p. ciliaris retinae
    p. iridica retinae
    p. marginalis musculi
      orbicularis oris
    p. optica retinae
    p. orbitalis glandulae
      lacrimalis
    p. orbitalis musculi
      orbicularis oculi
    p. palpebralis glandulae
      lacrimalis
    p. palpebralis musculi
      orbicularis oculi
    p. plana corporis ciliaris
    p. planitis
    p. plicata corporis ciliaris
PAS – peripheral anterior
    synechia
Pascheff's conjunctivitis
PAT – prism adaption test
patch
Paton's needle holder
Paufique's
    operation
    trephine
PD – interpupillary distance
    prism diopter
PDR – proliferative diabetic
    retinopathy
pectinate
pediculosis

pedunculated
Pel's crises
pemphigoid
pemphigus
penalization
pendular
perception
    light and color p.
periarteritis
    p. nodosa
peribulbar
perichiasmal
perifoveal
perihilar
perilenticular
perimeter
    Ferree-Rand p.
perimetry
perineuritis
periocular
periophthalmitis
periorbita
periorbital
periorbititis
periosteum
periostitis
peripapillary
periphacitis
peripheral
    p. anterior synechia
    p. curve
    p. fusion
    p. iridectomy
    p. retina
    p. uveitis
    p. vision
peripheraphose
periphlebitis
periscleral
peritectomy
peritomize
peritomy
perivasculitis
Perkins' tonometer
PERLA – pupils equal, react to
    light and accommodation

Perlia's nucleus
Perritt's forceps
PERRLA – pupils equal, round,
    regular, react to light and
    accommodation
Peter's
    anomaly
    operation
Petit's canal
Petzetakis-Takos syndrome
PGC – pontine gaze center
phacoanaphylaxis
phacocele
phacocyst
phacocystectomy
phacocystitis
phacodonesis
phacoemulsification
phacoerysis
phacoglaucoma
phacohymenitis
phacoiditis
phacoidoscope
phacolysis
phacolytic
phacomalacia
phacometachoresis
phacometer
phacopalingenesis
phacoplanesis
phacosclerosis
phacoscope
phacoscopy
phacoscotasmus
phacotoxic
phacozymase
phakitis
phakoma
phakomatosis
phenomenon
    Bell's p.
    Marcus-Gunn p.
    Pulfrich's p.
phlyctena
phlyctenar
phlyctenoid

phlyctenosis
phlyctenular
phlyctenule
PHM – posterior hyaloid
    membrane
phoria
phoriascope
phorometer
phorometry
phoropter
phoroscope
phorotone
photism
photochemistry
photochromic
photocoagulation
photocoagulator
    Mira's p.
    Zeiss' p.
photography
    fluorescence retinal p.
photo-ophthalmia
photophobia
photophthalmia
photopia
photopic
photopsia
photoptometer
photoptometry
photoreceptor
phthiriasis
phthisis
    p. bulbi
    p. corneae
    ocular p.
Physick's operation
physiologic
PI – peripheral iridectomy
pick
    Burch's p.
Pick's
    retinitis
    vision
"pie in the sky" defect
pigmentary
pigmentation

pigmentum
    p. nigrum
Pillat's dystrophy
pin
    Pischel's p.
    Walker's p.
pinguecula
pinhole
"pink eye"
Pischel's
    electrode
    pin
pituitary
PKP – penetrating keratoplasty
Placido's disc
pladarosis
planoconcave
planoconvex
plaque
    Hollenhorst's p.
plate
    Hardy-Rand-Ritter p's
    Ishihara's p.
    tarsal p.
plateau iris
pleoptics
Plexiglas implant
plexus
    annular p.
    intraepithelial p.
    ophthalmic p.
    p. ophthalmicus
    subepithelial p.
Pley's forceps
plica
    p. lacrimalis
    p. palpebronasalis
    p. semilunaris
      conjunctivae
plicae
    p. ciliares
    p. iridis
PN – periarteritis nodosa
pneumotonometer
poliosis
Polyak's operation
polyarteritis

polycoria
    p. spuria
    p. vera
polyopia, polyopsia
    binocular p.
    p. monophthalmica
polyp
pontine
    p. gaze
    p. lesion
Posner-Schlossman
    syndrome
posterior chamber
Post-Harrington erysiphake
Poulard's operation
Power's operation
Pr. – presbyopia
preauricular
prechiasmal
precorneal
preretinal
presbyope
presbyopia
presbyopic
presenile
    p. melanosis
Prince's forceps
prism
    p. diopter
    Maddox p.
    Risley's p.
prismatic
Pritikin's punch
probe
    Bowman's p.
    Theobald's p.
    Williams' p.
    Ziegler's p.
procedure
    Faden's p.
    Girard p.
    Hummelsheim p.
    Jensen p.
    Kestenbaum's p.
    Knapp's p.
prolapse
proliferative

prophylaxis
  Credé's p.
proptometer
proptosis
prosthesis
protanomalopia
protanomalous
protanomaly
protanopia
protanopic
protanopsia
protector
  Arruga's p.
protrusion
Prowazek-Greeff bodies
PRP–panretinal
  photocoagulation
PRRE–pupils round, regular,
  and equal
pseudoexfoliation
pseudoglioma
pseudoisochromatic chart
pseudomembrane
pseudomyopia
pseudoneuritis
pseudonystagmus
pseudopapilledema
pseudophakia
  p. adiposa
  p. fibrosa
pseudopterygium
pseudoptosis
pseudoretinitis pigmentosa
pseudostrabismus
pterion
pterygium
ptosis
  p. adiposa
  Horner's p.
  p. lipomatosis
  p. sympathica
ptotic
Pulfrich's phenomenon
punch
  Berens' p.
  Castroviejo's p.
  Holth's p.

punch (continued)
  Pritikin's p.
  Rubin-Holth p.
  Walton's p.
puncta
punctate
punctum
  p. caecum
  lacrimal p.
  p. lacrimale
pupil
  Adie's p.
  Argyll-Robertson p.
  Behr's p.
  bounding p.
  Bumke's p.
  cat's eye p.
  cornpicker's p.
  fixed p.
  Horner's p.
  Hutchinson's p.
  keyhole p.
  pinhole p.
  skew p's
  stiff p.
  tonic p.
pupilla
pupillary
pupillatonia
pupillograph
pupillometer
pupillometry
pupillomotor
pupilloplegia
pupilloscope
pupilloscopy
pupillostatometer
pupillotonia
Purkinje-Sanson images
Purkinje's image
Purtscher's
  angiopathic retinopathy
  disease
"push plus"
quadrantanopia
quadrantanopsia
quadrantic

Quaglino's operation
Quevedo's forceps
quiescent
rabdomiomah. See
   rhabdomyoma.
ramollitio
   r. retinae
Randolph's cannula
raphe
Raverdino's operation
Rayner-Choyce implant
RD–retinal detachment
recession
reciprocal
   r. innervation
Recklinghausen's disease
reclination
Reese's
   forceps
   syndrome
refixation
reflex
   Gifford-Galassi r.
   Gifford's r.
   red r.
   tapetal light r.
   Weiss's r.
reflexion
refract
refraction
   double r.
   dynamic r.
   homatropine r.
   static r.
refractionist
refractive
refractometer
refractometry
refractor
Reis-Bücklers disease
Reiter's
   disease
   syndrome
Rekoss' disc
Remy's separator
replacer
   Green's r.

resection
retina
   coarctate r.
   leopard r.
   nasal r.
   physiological r.
   shot silk r.
   temporal r.
   tigroid r.
   watered silk r.
retinal
   r. detachment
retinascope
retinitis
   actinic r.
   r. albuminurica
   apoplectic r.
   central angiospastic r.
   r. centralis serosa
   r. circinata
   circinate r.
   Coats' r.
   diabetic r.
   r. disciformans
   exudative r.
   r. gravidarum
   gravidic r.
   r. haemorrhagica
   hypertensive r.
   Jacobson's r.
   Jensen's r.
   leukemic r.
   metastatic r.
   r. nephritica
   Pick's r.
   r. pigmentosa
   r. proliferans
   r. punctata albescens
   punctate r.
   renal r.
   serous r.
   solar r.
   splenic r.
   r. stellata
   striate r.
   suppurative r.
   r. syphilitica

retinitis (continued)
    uremic r.
    Wagener's r.
retinoblastoma
retinochoroid
retinochoroiditis
    r. juxtapapillaris
retinocytoma
retinodialysis
retinograph
retinography
retinoid
retinomalacia
retinopapillitis
retinopathy
    arteriosclerotic r.
    background r.
    central disc-shaped r.
    central serous r.
    circinate r.
    diabetic r.
    exudative r.
    hemorrhagic r.
    hypertensive r.
    Keith-Wagener r.
    leukemic r.
    nonproliferative r.
    pigmentary r.
    Purtscher's angiopathic r.
    renal r.
    stellate r.
retinopexy
    pneumatic r.
retinoschisis
retinoscope
    Copeland's r.
retinoscopy
retinosis
retinotopic
retinotoxic
retractor
    Agrikola's r.
    Amoils' r.
    Berens' r.
    Brawley's r.
    Bronson-Turz r.
    Campbell's r.

retractor (continued)
    Castallo's r.
    Castroviejo's r.
    Desmarres' r.
    Elschnig's r.
    Ferris-Smith r.
    Ferris-Smith-Sewall r.
    Fink's r.
    Goldstein's r.
    Gradle's r.
    Groenholm's r.
    Hartstein's r.
    Hillis' r.
    Kirby's r.
    Knapp's r.
    Kronfeld's r.
    McGannon's r.
    Meller's r.
    Mueller's r.
    Rizzuti's r.
    Rollet's r.
    Stevenson's r.
retrobulbar
retroillumination
retroiridian
retrolental
retrolenticular
retro-ocular
retro-orbital
retrotarsal
Reuss'
    color charts
    tables
rhabdomyoma
rhabdomyosarcoma
rhegmatogenous
rheumatoid arthritis
rhinommectomy
rhinoptia
rhytidosis
Richet's operation
Riddoch's syndrome
Rieger's syndrome
Rifkind's sign
Riley-Day syndrome
rima
    r. cornealis

ring
 Bonaccolto's scleral r.
 ciliary r.
 Coats' r.
 common tendinous r.
 conjunctival r.
 Fleischer's r.
 Flieringa's r.
 glaucomatous r.
 Kayser-Fleischer r.
 Lowe's r.
 Maxwell's r.
 r. scotoma
 Soemmering's r.
 Vossius' lenticular r.
rinommektome. See
 rhinommectomy.
Riolan's muscle
Risley's prism
ritidosis. See *rhytidosis.*
rivus
 r. lacrimalis
Rizzuti's retractor
RK – radial keratotomy
RLF – retrolental fibroplasia
rod
 Maddox r.
 retinal r's
Rolf's
 forceps
 lance
Rollet's
 irrigator
 retractor
 syndrome
Romana's sign
Rommel-Hildreth cautery
Rommel's cautery
Rönne's nasal step
Roper's cannula
rosacea
Rosenmüller's gland
Rot-Bielschowsky syndrome
Rothmund's syndrome
Roth's spot
rotoextraction

rotoextractor
 Douvas' r.
Rowinski's operation
RP – retinitis pigmentosa
Rubbrecht's operation
rubeosis
 r. iridis
 r. retinae
Rubin-Holth punch
rule
 Kestenbaum's r.
 Knapp's r.
rupture
Rutherfurd's syndrome
sac
 lacrimal s.
 tear s.
saccade
saccadic
sacculus
 s. lacrimalis
Saemisch's
 operation
 ulcer
sagittal
 s. axis
 s. depth
Sakler's erysiphake
Salus' arch
Salzmann's dystrophy
Samoan conjunctivitis
Sanyal's conjunctivitis
Sappey's fibers
sarcoid
 Boeck's s.
sarcoma
 Kaposi's s.
satellite lesion
Sattler's veil
Sauer's
 debrider
 forceps
 speculum
Sauvineau's ophthalmoplegia
scalpel

scan
    A-s.
    CT s.
scaphoid
scarifier
    Desmarres' s.
Scarpa's staphyloma
Schäfer's syndrome
Scheie's
    cautery
    knife
    operation
schematic
Schilder's disease
Schiøtz's tonometer
Schirmer's test
Schlemm's canal
Schlichting's dystrophy
Schmalz's operation
Schmidt's keratitis
Schnabel's atrophy
Schnyder's dystrophy
Schöbl's scleritis
Schöler's treatment
Schön's theory
Schwalbe's line
Schweigger's forceps
scimitar
scirrhoblepharoncus
scirrhophthalmia
scissors
    Aebli's s.
    Barraquer-DeWecker s.
    Barraquer's s.
    Berens' s.
    canalicular s.
    Castroviejo's s.
    corneoscleral s.
    DeWecker-Pritikin s.
    DeWecker's s.
    Harrison's s.
    Huey's s.
    iris s.
    Irvine's s.
    Katzin's s.
    Kirby's s.

scissors (continued)
    Knapp's s.
    Lagrange's s.
    McClure's s.
    McGuire's s.
    McLean's s.
    McPherson-Castroviejo s.
    McPherson's s.
    McPherson-Vannas s.
    Nugent-Gradle s.
    Smart's s.
    Spencer's s.
    Stevens' s.
    Thorpe-Castroviejo s.
    Thorpe's s.
    Thorpe-Westcott s.
    Vannas' s.
    Verhoeff's s.
    Walker's s.
    Westcott's s.
    Wilmer's s.
sclera
scleral
    s. buckle
    s. crescent
    s. icterus
    s. lens
    s. plexus
    s. rigidity
    s. spur
    s. trabecula
scleratitis
sclerectasia
sclerectasis
sclerectoiridectomy
sclerectoiridodialysis
sclerectome
sclerectomy
scleriasis
scleriritomy
scleritis
    Schöbl's s.
sclerocataracta
sclerochoroiditis
scleroconjunctival
scleroconjunctivitis

sclerocornea
sclerocorneal
scleroderma
scleroiritis
sclerokeratitis
sclerokeratoiritis
sclerokeratosis
scleromalacia
    s. perforans
scleronyxis
sclero-optic
sclerophthalmia
scleroplasty
sclerostomy
scleroticectomy
scleroticochoroiditis
scleroticonyxis
scleroticopuncture
scleroticotomy
sclerotitis
sclerotome
    Curdy's s.
    Lundsgaard-Burch s.
sclerotomy
scoop
    Arlt's s.
    Daviel's s.
    Knapp's s.
    Lewis' s.
    Mules' s.
    Wilder's s.
scotoma
    arcuate s.
    Bjerrum's s.
    centrocecal s.
    paracentral s.
    peripapillary s.
    ring s.
    scintillating s.
    Seidel's s.
scotomagraph
scotomameter
scotomatous
scotometer
    Bjerrum's s.
scotometry
scotopia

scotopic
screen
    Bjerrum's s.
    Hess-Lees s.
    tangent s.
Searcy's erysiphake
sebaceous
Seidel's scotoma
sella turcica
semilunar
senile
separator
    Remy's s.
septum
    orbitale s.
    s. orbitale
sequela
serous
serpiginous
s. gl. – without correction
Shaaf's forceps
Shafer's sign
Shearing's lens
sheath syndrome
Sheets' lens
Sherrington's law
shield
    Buller's s.
    Fox's s.
shingles
shogrenz. See *Sjögren's.*
Sichel's disease
siderosis
    s. bulbi
    s. conjunctivae
Sidler-Huguenin endothelioma
Siegrist-Hutchinson syndrome
sign
    Abadie's s.
    Arroyo's s.
    Barany's s.
    Cantelli's s.
    Collier's s.
    Dalrymple's s.
    Gifford's s.
    Gowers' s.
    Graefe's s.

sign (continued)
    Jendrassik's s.
    Larcher's s.
    May's s.
    Möbius' s.
    Rifkind's s.
    Romana's s.
    Shafer's s.
    Stellwag's s.
    von Graefe's s.
    Weber's s.
    Wilder's s.
Silastic implant
siliquose
sillonneur
Silva-Costa operation
Simcoe lens
sinistrocular
sinistrocularity
sinistrogyration
sinistrotorsion
Sinskey lens
sinus
    Arlt's s.
    s. of Maier
    s. venosus sclerae
    venous s. of sclera
Sjögren's
    disease
    syndrome
Skeele's curet
skew deviation
skiametry
skiascopy
Sklar-Schiøtz tonometer
sleeve
    Watzke's s.
slit lamp
Smart's
    forceps
    scissors
SMD – senile macular
    degeneration
Smith-Green knife
Smith-Kuhnt-Szymanowski
    operation

Smith's
    expressor
    hook
    operation
Snellen's
    chart
    implant
    operation
    reform eye
Snell's law
"snowballs"
Soemmering's
    ring
    spot
Sondermann's canals
Soria's operation
Sourdille's operation
space
    Fontana's s.
    periscleral s.
    Tenon's s.
    zonular s's
Spaeth's operation
Spanlang-Tappeiner syndrome
spatia zonularia
spatula
    Berens' s.
    Castroviejo's s.
    Elschnig's s.
    Knapp's s.
    Lindner's s.
    McPherson's s.
    Wheeler's s.
Speas' operation
spectacles
    aspheric lenticular s.
    Masselon's s.
speculum
    Barraquer-Colibri s.
    Barraquer's s.
    Berens' s.
    Castroviejo's s.
    Guyton-Maumenee s.
    Guyton-Park s.
    Knapp's s.
    Lancaster's s.
    Lange's s.

speculum (continued)
    lid s.
    Lister-Burch s.
    Maumenee-Park s.
    McPherson's s.
    Mellinger's s.
    Mueller's s.
    Murdock-Wiener s.
    Park's s.
    Sauer's s.
    Weeks' s.
    Wiener's s.
    Williams' s.
Spencer's scissors
Spencer-Watson operation
Spero's forceps
sph. – spherical lens
sphenoid
sphere
spherical
sphincter
    s. iridis
    s. oculi
    s. oris
    s. pupillae
sphincterectomy
sphincterolysis
spindle
    Krukenberg's s.
sponge
    Lincoff's s.
    Weck-cel s.
spoon
    Bunge's s.
    Daviel's s.
    Elschnig's s.
    Hess' s.
    Kirby's s.
    Knapp's s.
sporotrichosis
spot
    Bitot's s.
    blind s.
    Brushfield's s.
    cherry red s.
    cotton-wool s's
    Elschnig's s's

spot (continued)
    Forster-Fuchs black s.
    Fuchs' s.
    Gaule's s's
    histo s's
    Horner-Trantas s's
    Mariotte's s.
    Maxwell's s.
    Roth's s.
    Soemmering's s.
    Tay's s.
spud
    Bahn's s.
    Corbett's s.
    Davis' s.
    Dix's s.
    Fisher's s.
    Francis' s.
    Hosford's s.
    LaForce's s.
    Walter's s.
spur
    scleral s.
squid
squint
    comitant s.
    convergent s.
    divergent s.
    noncomitant s.
    upward and downward s.
Stahli's line
stain
    Giemsa s.
staining
    corneal s.
Stallard's operation
staphyloma
    s. corneae
    s. cornea racemosum
    equatorial s.
    intercalary s.
    s. posticum
    Scarpa's s.
    scleral s.
    uveal s.
staphylomatous
Stargardt's syndrome

Stellwag's
    brawny edema
    sign
stenocoriasis
stenosis
step
    Rönne's nasal s.
stereocampimeter
stereogram
stereo-ophthalmoscope
Stereo-orthopter
stereopsis
stereoscope
stereoscopic
Stevens'
    forceps
    hook
    scissors
Stevens-Johnson syndrome
Stevenson's retractor
Stilling-Türk-Duane syndrome
Stocker's needle
Stock's operation
Stokes' lens
Stones' implant
Storz's magnet
strabismic
strabismometer
strabismus
    Braid's s.
    comitant s.
    concomitant s.
    s. deorsum vergens
    s. fixus
    kinetic s.
    noncomitant s.
    s. sursum vergens
strabometer
strabometry
strabotome
strabotomy
streak
    Knapp's s's
    s. retinoscope
streptotrichosis
striae
    s. ciliares

striae (continued)
    Haab's s.
    Knapp's s.
striascope
striated
stroboscopic
    s. disc
stroma
    s. iridis
    s. of cornea
    s. of iris
    vitreous s.
    s. vitreum
Sturge-Weber syndrome
Sturm's conoid
stye
    meibomian s.
    zeisian s.
Suarez-Villafranca operation
subcapsular
subconjunctival
subcutaneous
subendothelial
subepithelial
    s. plexus
subhyaloid
sublatio
    s. retinae
subluxation
subretinal
substantia
    s. propria corneae
sulcus
superblade
superciliary
supercilium
superimposition
supernumerary
suppression
suprachoroid
supraduction
supranuclear
supraocular
supraorbital
supratrochlear
surgical procedures. See
    operation.

sursumduction
sursumvergence
sursumversion
suture. See *General Surgical Terms* section.
Swan's syndrome
Sylva's irrigator
symblepharon
symblepharopterygium
symmetric
sympathetic
    s. nervous system
    s. ophthalmia
    s. uveitis
symptom
    Anton's s.
    halo s.
    Liebreich's s.
synathroisis
syncanthus
synchesis
synchysis
    s. scintillans
syndectomy
syndrome
    Adie's s.
    Alezzandrini's s.
    Alport's s.
    Alström-Olsen s.
    Andogsky's s.
    Angelucci's s.
    Anton-Babinski s.
    Axenfeld's s.
    Basmatter's s.
    Bassen-Kornzweig s.
    Beal's s.
    Behçet's s.
    Behr's c.
    Benedikt's s.
    Bielschowsky-Lutz-
      Cogan s.
    Bietti's s.
    Bloch-Stauffer s.
    Bloch-Sulzberger s.
    Bonnet-Dechaume-
      Blanc s.
    Brown's s.

syndrome (continued)
    Chandler's s.
    chiasma s.
    Claude's s.
    Cogan's s.
    Dejean's s.
    Duane's s.
    Elschnig's s.
    Foix's s.
    Foster-Kennedy s.
    Foville's s.
    Foville-Wilson s.
    Franceschetti's s.
    Friedenwald's s.
    Fuchs' s.
    Fuchs-Kraupa s.
    Gerstmann's s.
    Gradenigo's s.
    Graefe's s.
    Gregg's s.
    Greig's s.
    Guillain-Barré s.
    Gunn's s.
    Hallermann-Streiff s.
    Harada's s.
    Hertwig-Magendie s.
    Hippel-Lindau s.
    Horner-Bernard s.
    Horner's s.
    Hutchinson's s.
    Irvine-Gass s.
    Johnson's s.
    Kennedy's s.
    Kiloh-Nevin s.
    Kimmelstiel-Wilson s.
    Koerber-Salus-Elschnig s.
    Krause's s.
    Kurz's s.
    Laurence-Moon-Biedl s.
    Louis-Bar s.
    Lowe's s.
    Lyle's s.
    Marfan's s.
    Mikulicz's s.
    Millard-Gubler s.
    Miller's s.
    Möbius' s.

syndrome (continued)
    Parinaud's s.
    Petzetakis-Takos s.
    pigment dispersion s.
    Posner-Schlossman s.
    Reese's s.
    Reiter's s.
    Riddoch's s.
    Rieger's s.
    Riley-Day s.
    Rollet's s.
    Rot-Bielschowsky s.
    Rothmund's s.
    Rutherfurd's s.
    Schäfer's s.
    Siegrist-Hutchinson s.
    Sjögren's s.
    Spanlang-Tappeiner s.
    Stargardt's s.
    Stevens-Johnson s.
    Stilling-Türk-Duane s.
    Sturge-Weber s.
    Swan's s.
    Terry's s.
    Thompson's s.
    Tolosa-Hunt s.
    Touraine's s.
    Uyemura's s.
    Vogt-Koyanagi s.
    Vogt's s.
    Weber's s.
    Werner's s.
    Wernicke's s.
    Wolf's s.
synechia
synechotome
synechotomy
synergist
synkinesis
synophrys
synophthalmia
synoptophore
synoptoscope
syphilis
    s. of conjunctiva
    s. of iris

system
    McIntire aspiration-
      irrigation s.
systemic
    s. lupus erythematosus
    s. sclerosis
Szymanowski-Kuhnt operation
Szymanowski's operation
table
    Reuss t's
Tansley's operation
tantalum
TAP–tension by applanation
tapetum
    t. choroideae
    t. lucidum
    t. nigrum
    t. oculi
tarsadenitis
tarsal
tarsectomy
tarsi
tarsitis
tarsocheiloplasty
tarsomalacia
tarsoplasty
tarsorrhaphy
tarsotomy
tarsus
    t. inferior palpebrae
    t. superior palpebrae
tattooing
    t. of cornea
Tay's
    choroiditis
    spot
technique
    Atkinson's t.
    Van Lint t.
Teflon implant
teichopsia
telangiectasia
telangiectasis
telebinocular
telecanthus
temporal
    t. arteritis

temporal (continued)
    t. crescent
    t. loop
    t. pallor
tendon
    Lockwood's t.
    superior oblique t.
    Zinn's t.
tendotomy
Tenner's cannula
tenonitis
tenonometer
Tenon's
    capsule
    fascia
    space
tenontotomy
tenotome
tenotomist
tenotomize
tenotomy
tension
    intraocular t.
tereon. See pterion.
terijeum. See pterygium.
Terrien's ulcer
Terry's syndrome
Terson's operation
tertiary
test
    Bielschowsky's t.
    Bruchner's t.
    color vision t.
    complement fixation t.
    confrontation field t.
    cover t.
    duction t.
    duochrome t.
    "E" t.
    Farnsworth D-15 t.
    Farnsworth D-100 t.
    fluorescein dye
      disappearance t.
    four-prism-diopter t.
    head-tilt t.
    Hering's t.
    Holmgren's t.

test (continued)
    Ishihara's t.
    Jaeger's t.
    Jones' t.
    Lancaster red-green t.
    limulus lysate t.
    Marlow's t.
    Mauthner's t.
    prism adaption t.
    red glass t.
    Schirmer's t.
    shadow t.
    Titmus t.
    transillumination t.
    W4D – Worth four-dot t.
tetartanopia
tetartanopic
tetartanopsia
tetrastichiasis
thalamus
Theobald's probe
theory
    Hering's t.
    Schön's t.
    Young-Helmholtz t.
thermosector
thiriahsis. See phthiriasis.
Thomas'
    cryoptor
    operation
Thompson's syndrome
Thorpe-Castroviejo scissors
Thorpe's
    caliper
    forceps
    scissors
Thorpe-Wescott scissors
Thygeson's keratitis
thyroid
thyrotoxic
thyrotrophic, thyrotropic
TIA – transient ischemic attack
tic douloureux
tikopseah. See teichopsia.
tisis. See phthisis.
Titmus test
Todd's gouge

Tolosa-Hunt syndrome
tonogram
tonograph
tonographer
tonography
tonometer
    Draeger t.
    Goldmann's applanation
      t.
    indentation t.
    Mackay-Marg t.
    McLean's t.
    Perkins' t.
    pneumatic t.
    Schiøtz' t.
    Sklar-Schiøtz t.
tonometry
    applanation t.
    indentation t.
Tooke's knife
toric lens
torpor
    t. retinae
torsion
tortuous
tosis. See *ptosis.*
totic. See *ptotic.*
Toti-Mosher operation
Toti's operation
Touraine's syndrome
toxoplasmic
toxoplasmosis
trabecular
    t. meshwork
trabeculectomy
trabeculoplasty
    argon laser t.
trabeculotomy
trachoma
    Arlt's t.
    brawny t.
trachomatous
transcorneal
transient
    t. ischemia
    t. obscuration
transillumination

transilluminator
    Finnoff's t.
transplant
    corneal t.
transplantation
transposition
Trantas'
    dots
    operation
treatment
    Imre's t.
    Schöler's t.
trepanation
    corneal t.
trephination
trephine
    Arruga's t.
    Barraquer's t.
    Castroviejo's t.
    Elliot's t.
    Grieshaber's t.
    Paufique's t.
Tretherm
trichiasis
trichromat
trichromatopsia
trichromic
trifocal
trigeminal
    t. neuralgia
trigone
    Müller's t.
triplokoria
triplopia
tritanopia
tritanopic
tritanopsia
trochlea
tropia
tropometer
troposcope
Troutman's
    implant
    operation
tuck
tucker
    Burch-Greenwood t.

tunica
  t. adnata oculi
  t. conjunctiva
  t. conjunctiva bulbi
  t. conjunctiva bulbi oculi
  t. conjunctiva
    palpebrarum
  t. fibrosa oculi
  t. interna bulbi
  t. nervea of Bruecke
  t. vasculosa bulbi
  t. vasculosa lentis
  t. vasculosa oculi
tunicary
tunnel vision
Tyndall's effect
Tyrell's hook
ulcer
  Mooren's u.
  Saemisch's u.
  Terrien's u.
ulcus
  u. serpens corneae
ulectomy
ultrasonic
ultrasonogram
  B scan u.
ultrasonography
Undine's dropper
unit
  Bovie u.
  Mira u.
up-gaze
uvea
uveal
uveitic
uveitis
  Förster's u.
  heterochromic u.
  sympathetic u.
uveoparotid
uveoparotitis
uveoplasty
uveoscleritis
Uyemura's syndrome
VA – visual acuity
vaginae bulbi

valve
  Foltz's v.
  Hasner's v.
Van Lint
  akinesia
  block
  technique
Vannas' scissors
variation
  diurnal v.
varicoblepharon
Varilux
vasa sanguinea retinae
vascular
  v. insufficiency
vascularization
vasculitis
vectograph
veil
  Sattler's v.
vein
  ciliary v.
  cilioretinal v.
  posterior conjunctival v.
  retinal v.
  vorticose v.
venae
  v. centralis retinae
  v. vorticosae
venostasis
venula
  v. macularis inferior
  v. macularis superior
  v. medialis retinae
  v. nasalis retinae inferior
  v. nasalis retinae superior
  v. retinae medialis
  v. temporalis retinae
    inferior
  v. temporalis retinae
    superior
venule
  medial v. of retina
  nasal v. of retina, inferior
    and superior
  temporal v. of retina,
    inferior and superior

VEP – visual evoked potential
VER – visual evoked response
vergence
Verhoeff's
    forceps
    operation
    scissors
vernal
    v. catarrh
    v. conjunctivitis
vernier
version
vertebrobasilar
vertex
Verwey's operation
vesicle
    ocular v.
    ophthalmic v.
    optic v.
vesicula
    v. ophthalmica
vestibular
vestibulo-ocular
VF – visual field
Viers' erysiphake
Vieth-Muller horopter
VISC – vitreous infusion suction
    cutter
vision
    achromatic v.
    binocular v.
    chromatic v.
    color c.
    dichromatic v.
    foveal v.
    halo v.
    haploscopic v.
    iridescent v.
    monocular v.
    v. nul
    oscillating v.
    peripheral v.
    photopic v.
    Pick's v.
    pseudoscopic v.
    rod v.
    scoterythrous v.

vision (continued)
    scotopic v.
    stereoscopic v.
    tunnel v.
visual
    v. acuity
    v. axis
    v. cortex
    v. evoked potential
    v. field examination
    v. purple
visualization
visualize
visuometer
visuoscope
visuosensory
Vitallium implant
vitiligo
    v. iridis
vitrectomy
    "open sky" v.
    pars plana v.
vitrector
    Kaufman's v.
vitreocapsulitis
vitreous
    v. base
    v. body
    v. bulge
    detached v.
    v. floater
    v. hemorrhage
    v. humor
    v. opacity
    primary persistent
      hyperplastic v.
    secondary v.
    v. tap
    tertiary v.
    v. touch
vitreum
vitritis
VOD – visio oculus dextra –
    vision, right eye
Vogt-Koyanagi syndrome
Vogt's
    cataract

Vogt's (continued)
    cornea
    degeneration
    disease
    syndrome
Vogt-Spielmeyer disease
von Graefe's
    cautery
    cystotome
    forceps
    hook
    knife
    knife needle
    operation
    sign
von Hippel-Lindau disease
von Monakow's fibers
von Mondak's forceps
von Recklinghausen's disease
vortex
    v. dystrophy
    v. lentis
VOS – visio oculus sinister –
    vision, left eye
Vossius' lenticular ring
VOU – visio oculus uterque –
    vision of each eye
Wadsworth-Todd cautery
Wagener's retinitis
Wagner's disease
Waldeau's forceps
Waldhauer's operation
Walker's
    lid everter
    pin
    scissors
walleye
Walter's spud
Walton's punch
wart
    Hassall-Henle w's
Watzke's sleeve
Weber's
    knife
    sign
    syndrome
Weck-cel sponge

Weekers' operation
Weeks'
    bacillus
    needle
    operation
    speculum
Weil's disease
Weiss's reflex
Werner's syndrome
Wernicke's syndrome
Westcott's scissors
Westphal-Strumpell disease
West's operation
Weve's
    electrode
    operation
Wheeler's
    cystotome
    implant
    knife
    operation
    spatula
Wicherkiewicz' operation
Widmark's conjunctivitis
Wiener's
    hook
    operation
    speculum
Wilder's
    scoop
    sign
Williams'
    probe
    speculum
Willis' circle
Wilmer's
    operation
    scissors
Wilson's disease
wing
    Maddox w.
"wipe-out" syndrome
Wolfe's operation
Wolfring's gland
Wolf's syndrome
Worth four-dot test
Worth's operation

Wucherer's conjunctivitis
xanthelasma
    x. palpebrarum
xanthelasmatosis
xanthoma
    x. palpebrarum
xanthomatosis
    x. bulbi
    x. iridis
xanthophane
xanthopia
xanthopsia
xeroma
xerophthalmia
xerophthalmus
xeroradiography
xerosis
    x. conjunctivae
    x. superficialis
YAG laser
Young-Helmholtz theory
YS – yellow spot of the retina
zan-. See words beginning *xan-.*
Zeis
    glands of Z.
zeisian gland
Zeiss'
    microscope
    photocoagulator
zero-. See words beginning *xero-.*

zeromah. See *xeroma.*
Ziegler's
    cautery
    forceps
    knife
    operation
    probe
Zinn's
    annulus
    circlet
    corona
    ligament
    tendon
    zonule
zonula
    z. ciliaris
zonulae
zonular
    z. fibers
    z. space
zonule
    ciliary z.
    z. of Zinn
zonulitis
zonulolysis
    enzymatic z.
zonulotomy
zonulysis
zygoma
zygomatic

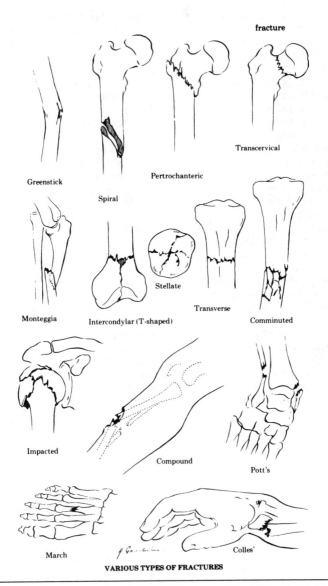

fracture

Greenstick

Spiral

Pertrochanteric

Transcervical

Monteggia

Intercondylar (T-shaped)

Stellate

Transverse

Comminuted

Impacted

Compound

Pott's

March

Colles'

VARIOUS TYPES OF FRACTURES

(Courtesy of Dorland's Illustrated Medical Dictionary, 27th ed. Plate 17. Philadelphia, W. B. Saunders Company, 1988).

Orthopedics

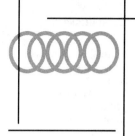

AAOS – American Academy of
    Orthopaedic Surgeons
abarthrosis
abarticular
abarticulation
abasia
Abbott-Lucas operation
Abbott's
    method
    operation
abduction
abductor
ablation
abscess
    Brodie's a.
abscise
absconsio
AC – acromioclavicular
acampsia
acantha
accessiflexor
acetabular
acetabulectomy
acetabuloplasty
acetabulum
acetylcholine
acetylcholinesterase
Achilles
    bursa
    bursitis
    jerk
    reflex
    tendon
achillobursitis
achillodynia
achillorrhaphy
achillotenotomy
    plastic a.

achondrogenesis
achondroplasia
acidosteophyte
aclasia
aclasis
    diaphyseal a.
    tarsoepiphyseal a.
acoustogram
acral
acrocontracture
acrocyanosis
acroesthesia
acromial
acromioclavicular
acromiocoracoid
acromiohumeral
acromion
acromionectomy
acromioneurosis
acromioscapular
acromiothoracic
acromyotonia
acro-osteolysis
acropachy
acroparalysis
acroparesthesia
acropathy
acrosclerosis
acrostealgia
acrosyndactyly
ACSM – American College of
    Sports Medicine
actin
actinomycosis
actomyosin
acusection
Adams'
    operation

Adams' (continued)
    saw
adapter
    McReynolds' a.
adducent
adduct
adduction
adductor
Adelmann's operation
adenomyoma
adhesive
adromia
advancement
adventitious
AE-above elbow
Agnew's splint
AJ-ankle jerk
AK-above knee
akilez. See *Achilles.*
akilo-. See words beginning
    achillo-.
akinesia
Akin's bunionectomy
akondroplazea. See
    achondroplasia.
ala (alae)
    a. ilii
    a. ossis ilii
    a. ossis ilium
Alanson's amputation
Albee-Delbet operation
Albee's
    operation
    osteotome
Albers-Schönberg
    bone
    disease
Albert's operation
Albright's
    disease
    syndrome
Alexander-Farabeuf
    periosteotome
Alexander's
    osteotome
    periosteotome

algodystrophy
alignment
Allen's maneuver
Allis' sign
Alouette's
    amputation
    operation
ambulation
ambulatory
American Academy of
    Orthopaedic Surgeons
American College of Sports
    Medicine
American Physical Therapy
    Association
Amoss' sign
amphiarthrosis
amputation
    AK (above knee) a.
    Alanson's a.
    Alouette's a.
    aperiosteal a.
    Béclard's a.
    Bier's a.
    BK (below knee) a.
    Bunge's a.
    Callander's a.
    Carden's a.
    chop a.
    Chopart's a.
    cineplastic a.
    circular a.
    coat sleeve a.
    cutaneous a.
    diaclastic a.
    double flap a.
    Dupuytren's a.
    eccentric a.
    elliptic a.
    Farabeuf's a.
    Forbes' a.
    forequarter a.
    Gritti's a.
    Gritti-Stokes a.
    guillotine a.
    Guyon's a.

amputation (continued)
    Hancock's a.
    Hey's a.
    hindquarter a.
    a. in contiguity
    interilioabdominal a.
    interinnominoabdominal a.
    interpelviabdominal a.
    interscapulothoracic a.
    Jaboulay's a.
    Kirk's a.
    Langenbeck's a.
    Larrey's a.
    Le Fort's a.
    Lisfranc's a.
    MacKenzie's a.
    Maisonneuve's a.
    major a.
    Malgaigne's a.
    mediotarsal a.
    musculocutaneous a.
    oblique a.
    osteoplastic a.
    periosteoplastic a.
    phalangophalangeal a.
    Pirogoff's a.
    racket a.
    rectangular a.
    Ricard's a.
    Stokes' a.
    subastragalar a.
    subperiosteal a.
    Syme's a.
    Teale's a.
    transfixation a.
    Tripier's a.
    Vladimiroff-Mikulicz a.
amyloid
amyoplasia
    a. congenita
amyotonia
anapophysis
anarrhexis
anconagra
anconeal

anconitis
Anderson's
    operation
    splint
anesthesia. See *General Surgical Terms* section.
Anghelescu's sign
Angle's splint
angulation
ankle
    tailors' a.
ankylodactyly
ankylosis
Annandale's operation
anosteoplasia
anostosis
antagonist
antebrachium
antecubital
anteflexion
anteroinferior
anteroposterior
anterosuperior
anteroventral
anteversion
anti-inflammatory
anulus
anvil
    Bunnell's a.
AP – anteroposterior
aperture
apocope
apocoptic
apofi-. See words beginning *apophy-*.
aponeurectomy
aponeurorrhaphy
aponeurosis
aponeurotomy
apophyseal
apophysis (apophyses)
apophysitis
    a. tibialis adolescentium
apparatus
    Kirschner's a.
    Sayre's a.

appendage
apprehension test
APTA – American Physical
    Therapy Association
arachnodactyly
arachnoid
arachnoidal
arch
    neural a.
    vertebral a.
arciform
arcuate
areflexia
areten-. See words beginning
    aryten-.
Arnold-Chiari
    deformity
    malformation
    syndrome
artery
    basilic a.
    brachial a.
    cephalic a.
    femoral a.
    genicular a.
    gluteal a.
    interosseous a.
    obturator a.
    peroneal a.
    popliteal a.
    princeps pollicis a.
    profunda brachii a.
    pudendal a.
    radial a.
    radialis indicis a.
    saphenous a.
    ulnar a.
    vesical a.
    volar a.
arthragra
arthralgia
arthrectomy
arthrempyesis
arthritic
arthritis
    Bekhterev's a.
    chronic villous a.

arthritis (continued)
    degenerative a.
    exudative a.
    gouty a.
    hypertrophic a.
    juvenile rheumatoid a.
    Lyme a.
    a. mutilans
    navicular a.
    nonarticular a.
    rheumatoid a.
    suppurative a.
    vertebral a.
arthrocentesis
arthrochalasis
arthrochondritis
arthroclasia
arthrodesis
    Charnley's a.
    Moberg's a.
arthrodynia
arthrodysplasia
arthroempyesis
arthroereisis
arthrogram
arthrography
arthrogryposis
arthrokatadysis
arthrokleisis
arthrolith
arthrolithiasis
arthrology
arthrolysis
arthromeningitis
arthrometer
arthrometry
arthroncus
arthroneuralgia
arthronosos
arthro-onychodysplasia
arthropathy
arthrophyma
arthrophyte
arthroplasty
    Bechtol's a.
    Charnley-Mueller a.
arthropneumoroentgenography

arthropyosis
arthrorheumatism
arthrosclerosis
arthroscope
arthroscopy
arthrosis
    Charcot's a.
    a. deformans
arthrosteitis
arthrostomy
arthrosynovitis
arthrotome
arthrotomy
arthroxerosis
arthroxesis
articular
articulated
articulatio
    a. acromioclavicularis
    a. atlantoaxialis mediana
    a. bicondylaris
    a. calcaneocuboidea
    a. capitis costae
    a. carpometacarpea
      pollicis
    a. costotransversaria
    a. coxae
    a. cricoarytenoidea
    a. cubiti
    a. ellipsoidea
    a. genu
    a. humeri
    a. humeroradialis
    a. ossis pisiformis
    a. radiocarpea
    a. sacroiliaca
    a. sternoclavicularis
    a. tarsi transversa
    a. tibiofibularis
    a. trochoidea
articulation
    acromioclavicular a.
    brachioulnar a.
    calcaneocuboid a.
    carpal a's
    carpometacarpal a's
    chondrosternal a's

articulation (continued)
    costocentral a.
    costosternal a's
    costotransverse a.
    costovertebral a's
    ellipsoidal a.
    humeroradial a.
    humeroulnar a.
    iliosacral a.
    intermetacarpal a's
    intermetatarsal a's
    interphalangeal a's
    metacarpophalangeal a's
    metatarsophalangeal a's
    phalangeal a's
    radiocarpal a's
    sacrococcygeal a.
    sacroiliac a.
    sternoclavicular a.
    talocalcaneonavicular a.
    talonavicular a.
    tarsometatarsal a's
    tibiofibular a.
    trochoidal a.
arytenoidectomy
arytenoiditis
arytenoidopexy
Ashhurst's splint
aspirate
aspiration
astragalar
astragalectomy
astragalocalcanean
astragalocrural
astragaloscaphoid
astragalotibial
astragalus
ataxia
atelomyelia
atelopodia
atelorachidia
atraumatic
atrophy
    Sudeck's a.
Aufranc-Turner prosthesis
Augustine's nail
Austin-Moore prosthesis

Avila's operation
avulsion
awl
    Wilson's a.
Axer's operation
axis
axon
Baastrup's syndrome
Babinski's sign
Badgley's
    operation
    plate
Baker's cyst
Bakwin-Eiger syndrome
Balkan splint
band
    iliotibial b.
    Parham's b.
    periosteal b.
bandage. See *General Surgical Terms* section.
Bankhart's
    operation
    retractor
Bardenheuer's extension
Barker's operation
Barré-Liéou syndrome
Barsky's operation
Barton's
    fracture
    operation
    tong
Barwell's operation
Basile's screw
basioccipital
basioglossus
basisphenoid
basitemporal
basivertebral
Bateman's
    operation
    prosthesis
Baylor's splint
Bechterew-Mendel reflex
Bechterew's reflex
Bechtol's
    arthroplasty

Bechtol's (continued)
    prosthesis
Beckman-Adson retractor
Béclard's amputation
bed
    CircOlectric b.
Beevor's sign
Bekhterev's
    arthritis
    spondylitis
    test
belly
Bennett's
    elevator
    fracture
    retractor
Bent's operation
Berger's
    operation
    paresthesia
Bertin's
    bone
    ligament
Bertolotti's syndrome
Besnier's rheumatism
biarticular
biceps
    b. brachii
    b. femoris
bicipital
Bier's amputation
bifurcate
Bigelow's ligament
biopsy
    muscle b.
biparietal
bipedal
bipenniform
Bishop-Black tendon tucker
Bishop-DeWitt tendon tucker
Bishop-Peter tendon tucker
Bishop's tendon tucker
BK – below knee
block
    parasacral b.
    paravertebral b.
    perineural b.

block (continued)
    presacral b.
    pudendal b.
    sacral b.
    stellate b.
    subarachnoid b.
    sympathetic b.
    transsacral b.
Blount's
    disease
    operation
    osteotome
    plate
    retractor
    stapler
Blundell-Jones operation
Bobroff's operation
body
    Schmorl's b.
    vertebral b.
Böhler-Braun splint
Böhler's
    clamp
    splint
Bohlman's pin
bolt
    Webb's b.
    Wilson's b.
Bond's splint
bone
    accessory b.
    acetabular b.
    acromial b.
    alar b.
    Albers-Schönberg b's
    alisphenoid b.
    ankle b.
    astragaloid b.
    astragaloscaphoid b.
    basihyal b.
    basilar b.
    Bertin's b.
    breast b.
    bregmatic b.
    brittle b's
    calcaneal b.
    cancellated b.

bone (continued)
    cancellous b.
    capitate b.
    carpal b's
    chalky b's
    coccygeal b.
    collar b.
    compact b.
    cortical b.
    costal b.
    cranial b's
    cuneiform b.
    ectethmoid b's
    ectocuneiform b.
    endochondral b.
    entocuneiform b.
    epactal b's
    ethmoid b.
    exoccipital b.
    femoral b.
    fibular b.
    flank b.
    frontal b.
    hamate b.
    haunch b.
    humeral b.
    hyoid b.
    iliac b.
    incarial b.
    intermaxillary b.
    interparietal b.
    intrachondrial b.
    ischial b.
    ivory b's
    lacrimal b.
    lenticular b.
    lunate b.
    maxillary b.
    mesocuneiform b.
    metacarpal b's
    metatarsal b's
    multangular b.
    nasal b.
    navicular b.
    occipital b.
    orbitosphenoidal b.
    parietal b.

bone (continued)
    pelvic b.
    periosteal b.
    petrous b.
    phalangeal b's
    Pirie's b.
    pisiform b.
    pubic b.
    radial b.
    replacement b.
    rider's b.
    sacral b.
    scaphoid b.
    scapular b.
    sesamoid b's
    shin b.
    shoulder b.
    sphenoid b.
    spongy b.
    supernumerary b.
    tarsal b's
    temporal b.
    tibia b.
    trapezium b.
    trapezoid b.
    triangular b.
    triquetral b.
    turbinate b.
    ulna b.
    ulnar styloid b.
    unciform b.
    uncinate b.
    vesalian b.
    vomer b.
    whettle b's
    wormian b.
    xiphoid b.
    zygomatic b.
bone depression
bone graft
    diamond inlay b.g.
    dual inlay b.g.
    hemicylindrical b.g.
    inlay b.g.
    intramedullary b.g.
    medullary b.g.
    onlay b.g.

bone graft (continued)
    osteoperiosteal b.g.
    peg b.g.
    sliding inlay b.g.
bone head
bone processes
bone wax
Bonnet's sign
boot
    Gibney's b.
    Jobst's b.
    Unna's paste b.
bootonyar. See *boutonnière.*
boss
    parietal b's
Bosworth's
    operation
    screw
Bouchard's nodes
boutonnière
Bowen-Grover meniscotome
Bowen's osteotome
Bowlby's splint
bowleg
Boyd's operation
Boyes-Goodfellow hook
brace
    drop foot b.
    ischial weight-bearing b.
    Knight's b.
    longleg b.
    Lyman-Smith b.
    Milwaukee b.
    Taylor's b.
    toe drop b.
    weight-bearing b.
brachial
brachialgia
brachiocephalic
brachiocrural
brachiocubital
brachiocyllosis
brachiocyrtosis
brachiogram
brachium
brachymetacarpia
brachymetapody

brachymetatarsia
brachyphalangia
brachyskelous
brachystasis
Bradford's frame
Bragard's sign
Brant's splint
Brett's operation
brevicollis
breviflexor
brisement
    b. forcé
Brissaud's scoliosis
Bristow's operation
Brittain's operation
Brockman's operation
Brodie's
    abscess
    disease
    knee
    ligament
Brown's dermatome
Brudzinski's sign
Bryant's
    sign
    traction
Buck's
    extension
    hook
    operation
    splint
    traction
Büdinger-Ludloff-Laewen disease
Budin's joint
Bunge's amputation
bunion
bunionectomy
    Akin's b.
    Keller's b.
    Mitchell's b.
    Silver's b.
    Stone's b.
bunionette
Bunnell's
    anvil
    drill
    needle

Bunnell's (continued)
    operation
    probe
bur
    Jordan-Day b.
    Lempert's b.
Burch-Greenwood tendon tucker
bursa
    Achilles b.
    anserine b.
    ischiogluteal b.
    b. of iliopsoas muscle
    olecranon b.
    patellar b.
    prepatellar b.
    radiohumeral b.
    retrocalcaneal b.
    scapulohumeral b.
    subacromial b.
    subdeltoid b.
bursae
bursectomy
bursitis
    Achilles b.
    Duplay's b.
    prepatellar b.
    radiohumeral b.
    subacromial b.
    subdeltoid b.
bursolith
bursopathy
bursotomy
Butcher's saw
buttock
C-1, C-2, etc.–cervical vertebrae
Ca–calcium
Cabot's splint
cacomelia
CAD (computerized assisted
    design) prosthesis
calcaneal
calcaneitis
calcaneoapophysitis
calcaneoastragaloid
calcaneocavus
calcaneocuboid
calcaneodynia

calcaneofibular
calcaneonavicular
calcaneoplantar
calcaneoscaphoid
calcaneotibial
calcaneovalgocavus
calcaneus
calcar
    c. femorale
    c. pedis
calcification
calcinosis
    c. intervertebralis
    tumoral c.
calcium
Caldani's ligament
Callahan's operation
Callander's amputation
Callaway's test
callosity
callus
    definitive c.
    ensheathing c.
    intermediate c.
    medullary c.
    myelogenous c.
    permanent c.
    provisional c.
calvaria
calvarial
calvarium
Calvé-Perthes disease
cambium
Campbell's
    ligament
    operation
    osteotome
camptocormia
camptodactyly
camptomelia
camptospasm
Canadian crutch
canal
    Guyon's c.
    haversian c.
    Hunter's c.
    neural c.

canal (continued)
    tarsal c.
cancellated
cancelli
cancellous
cancellus
cane
    adjustable c.
    English c.
    quadripod c.
    tripod c.
cannula
cannulate
cannulation
capeline
capital
capitatum
capitellum
capitular
capitulum
capsula
capsular
capsule
    articular c.
    joint c.
capsulectomy
capsulitis
    adhesive c.
capsuloplasty
capsulorrhaphy
capsulotomy
caput
    c. radii
    c. tali
Carden's amputation
Carleton's spots
caro
    c. quadrata manus
    c. quadrata sylvii
carpal
    c. tunnel
carpectomy
carpocarpal
carpometacarpal
carpopedal
carpophalangeal
carpoptosis

carpus
    c. curvus
Carrell's operation
Carroll-Legg osteotome
Carroll-Smith-Petersen
    osteotome
Carroll's osteotome
cartilage
    articular c.
    ensiform c.
    falciform c.
    floating c.
    interarticular c.
    interosseous c.
    intervertebral c.
    tendon c.
cartilaginous
cast
    Cotrel's c.
    long-arm c.
    long-leg c.
    Pietrie's c.
    Risser's c.
    short-arm c.
    short-leg c.
CAT scan – computerized axial
    tomography scan
cauda (caudae)
    c. equina
caudad
caudocephalad
cavernous
Cave-Rowe operation
Cave's operation
cavity
    medullary c.
    synovial c.
cavus
cephalad
cephalic
cephalocaudad
cervical
cervicalis
cervicoaxillary
cervicobrachial
cervicobrachialgia
cervicodorsal

cervicodynia
cervico-occipital
cervicoplasty
cervicoscapular
cervicothoracic
Chaddock's reflex
Chandler's
    disease
    elevator
    splint
Chaput's method
Charcot's
    arthrosis
    foot
    joint
charley horse
Charnley-Mueller
    arthroplasty
    prosthesis
Charnley's arthrodesis
Charrière's saw
cheilectomy
cheiragra
cheiralgia
    c. paresthetica
cheirobrachialgia
cheiromegaly
cheiroplasty
cheiropodalgia
cheirospasm
chemotherapy
Cherry's osteotome
chiasm
chiasma
    c. tendinum digitorum
        manus
Chiene's
    operation
    test
chisel
    Moore's c.
chondral
chondrectomy
chondric
chondrification
chondritis
    c. intervertebralis calcanea

chondroblast
chondroblastoma
chondrocalcinosis
chondrocarcinoma
chondroclast
chondrocostal
chondrydynia
chondrodysplasia
chondrodystrophia
chondrodystrophy
   c. malacia
chondroepiphyseal
chondroepiphysitis
chondrogenesis
chondrogenic
chondroglossus
chondroid
chondroitic
chondrolipoma
chondrylysis
chondroma
chondromalacia
chondromatosis
   Reichel's c.
   synovial c.
chondromatous
chondrometaplasia
   tenosynovial c.
chondromyxoma
chondromyxosarcoma
chondronecrosis
chondro-osseous
chondrophyte
chondroplasia
chondroplastic
chondroplasty
chondroporosis
chondrosarcoma
chondrosarcomatosis
chondroskeleton
chondrosternal
chondrosternoplasty
chondrotome
chondrotomy
chondroxiphoid
chonechondrosternon

Chopart's
   amputation
   joint
chorda
   c. dorsalis
chorda-mesoderm
chordotomy
Chvostek sign
Chvostek-Weiss sign
chymopapain
cineplasty
cineradiography
CircOlectric bed
circumduction
circumflex
CK – creatine kinase
clamp
   Böhler's c.
   Forrester's c.
   Humphries' c.
   Jackson's c.
   Lambotte's c.
   Lowman's c.
   Verbrugge's c.
   Wester's c.
   Williams' c.
   Wilman's c.
   Wilson's c.
claudication
clavicle
clavicotomy
clavicula
clavicular
claviculus
clavipectoral
clavus
clawfoot
clawhand
Clayton's osteotome
Cleeman's sign
cleidagra
cleidal
cleidarthritis
cleidocostal
cleidocranial
clinodactyly
clinostatism

clinotherapy
clonus
Cloward's
    drill
    operation
    osteotome
    rongeur
clubbing
clubfoot
clubhand
cluneal
clunis
Clutton's joint
coapt
Cobb's
    elevator
    gouge
    osteotome
coccygeal
coccygectomy
coccygerector
coccygeus
coccygodynia
coccygotomy
coccyx
Codivilla's
    extension
    operation
Codman's
    exercise
    sign
cogwheel phenomenon
Cole's operation
collar
    Thomas' c.
collateral
Colles'
    fracture
    splint
Collin's osteoclast
Collison's screw
collum
    c. anatomicum
      humeri
    c. chirurgicum humeri
    c. costae
    c. distortum

collum (continued)
    c. femoris
    c. mallei
    c. processus condyloidei
      mandibulae
    c. radii
    c. scapulae
    c. tali
    c. valgum
Colonna's operation
column
    spinal c.
    vertebral c.
comminuted
comminution
Comolli's sign
compact
Compere's
    operation
    pin
compression
computerized axial tomography
    scan
concave
concavity
concavoconcave
concavoconvex
concussion
condylar
condyle
condylectomy
condylion
condylotomy
condylus
congenerous
connexus
    c. intertendineus
Conn's operation
contractility
    idiomuscular c.
contraction
contracture
    Dupuytren's c.
    ischemic c.
    Volkmann's c.
contralateral
contrecoup

contusion
conus
    c. medullaris
Converse's osteotome
convexity
convexobasia
Conzett's goniometer
Coopernail's sign
coracoacromial
coracoclavicular
coracohumeral
coracoid
coracoiditis
coracoradialis
coracoulnaris
Corbett's forceps
cordotomy
cornoid
cornu (cornua)
cornual
cornuate
cornucopia
coronoid
corticospinal
corticosteroid
costa (costae)
    c. cervicalis
    c. fluctuans
    c. fluctuans decima
    c. fluitantes
    c. prima
    c. spuriae
    c. verae
costal
costalgia
costalis
costectomy
costicartilage
costicervical
costiform
costispinal
costocentral
costocervicalis
costochondral
costochondritis
costoclavicular

costocoracoid
costogenic
costoinferior
costopleural
costoscapular
costoscapularis
costosternal
costosternoplasty
costosuperior
costotome
costotomy
costotransverse
costotransversectomy
costovertebral
costoxiphoid
Cotrel's cast
Cottle's osteotome
Cotton's fracture
cotyloid
cotylosacral
counterextension
countertraction
Coventry's
    osteotomy
    screw
coxa
    c. adducta
    c. flexa
    c. magna
    c. plana
    c. valga
    c. vara
    c. vara luxans
coxalgia
coxankylometer
coxarthria
coxarthritis
coxarthrocace
coxarthropathy
coxarthrosis
coxitis
    c. fugax
    senile c.
coxodynia
coxofemoral
coxotomy

coxotuberculosis
Crane's
    mallet
    osteotome
craniad
cranial
cranialis
cranioacromial
craniosacral
craniospinal
craniotome
craniotomy
cranium
craterization
Credo's operation
cremaster
cremasteric
crena
    c. ani
crepitation
crepitus
cricoid
cricoidectomy
cruciate
crural
crus (crura)
crutch
    Canadian c.
    jocked stand c.
Crutchfield's
    operation
    tong
Cruveilhier's joint
cryosurgery
cryotherapy
Cubbins' operation
cubital
cubitocarpal
cubitoradial
cubitus
    c. valgus
    c. varus
cuboid
cuboidal
cuff
    musculotendinous c.

cuff (continued)
    rotator c.
cuneiform
cuneocuboid
cuneonavicular
cuneoscaphoid
curet
    Spratt's c.
Curry's splint
curvature
CVA – costovertebral angle
Cybex test
cyst
    Baker's c.
Czerny's disease
dactylitis
dactylolysis
dactylospasm
Darrach's operation
Davies-Colley operation
Davis' splint
Dawbarn's sign
débridement
decalcification
decapitation
decompression
decubitus
deformity
    Arnold-Chiari d.
    boutonnière d.
    buttonhole d.
    Ilfeld-Holder d.
    lobster-claw d.
    Madelung's d.
    recurvatum d.
    seal-fin d.
    silver fork d.
    Sprengel's d.
    swan-neck d.
    ulnar drift d.
    valgus d.
    varus d.
    Velpeau's d.
    Volkmann's d.
degeneration
    Zenker's d.

degenerative
dehiscence
    Zuckerkandl's d.
Dejerine's sign
Delore's method
delta
    d. mesoscapulae
deltoid
Demianoff's sign
demifacet
demigauntlet
denervation
Denis-Browne clubfoot splint
denudation
Denuse's operation
deossification
DePalma's prosthesis
DePuy's
    prosthesis
    splint
de Quervain's disease
derangement
    Hey's internal d.
dermatome
    Brown's d.
dermatomyositis
Desault's sign
desmalgia
desmectasis
desmodynia
desmoid
desmology
desmoma
desmoneoplasm
desmopathy
desmoplasia
desmoplastic
desmorrhexis
desmosis
desmotomy
Deutschländer's disease
dextroverted
Deyerle's
    drill
    plate
    punch
diaclasis

diaphyseal
diaphysectomy
diaphysis (diaphyses)
diaphysitis
    tuberculous d.
diaplasis
diaplastic
diapophysis
diarthric
diarthrosis (diarothroses)
diastasis
diastematomyelia
diastrophic
Dickson-Diveley operation
Dickson's operation
Dieffenbach's operation
digit
digital
digitation
Dingman's
    forceps
    osteotome
DIP–distal interphalangeal
DIPJ–distal interphalangeal joint
diplegia
diploë
diploetic
diploic
dis-. See also words beginning
    dys-.
disarticulation
disc (also disk)
disciform
discogenic
discoid
discoidectomy
discopathy
disease
    Albers-Schönberg d.
    Albright's d.
    Blount's d.
    Brodie's d.
    Büdinger-Ludloff-
      Laewen d.
    Calvé-Perthes d.
    Chandler's d.
    Czerny's d.

disease (continued)
  degenerative joint d.
  de Quervain's d.
  Deutschländer's d.
  Duplay's d.
  Erb-Goldflam d.
  Erb's d.
  Erichsen's d.
  Freiberg's d.
  Haglund's d.
  Hand-Schüller-
    Christian d.
  Inman's d.
  Jüngling's d.
  Kashin-Bek d.
  Köhler's d.
  Kümmell's d.
  Kümmell-Verneuil d.
  Larsen-Johansson d.
  Legg-Calvé-
    Waldenström d.
  Marie-Strümpell d.
  Marie-Tooth d.
  McArdle's d.
  Morquio's d.
  Ollier's d.
  Osgood-Schlatter d.
  Otto's d.
  Paget's d.
  Pauzat's d.
  Pellegrini-Stieda d.
  Perrin-Ferraton d.
  Perthes' d.
  Pott's d.
  Poulet's d.
  Preiser's d.
  Quervain's d.
  Recklinghausen's d.
  Schanz's d.
  Scheuermann's d.
  Schlatter's d.
  Schmorl's d.
  Sever's d.
  Steinert's d.
  Swediaur's d.
  Talma's d.
  Volkmann's d.

disease (continued)
  von Recklinghausen's d.
  Waldenström's d.
  Wartenberg's d.
DISI – dorsiflexion intercalated
    segment instability
disk (also disc)
  cartilaginous d's
  herniated d.
  intervertebral d's
diskectomy
diskiform
diskitis
diskogram
diskography
dislocatio
  d. erecta
dislocation
  divergent d.
  Kienböck's d.
  Monteggia's d.
  Nélaton's d.
  Smith's d.
  subastragalar d.
  subcoracoid d.
  subglenoid d.
dismemberment
dissector
  Lewin's d.
distraction
DJD – degenerative joint disease
dolichostenomelia
dolor
  d. coxae
dorsa
dorsad
dorsal
dorsalgia
dorsalis
dorsiflexion
dorsintercostal
dorsispinal
dorsolateral
dorsolumbar
dorsomedian
dorsomesial
dorsonuchal

dorsoradial
dorsoscapular
dorsoventrad
dorsoventral
dorsum (dorsa)
Downing's knife
drain
> Redivac d.

drill
> Bunnell's d.
> Cloward's d.
> Deyerle's d.
> Hall's air d.
> intramedullary d.
> Smedberg's d.
> Vitallium d.

driver
> Küntscher's d.

drop
> foot d.
> d. phalangette

drugs. See *Drugs and Chemistry* section.
DTR – deep tendon reflex
Duchenne's-type muscular dystrophy
Dugas' test
Dunn-Brittain operation
Duplay's
> bursitis
> disease

Dupuytren's
> amputation
> contracture
> fracture
> sign
> splint

dura
dural
dura mater
> d.m. spinalis

duraplasty
Durman's operation
duroarachnitis
Duverney's fracture
dynamometer
> squeeze d.

dysarthrosis
dyschondroplasia
> Ollier's d.

dysesthesia
dyskinesia
dysmetria
dysostosis
dysplasia
> diaphyseal d.
> metaphyseal d.

dysplastic
dystonia
dystrophic
dystrophy
> Duchenne's-type muscular d.
> muscular d.

ebonation
eburnation
eccentro-osteochondrodysplasia
ecchondrotome
ectocondyle
ectromelia
ectromelus
ectrometacarpia
ectrometatarsia
ectrophalangia
ectrosyndactyly
Eden-Hybbinette operation
Eggers'
> operation
> plate
> screw
> splint

Eicher's prosthesis
elastin
elbow
> capped e.
> tennis e.

electroanalgesia
electromyogram
electromyography
elevator
> Bennett's e.
> Chandler's e.
> Cobb's e.
> Farabeuf's e.

elevator (continued)
    joker e.
    Lane's e.
    Langenbeck's e.
Elliott's plate
Ellis-Jones operation
Elmslie-Cholmeley operation
Ely's test
EMG – electromyogram
eminence
    thenar e.
eminentia
enarthrosis
enchondroma
enchondromatosis
enchondromatous
enchondrosarcoma
enchondrosis
endochondral
endoscope
endoskeleton
endosteal
endosteitis
endosteoma
endosteum
Engelmann's splint
Engen extension orthosis
English cane
enostosis
entepicondyle
enthesis
ependyma
epicondylagia
epicondyle
epicondylitis
epicondylus (epicondyli)
epifizeal. See *epiphyseal;*
    epiphysial.
epifizee-. See words beginning
    epiphysi-.
epimysium
epiphyseal
epiphysial
epiphysiodesis
epiphysioid
epiphysiolysis
epiphysiometer

epiphysiopathy
epiphysis (epiphyses)
    capital e.
    e. cerebri
    slipped e.
    stippled e.
epiphysitis
    vertebral e.
epipyramis
epirotulian
epistropheus
epitendineum
epitenon
epithesis
epitrochlea
Epstein's osteotome
equinovalgus
equinovarus
equinus
erasion
    e. of joint
Erb-Goldflam disease
Erb's disease
ergogram
ergograph
    Mosso's e.
Erichsen's
    disease
    sign
Esmarch's tourniquet
ESR – erythrocyte sedimentation
    rate
Essex-Lopresti method
Evans' operation
eversion
evertor
Ewing's
    sarcoma
    tumor
exarticulation
exercise
    Codman's e.
    Williams' e.
exoskeleton
exostosectomy
exostosis
    e. bursata

exostosis (continued)
    e. cartilaginea
    e. osteocartilaginous
exsanguinate
extension
    Bardenheuer's e.
    Buck's e.
    Codivilla's e.
extensor
extracarpal
extractor
    Jewett's e.
    Moore's e.
extradural
extraepiphyseal
extraligamentous
extramalleolus
extraosseous
extremities
extremity
Eyler's operation
fabella (fabellae)
fabere sign
facet
facetectomy
facial
facioscapulohumeral
Fahey's operation
Fajersztajn's sign
falan-. See words beginning
    phalan-.
falanks. See *phalanx*.
falx
    f. inguinalis
    f. ligamentosa
Farabeuf-Lambotte forceps
Farabeuf's
    amputation
    elevator
    forceps
faradization
    galvanic f.
faradomuscular
fascia (fasciae)
    f. lata femoris
fascial

fasciaplasty
fasciatome
    Luck's f.
fascicle
fascicular
fasciculated
fasciculation
fasciculus (fasciculi)
fasciectomy
fasciitis
    pseudosarcomatous f.
fasciodesis
fascioplasty
fasciorrhaphy
fasciotomy
felon
femoral
femoroiliac
femorotibial
femur (femora)
Ferguson's forceps
fiber
    Sharpey's f's
fiberoptic
fibril
    muscle f.
fibrillation
fibrocartilage
fibrocartilaginous
fibroma
    chondromyxoid f.
    nonosteogenic f.
    osteogenic f.
fibromatosis
fibromuscular
fibromyitis
fibromyositis
fibrosarcoma
fibrosis
fibrositis
fibrotic
fibrous
fibula
fibular
fibularis
fibulocalcaneal

filum (fila)
    f. spinale
    f. terminale
finger
    baseball f.
    clubbed f.
    drumstick f.
    hammer f.
    hippocratic f's
    mallet f.
    trigger f.
    webbed f's
Finkelstein's test
Fink's tendon tucker
fissure
fixation
fizeotherape. See *physiotherapy.*
flail
flatfoot
    spastic f.
flex
flexible
flexion
    plantar f.
flexor
    f. retinaculum
flexorplasty
fluid
    synovial f.
fluoroscopy
fontanelle
foot
    Charcot's f.
    cleft f.
    club f.
    drop f.
    Friedreich's f.
    Madura f.
    Morand's f.
    rocker-bottom f.
    tabetic f.
footdrop
foramen
    f. magnum
foramina
foraminotomy

Forbes' amputation
forceps
    bayonet f.
    Corbett's f.
    Dingman's f.
    Farabeuf-Lambotte f.
    Farabeuf's f.
    Ferguson's f.
    Hibbs' f.
    Horsley's f.
    Kern's f.
    Lambotte's f.
    Lane's f.
    Liston-Stille f.
    Littauer-Liston f.
    Martin's f.
    Van Buren's f.
forearm
forefoot
Forrester's clamp
fossa (fossae)
Foster frame
fovea
    f. capitis femoris
Fowler's operation
Fox's splint
fracture
    agenetic f.
    apophyseal f.
    articular f.
    atrophic f.
    avulsion f.
    Barton's f.
    Bennett's f.
    bimalleolar f.
    boxer's f.
    bucket-handle f.
    bumper f.
    bursting f.
    butterfly f.
    buttonhole f.
    chisel f.
    "clay-shoveler" f.
    cleavage f.
    closed f.
    Colles' f.

fracture (continued)
    comminuted f.
    compound f.
    compression f.
    condylar f.
    congenital f.
    Cotton's f.
    depressed f.
    diacondylar f.
    displaced f.
    Dupuytren's f.
    Duverney's f.
    dyscrasic f.
    f. en coin
    endocrine f.
    f. en rave
    epiphysial f.
    extracapsular f.
    fatigue f.
    Galeazzi's f.
    Gosselin's f.
    greenstick f.
    Guérin's f.
    hangman's f.
    impacted f.
    intercondylar f.
    intertrochanteric f.
    intra-articular f.
    intracapsular f.
    intraperiosteal f.
    Jefferson's f.
    lead pipe f.
    LeFort's f.
    linear f.
    longitudinal f.
    march f.
    Monteggia's f.
    Moore's f.
    neoplastic f.
    oblique f.
    open f.
    pathologic f.
    pertrochanteric f.
    pillion f.
    Pott's f.
    Quervain's f.
    segmental f.

fracture (continued)
    Shepherd's f.
    silver-fork f.
    Skillern's f.
    Smith's f.
    spiral f.
    splintered f.
    spontaneous f.
    sprinter's f.
    stellate f.
    Stieda's f.
    subcapital f.
    subperiosteal f.
    supracondylar f.
    torsion f.
    torus f.
    transcervical f.
    transcondylar f.
    transverse f.
    trimalleolar f.
    tuft f.
    Wagstaffe's f.
    willow f.
fracture-dislocation
fragilitas
    f. ossium
frame
    Bradford's f.
    Foster f.
    Hibbs' f.
    Stryker's f.
    Whitman's f.
Frankel's sign
Frazier's osteotome
Freiberg's
    disease
    infraction
    knife
Frejka's splint
Friedreich's foot
Fritz-Lange operation
Froment's sign
funnel chest
fusiform
fusimotor
fusion
    diaphyseal-epiphyseal f.

fusion (continued)
    spinal f.
Futura splint
Gaenslen's sign
gait
    antalgic g.
    ataxic g.
    calcaneous g.
    drag-to g.
    four-point g.
    gluteal g.
    heel-toe g.
    hemiplegic g.
    scissor g.
    steppage g.
    swing-through g.
    swing-to g.
    three-point g.
    Trendelenburg g.
    two-point g.
    waddling g.
Galeazzi's
    fracture
    sign
galvanic
galvanization
gampsodactylia
ganglion
ganglionectomy
ganglioneuroma
gangrene
    Pott's g.
gangrenous
Gant's operation
Garré's osteomyelitis
Gatellier's operation
Gelfoam packing
Gelpi's retractor
genicula
genicular
geniculate
geniculum
genu
    g. impressum
    g. recurvatum
    g. valgum
    g. varum

Geomedic prosthesis
Ghormley's operation
gibbosity
gibbous
gibbus
Gibney's
    boot
    perispondylitis
Gibson's operation
Gigli's saw
Giliberty's prosthesis
Gillespie's operation
Gill's operation
ginglymoid
ginglymus
Girdlestone's operation
glenohumeral
glenoid
Glisson's sling
gluteal
gluteofemoral
gluteoinguinal
Goldthwait's
    operation
    sign
gonarthritis
gonarthromeningitis
gonarthrosis
gonarthrotomy
gonatocele
goniometer
    Conzett's g.
gonitis
    fungous g.
    g. tuberculosa
gonocampsis
Gordon's splint
Gosselin's fracture
gouge
    Cobb's g.
    Moore's g.
goundou
gout
Graber-Duvernay operation
graft
    allogeneic g.
    autogenous g.

graft (continued)
    autoplastic g.
    full-thickness g.
    heterogenous g.
    homogenous g.
    homoplastic g.
    onlay bone g.
    Russe's bone g.
    split-thickness g.
Grice-Green operation
Gritti's amputation
Gritti-Stokes amputation
Guepar's prosthesis
Guérin's fracture
Guillain-Barré syndrome
Guilland's sign
guillotine
Guleke-Stookey operation
Guyon's
    amputation
    canal
Haas' operation
Hagie's pin
Haglund's disease
Hall's air drill
hallux
    h. dolorosa
    h. flexus
    h. malleus
    h. rigidus
    h. valgus
    h. varus
hamate
hamatum
Hamilton's test
hammertoe
Hammond's operation
hamstring
hamulus
Hancock's amputation
hand
    claw h.
    cleft h.
    club h.
    Krukenberg's h.
    lobster-claw h.
    mitten h.
    opera-glass h.

hand (continued)
    trident h.
    writing h.
Hand-Schüller-Christian
    disease
Hansen-Street
    nail
    pin
Hark's operation
Harmon's operation
Harrington's
    nail
    rod
Harris-Beath operation
Hart's splint
Hatcher's pin
Hauser's operation
haversian
Heberden's nodes
Hector's tendon
Hefke-Turner sign
Heifitz's operation
Helbing's sign
hemapophysis
hemarthrosis
hematoma
hematomyelia
hemiarthrosis
hemilaminectomy
hemimelia
hemiparesis
hemipelvectomy
hemiphalangectomy
hemiplegia
hemivertebra
Henderson's operation
Hendry's operation
Henry-Geist operation
herniated
herniation
    h. of nucleus pulposus
hetero-osteoplasty
Heuter's operation
Heyman's operation
Hey's
    amputation
    internal derangement

Hibbs'
   forceps
   frame
   operation
   osteotome
   retractor
hindfoot
hip
   snapping h.
Hirschberg's sign
Hodgen's splint
Hoen's plate
Hoffa-Lorenz operation
Hoffa's operation
Hoffmann's sign
Hohmann's
   operation
   retractor
Hoke's osteotome
Holmes' operation
Homans' sign
hook
   Boyes-Goodfellow h.
   Buck's h.
Horsley's forceps
Horwitz-Adams operation
Houston's operation
Howorth's
   operation
   osteotome
Hubbard's tank
Hueter's sign
humeral
humeroradial
humeroscapular
humeroulnar
humerus (humeri)
humpback
Humphries' clamp
Hunter's canal
hydrarthrosis
hydrocollator
hydromyelia
hydroxyapatite
hygroma
hypalgesia
hypercalcemia
hyperesthesia

hyperextension
hyperflexion
hyperostosis
hypertrophic
hypertrophy
   Marie's h.
hyperuricemia
hypesthesia
hypolemmal
hypoplasia
hypothenar
idiomuscular
iksomielitis. See
   ixomyelitis.
Ilfeld-Holder deformity
iliac
iliococcygeal
iliocostal
iliofemoral
iliofemoroplasty
ilioinguinal
iliolumbar
iliolumbocostoabdominal
iliometer
iliopectineal
iliopectinal
iliopelvic
iliopsoas
iliopubic
iliosacral
iliosciatic
iliospinal
iliotibial
iliotrochanteric
ilioxiphopagus
ilium (ilia)
IM – intramuscularly
immobilization
incision. See *General Surgical*
   Terms section.
induction
   spinal i.
inflammation
inflammatory
infra-axillary
infraclavicular
infracostal

infraction
    Freiberg's i.
infraglenoid
infrapatellar
infrascapular
infraspinous
infrasternal
infratrochlear
Inman's disease
innervation
innominate
inochondritis
inotropic
inotropism
instability
    lumbosacral i.
instep
insufficientia
    i. vertebrae
interarticular
intercarpal
intercartilaginous
intercellular
interchondral
interclavicular
intercondylar
intercostal
intercostohumeral
interdigital
intergluteal
intermetacarpal
interosseal
interosseous
interpediculate
interphalangeal
interscapular
interspace
interspinal
intertrochanteric
intervertebral
intramedullary
involucrum
ischial
ischialgia
ischiectomy
ischiocapsular
ischiococcygeal

ischiococcygeus
ischiofemoral
ischiofibular
ischiohebotomy
ischiopubic
ischiopubiotomy
ischiosacral
ischiovertebral
ischium
iskeal. See *ischial.*
iskealjea. See *ischialgia.*
iskeo-. See words beginning
    ischio-.
iskeum. See *ischium.*
ithyokyphosis
ixomyelitis
Jaboulay's amputation
jacket
    Kydex body j.
    Minerva's j.
    plaster-of-Paris j.
    Royalite body j.
    Sayre's j.
Jackson's clamp
Jansen's test
Jefferson's fracture
Jendrassik's maneuver
jerk
    Achilles j.
    ankle j.
    quadriceps j.
    triceps surae j.
Jewett's
    extractor
    nail
    plate
Jobst's
    boot
    stocking
joint. See also *articulation.*
    amphidiarthrodial j.
    ankle j.
    apophyseal j's
    arthrodial j.
    ball-and-socket j.
    biaxial j.
    bilocular j.

joint (continued)
    Budin's j.
    cartilaginous j.
    Charcot's j.
    Chopart's j.
    Clutton's j.
    cochlear j.
    composite j.
    compound j.
    condyloid j.
    Cruveilhier's j.
    diarthrodial j.
    dry j.
    elbow j.
    ellipsoidal j.
    enarthrodial j.
    false j.
    fibrocartilaginous j.
    fibrous j.
    flail j.
    freely movable j.
    fringe j.
    hinge j.
    hip j.
    hysteric j.
    immovable j.
    intercarpal j's
    irritable j.
    knee j.
    ligamentous j.
    Lisfranc's j.
    Luschka's j's
    j. mice
    midcarpal j.
    mixed j.
    multiaxial j.
    pivot j.
    plane j.
    polyaxial j.
    rotary j.
    sacrococcygeal j.
    saddle j.
    scapuloclavicular j.
    shoulder j.
    simple j.
    spheroidal j.
    spiral j.

joint (continued)
    stifle j.
    synarthrodial j.
    synovial j.
    tarsal j.
    trochoid j.
    uniaxial j.
    unilocular j.
    von Gies' j.
joint mice
Jones' splint
Joplin's operation
Jordan-Day bur
Judet's prosthesis
Jüngling's disease
Jung's muscle
juxta-articular
juxtaepiphyseal
juxtaposition
juxtaspinal
Kanavel's
    sign
    splint
Kapel's operation
Kashin-Bek disease
Keen's sign
Keith's needle
Keller-Blake splint
Keller's bunionectomy
Kellogg-Speed operation
Kernig's sign
Kern's forceps
Kerrison's rongeur
Kerr's sign
Kessel's plate
Kessler's operation
Kezerian's osteotome
Kidner's operation
Kienböck's dislocation
kifo-. See words beginning
    kypho-.
kineplasty
kinesalgia
King-Richards operation
Kirkaldy-Willis operation
Kirk's amputation

Kirmisson's
    operation
    raspatory
kirospazm. See *cheirospasm.*
Kirschner's
    apparatus
    splint
    wire
KJ – knee jerk
KK – knee kick
Klippel-Feil syndrome
knee
    Brodie's k.
knife
    Downing's k.
    Freiberg's k.
    Liston's k.
    Lowe-Breck k.
    Smillie's k.
Knight's brace
knock-knee
Knowles' pin
knuckle
Kocher's operation
Koenig-Wittek operation
Köhler's disease
kokse-. See words beginning
    coccy-.
Kolomnin's operation
kon-. See words beginning *chon-.*
König's operation
Kreuscher's
    operation
    scissors
Kristiansen's screw
Krukenberg's hand
Kümmell's
    disease
    spondylitis
Kümmell-Verneuil disease
Küntscher's
    driver
    nail
    reamer
Kydex body jacket
kyllosis

kyphos
kyphoscoliosis
kyphosis
    Scheuermann's k.
kyphotic
kyrtorrhachic
L-1, L-2, etc. – lumbar vertebrae
labrum
    l. acetabulare
    l. glenoidale
laceration
lacertus
lacuna (lacunae)
Laing's plate
Lambotte-Henderson osteotome
Lambotte's
    clamp
    forceps
    osteotome
Lambrinudi's operation
lamella (lamellae)
lamellar
lamina (laminae)
laminagram
laminar
laminectomy
    lumbar l.
    thoracic l.
laminotomy
lancinating
Lane's
    elevator
    forceps
    plate
Langenbeck's
    amputation
    elevator
    saw
Lange's operation
Langoria's sign
Lapidus' operation
Larrey's amputation
Larsen-Johansson disease
Lasègue's sign
laser
lateral

lateralis
latissimus
Laugier's sign
Lawson-Thorton plate
LE–lupus erythematosus
Le Fort's
    amputation
    fracture
Legg-Calvé-Perthes syndrome
Legg-Calvé-Waldenström disease
Legg's osteotome
Leichtenstern's sign
Leinbach's
    osteotome
    screw
leiomyoma
leiomyosarcoma
Leksell's rongeur
Lempert's bur
L'Episcopo's operation
Leri's sign
levator
Levine's operation
Lewin's
    dissector
    splint
Lewin-Stern splint
Lhermitte's sign
ligament
    accessory l.
    acromioclavicular l.
    acromiocoracoid l.
    adipose l.
    annular l.
    anterior l.
    arcuate l.
    Bertin's l.
    Bigelow's l.
    Brodie's l.
    calcaneofibular l.
    calcaneonavicular l.
    Caldani's l.
    Campbell's l.
    capsular l.
    carpometacarpal l.
    collateral l.

ligament (continued)
    coracoacromial l.
    coracoclavicular l.
    coracohumeral l.
    costoclavicular l.
    cruciate l's
    crural l.
    cuboideonavicular l.
    cuneonavicular l.
    deltoid l.
    dentate l.
    fabellofibular l.
    falciform l.
    flaval l.
    hamatometacarpal l.
    iliofemoral l.
    iliotrochanteric l.
    inguinal l.
    laciniate l.
    lateral l.
    medial l.
    olecranon l.
    patellar l.
    pisohamate l.
    pisometacarpal l.
    plantar l.
    popliteal l.
    posterior l.
    pubocapsular l.
    pubofemoral l.
    radiocarpal l.
    rhomboid l.
    sacrospinous l.
    sacrotuberous l.
    sternoclavicular l.
    sternocostal l.
    talocalcaneal l.
    talofibular l.
    talonavicular l.
    tendinotrochanteric l.
    transverse l.
    trapezoid l.
    ulnar l.
    ulnocarpal l.
    volar l.
    Wrisberg's l.

ligamentous
ligamentum
    l. flavum
    l. teres femoris
ligature
Linder's sign
line
    Nélaton's l.
    Ogston's l.
    Schoemaker's l.
    Shenton's l.
    Ullmann's l.
linea
    l. alba cervicalis
    l. arcuata ossis ilii
    l. aspera femoris
    l. epiphysialis
    l. glutea
    l. pectinea femoris
    l. terminalis pelvis
    l. trapezoidea
linear
lipoma
lipomatous
lipomeningocele
liposarcoma
Lippman's prosthesis
Lisfranc's
    amputation
    joint
Lissauer's zone
Liston's
    knife
    splint
Liston-Stille forceps
Littauer-Liston forceps
Littler's operation
Littlewood's operation
locomotion
locomotor
LOM—limitation of motion
    loss of motion
longitudinal
Looser-Milkman syndrome
Looser's zone
lordoscoliosis
lordosis

lordotic
Lorenz's
    osteotomy
    sign
Lottes'
    nail
    operation
Lowe-Breck knife
Lowman's clamp
LS—lumbosacral
Lucae's mallet
Lucas-Cottrell operation
Luck's
    fasciatome
    operation
Ludloff's
    operation
    sign
lumbago
lumbar
lumbarization
lumbodorsal
lumbodynia
lumboiliac
lumbosacral
lumbrical
lumbricus (lumbrici)
lumbus
Lund's operation
Luschka's joints
luxatio
    l. coxae congenita
    l. erecta
    l. imperfecta
    l. perinealis
luxation
    Malgaigne's l.
Lyman-Smith brace
Lyme arthritis
lytic
Lytle's splint
MacAusland's operation
Macewen's osteotomy
MacIntosh's prosthesis
MacKenzie's amputation
MacLeod's capsular rheumatism
Madelung's deformity

Madura foot
magnetic resonance imaging
Magnuson's operation
Magnuson-Stack operation
Mahorner-Mead operation
main
        m. en crochet
        m. en griffe
        m. en lorgnette
        m. en pince
        m. fourché
Maisonneuve's
        amputation
        sign
malacia
malformation
        Arnold-Chiari m.
Malgaigne's
        amputation
        luxation
malleolar
malleolus (malleoli)
malleotomy
mallet
        Crane's m.
        m. finger
        Lucae's m
        Meyerding's m.
        Rush's m.
        m. toe
malum
        m. articulorum senilis
        m. coxae senilis
malunion
mandible
mandibular
maneuver
        Allen's m.
        Jendrassik's m
manipulation
manubrium
        m. sterni
manus
        m. cava
        m. extensa
        m. flexa
        m. plana

manus (continued)
        m. superextensa
        m. valga
        m. vara
Marfan's syndrome
Marie-Foix sign
Marie's hypertrophy
Marie-Strümpell
        disease
        spondylitis
Marie-Tooth disease
marrow
        red bone m.
        yellow bone m.
Martin's forceps
Mason-Allen splint
Massie's nail
Matchett-Brown prosthesis
matrix
Mauck's operation
maxilla
maxillary
Mayer's reflex
Mayfield's osteotome
Mayo's operation
Mazur's operation
McArdle's disease
McAtee's screw
McBride's operation
McCarroll's operation
McKee-Farrar prosthesis
McKeever's
        operation
        prosthesis
McLaughlin's
        operation
        plate
        screw
McMurray's
        sign
        test
McReynolds' adapter
mechanoreceptor
medial
medialis
median
mediastinal

mediastinum
medications. See *Drugs and Chemistry* section.
medulla (medullae)
    m. ossium
    m. spinalis
medullary
medullitis
medullization
medulloarthritis
megalodactyly
melorheostosis
melosalgia
membrane
    synovial m.
membranocartilaginous
membranous
meninges
meningitis
meningocele
meningomyelitis
meningomyelocele
meningomyeloradiculitis
meningoradiculitis
meningosis
meninx
meniscal
meniscectomy
    medial m.
menisci
meniscitis
meniscosynovial
meniscotome
    Bowen-Grover m.
    Smillie's m.
meniscus (menisci)
    m. articularis
    m. articulationis genus, lateralis, medialis
    medial m. of knee joint
    m. of acromioclavicular joint
    m. of temporomaxillary joint
Mennell's sign

meralgia
    m. paresthetica
meromelia
mesh
    Vitallium m.
mesomelic
mesomorphic
mesomorphy
mesotendineum
metacarpal
metacarpectomy
metacarpophalangeal
metacarpus
metaphyseal
metaphysis (metaphyses)
metaphysitis
metapodialia
metapophysis
metatarsal
metatarsalgia
metatarsectomy
metatarsophalangeal
metatarsus
    m. adductocavus
    m. adductovarus
    m. adductus
    m. atavicus
    m. brevis
    m. latus
    m. primus varus
    m. varus
method
    Abbott's m.
    Chaput's m.
    Delore's m.
    Essex-Lopresti m.
methyl
    m. methacrylate
Meyerding's
    mallet
    osteotome
    retractor
Michaelis's rhomboid
Michele's trephine
micromelia
midcarpal

midfoot
midtarsal
mielo-. See words beginning
　myelo-.
Mikulicz's operation
Milch's operation
Milkman's syndrome
Mills' test
Milwaukee brace
Miner's osteotome
Minerva's jacket
Minor's sign
Mitchell's
　bunionectomy
　operation
Moberg's arthrodesis
mobilization
Moe's plate
monarthritis
　m. deformans
monoplegia
monostotic
Monteggia's
　dislocation
　fracture
Moore's
　chisel
　extractor
　fracture
　gouge
　nail
　osteotome
　pin
　prosthesis
　reamer
　template
Morand's foot
Morestin's operation
Morquio's
　disease
　sign
Morton's
　neuralgia
　neuroma
　toe
Mosso's ergograph

MP – metacarpophalangeal
MPJ – metacarpophalangeal joint
MRI – magnetic resonance
　imaging
Mueller's prosthesis
multifidus
Mumford-Gurd operation
muscle
　abductor digiti minimi
　　manus m.
　abductor digiti minimi
　　pedis m.
　abductor digiti quinti m.
　abductor hallucis m.
　abductor pollicis brevis m.
　abductor pollicis longus
　　m.
　adductor brevis m.
　adductor hallucis m.
　adductor longus m.
　adductor magnus m.
　adductor minimus m.
　adductor pollicis m.
　anconeus m.
　appendicular m's
　biceps brachii m.
　biceps femoris m.
　brachialis m.
　brachioradialis m.
　coracobrachialis m.
　deltoid m.
　erector m. of spine
　extensor carpi radialis
　　brevis m.
　extensor carpi radialis
　　longus m.
　extensor carpi ulnaris m.
　extensor digiti minimi m.
　extensor digiti quinti
　　proprius m.
　extensor digitorum brevis
　　m.
　extensor digitorum
　　communis m.
　extensor digitorum longus
　　m.

muscle (continued)
    extensor hallucis brevis m.
    extensor hallucis longus
      m.
    extensor indicis m.
    extensor pollicis brevis m.
    extensor pollicis longus m.
    flexor carpi radialis m.
    flexor carpi ulnaris m.
    flexor digitorum brevis m.
    flexor digitorum longus m.
    flexor digitorum
      profundus m.
    flexor digitorum sublimis
      m.
    flexor digitorum
      superficialis m.
    flexor hallucis brevis m.
    flexor hallucis longus m.
    flexor pollicis brevis m.
    flexor pollicis longus m.
    gastrocnemius m.
    gemellus m.
    gluteus maximus m.
    gluteus medius m.
    gluteus minimus m.
    gracilis m.
    greater trochanter m.
    hamstring m's
    m. iliacus
    iliococcygeal m.
    iliocostalis cervicis m.
    iliocostalis lumborum m.
    iliocostalis thoracis m.
    iliopsoas m.
    interosseous m.
    involuntary m's
    Jung's m.
    lateral malleolus m.
    latissimus dorsi m.
    levator m's
    nonstriated m.
    m. opponens pollicis
    palmaris brevis m.
    palmaris longus m.
    paraspinal m.
    pectineus m.

muscle (continued)
    pectoralis major m.
    pectoralis minor m.
    peroneus brevis m.
    peroneus longus m.
    peroneus tertius m.
    piriform m.
    m. piriformis
    plantar m.
    popliteal m.
    pronator quadratus m.
    pronator teres m.
    psoas m.
    quadriceps femoris m.
    rectus m.
    sartorius m.
    scalenus m.
    semimembranosus m.
    semispinalis m.
    semitendinosus m.
    serratus m.
    skeletal m's
    smooth m's
    soleus m.
    spinalis m.
    splenius m.
    sternocleidomastoid m.
    striated m's
    subscapular m.
    supinator m.
    supraspinous m.
    tensor fasciae latae m.
    teres m.
    tibialis m.
    transverse m.
    trapezius m.
    triceps brachii m.
    triceps surae m.
    m. unipennatus
    vastus intermedius m.
    vastus lateralis m.
    vastus medialis m.
    visceral m's
    voluntary m's
muscular
muscularis
muscularity

musculature
musculoaponeurotic
musculocutaneous
musculoelastic
musculointestinal
musculomembranous
musculophrenic
musculoskeletal
musculospiral
musculotendinous
musculus (musculi)
myalgia
myasthenia
    m. gravis
myatonia
myectomy
myelin
myelinated
myelitis
myelocele
myelocystomeningocele
myelodysplasia
myelofugal
myelogenesis
myelogram
myelography
myeloid
myeloma
myelomalacia
myelomenia
myelomeningitis
myelomeningocele
myelon
myeloneuritis
myelo-opticoneuropathy
myeloparalysis
myelopathy
myelopetal
myelophthisis
myeloplegia
myelopoiesis
myelopore
myeloradiculitis
myeloradiculodysplasia
myeloradiculopathy
myelorrhagia
myeloschisis

myelosclerosis
myelospasm
myelosyphilis
myelotome
myelotomy
    commissural m.
myesthesia
myoblastoma
myocele
myocerosis
myoclonia
myoclonic
myoclonus
myocrismus
myocytoma
myodemia
myodiastasis
myodynia
myodystonia
myoedema
myoelastic
myoelectric
myofascitis
myofibril
myofibroma
myofibrosis
myofibrositis
myofilament
myogelosis
myogenic
myoglobin
myoglobinuria
myography
myohypertrophia
myokerosis
myokinesis
myokymia
myologia
myology
myolysis
myoma (myomata)
    m. striocellulare
myomalacia
myomectomy
myomelanosis
myometer
myonecrosis

myoneural
myoneuralgia
myoneurectomy
myoparalysis
myopathia
    m. infraspinata
myopathy
myoplastic
myoplasty
myorrhaphy
myorrhexis
myosarcoma
myosclerosis
myoscope
myoseism
myoserum
myosin
myositis
    acute progressive m.
    m. fibrosa
    m. ossificans
    progressive ossifying m.
    rheumatoid m.
    m. serosa
    suppurative m.
myospasia
myospasm
myospasmia
myosteoma
myosthenic
myosthenometer
myotasis
myotatic
myotenositis
myotenotomy
myotome
myotomy
myotonia
    m. acquisita
    m. atrophica
    m. congenita
    m. dystrophica
myotonic
myotonoid
myotonometer
myotonus
myxoma

Naffziger's syndrome
nail
    Augustine's n.
    Hansen-Street n.
    Harrington's n.
    Jewett's n.
    Küntscher n.
    Lottes' n.
    Massie's n.
    Moore's n.
    Neufeld's n.
    Pugh's n.
    Schneider's n.
    Smillie's n.
    Smith-Petersen n.
    Thornton's n.
    Venable-Stuck n.
    Zickle's n.
nailing
    intramedullary n.
nates
navicula
navicular
nearthrosis
neck
    surgical n.
necrosis
    aseptic n.
    Paget's quiet n.
    Zenker's n.
needle
    Bunnell's n
    Keith's n.
    Turkel's n.
Neer's prosthesis
Nélaton's
    dislocation
    line
    operation
nerve
    peroneal n.
Neufeld's nail
neuralgia
    Morton's n.
neurapraxia
neurofibroma
neurofibromatosis

neurofibrositis
neurologic
neurolysis
neuroma
    Morton's n.
neuromuscular
neuropathy
neurorrhaphy
neuroskeletal
Neviaser's operation
Nicola's operation
nociceptor
    polymodal n.
node
    Bouchard's n's
    Heberden's n's
nodular
nodule
    Schmorl's n.
nomogram
nonunion
notch
    clavicular n.
    coracoid n.
    interclavicular n.
    intercondylar n.
    intervertebral n.
    semilunar n.
    trochlear n.
    vertebral n.
NSAIDs – nonsteroidal anti-
    inflammatory drugs
nuchal
nucleus
    n. pulposus
Ober's
    operation
    test
Ogston's
    line
    operation
olecranal
olecranarthritis
olecranarthrocace
olecranarthropathy
olecranoid
olecranon

olisthy
Ollier's
    disease
    dyschondroplasia
    operation
omoclavicular
omodynia
omohyoid
omoplata
omosternum
operation
    Abbott-Lucas o.
    Abbott's o.
    Adams' o.
    Adelmann's o.
    Albee-Delbet o.
    Albee's o.
    Albert's o.
    Alouette's o.
    Anderson's o.
    Annandale's o.
    Avila's o.
    Axer's o.
    Badgley's o.
    Bankhart's o.
    Barker's o.
    Barsky's o.
    Barton's o.
    Barwell's o.
    Bateman's o.
    Bent's o.
    Berger's o.
    Blount's o.
    Blundell-Jones o.
    Bobroff's o.
    Bosworth's o.
    Boyd's o.
    Brett's o.
    Bristow's o.
    Brittain's o.
    Brockman's o.
    Buck's o.
    Bunnell's o.
    Callahan's o.
    Campbell's o.
    Carrell's o.
    Cave-Rowe o.

operation (continued)
    Cave's o.
    Chiene's o.
    Cloward's o.
    Codivilla's o.
    Cole's o.
    Colonna's o.
    Compere's o.
    Conn's o.
    Credo's o.
    Crutchfield's o.
    Cubbins' o.
    Darrach's o.
    Davies-Colley o.
    Denuse's o.
    Dickson-Diveley o.
    Dickson's o.
    Dieffenbach's o.
    Dunn-Brittain o.
    Durman's o.
    Eden-Hybbinette o.
    Eggers' o.
    Ellis-Jones o.
    Elmslie-Cholmeley o.
    Evans' o.
    Eyler's o.
    Fahey's o.
    Fowler's o.
    Fritz-Lange o.
    Gant's o.
    Gatellier's o.
    Ghormley's o.
    Gibson's o.
    Gillespie's o.
    Gill's o.
    Girdlestone's o.
    Goldthwait's o.
    Graber-Duvernay o.
    Grice-Green o.
    Guleke-Stookey o.
    Haas' o.
    Hammond's o.
    Hark's o.
    Harmon's o.
    Harris-Beath o.
    Hauser's o.
    Heifitz's o.

operation (continued)
    Henderson's o.
    Hendry's o.
    Henry-Geist o.
    Heuter's o.
    Heyman's o.
    Hibbs' o.
    Hoffa-Lorenz o.
    Hoffa's o.
    Hohmann's o.
    Holme's o.
    Horwitz-Adams o.
    Houston's o.
    Howorth's o.
    Joplin's o.
    Kapel's o.
    Kellogg-Speed o.
    Kessler's o.
    Kidner's o.
    King-Richards o.
    Kirkaldy-Willis o.
    Kirmisson's o.
    Kocher's o.
    Koenig-Wittek o.
    Kolomnin's o.
    König's o.
    Kreuscher's o.
    Lambrinudi's o.
    Lange's o.
    Lapidus o.
    L'Episcopo's o.
    Levine's o.
    Littler's o.
    Littlewood's o.
    Lottes' o.
    Lucas-Cottrell o.
    Luck's o.
    Ludloff's o.
    Lund's o.
    MacAusland's o.
    Magnuson's o.
    Magnuson-Stack o.
    Mahorner-Mead o.
    Mauck's o.
    Mayo's o.
    Mazur's o.
    McBride's o.

operation (continued)
> McCarroll's o.
> McKeever's o.
> McLaughlin's o.
> Mikulicz's o.
> Milch's o.
> Mitchell's o.
> Morestin's o.
> Mumford-Gurd o.
> Nélaton's o.
> Neviaser's o.
> Nicola's o.
> Ober's o.
> Ogston's o.
> Ollier's o.
> Osborne's o.
> Osgood's o.
> Overholt's o.
> Paci's o.
> Palmer-Widen o.
> Pauwels' o.
> Pheasant's o.
> Phelps' o.
> Phemister's o.
> Pollock's o.
> Poncet's o.
> Putti-Platt o.
> Puusepp's o.
> Reichenheim-King o.
> Reverdin's o.
> Ridlon's o.
> Routier's o.
> Roux-Goldthwait o.
> Salter's o.
> Sayre's o.
> Schanz's o.
> Schede's o.
> shelf o.
> Slocum's o.
> Smith-Petersen o.
> Sofield's o.
> Speed-Boyd o.
> Stamm's o.
> Steindler's o.
> Swanson's o.
> Thomson's o.
> Turko's o.

operation (continued)
> Van Gorder's o.
> Vladimiroff's o.
> Wagoner's o.
> Watson-Jones o.
> Whitman's o.
> Wilson-McKeever o.
> Wyeth's o.
> Yount's o.
> Zahradnicek's o.
> Zancolli's o.

Oppenheim's sign
opponens
ortho. – orthopedics
orthopaedics (Br.)
orthopedic
orthopercussion
orthopraxy
orthosis
> Engen extension o.

orthotic
os
> o. calcis
> o. coxae
> o. cuboideum
> o. lunatum
> o. magnum
> o. naviculare
> o. peroneum
> o. pisiforme
> o. trapezium
> o. trigonum tarsi
> o. triquetrum
> o. vesalianum pedis

Osborne's operation
osfe-. See words beginning *osphy-.*
Osgood's operation
Osgood-Schlatter disease
osphyarthrosis
osphyomyelitis
osphyotomy
ossa
> o. suturarum

ossature
ossein
osseoaponeurotic
osseocartilaginous

osseofibrous
osseomucin
osseomucoid
osseosonometer
ooseosonometry
osseous
ossicle
ossicula
ossiculum
ossiferous
ossific
ossification
ossifluence
ossifying
osteal
ostealgia
osteanabrosis
ostearthrotomy
ostectomy
osteectopia
osteitis
    alveolar o.
    o. condensans ilii
    o. deformans
    o. fibrosa cystica
    o. fragilitans
    o. ossificans
    o. pubis
ostempyesis
osteoanagenesis
osteoanesthesia
osteoaneurysm
osteoarthritis
osteoarthropathy
osteoarthrosis
osteoarticular
osteoblast
osteoblastic
osteoblastoma
osteocachectic
osteocachexia
osteocampsia
osteocartilaginous
osteochondral
osteochondritis
    o. deformans juvenilis
    o. dissecans

osteochondritis (continued)
    o. ischiopubica
    o. necroticans
osteochondrodystrophy
osteochondrofibroma
osteochondrolysis
osteochondroma
osteochondromatosis
    synovial o.
osteochondromyxoma
osteochondropathia
osteochondropathy
osteochondrosarcoma
osteochondrosis
osteochondrous
osteoclasis
osteoclast
    Collin's o.
    Phelps-Gocht o.
    Rizzoli's o.
osteoclastic
osteoclastoma
osteocomma
osteocope
osteocystoma
osteocyte
osteodesmosis
osteodiastasis
osteodynia
osteodysplasty
osteodystrophia
    o. cystica
    o. fibrosa
osteodystrophy
osteoectasia
osteoepiphysis
osteofibrochondrosarcoma
osteofibroma
osteofibromatosis
osteogenesis
    o. imperfecta
    o. imperfecta cystica
osteogenic
osteogram
osteography
osteohydatidosis
osteoid

osteology
osteolysis
osteoma
      cavalryman's o.
      o. durum
      osteoid o.
      o. sarcomatosum
      o. spongiosum
osteomalacia
osteometry
osteomiosis
osteomyelitis
      Garré's o.
osteomyelodysplasia
osteomyelography
osteon
osteoneuralgia
osteopathy
osteopenia
osteoperiosteal
osteoperiostitis
osteopetrosis
osteophlebitis
osteophore
osteophyma
osteophyte
osteophytosis
osteoplastica
osteoplasty
osteopoikilosis
osteoporosis
osteoporotic
osteopsathyrosis
osteoradionecrosis
osteorrhagia
osteorrhaphy
osteosarcoma
osteosarcomatous
osteosclerosis
osteosclerotic
osteoscope
osteosis
osteostixis
osteosynovitis
osteosynthesis
osteothrombosis

osteotome
      Albee's o.
      Alexander's o.
      Blount's o.
      Bowen's o.
      Campbell's o.
      Carroll-Legg o.
      Carroll's o.
      Carroll-Smith-Petersen o.
      Cherry's o.
      Clayton's o.
      Cloward's o.
      Cobb's o.
      Converse's o.
      Cottle's o.
      Crane's o.
      Dingman's o.
      Epstein's o.
      Frazier's o.
      Hibbs' o.
      Hoke's o.
      Howorth's o.
      Kezerian's o.
      Lambotte-Henderson o.
      Lambotte's o.
      Legg's o.
      Leinbach's o.
      Mayfield's o.
      Meyerding's o.
      Miner's o.
      Moore's o.
      Rowland's o.
      Sheehan's o.
      Smith-Petersen o.
      Stille's o.
osteotomoclasis
osteotomy
      angulation o.
      block o.
      Coventry's o.
      cuneiform o.
      cup-and-ball o.
      displacement o.
      innominate o.
      linear o.
      Lorenz's o.
      Macewen's o.

osteotomy (continued)
    subtrochanteric o.
    transtrochanteric o.
osteotribe
osteotylus
Otto's
    disease
    pelvis
Overholt's operation
P–phosphorus
Paci's operation
packing
    Gelfoam p.
Paget's
    disease
    quiet necrosis
palm
palma
    p. manus
palmar
palmaris
Palmer-Widen operation
panarthritis
pannus
panosteitis
parallagma
paralysis
    Pott's p.
parameniscus
paramyoclonus
    p. multiplex
paramyotonia
    ataxia p.
    p. congenita
paramyotonus
paraplegia
parapophysis
parasacrum
parasternal
paratarsium
paratenon
paravertebral
paraxial
paresis
paresthesia
    Berger's p.
Parham's band

parietal
Parona's space
paronychia
    p. tendinosa
parosteal
parosteitis
parosteosis
patella
    p. bipartita
    p. cubiti
    floating p.
    p. partita
    slipping p.
patellapexy
patellar
patellectomy
patellofemoral
patellometer
Patrick's test
Pauwels' operation
Pauzat's disease
pectoral
pectoralgia
pectoralis
pectus
    p. carinatum
    p. excavatum
    p. gallinatum
    p. recurvatum
pedal
pedicle
    p. of vertebral arch
pediculus
    p. arcus vertebrae
Pellegrini-Stieda disease
pelvic
pelvifemoral
pelvimetry
pelviotomy
pelvis (pelves)
    Otto's p.
pelvisacral
pelvisacrum
pelvisection
pelvitrochanterian
pelvospondylitis
    p. ossificans

percuss
percussible
percussion
periarthritis
periarticular
peribursal
pericapsular
perichondrial
perichondritis
perichondrium
perichondroma
perichord
perichordal
pericoxitis
peridesmium
perimysium (perimysia)
perineum
perineuritis
perineurium
periosteal
periosteomyelitis
periosteophyte
periosteorrhaphy
periosteotome
    Alexander-Farabeuf p.
    Alexander's p.
periosteotomy
periosteum
periostitis
periostosis
peripatellar
perispondylitis
    Gibney's p
peritendineum
peritendinitis
    p. calcarea
    p. crepitans
peritenon
peritenoneum
peritenonitis
perivertebral
peroneal
peroneotibial
Perrin-Ferraton disease
Perthes' disease
pes
    p. abductus

pes (continued)
    p. adductus
    p. anserinus
    p. cavus
    congenital convex p.
      valgus
    p. equinovalgus
    equinovarus p.
    p. planovalgus
    p. planus
    p. pronatus
    p. supinatus
    p. valgus
    p. varus
petechia (petechiae)
phalangeal
phalangectomy
phalanges
phalangette
phalangitis
phalangization
phalangophalangeal
phalanx (phalanges)
    distal p.
    proximal p.
Pheasant's operation
Phelps-Gocht osteoclast
Phelps' operation
Phemister's operation
phocomelia
phonomyoclonus
phonomyogram
phonomyography
phosphorus
physeal
physiotherapy
physis
Pietrie's cast
pillion
pin
    Bohlman's p.
    Compere's p.
    Hagie's p.
    Hansen-Street p.
    Hatcher's p.
    Knowles' p.
    Moore's p.

pin (continued)
    Rush's p.
    Steinmann's p.
    Street's p.
    Turner's p.
    von Saal's p.
    Zimmer's p.
Piotrowski's sign
PIP – proximal interphalangeal
PIPJ – proximal interphalangeal
    joint
Pirie's bone
piriform
Pirogoff's amputation
piroxicam
plantar
plantaris
plantigrade
plate
    Badgley's p.
    Blount's p.
    Deyerle's p.
    Eggers' p.
    Elliott's p.
    epiphyseal p.
    Hoen's p.
    Jewett's p.
    Kessel's p.
    Laing's p.
    Lane's p.
    Lawson-Thornton p.
    McLaughlin's p.
    Moe's p.
    Sherman's p.
    Thornton's p.
    Wilson's p.
    Wright's p.
platypodia
pleurapophysis
plica (plicae)
plication
plombage
plombierung
pneumarthrogram
pneumarthrography
pneumarthrosis
pneumatorrhachis

pneumatoscope
pneumoencephalogram
pneumoencephalomyelogram
poculum
    p. diogenis
podagra
pododynia
pollicization
Pollock's operation
polyarthric
polyarthritis
polyarticular
polychondritis
polychondropathy
polydactylia
polydactylism
polydactyly
polydysspondylism
polydystrophy
polymetacarpia
polymetatarsia
polymyalgia
    p. rheumatica
polymyoclonus
polymyopathy
polymyositis
polyostotic
polyperiostitis
polyphalangia
polyphasic
polysyndactyly
polytendinitis
polytendinobursitis
Poncet's operation
poples
popliteal
position. See *General Surgical Terms* section.
Pott's
    disease
    fracture
    gangrene
    paralysis
Poulet's disease
prehallux
Preiser's disease
prepatellar

prescapular
prespondylolisthesis
presternum
pretarsal
pretibial
probe
    Bunnell's p.
process
    acromion p.
    articular p.
    capitular p.
    condyloid p.
    conoid p.
    coracoid p.
    intercondylar p.
    mastoid p.
    odontoid p.
    olecranon p.
    spinous p.
    styloid p.
    ungual p.
    xiphoid p.
processus
    p. spinosus vertebrarum
    p. transversus vertebrarum
pronation
pronatoflexor
pronator
propriospinal
prosthesis
    Aufranc-Turner p.
    Austin-Moore p.
    Bateman's p.
    Bechtol's p.
    CAD (computerized
      assisted design) p.
    Charnley-Mueller p.
    DePalma's p.
    DePuy's p.
    Eicher's p.
    Geomedic p.
    geometric p.
    Giliberty's p.
    Guepar's p.
    Judet's p.
    Lippman's p.
    MacIntosh's p.

prosthesis (continued)
    Matchett-Brown p.
    McKee-Farrar p.
    McKeever's p.
    Moore's p.
    Mueller's p.
    Neer's p.
    Shier's p.
    Smith-Petersen p.
    Swanson's p.
    Thompson's p.
    Townley's p.
    Vitallium p.
    Walldius' p.
    Zimaloy's p.
    Zimmer's p.
prosthetic
protovertebra
protractor
    Robinson's p.
protrusion
pseudoarthrosis
pseudoepiphysis
pseudofracture
pseudogout
pseudohypertrophic
pseudoluxation
psoas muscle
pubetrotomy
pubic
pubioplasty
pubiotomy
pubis (pubes)
pubofemoral
pubotibial
Pugh's nail
pulvinar
punch
    Deyerle's p.
Putti-Platt operation
Putti's rasp
Puusepp's operation
pyarthrosis
pyknotic
pylon
pyogenic
quadrant

quadratipronator
quadriceps
quadricepsplasty
quadriplegia
Queckenstedt's sign
Quervain's
    disease
    fracture
RA – rheumatoid arthritis
rabdo-. See words beginning
   rhabdo-.
rachialgia
rachicentesis
rachidial
rachidian
rachigraph
rachilysis
rachiocampsis
rachiocentesis
rachiochysis
rachiodynia
rachiokyphosis
rachiometer
rachiomyelitis
rachiopathy
rachioscoliosis
rachiotome
rachiotomy
rachis
rachisagra
rachischisis
rachitic
rachitis
rachitome
rachitomy
radial
radicular
radiculectomy
radiculitis
radiculoganglionitis
radiculomedullary
radiculomeningomyelitis
radiculomyelopathy
radiculoneuritis
radiculoneuropathy
radiculopathy
radiobicipital

radiocarpal
radiocarpus
radiodigital
radiohumeral
radiolucent
radiomuscular
radiopalmar
radioulnar
radius
ragocyte
rake. See words beginning *rachi-.*
rakealjea. See *rachialgia.*
rakeo-. See words beginning
   rachio-.
rakitis. See *rachitis.*
ramus (rami)
    r. of pubis
Raney-Crutchfield tong
range of motion
rasp
    Putti's r.
raspatory
    Kirmisson's r.
Rauchfuss's sling
ray
    digital r.
reamer
    Küntscher's r.
    Moore's r.
    Rush's r.
Recklinghausen's disease
recurvation
Redivac drain
reducible
reduction
    closed r.
    open r.
reef
reefing
reflex
    Achilles tendon r.
    adductor r.
    antagonistic r's
    Bechterew-Mendel r.
    Bechterew's r.
    Chaddock's r.
    cremasteric r.

reflex (continued)
    Mayer's r.
    patellar r.
    patelloadductor r.
    scapulohumeral r.
    Stookey r.
    Strümpell's r.
    triceps r.
refracture
Reichel's chondromatosis
Reichenheim-King operation
rete
    r. articulare genus
    r. calcaneum
    r. carpi dorsale
retinaculum
retractor
    Bankhart's r.
    Beckman-Adson r.
    Bennett's r.
    Blount's r.
    cobra r.
    Gelpi's r.
    Hibb's r.
    Hohmann's r.
    Meyerding's r.
    Rizzo's r.
    Senn's r.
    Sweet's r.
retrocalcaneobursitis
retropatellar
retropulsion
retrosternal
Reverdin's operation
RF - rheumatoid factor
rhabdomyoma
rhabdomyosarcoma
rheumatism
    Besnier's r.
    MacLeod's capsular r.
    palindromic r.
rheumatoid
rheumatologist
rhizomelic
rhizotomy
rhomboid
    Michaelis's r.

rib
    bicipital r.
    cervical r.
    false r's
    floating r's
    slipping r.
    spurious r's
    Stiller's r.
    true r's
    vertebral r's
    vertebrocostal r's
    vertebrosternal r's
Ricard's amputation
Richard's screw
rickets
Ridlon's operation
RIF - right iliac fossa
rigidity
    cogwheel r.
risomelik. See *rhizomelic.*
Risser's cast
Rizzoli's osteoclast
Rizzo's retractor
Robinson's protractor
rod
    Harrington's r.
    Rush's r.
ROM - range of motion
Romberg's sign
romboid. See *rhomboid.*
rongeur
    Cloward's r.
    Kerrison's r.
    Leksell's r.
    Schlesinger's r.
roomatizm. See *rheumatism.*
rotation
Routier's operation
Roux-Goldthwait operation
Rowland's osteotome
Royalite body jacket
Rush's
    mallet
    pin
    reamer
    rod
Russell's traction

Russe's bone graft
Ryerson's tenotome
sacral
sacralgia
sacralization
sacrathrogenic
sacrectomy
sacroanterior
sacrococcygeal
sacrococcyx
sacrocoxalgia
sacrocoxitis
sacrodynia
sacroiliac
sacroiliitis
sacrolisthesis
sacrolumbar
sacroperineal
sacroposterior
sacropromontory
sacrosciatic
sacrospinal
sacrotomy
sacrovertebral
sacrum
    assimilation s.
    tilted s.
sagittal
Salter's operation
Sarbó's sign
sarcoblast
sarcoidosis
    muscular s.
sarcolemma
sarcoma (sarcomata)
    Ewing's s.
    osteogenic s.
    reticulum cell s.
sarcomere
sarcoplasm
sarcoplast
Satterlee's saw
saucerization
saw
    Adams' s.
    Butcher's s.

saw (continued)
    Charrière's s.
    Gigli's s.
    Langenbeck's s.
    Satterlee's s.
    Stryker's s.
Sayre's
    apparatus
    jacket
    operation
    splint
scalene
scalenectomy
scalenotomy
scan
    bone s.
scaphoid
scaphoiditis
    tarsal s.
scapula
scapulalgia
scapular
scapulectomy
scapuloclavicular
scapulodynia
scapulohumeral
scapulopexy
scapuloposterior
scapulothoracic
Scarpa's triangle
Schanz's
    disease
    operation
    syndrome
Schede's operation
Scheuermann's
    disease
    kyphosis
Schlatter's disease
Schlesinger's
    rongeur
    sign
Schmorl's
    body
    disease
    nodule

Schneider's nail
Schoemaker's line
sciatic
sciatica
scissors
    Kreuscher's s.
    Wester's s.
scoliokyphosis
scoliosis
    Brissaud's s.
    cicatricial s.
    coxitic s.
    empyematic s.
    inflammatory s.
    ischiatic s.
    myopathic s.
    ocular s.
    ophthalmic s.
    osteopathic s.
    paralytic s.
    rachitic s.
    rheumatic s.
    sciatic s.
    static s.
scoliosometer
scoliotic
scoliotone
scolopsia
screw
    Basile's s.
    Bosworth's s.
    Collison's s.
    Coventry's s.
    Eggers' s.
    Kristiansen's s.
    Leinbach's s.
    McAtee's s.
    McLaughlin's s.
    Richards' s.
    Sherman's s.
    Thornton's s.
    Vitallium s.
    Zimmer's s.
scurvy
sella (sellae)
    s. turcica

semilunar
semilunare
Senn's retractor
sensorimuscular
sequestrectomy
sequestrum (sequestra)
sesamoid
sesamoiditis
Sever's disease
sfirektome. See *sphyrectomy.*
sfirotome. See *sphyrotomy.*
Sharpey's fibers
Sheehan's osteotome
Shenton's line
Shepherd's fracture
Sherman's
    plate
    screw
Shier's prosthesis
SI – sacroiliac
siatik. See *sciatic.*
siatika. See *sciatica.*
sign
    Allis' s.
    Amoss' s.
    Anghelescu's s.
    anterior tibial s.
    Babinski's s.
    Beevor's s.
    Bonnet's s.
    Bragard's s.
    Brudzinski's s.
    Bryant's s.
    Chvostek's s.
    Chvostek-Weiss s.
    Cleeman's s.
    Codman's s.
    Comolli's s.
    Coopernail's s.
    Dawbarn's s.
    Dejerine's s.
    Demianoff's s.
    Desault's s.
    drawer s.
    Dupuytren's s.
    Erichsen's s.

sign (continued)
    fabere s.
    Fajersztajn's s.
    Fränkel's s.
    Froment's s.
    Gaenslen's s.
    Galeazzi's s.
    Goldthwait's s.
    Guilland's s.
    Hefke-Turner s.
    Helbing's s.
    Hirschberg's s.
    Hoffmann's s.
    Homans' s.
    Hueter's s.
    Kanavel's s.
    Keen's s.
    Kernig's s.
    Kerr's s.
    Langoria's s.
    Lasègue's s.
    Laugier's s.
    Leichtenstern's s.
    Leri's s.
    Lhermitte's s.
    Linder's s.
    Lorenz's s.
    Ludloff's s.
    Maisonneuve's s.
    Marie-Foix s.
    McMurray's s.
    Mennell's s.
    Minor's s.
    Morquio's s.
    Oppenheim's s.
    Piotrowski's s.
    pronation s.
    Queckenstedt's s.
    radialis s.
    Romberg's s.
    sail s.
    Sarbó's s.
    Schlesinger's s.
    Soto-Hall s.
    Strümpell's s.
    Strunsky's s.
    Thomas' s.

sign (continued)
    tibialis s.
    Tinel's s.
    Turyn's s.
    Vanzetti's s.
    Wartenberg's s.
    Westphal's s.
Silver's bunionectomy
simphysis. See *symphysis.*
sin-. See words beginning *syn-.*
sinew
sino-. See words beginning *syno-.*
sinus
    tarsal s.
skeletal
skeleton
skewfoot
Skillern's fracture
SLE – systemic lupus
    erythematosus
sling
        Glisson's s.
        Rauchfuss' s.
        Teare's s.
Slocum's operation
SLR – straight leg raising
Smedberg's drill
Smillie's
    knife
    meniscotome
    nail
Smith-Petersen
    nail
    operation
    osteotome
    prosthesis
Smith's
    dislocation
    fracture
soas-. See *psoas.*
Sofield's operation
Soto-Hall sign
space
    palmar s.
    Parona's s.
    thenar s.
    web s's

Spanish windlass
spasmus
    s. nutans
spastic
Speed-Boyd operation
sphenoid
sphyrectomy
sphyrotomy
spica
    hip s.
spina
    s. bifida occulta
spinal
spinalgia
spine
    bamboo s.
    cervical s.
spinifugal
spinipetal
spinobulbar
spinocerebellar
spinocostalis
spinogalvanization
spinoglenoid
spinogram
spinous
splayfoot
splint
    Agnew's s.
    airplane s.
    Anderson's s.
    Angle's s.
    Ashhurst's s.
    Balkan s.
    banjo s.
    Baylor's s.
    Böhler-Braun s.
    Böhler's s.
    Bond's s.
    Bowlby's s.
    Brant's s.
    Buck's s.
    buddy s.
    Cabot's s.
    Chandler's s.
    coaptation s.
    cock-up s.

splint (continued)
    Colles' s.
    Curry's s.
    Davis' s.
    Denis-Browne clubfoot s.
    DePuy's s.
    drop-foot s.
    Dupuytren's s.
    Eggers' s.
    Englemann's s.
    Fox's s.
    Frejka's s.
    Futura s.
    Gordon's s.
    Hart's s.
    Hodgen's s.
    Jones' s.
    Kanavel's s.
    Keller-Blake s.
    Kirschner wire s.
    Lewin's s.
    Lewin-Stern s.
    Liston's s.
    Lytle's s.
    Mason-Allen s.
    opponens s.
    plaster s.
    Protecto s.
    Sayre's s.
    Stader's s.
    Taylor's s.
    Thomas' s.
    Tobruk s.
    Valentine's s.
    Volkmann's s.
    Wertheim's s.
    Zimmer's s.
spondylalgia
spondylarthritis
    s. ankylopoietica
spondylarthrocace
spondylexarthrosis
spondylitic
spondylitis
    ankylosing s.
    Bekhterev's s.
    s. deformans

spondylitis (continued)
    hypertrophic s.
    s. infectiosa
    Kümmell's s.
    Marie-Strümpell s.
    rheumatoid s.
    rhizomelic s.
    tuberculous s.
    s. typhosa
spondylizema
spondyloarthropathy
spondylocace
spondylodesis
spondylodynia
spondylolisthesis
spondylolisthetic
spondylolysis
spondylomalacia
    s. traumatica
spondylopathy
    traumatic s.
spondylopyosis
spondyloschisis
spondylosis
    cervical s.
    s. chronica ankylopoietica
    rhizomelic s.
    s. uncovertebralis
spondylosyndesis
spondylotherapy
spondylotic
spondylotomy
spondylous
spongiosa
spongiosaplasty
spot
    Carleton's s's
sprain
    riders' s.
Spratt's curet
Sprengel's deformity
spur
    calcaneal s.
    occipital s.
    olecranon s.
Spurling's test

Stader's splint
Stamm's operation
stapler
    Blount's s.
Steindler's operation
Steinert's disease
Steinmann's pin
stellate
stenosed
sternal
sternebra
sternoclavicular
sternocleidal
sternocleidomastoid
sternocostal
sternoscapular
sternoschisis
sternotomy
sternovertebral
sternum
Stieda's fracture
Stiller's rib
Stille's osteotome
stimulator
stockinette
stocking
    Jobst's s.
    thromboembolic s.
Stokes' amputation
Stone's bunionectomy
Stookey reflex
stratification
Street's pin
striated
Strümpell's
    reflex
    sign
Strunsky's sign
Stryker's
    frame
    saw
styloid
styloiditis
stylopodium
subacromial
subaponeurotic

subarachnoid
subastragalar
subcapsuloperiosteal
subchondral
subclavicular
subcostal
subdeltoid
subdiaphragmatic
subdural
subhumeral
subluxation
    Volkmann's s.
submaxillary
subparietal
subperiosteal
subscapular
substantia
    s. spongiosa ossium
subsultus
    s. tendinum
subtalar
subtarsal
subvertebral
Sudeck's atrophy
sudoluxation. See
    pseudoluxation.
sulcus
supinate
supination
supinator
supine
supraclavicular
supracondylar
supracostal
supraepicondyle
supraepitrochlear
supraglenoid
supralumbar
supramalleolar
suprapatellar
suprapubic
suprascapular
supraspinal
supraspinous
suprasternal
supratrochlear

sura
sural
surgical procedures. See
    operation.
suspensory
sustentacular
sustentaculum
suture. See *General Surgical*
    Terms section.
Swanson's
    operation
    prosthesis
swayback
Swediaur's disease
Sweet's retractor
symbrachydactyly
Syme's amputation
symphalangia
symphysis
    s. pubis
synarthrophysis
synarthrosis
synchondrectomy
synchondroses
synchondrosis
synchondrotomy
synclonus
syndactyly
syndesis
syndesmectomy
syndesmectopia
syndesmitis
    s. metatarsea
syndesmography
syndesmology
syndesmoma
syndesmo-odontoid
syndesmopexy
syndesmophyte
syndesmoplasty
syndesmorrhaphy
syndesmosis
syndesmotomy
syndrome
    Albright's s.
    Arnold-Chiari s.

syndrome (continued)
    Baastrup's s.
    Bakwin-Eiger s.
    Barré-Liéou s.
    Bertolotti's s.
    carpal tunnel s.
    cervical s.
    Guillain-Barré s.
    Klippel-Feil s.
    Legg-Calvé-Perthes s.
    Looser-Milkman s.
    Marfan's s.
    Milkman's s.
    Naffziger's s.
    scalenus anticus s.
    Schanz's s.
    Tietze's s.
synosteology
synosteotomy
synostosis
    radioulnar s.
    tarsal s.
synovectomy
synovia
synovial
synovioma
synoviosarcoma
synoviparous
synovitis
synovium
syntenosis
synthesis
    s. of continuity
synthetism
syntripsis
syringocele
syringomyelia
syringomyelitis
syringomyelocele
systemic lupus erythematosus
T-1, T-2, etc.–thoracic vertebrae
tabatière anatomique
tailbone
talar
taliped
talipes
    t. calcaneovalgus

talipes (continued)
    t. calcaneovarus
    t. calcaneus
    t. cavovalgus
    t. cavus
    t. equinovalgus
    t. equinovarus
    t. equinus
    t. planovalgus
    t. valgus
    t. varus
talipomanus
Talma's disease
talocalcaneal
talocrural
talofibular
talonavicular
taloscaphoid
talotibial
talus
tank
    Hubbard's t.
tarsal
tarsalgia
tarsectomy
tarsectopia
tarsoclasis
tarsomegaly
tarsometatarsal
tarsophalangeal
tarsoptosis
tarsotarsal
tarsotibial
tarsus
Taylor's
    brace
    splint
Teale's amputation
tear
    bucket-handle t.
Teare's sling
TED–thromboembolic disease
teerfo. See *tirefond*.
template
    Moore's t.
tendines
tendinitis

tendinoplasty
tendinosuture
tendinous
tendo
  t. Achillis
  t. calcaneus
tendolysis
tendon
  Achilles t.
  calcaneal t.
  flexor carpi radialis t.
  flexor digitorum
    profundus t.
  flexor digitorum sublimis
    t.
  t. of Hector
  palmaris longus t.
  patellar t.
  rider's t.
tendoplasty
tenectomy
tenodesis
tenodynia
tenolysis
tenomyoplasty
tenomyotomy
tenonectomy
tenontagra
tenontitis
  t. prolifera calcarea
tenontodynia
tenontophyma
tenontothecitis
tenophyte
tenoplasty
tenorrhaphy
tenositis
tenostosis
tenosuspension
tenosynovectomy
tenosynovitis
tenotome
  Ryerson's t.
tenotomy
tenovaginitis
TENS – transcutaneous electrical
  nerve stimulator

Tensilon test
tensor
teres
test
  apprehension t.
  Bekhterev's t.
  Callaway's t.
  Chiene's t.
  Cybex t.
  Dugas' t.
  Ely's t.
  erythrocyte sedimentation
    rate t.
  fabere (fixation,
    abduction, external
    rotation, extension) t.
  Finklestein's t.
  Hamilton's t.
  Jansen's t.
  latex fixation t.
  lupus erythematosus (LE)
    cell t.
  McMurray's t.
  Mills' t.
  Ober's t.
  Patrick's t.
  rheumatoid factor t.
  serum calcium t.
  serum creatine kinase t.
  serum phosphorus t.
  Spurling's t.
  straight leg raising t.
  Tensilon t.
  Thomas' t.
  thumbnail t.
  Tinel's t.
  Trendelenburg's t.
  uric acid t.
theca (thecae)
thecal
thecitis
thecostegnosis
thenar
thermophore
Thomas'
  collar
  sign

Thomas' (continued)
    splint
    test
Thompson's prosthesis
Thomson's operation
thoracic
thoracicohumeral
thoracispinal
thoracolumbar
thorax
Thornton's
    nail
    plate
    screw
thrust
    paraspinal t.
thrypsis
thumb
    bifid t.
    tennis t.
    trigger t.
tibia
    saber t.
    t. valga
    t. vara
tibiad
tibial
tibialgia
tibialis
tibiocalcanean
tibiofemoral
tibiofibular
tibionavicular
tibioperoneal
tibioscaphoid
tibiotarsal
Tietze's syndrome
Tinel's
    sign
    test
tirefond
tiring
tissue
    osseous t.
Tobruk splint
toe
    hammer t.

toe (continued)
    Morton's t.
tong
    Barton's t.
    Crutchfield's t.
    Raney-Crutchfield t.
tonoclonic
tonus
tophaceous
tophi
tophus
torsion
torsionometer
torticollis
tourniquet
    Esmarch's t.
    pneumatic t.
Townley's prosthesis
trabecula (trabeculae)
trabecular
trabeculation
traction
    Bryant's t.
    Buck's t.
    halo-pelvic t.
    Russell's t.
    skeletal t.
transfix
transfixion
transiliac
transischiac
translateral
transplantation
transposition
transpubic
transsacral
transsection
transsphenoidal
transsternal
transversalis
transverse
transversectomy
transversotomy
trapezial
trapeziform
trapeziometacarpal
trapezium

trapezoid
Trendelenburg's
        gait
        test
trephine
        Michele's t.
        Turkel's t.
triangle
        Scarpa's t.
        Ward's t.
triceps
triphalangeal
triphasic
Tripier's amputation
triquetrum
trochanter
trochanteric
trochanterplasty
trochlea
trochlear
tubercle
tuberculosis
        t. of bone
tuberositas
tuberosity
tucker
        Bishop-Black tendon t.
        Bishop-DeWitt tendon t.
        Bishop-Peter tendon t.
        Bishop's tendon t.
        Burch-Greenwood
          tendon t.
        Fink's tendon t.
tumefacient
tumefaction
tumor
        Ewing's t.
        giant cell t.
tumorous
turgid
Turkel's
        needle
        trephine
Turko's operation
Turner's pin
Turyn's sign
Ullmann's line

ulna
ulnad
ulnar
ulnare
ulnaris
ulnocarpal
ulnoradial
ultrasonics
ultrasound
uncovertebral
uncus
        u. corporis
        u. of hamate bone
uniarticular
unilateral
unmyelinated
Unna's paste boot
Valentine's splint
valgus
Van Buren's forceps
Van Gorder's operation
Vanzetti's sign
varus
vein
        antebrachial cephalic v.
        cephalic v.
        saphenous v.
Velpeau's deformity
Venable-Stuck nail
Verbrugge's clamp
vertebra (vertebrae)
        cervical v. (C1-C7)
        coccygeal v.
        lumbar v. (L1-L5)
        sacral v.
        thoracic v. (T1-T12 or
          D1-D12)
vertebral
vertebrectomy
vertebrochondral
vertebrocostal
vertebrofemoral
vertebrogenic
vertebroiliac
vertebrosacral
vertebrosternal
vesalianum

vinculum
    v. breve
    v. longum
visceral
Vitallium
    drill
    mesh
    prosthesis
    screw
Vladimiroff-Mikulicz
    amputation
Vladimiroff's operation
volar
volardorsal
volaris
Volkmann's
    contracture
    deformity
    disease
    splint
    subluxation
vomer
von Gies' joint
von Recklinghausen's disease
von Saal's pin
Wagoner's operation
Wagstaffe's fracture
Waldenström's disease
Walldius' prosthesis
Ward's triangle
Wartenberg's
    disease
    sign
Watson-Jones operation
webbed
Webb's bolt
weight-bearing
Wertheim's splint
Wester's
    clamp
    scissors
Westphal's
    sign
    zone
whitlow
    herpetic w.
    thecal w.

Whitman's
    frame
    operation
Williams'
    clamp
    exercise
Wilman's clamp
Wilson-McKeever operation
Wilson's
    awl
    bolt
    clamp
    plate
    wrench
windlass
    Spanish w.
wire
    Kirschner's w.
wormian bone
wrench
    Wilson's w.
Wright's plate
Wrisberg's ligament
wrist
wristdrop
wryneck
Wyeth's operation
xanthoma
    x. disseminatum
xanthomatosis
xanthosarcoma
xiphisternum
xiphocostal
xiphoid
xiphoiditis
xiphopagotomy
Yount's operation
Zahradnicek's operation
Zancolli's operation
zanthoma. See *xanthoma.*
zanthomatosis. See
    xanthomatosis.
zanthosarkoma. See
    xanthosarcoma.
Zenker's
    degeneration
    necrosis

Zickle's nail
zifisternum. See *xiphisternum.*
zifo-. See words beginning *xipho-.*
zifoid. See *xiphoid.*
Zimaloy's prosthesis
Zimmer's
    pin
    prosthesis
    screw

Zimmer's (continued)
    splint
zone
    cornuradicular z.
    Lissauer's z.
    Looser's z.
    orbicular z. of hip
    Westphal's z.
Zuckerkandl's dehiscence

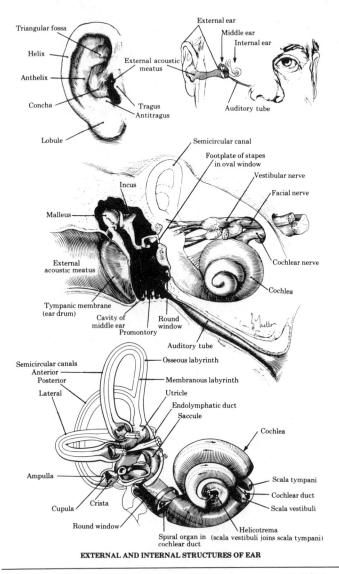

EXTERNAL AND INTERNAL STRUCTURES OF EAR

(Courtesy of Dorland's Illustrated Medical Dictionary, 27th ed. Plate 15. Philadelphia, W. B. Saunders Company, 1988.)

Otorhinolaryngology

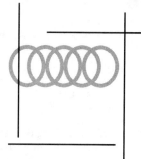

Abelson's adenotome
ablation
ABR – auditory brain stem
    evoked response
Abraham's cannula
abscess
    alveolar a.
    Bezold's a.
    dural a.
    extradural a.
    masticator a.
    orbital a.
    peritonsillar a.
    retropharyngeal a.
    subdural a.
    subperiosteal a.
AC – air conduction
achalasia
acouesthesia
acoumeter
acoumetry
acouometer
acouophone
acouophonia
acoustic
    a. immitance
    a. neuroma
    a. reflex
acousticofacial
acousticon
acoustics
acquired immunodeficiency
    syndrome
acrocephalosyndactyly
AD – right ear (auris dextra)
Adam's apple
Adams' operation
adaptor
    House's a.

adenocaracinoma
adenofibroma
    a. edematodes
adenoid
adenoidectomy
adenoidism
adenoiditis
adenoma
    oxyphil a.
    pleomorphic a.
    serous cell a.
adenopathy
adenotome
    Abelson's a.
    Kelley's a.
    Laforce-Grieshaber a.
    Laforce's a.
    Shambaugh's a.
    Sluder's a.
adenotomy
adenotonsillectomy
adenovirus
aditus
    a. ad antrum
    a. ad antrum mastoideum
    a. ad antrum tympanicum
    a. laryngis
Adler's punch
Adson's forceps
afagopraksea. See *aphagopraxia.*
aftha. See *aphtha.*
aftho-. See words beginning
    aphtho-.
agger
    a. nasi
AIDS – acquired
    immunodeficiency
    syndrome
air bone gap

661

ala
   a. auris
   a. nasi
alae
alaryngeal
Albers-Schönberg disease
Albert-Andrews laryngoscope
albinism
Alexander's
   chisel
   gouge
allergen
allergenic
allergy
Allport's
   retractor
   searcher
Almoor's operation
Alport's disease
Alstrom's disease
alveolonasal
ama
Ameslan – American Sign
   Language
amplification
ampulla
anaerobe
anakusis
anastomosis
   Galen's a.
   Jacobson's a.
Andrews'
   applicator
   gouge
Andrews-Hartmann forceps
anesthesia. See *General Surgical
   Terms* section.
aneurysm
angina
   Ludwig's a.
   Plaut-Vincent a.
angiofibroma
   nasopharyngeal a.
angle
   olfactive a.
   olfactory a.
   ophryospinal a.

angle (continued)
   orifacial a.
   Topinard's a.
angulus
   a. mastoideus ossis
      parietalis
ankyloglossia
ankylosis
   cricoarytenoid joint a.
ankylotia
ankylotome
ankylotomy
annulus
   a. tracheae
   tympanic a.
   a. tympanicus
   Vieussen's a.
anosmatic
anosmia
   a. gustatoria
   preferential a.
   a. respiratoria
anosphrasia
anotia
anthelix
Anthony's tube
antibody
antigen
antihelix
antihistamine
antihistaminic
antitragus
antral
antrectomy
antritis
antroatticotomy
antrocele
antronalgia
antronasal
antroscope
antroscopy
antrostomy
antrotomy
antrotympanic
antrotympanitis
antrum
   attic-aditus a.

antrum (continued)
    a. auris
    ethmoid a.
    a. ethmoidale
    frontal a.
    a. highmori
    mastoid a.
    a. mastoideum
    a. maxillare
    maxillary a.
    a. of Highmore
    tympanic a.
    a. tympanicum
anulus tympanicus
anvil
Apert's syndrome
apertura
    a. chordae tympani
    a. externa aqueductus
      vestibuli
    a. sinus frontalis
    a. sinus sphenoidalis
    a. tympanica canaliculi
aperture
    a. of frontal sinus
    a. of larynx
    a. of sphenoid sinus
    tympanic a. of canaliculus
      of chorda tympani
apex
    a. auriculae
    a. linguae
    a. nasi
aphagopraxia
aphasia
aphonia
    a. paralytica
    spastic a.
aphtha
aphthosis
aphthous
apnea
    sleep a.
aponeurosis
applicator
    Andrews' a.
    Brown's a.

applicator (continued)
    Dean's a.
    Holinger's a.
    Lathbury's a.
    Lejeune's a.
    Pynchon's a.
    Roberts' a.
apraxia
aqueduct
    a. of cochlea
    a. of Cotunnius
    fallopian a.
    a. of Fallopius
    a. of the vestibule
aqueductus
    a. endolymphaticus
    a. vestibuli
arachnorhinitis
Arbuckle's probe
arch
    auricular a.
    a's of Corti
    palatine a.
arcus
    a. glossopalatinus
    a. lipoides myringis
    a. palatini
    a. palatoglossus
    a. palatopharyngeus
    a. pharyngopalatinus
area
    Kiesselbach's a.
areepi-. See words beginning
    aryepi-.
aretenoid. See *arytenoid.*
argyria
    a. nasalis
arhinia
ariteno-. See words beginning
    aryteno-.
arjirea. See *argyria.*
Arnold's nerve
Arslan's operation
arteritis
artery
    carotid a.
    occipital a.

artery (continued)
    pharyngeal a.
    thyroid a.
arthritis
    cricoarytenoid a.
    rheumatoid a.
articulation
    a's of auditory ossicles
aryepiglottic
aryepiglotticus
aryepiglottidean
arytenoepiglottic
arytenoid
arytenoidectomy
arytenoideus
arytenoiditis
arytenoidopexy
AS–left ear (auris sinistra)
Asch's
    operation
    splint
aspergillosis
Aspergillus
asphyxia
aspiration
aspirator
    Gottschalk's a.
asterion
asthma
ataxia
atelectasis
Atkins-Tucker laryngoscope
atomizer
    Devilbiss' a.
atresia
atrium
    a. glottidis
    a. laryngis
    a. matus medii
    a. of glottis
    a. of larynx
attic
atticitis
atticoantrotomy
atticomastoid
atticotomy
    transmeatal a.

AU–both ears (aures unitas)
    each ear (auris uterque)
audiogram
audiologist
audiology
audiometer
audiometric
audiometrician
audiometry
audiosurgery
audiphone
audition
auditive
auditognosis
auditory
    a. canal
    a. meatus
Aufricht-Lipsett rasp
Aufricht's
    rasp
    retractor
    speculum
aura
    a. asthmatica
aural
aures
auricle
auricula
auricular
auriculare
auricularis
auriculocranial
auriculotemporal
auriculoventricular
aurilave
aurinarium
aurinasal
auriphone
auripuncture
auris
    a. externa
    a. interna
    a. media
auriscalpium
auriscope
auris dextra
auris sinistra

aurist
auristics
auristilla
auristillae
auris uterque
aurogauge
aurometer
autophony
Avellis' syndrome
avulsion
axoneme
axonotmesis
axoplasm
Baelz's syndrome
bag
    Politzer's b.
Ballenger's
    curet
    elevator
    forceps
    knife
Ballenger-Sluder tonsillectome
balloon
    intranasal b.
Bane's forceps
Bárány's
    symptom
    syndrome
    test
Barlow's forceps
Barnhill's curet
barosinusitis
barotitis
    b. media
barotrauma
BC–bone conduction
Bechterew's nucleus
Becker's operation
Beckman-Colver speculum
Beck-Mueller tonsillectome
Beck-Schenck tonsillectome
Beck's knife
Bellocq's cannula
Bell's palsy
Bellucci's scissors
Bermingham's nasal
    douche

Berne's
    forceps
    rasp
Bespaloff's sign
Beyer's
    forceps
    rongeur
Bezold's
    abscess
    mastoiditis
    perforation
Biderman's sign
Bieg's sign
Billeau's curet
Billroth's operation
binaural
binauricular
Bing's test
binotic
Bizzarri-Guiffrida
    laryngoscope
black hairy tongue
Blakemore's tube
Blake's forceps
Blakesley's forceps
blennorrhea
    Stoerk's b.
Blom-Singer prosthesis
Boettcher's
    forceps
    hook
    scissors
bone
    b. conduction
    hyoid b.
    petrous b.
    squamosal b.
    temporal b.
    tympanic b.
    zygomatic b.
border
    vermilion b.
Boro's esophagoscope
Bostock's catarrh
Bosworth's snare
Boucheron's speculum
Bouchut's tube

bougie
  Hurst's b.
  Jackson's b.
  Plummer's b.
Boyle's law
branchia
branchial
  b. arch
  b. cleft
branchiogenic
branchiogenous
branchioma
branchiomere
branchiomeric
branchiomerism
Branhamella
  B. catarrhalis
breathiness
Breslow's classification
bronchi
bronchial
bronchiectasis
bronchogram
bronchography
bronchoscope
bronchoscopy
bronchus
Brown's
  applicator
  needle
  retractor
  snare
  tonsillectome
Broyles'
  esophagoscope
  laryngoscope
  nasopharyngoscope
Bruening's
  esophagoscope
  forceps
  otoscope
  snare
Brun's curet
Brunton's otoscope
bruxism
BTE – behind the ear

bucca
  b. cavi oris
buccal
buccoglossopharyngitis
buccomaxillary
buccopharyngeal
Buck's
  curet
  knife
bulla
  b. ethmoidalis cavi
    nasi
  b. ethmoidalis ossi
    ethmoidalis
  b. ossea
bullous
bur
  diamond b.
  Hall's b.
  Jordan-Day b.
  Lempert's b.
  Wullstein's b.
bursa
  nasopharyngeal b.
  pharyngeal b.
bursitis
  Tornwaldt's b.
button
  polyethylene collar b.
calcification
calculus
  salivary c.
Caldwell-Luc operation
caliculus
  c. gustatorius
canal
  alveolar c's
  auditory c.
  carotid c.
  eustachian c.
  Huschke's c.
  c. of Corti
  palatine c's
  semicircular c.
canaliculus
  c. chordae tympani
  c. cochleae
  mastoid c.

canaliculus (continued)
    c. mastoideus
    c. of chorda tympani
    c. of cochlea
    tympanic c.
    c. tympanicus
canaloplasty
cancrum
    c. nasi
    c. oris
Candida
    C. albicans
candidiasis
Canfield's
    knife
    operation
cannula
    Abraham's c.
    Bellocq's c.
    Coakley's c.
    Day's c.
    Goodfellow's c.
    Kos' c.
    Krause's c.
    Paterson's c.
    Scott's c.
cannulization
capitulum
    c. stapedis
capsule
    articular c.
caput stapedis
carcinoma
    acinic cell c.
    adenocystic c.
    basal cell c.
    epidermoid c.
    laryngeal c.
    mucoepidermoid c.
    nasopharyngeal c.
    schneiderian c.
    squamous cell c.
    tonsillar c.
Carhart notch
Carmack's curet
caroticotympanic
carotid
    c. artery

carotidynia
Carpenter's knife
Carpue's
    operation
    rhinoplasty
Carter's
    operation
    splint
cartilage
    alar c.
    arytenoid c.
    corniculate c.
    cricoid c.
    cuneiform c.
    epiglottic c.
    hyaline c.
    intrathyroid c.
    laryngeal c. of Luschka
    Santorini's c.
    thyroid c.
    Wrisberg's c.
cartilagines
    c. alares minores
    c. laryngis
    c. nasales accessoriae
    c. nasi
    c. sesamoideae nasi
    c. tracheales
cartilaginous
cartilago
    c. alaris major
    c. arytenoidea
    c. auriculae
    c. corniculata
    c. cricoidea
    c. cuneiformis
    e. epiglottica
    c. meatus acustici
    c. nasi lateralis
    c. santorini
    c. septi nasi
    c. sesamoidea laryngis
    c. sesamoidea ligamenti
        vocalis
    c. thyroidea
    c. triquetra

cartilago (continued)
    c. tubae auditivae
    c. wrisbergi
caruncle
    sublingual c.
caruncula
    c. salivaris
    c. sublingualis
Cassel's operation
Castelli's tube
catarrh
    Bostock's c.
catarrhal
catheter
    Yankauer's c.
catheterization
    laryngeal c.
cauda
    c. helicis
cavity
    tympanic c.
cavum
    c. conchae
    c. infraglotticum
    c. laryngis
    c. nasi
    c. nasi osseum
    c. oris
    c. oris externum
    c. pharyngis
    c. tympani
cecum
    cupular c. of cochlear duct
    c. cupulare ductus
      cochlearis
    vestibular c. of cochlear
      duct
    c. vestibulare ductus
      cochlearis
cellulae
    c. ethmoidales osseae
    c. mastoideae
    c. pneumaticae tubae
      auditivae
    c. pneumaticae tubariae
    c. tympanicae

cellulitis
    cervical c.
    orbital c.
    peritonsillar c.
cephalalgia
    histamine c.
    pharyngotympanic c.
cephalgia
cerebellopontine
    c. angle
cerumen
    inspissated c.
ceruminal
ceruminolysis
ceruminolytic
ceruminosis
ceruminous
cervical
chain
    ossicular c.
Chausse III projection
Cheever's operation
cheilectropion
cheilitis
cheilognathoprosoposchisis
cheilognathoschisis
cheilognathouranoschisis
cheiloplasty
cheiloschisis
cheilosis
chemodectoma
chemotherapy
Chevalier Jackson
    esophagoscope
    laryngoscope
    operation
    speculum
    tube
chisel
    Alexander's c.
    Converse's c.
    Derlacki's c.
    Derlacki-Shambaugh c.
    Fomon's c.
    Freer's c.
    guarded c.

chisel (continued)
    Hajek's c.
    House's c.
    Killian's c.
    Sewall's c.
    Shambaugh-Derlacki c.
    Sheehan's c.
    Troutman's c.
choana
choanae
    c. osseae
choanal
    s. atresia
choanoid
cholesteatoma
    c. tympani
chondritis
chondroma
chorda
    c. tympani
chordectomy
chorditis
    c. cantorum
    c. fibrinosa
    c. nodosa
    c. tuberosa
    c. vocalis
chromorhinorrhea
cicatricial
cicatrix
    manometric c.
Cicherelli's forceps
cilia
ciliary
Citelli-Meltzer punch
clamp
    Cottle's c.
    Jesberg's c.
Clark's classification
classification
    Breslow's c.
    Clark's c.
    Jewett's c.
    Lennert's c.
    Lukes-Collins c.
    Rappaport's c.

cleft
    c. lip
    laryngotracheoesophageal
      c.
    c. palate
Clerf's
    laryngoscope
    saw
Cloquet's ganglion
Coakley's
    cannula
    curet
    forceps
    operation
    speculum
    trocar
cochlea
cochleae
cochlear
    c. duct
    c. implant
    c. nerve
cochleariform
cochleitis
cochleovestibular
cochlitis
Cody's operation
cog-tooth
Cohen's forceps
collum
collunarium
columella
    c. cochleae
    c. nasi
columna
    c. nasi
columnae
Colver's
    forceps
    knife
Commando's operation
commissure
    laryngeal c.
commissurorrhaphy
Communitrach tube
compliance

computed tomography
concha
    c. auriculae
    c. bullosa
    ethmoidal c.
    c. nasalis inferior ossea
    c. nasalis media ossea
    c. nasalis superior ossea
    c. nasalis suprema ossea
    nasoturbinal c.
    c. of auricle
    sphenoidal c.
    c. sphenoidalis
conchae
conchitis
conchoscope
conchotome
conchotomy
concussion
conduction
    air c.
    bone c.
conjunctiva
conjunctivorhinostomy
constriction
conus
    c. elasticus laryngis
Converse's
    chisel
    rongeur
    speculum
cord
    vocal c.
cordal
cordectomy
Cordes-New forceps
cordopexy
cordotomy
corniculate
cornu
    ethmoid c.
    c. majus ossis hyoidei
    c. minus ossis hyoidei
cornua
corona
coronae
coronal

coronale
coronalis
corone
coronion
coronoid
Corti's
    arches
    canal
    organ
    rods
    tunnel
Corwin's hemostat
coryza
    allergic c.
    c. oedematosa
cosmesis
Costen's syndrome
Cottle-Arruga forceps
Cottle-Jansen forceps
Cottle-Kazanjian forceps
Cottle-Neivert retractor
Cottle's
    clamp
    elevator
    forceps
    knife
    osteotome
    rasp
    retractor
    saw
    scissors
    speculum
    tenaculum
Cotunnius
    aqueduct of C.
CPAP–continuous positive
    airway pressure
Craig's forceps
cranioaural
craniofacial
craniopharyngeal
cretinism
cribriform
cricoarytenoid
cricoid
cricoidectomy
cricoidynia

cricopharyngeal
cricopharyngeus
cricothyreotomy
cricothyroid
cricothyroidotomy
cricothyrotomy
cricotomy
cricotracheotomy
crista
    c. ampullaris
    c. arcuata cartilaginis
      arytenoideae
    c. conchalis maxillae
    c. conchalis ossis palatini
    c. ethmoidalis maxillae
    c. ethmoidalis ossis
      palatini
    c. fenestrae cochleae
    c. frontalis
    c. galli
cristae
    c. nasalis maxillae
    c. tympanica
CROS – Contralateral Routing of
  Signals
cross hearing
croup
Crouzon's syndrome
crura
    c. anthelicis
    c. of anthelix
crus
    anterior c. of stapes
    c. anterius stapedis
    c. breve incudis
    c. helicis
    c. of helix
    posterior c. of stapes
    c. posterius stapedis
cryosurgery
CT – computed tomography
cuneiform
cupula (cupulae)
    c. cristae ampullaris
    c. of cochlea
    c. cochleae
cupulolithiasis

curet
    Ballenger's c.
    Barnhill's c.
    Billeau's c.
    Brun's c.
    Buck's c.
    Carmack's c.
    Coakley's c.
    Derlacki's c.
    Faulkner's c.
    Freimuth's c.
    Gross' c.
    Halle's c.
    Hartmann's c.
    Hayden's c.
    Hotz's c.
    House's c.
    Ingersoll's c.
    Jones' c.
    Lempert's c.
    McCaskey's c.
    Middleton's c.
    Mosher's c.
    Myles' c.
    Pratt's c.
    Richards' c.
    Ridpath's c.
    Rosenmüller's c.
    Schaeffer's c.
    Shapleigh's c.
    Shea's c.
    St. Clair-Thompson c.
    Spratt's c.
    Stubbs' c.
    Tabb's c.
    Vogel's c.
    Weisman's c.
    Whiting's c.
    Yankauer's c.
Cushing's forceps
cymba
    c. conchae auriculae
cyst
    dermoid c.
    epidermoid c.
    Klestadt's c.
    nasoalveolar c.

cyst (continued)
    nasopalatine c.
    odontogenic c.
    radicular c.
    retention c.
    sebaceous c.
cystic fibrosis
cytomegalovirus
dacryocystorhinostenosis
dacryocystorhinostomy
Daniels' tonsillectome
Davis-Crowe mouth gag
Davis' retractor
Day's
    cannula
    operation
deafness
    acoustic trauma d.
    apoplectiform d.
    cerebral d.
    ceruminous d.
    conduction d.
    congenital d.
    cortical d.
    genetic d.
    labyrinthine d.
    Michel's d.
    Mondini's d.
    neural d.
    paradoxic d.
    perceptive d.
    Scheibe's d.
    sensorineural d.
    toxic d.
    vascular d.
Dean's
    applicator
    forceps
    knife
    periosteotome
    scissors
decibel
decongestant
Dedo-Pilling laryngoscope
Dedo's laryngoscope
degeneration
deglutition

Deiters' nucleus
Demarquay's sign
Denhardt-Dingman mouth gag
Denhardt's mouth gag
Denker's operation
Denonvilliers' operation
Derlacki's
    chisel
    curet
    gouge
    knife
    mobilizer
    operation
Derlacki-Shambaugh chisel
dermatitis
    eczematous d.
dermatome
dermoplasty
desensitization
Devilbiss' atomizer
diapason
diastolization
dilation
dilator
    Maloney's d.
Dingman's
    elevator
    forceps
    osteotome
    retractor
diphtheria
diplacusis
    binaural d.
    d. binauralis
        dysharmonica
    d. binauralis echoica
    disharmonic d.
    echo d.
    monaural d.
diplopia
disease
    Albers-Schönberg d.
    Alport's d.
    Alstrom's d.
    attic d.
    Hunt's d.
    Legal's d.

disease (continued)
    Lyme d.
    Ménière's d.
    Mikulicz's d.
    Pendred's d.
    Ramsay-Hunt d.
    Refsum's d.
    Sutton's d.
    Thornwaldt's d.
    Usher's d.
    von Recklinghausen's d.
    Waardenburg's d.
dissector
    Fisher's d.
    Holinger's d.
    Hurd's d.
    McWhinnie's d.
    Pierce's d.
    Rogers' d.
    Walker's d.
diverticula
diverticulum
    Zenker's d.
dizziness
Doerfler Stewart Test
Donaldson's tube
dorsum
    d. nasi
Dott's operation
douche
    Bermingham's nasal d.
Douglas' knife
drill
    Jordan-Day d.
    Shea's d.
drooling
drugs. See *Drugs and Chemistry* section.
drumhead
duct
    cochlear d.
    endolymphatic d.
    lacrimal d.
    d's of Rivinus
    Stensen's d.
    Walther's d's
    Wharton's d.

ductus
    d. cochlearis
    d. endolymphaticus
    d. reuniens
Dufourmental's
    forceps
    rongeur
Duplay-Lynch speculum
Duplay's speculum
dura
dysacousia
dysarthria
dysaudia
dysfluency
dysfunction
    temporomandibular joint d.
dysosmia
dysostosis
    craniofacial d.
    mandibulofacial d.
dysphagia
dysphonia
    d. plicae ventricularis
    d. spastica
dysplasia
    fibrous d.
dyspnea
EAC – external auditory canal
EAM – external auditory meatus
earache
eardrum
Eaton's speculum
ecchymosis
edentulous
Eder-Hufford esophagoscope
EENT – eyes, ears, nose, and throat
electrocoagulation
electromyography
electroneuronography
electronystagmography
electropneumatotherapy
elevator
    Ballenger's e.
    Cottle's e.
    Dingman's e.

elevator (continued)
    Freer's e.
    Hajek-Ballenger e.
    Hamrick's e.
    House's e.
    Hurd's e.
    Killian's e.
    Lamont's e.
    Lempert's e.
    Mackenty's e.
    Pennington's e.
    periosteal e.
    Pierce's e.
    Proctor's e.
    Ray-Parsons-Sunday e.
    Shambaugh-Derlacki e.
    Shambaugh's e.
    Sunday's e.
eminence
    arytenoid e.
    nasal e.
    pyramidal e.
eminentia
    e. articularis ossis
       temporalis
    e. conchae
    e. fallopii
    e. fossae triangularis
       auriculae
emissarium
    e. mastoideum
enanthema
encephalitis
encephalocele
enchondroma
endolabyrinthitis
endolaryngeal
endolarynx
endolymph
endolympha
endolymphatic
    e. hydrops
endomastoiditis
endonasal
endoscope
endoscopy
    peroral e.

endotoscope
endotracheal
English rhinoplasty
ENT – ear, nose, and throat
entacoustic
entotic
entotympanic
enucleation
eparterial
epidermoid
epiglottectomy
epiglottic
epiglottidean
epiglottidectomy
epiglottiditis
epiglottis
epiglottitis
epiotic
epipharyngeal
epipharyngitis
epipharynx
epistaxis
epithelialization
epiturbinate
epitympanic
epitympanum
Epstein-Barr virus
Equen-Neuffer knife
equilibrium
Erhard's test
Erhardt's speculum
Erich's
    forceps
    splint
errhine
erysipelas
erythema
    e. multiforme
erythroplakia
esophageal
esophagectomy
esophagitis
esophagogram
esophaglolaryngectomy
esophagopharynx
esophagoscope
    Boros' e.

esophagoscope (continued)
  Broyles' e.
  Bruening's e.
  Chevalier Jackson e.
  Eder-Hufford e.
  fiberoptic e.
  full-lumen e.
  Haslinger's e.
  Holinger's e.
  Jackson's e.
  Jesberg's e.
  Lell's e.
  Moersch's e.
  Mosher's e.
  Moure's e.
  optical e.
  oval e.
  Roberts' e.
  Schindler's e.
  Tucker's e.
  Yankauer's e.
esophagoscopy
esophagostomy
esophagotomy
esophagus
espundia
esthesioneuroblastoma
ETF–eustachian tube function
ethmofrontal
ethmoid
ethmoidal
ethmoidectomy
ethmoideomaxillary
ethmoiditis
ethmoidotomy
ethmolacrimal
ethmomaxillary
ethmonasal
ethmopalatal
ethmosphenoid
ethmoturbinal
ethmovomerine
ethmyphitis
eustachian
  e. tube
eustachitis
eustachium

Eves' snare
Ewing's sign
excavator
  Schuknecht's e.
excernent
excochleation
exostosis
expectorant
expectoration
explorer
  Rosen's e.
extradural
extranodal
exudate
facial
fahringo-. See words beginning
  pharyngo-.
Fallopius
  aqueduct of F.
farin-. See words beginning
  pharyn-.
Farrington's forceps
Farrior's speculum
fasciitis
fauces
faucial
faucitis
Faulkner's curet
Fauvel's forceps
fenestra
  f. cochleae
  f. nov-ovalis
  f. of cochlea
  f. ovalis
  f. rotunda
  f vestibuli
fenestrae
fenestrated
fenestrater
  Rosen's f.
fenestration
Fergusson's operation
Ferris-Robb knife
Ferris-Smith
  forceps
  operation
Ferris-Smith-Kerrison forceps

Ferris-Smith-Sewall retractor
fibers
        Prussak's f's
fibroangioma
fibroma
fibromatosis
fibromyalgia
fibrosarcoma
fibrositis
Fick's operation
Fink's laryngoscope
Fisher's
    dissector
    knife
Fish's forceps
fissure
    entorbital f.
    ethmoid f.
    glaserian f.
    petrotympanic f.
fistula
    oroantral f.
    perilymph f.
Flagg's laryngoscope
Flannery's speculum
flap
    tympanomeatal f.
flebektazea. See *phlebectasia*.
flem. See *phlegm*.
Fletcher's knife
flu
fold
    aryepiglottic f.
    salpingopharyngeal f.
folium
    lingual f.
folliculitits
Fomon's
    chisel
    knife
    periosteotome
    rasp
    scissors
footplate
foramen
    Huschke's f.
    f. incisivum

foramen (continued)
    f. mastoideum
    rivinian f.
    Scarpa's f.
    f. sphenopalatinum
    Stensen's f.
    f. stylomastoideum
forceps
    Adson's f.
    Andrews-Hartmann f.
    Ballenger's f.
    Bane's f.
    Barlow's f.
    Berne's f.
    Beyer's f.
    Blake's f.
    Blakesley's f.
    Boettcher's f.
    Bruening's f.
    Cicherelli's f.
    Coakley's f.
    Cohen's f.
    Colver's f.
    Cordes-New f.
    Cottle-Arruga f.
    Cottle-Jansen f.
    Cottle-Kazanjian f.
    Cottle's f.
    Craig's f.
    Cushing's f.
    Dean's f.
    Dingman's f.
    Dufourmentel's f.
    Erich's f.
    Farrington's f.
    Fauvel's f.
    Ferris-Smith f.
    Ferris-Smith-Kerrison f.
    Fish's f.
    Fraenkel's f.
    Goldman-Kazanjian f.
    Goodhill's f.
    Gruenwald-Bryant f.
    Gruenwald's f.
    Guggenheim's f.
    Hajek-Koffler f.
    Hartmann-Citelli f.

forceps (continued)
    Hartmann-Gruenwald f.
    Hartmann's f.
    Hoffmann's f.
    House's f.
    Howard's f.
    Hurd's f.
    Imperatori's f.
    Jackson's f.
    Jansen-Middleton f.
    Jansen's f.
    Jansen-Struycken f.
    Juers-Lempert f.
    Jurasz's f.
    Kazanjian's f.
    Knight's f.
    Knight-Sluder f.
    Koffler-Lillie f.
    Koffler's f.
    Krause's f.
    Lempert's f.
    Lillie's f.
    Littauer's f.
    Lucae's f.
    Luc's f.
    Lutz's f.
    Lynch's f.
    Marshik's f.
    Martin's f.
    McHenry's f.
    McKay's f.
    Metzenbaum's f.
    Moritz-Schmidt f.
    Museholdt's f.
    Myerson's f.
    Myles' f.
    Noyes' f.
    Pang's f.
    Paterson's f.
    Reiner-Knight f.
    Robb's f.
    Robertson's f.
    Rowland's f.
    Ruskin's f.
    Sawtell's f.
    Scheinmann's f.
    Seiffert's f.

forceps (continued)
    Semken's f.
    Shearer's f.
    Struempel's f.
    Struyken's f.
    Takahashi's f.
    Tivnen's f.
    Tobold's f.
    Tydings' f.
    Tydings-Lakeside f.
    Van Struycken f.
    Walsham's f.
    Watson-Williams f.
    Weil's f.
    Weingartner's f.
    White-Lillie f.
    White's f.
    Wilde's f.
    Wullstein-House f.
    Wullstein's f.
    Yankauer-Little f.
    Yankauer's f.
Foregger's laryngoscope
formula
    Seiler's f.
fossa
    f. incudis
    f. ovalis
    pharyngomaxillary f.
    Rosenmüller's f.
    triangular f.
fovea
fracture
    blow-out f.
Fraenkel's forceps
Frazier's tube
Freer's
    chisel
    elevator
    knife
Freimuth's curet
frenotomy
frenulum
frenum
Friesner's knife
frontal
    f. bone

frontal (continued)
    f. lobe
frontoethmoidal
frontoethmoidectomy
frontolacrimal
frontomaxillary
frontonasal
fronto-occipital
frontoparietal
frontotemporal
frontozygomatic
Fröschel's symptom
fundus
    f. meatus acustica interni
    f. tympani
fungal
furcula
furuncular
furuncle
furunculosis
gag reflex
galea
    g. aponeurotica
    tendinous g
Galen's anastomosis
Gandhi's knife
ganglion
    acousticofacial g.
    Cloquet's g.
    geniculate g.
    g. geniculi nervi facialis
    nodose g.
    otic g.
gangosa
Garfield-Holinger laryngoscope
Gault's test
Gellé's test
geniohyoid
genioplasty
genyantralgia
genyantritis
genyantrum
genycheiloplasty
genyplasty
Gerzog's speculum
Gifford's retractor

Gillies'
    hook
    operation
Gillies-Dingman hook
glabella
glabellad
glabellum
gland
    parotid g.
    Rivinus g.
    salivary g.
    sublingual g.
    submandibular g.
    thyroid g.
glioma
glomangioma
glomus
    g. jugulare
    g. tympanicum
glossa
glossagra
glossal
glossalgia
glossanthrax
glossectomy
glossitis
    rhomboid g.
glossocele
glossocoma
glossodynamometer
glossodynia
glossoepiglottidean
glossoncus
glossopathy
glossopexy
glossopharyngeal
glossopharyngeum
glossoplasty
glossoplegia
glossopyrosis
glossorrhaphy
glossoscopy
glossotomy
glottic
glottides
glottis

goiter
Goldman-Kazanjian forceps
Goodfellow's cannula
Goodhill's forceps
Good's rasp
Goodyear's knife
Gottschalk's
    aspirator
    saw
gouge
    Alexander's g.
    Andrews' g.
    Derlacki's g.
    Holmes' g.
    Troutman's g.
goundou
Gradenigo's syndrome
graft
granulation
granuloma
granulomatosis
    Wegener's g.
granulomatous
groove
    Verga's lacrimal g.
Gross'
    curet
    spoon
    spud
Gruber's speculum
Gruenwald-Bryant forceps
Gruenwald's forceps
Guedel's laryngoscsope
Guggenheim's forceps
Guilford's stapedectomy
guillotine
    Sluder's g.
    Sluder-Sauer g.
gumma
Gundelach's punch
Hajek-Ballenger elevator
Hajek-Koffler forceps
Hajek's
    chisel
    retractor
Hajek-Skillern punch

halitosis
Halle's
    curet
    speculum
Halle-Tieck speculum
Hall's bur
hammer
    Quisling's h.
Hamrick's elevator
Harrison's knife
Hartmann-Citelli forceps
Hartmann-Dewaxer speculum
Hartmann-Gruenwald forceps
Hartmann-Herzfeld ronguer
Hartmann's
    curet
    forceps
    punch
    rongeur
    speculum
    tuning fork
Haslinger's
    esophagoscope
    laryngoscope
    retractor
Haverhill's operation
Hayden's curet
HD – hearing distance
headache
    "hat band" h.
    migraine h.
headrest
    Shambaugh's h.
Heath's operation
HEENT – head, eyes, ears, nose,
    and throat
Heerfordt's syndrome
Heerman's operation
Heffernan's speculum
Heimlich maneuver
helicotrema
helix
hemangioma
hematoma
    h. auris
hemiglossal

hemiglossectomy
hemiglossitis
hemilaryngectomy
hemorrhage
hemostat
    Corwin's h.
Henle's spine
Henner's retractor
herpes
    h. catarrhalis
    h. febrilis
    h. labialis
    h. oticus
    h. simplex
    h. zoster
    h. zoster oticus
herpesvirus
Hertz unit
hiatus
    h. hernia
    h. semilunaris
Highmore's antrum
highmori
    sinus maxillaris h.
highmoritis
Hilger's operation
hircus
histamine
histiocytoma
histiocytosis
histoplasmosis
HIV – human immunodeficiency
    virus
hoarseness
Hodgkin's lymphoma
hoe
    Hough's h.
Hoffmann's
    forceps
    punch
    rongeur
Holinger's
    applicator
    dissector
    esophagoscope
    laryngoscope

Holms'
    gouge
    nasopharyngoscope
hook
    Boettcher's h.
    Gillies' h.
    Gillies-Dingman h.
    House's h.
    Lillie's h.
    Schuknecht's h.
    Shambaugh's h.
    Shea's h.
Hopmann's polyp
Hopp's laryngoscope
Horgan's operation
Horner's syndrome
Hotz's curet
Hough's
    hoe
    stapedectomy
Hourin's needle
House-Barbara needle
House-Rosen needle
House's
    adaptor
    chisel
    curet
    elevator
    forceps
    hook
    irrigator
    knife
    needle
    prosthesis
    rod
    scissors
    separator
    stapedectomy
    tube
House-Urban retractor
Howard's forceps
Howorth's operation
Huguier's sinus
Hunt's disease
Hurd's
    dissector

Hurd's (continued)
    elevator
    forceps
Hurler's syndrome
Hurst's bougie
Huschke's
    canal
    foramen
    valve
Husks' rongeur
hydrocephalus
    otitic h.
hydrorrhea
    nasal h.
hydrotis
hydrotympanum
hygroma
hyothyroid
hypacusis
hyperacusis
hyperemic
hyperkeratosis
    h. lacunaris
hypernasal
hypernasality
hypernephroma
hyperostosis
hyperpigmentation
hyperptyalism
hyperrhinoplasty
hypertension
hyperthyroidism
hypertrophy
hyperventilation
hypoglossal
hypoglottis
hypoglycemia
hyponasal
hyponasality
hypopharyngectomy
hypopharyngoscope
hypopharyngoscopy
hypopharynx
hypoplasia
hypopnea
hypothyroidism

hypotympanotomy
hypotympanum
hypoxia
Hz – Hertz
IA – internal auditory
IAC – internal auditory canal
immune
    i. response
    i. system
immunization
immunosuppression
impairment
    hearing i.
Imperatori's forceps
implant
    cochlear i.
incision. See *General Surgical Terms* section.
incisura
    i. anterior auris
    i. intertragica
    i. mastoidea ossis temporalis
    Santorini's i.
    i. terminalis auris
    i. tympanica
incisure
    Rivinus' i.
incostapedial
incudal
incudectomy
incudomalleal
incudostapedial
incus
Indian
    operation
    rhinoplasty
infarction
infection
    fungal i.
    Vincent's i.
inflammation
influenza
infundibulum
    ethmoidal i.
    i. nasi

Ingals' speculum
Ingersoll's curet
innervation
interarytenoid
intercricothyrotomy
intermaxillary
internarial
internasal
intralaryngeal
intramastoiditis
intranarial
intranasal
intubation
irrigation
    antral i.
irrigator
    House's i.
    Shambaugh's i.
    Shea's i.
isthmus
Italian
    operation
    rhinoplasty
ITE–in the ear
iter
Ivy's rongeur
Jackson's
    bougie
    esophagoscope
    forceps
    laryngoscope
    scissors
Jacobson's
    anastomosis
    nerve
Jako's laryngoscope
Jansen-Middleton forceps
Jansen-Newhart probe
Jansen's
    forceps
    operation
    retractor
Jansen-Struycken forceps
Jarvis' operation
Jennings' mouth gag
Jesberg's
    clamp

Jesberg's (continued)
    esophagoscope
Jewett's classification
joint
    incudostapedial j.
Jones'
    curet
    splint
Jordan-Day
    bur
    drill
Joseph-Maltz saw
Joseph's
    knife
    periosteotome
    saw
    scissors
Juers-Lempert forceps
jugomaxillary
jugular
Jurasz's forceps
Kartagener's
    syndrome
    triad
Kazanjian's
    forceps
    splint
Keegan's operation
Kelley's adenotome
keloid
keratosis
    k. obturans
    k. pharyngeus
Kerrison's rongeur
kHz-kilohertz
Kiesselbach's
    area
    plexus
Killian's
    chisel
    elevator
    knife
    operation
    speculum
kilo-. See words beginning
    cheilo-.

Klebsiella
    K. rhinoscleromatis
Klestadt's cyst
Klippel-Feil syndrome
Knapp's scissors
knife
    Ballenger's k.
    Beck's k.
    Buck's k.
    Canfield's k.
    Carpenter's k.
    Colver's k.
    Cottle's k.
    Dean's k.
    Derlacki's k.
    Douglas' k.
    Equen-Neuffer k.
    Ferris-Robb k.
    Fisher's k.
    Fletcher's k.
    Fomon's k.
    Freer's k.
    Friesner's k.
    Gandhi's k.
    Goodyear's k.
    Harrison's k.
    House's k.
    Joseph's k.
    Killian's k.
    Leland's k.
    Lempert's k.
    Lothrop's k.
    Lynch's k.
    Maltz's k.
    McHugh's k.
    Robertson's k.
    Rosen's k.
    Schuknecht's k.
    Seiler's k.
    Sexton's k.
    Shambaugh-Lempert k.
    Shea's k.
    Sheehy's k.
    Tobold's k.
    Tydings' k.
    Wullstein's k.

Knight's
    forceps
    scissors
Knight-Sluder forceps
koanah. See *choana.*
Koffler-Lillie forceps
Koffler's forceps
kokle-. See words beginning
    cochle-.
koklea. See *cochlea.*
Koplik's spots
Kos' cannula
Kramer's speculum
Krause's
    cannula
    forceps
    snare
Kuhnt's operation
Kuster's operation
Kyle's speculum
labial
labium
    antgerius ostii pharyngei
        tubae auditivae
labyrinth
    acoustic l.
    ethmoidal l.
    membranous l.
    nonacoustic l.
    osseus l.
labyrinthectomy
labyrinthine
labyrinthitis
    suppurative l.
labyrinthosis
labyrinthotomy
lacrimation
lacrimoconchal
lacrimomaxillary
lacrimonasal
Laforce-Grieshaber
    adenotome
Laforce's
    adenotome
    tonsillectome
lahringo-. See words beginning
    laryngo-.

lamina
    l. spiralis ossea
    l. spiralis secundaria
Lamont's
    elevator
    saw
Lane's mouth gag
LaRocca's tube
laryngalgia
laryngeal
laryngect
laryngectomee
laryngectomy
laryngemphraxis
laryngendoscope
laryngismal
laryngismus
    l. paralyticus
    l. stridulus
laryngitic
laryngitis
    catarrhal l.
    croupous l.
    diphtheritic l.
    membranous l.
    phlegmonous l.
    l. sicca
    l. stridulosa
    subglottic l.
    syphilitic l.
    tuberculous l.
    vestibular l.
laryngocele
laryngocentesis
laryngofission
laryngofissure
laryngogram
laryngograph
laryngography
laryngohypopharynx
laryngology
larngomalacia
laryngometry
laryngoparalysis
laryngopathy
laryngophantom
laryngopharyngeal

laryngopharyngectomy
laryngopharyngeus
laryngopharyngitis
laryngopharyx
laryngophony
laryngophthisis
laryngoplasty
laryngoplegia
laryngoptosis
laryngopyocele
laryngorhinology
laryngorrhagia
laryngorrhaphy
laryngorrhea
laryngoscleroma
laryngoscope
    Albert-Andrews l.
    Atkins-Tucker l.
    Bizzarri-Guiffrida l.
    Broyles' l.
    Chevalier Jackson l.
    Clerf's l.
    commissure l.
    Dedo-Pilling l.
    Dedo's l.
    fiberoptic l.
    Fink's l.
    Flagg's l.
    Foregger's l.
    Garfield-Holinger l.
    Guedel's l.
    Haslinger's l.
    Holinger's l.
    Hopp's l.
    Jackson's l.
    Jako's l.
    Lewy's l.
    Lundy's l.
    Lynch's l.
    MacIntosh's l.
    Magill's l.
    Miller's l.
    reverse-bevel l.
    Roberts' l.
    rotating l.
    Rusch's l.
    Sanders' l.

laryngoscope (continued)
    self-retaining l.
    Siker's l.
    slotted l.
    suspension l.
    Tucker's l.
    Welch-Allyn l.
    Wis-Foregger's l.
    Wis-Hipple's l.
    Yankauer's l.
laryngoscopic
laryngoscopist
laryngoscopy
laryngospasm
laryngostasis
laryngostat
laryngostenosis
laryngostomy
laryngostroboscope
laryngotome
laryngotomy
    subhyoid l.
    thyrohyoid l.
laryngotracheal
laryngotracheitis
laryngotracheobronchitis
laryngotracheobronchoscopy
laryngotracheoesophageal
laryngotracheoscopy
laryngotracheotomy
laryngotyphoid
laryngovestibulitis
laryngoxerosis
larynx
    artificial l.
laser
Lathbury's applicator
Latrobe's retractor
Lauren's operation
law
    Boyle's l.
Law's
    position
    view
Legal's disease
Lejeune's
    applicator

Lejeune's (continued)
    scissors
Leland's knife
Lell's esophagoscope
Lempert-Colver speculum
Lempert's
    bur
    curet
    elevator
    forceps
    knife
    operation
    perforator
    retractor
Lennert's classification
leprosy
Lermoyez's
    punch
    syndrome
leukemia
leukoplakia
Lewis'
    rasp
    snare
    tube
Lewy's laryngoscope
lichen planus
ligament
    annular l.
    axis l.
    cricoarytenoid l.
    cricopharyngeal l.
    cricothyroarytenoid l.
    cricothyroid l.
    cricotracheal l.
    hypoepiglottic l.
    posterior l.
    superior l.
    thyroepiglottic l.
    thyrohyoid l.
ligation
Lillie's
    forceps
    hook
    scissors
    speculum

limen
    l. nasi
Lindeman-Silverstein tube
line
    cricoclavicular l.
    Topinard's l.
lingua
    l. dissecta
    l. fraenata
    l. geographica
    l. nigra
    l. plicata
    l. villosa nigra
lingual
linguale
lingualis
lingually
lingula
lingulectomy
lipoma
Littauer's forceps
lobule
lobulus
    l. auriculae
Lombard-Boies rongeur
Lombard's test
Lothrop's
    knife
    retractor
loupe
Love's
    retractor
    splint
Lucae's forceps
Luc's forceps
Ludwig's angina
Luer's retractor
Lukes-Collins classification
Lundy's laryngoscope
Luongo's retractor
Luschka's
    laryngeal cartilage
    tonsil
Lutz's forceps
Lyme disease
lymphadenectomy
lymphadenitis

lymphadenoid
lymphangioma
lymphatic
lymphoblastoma
lymphoepithelial
lymphoepithelioma
lymphoma
    Hodgkin's l.
    non-Hodgkin's l.
lymphomatosum
    papillary adenocystoma l.
lymphosarcoma
lymphotism
lymphotome
Lynch's
    forceps
    knife
    laryngoscope
    scissors
MacFee neck flap
MacIntosh's laryngoscope
Mackenty's
    choanal plug
    elevator
    tube
Mack's tonsillectome
Maclay's scissors
macrocephalia
macrocheilia
macroglossia
macrognathia
macrostomia
macrotia
macula
    m. acustica sacculi
    m. acustica utriculi
    m. sacculi
    m. utriculi
Magill's laryngoscope
magnetic resonance imaging
Mahoney's speculum
malar
malformation
    arteriovenous m.
malleoincudal
malleolar
malleotomy

malleus
malocclusion
Maloney's dilator
Maltz-Lipsett rasp
Maltz's
    knife
    rasp
    saw
mandible
mandibula
mandibulae
mandibular
mandibulofacial
mandibulopharyngeal
Mandl's paint
maneuver
    Heimlich m.
manubrium (manubria)
    m. mallei
    m. of malleus
Marshik's forceps
Martin's forceps
mastoid
mastoidal
mastoidale
mastoidalgia
mastoidea
mastoidectomy
    radical m.
    simple m.
mastoideocentesis
mastoideum
mastoiditis
    Bezold's m.
    coalescent m.
    m. externa
    m. interna
    sclerosing m.
    silent m.
mastoidotomy
mastoidotympanectomy
maxilla
maxillary
maxillofacial
Mayer
    position

Mayer (continued)
    splint
McCaskey's curet
McCurdy's needle
McGee's operation
McHenry's forceps
McHugh's
    knife
    speculum
McIvor's mouth gag
McKay's forceps
McWhinnie's dissector
measles
meatoantrotomy
meatus
    auditory m.
    m. conchae
      ethmoturbinalis minoris
    external acoustic m.
    m. nasi communis osseus
    m. nasopharyngeus osseus
mediastinoscopy
mediastinum
medications. See *Drugs and*
    Chemistry section.
melanoma
Meltzer's
    nasopharyngoscope
    punch
membrana
    m. basilaris ductus
      cochlearis
    m. elastica laryngis
    m. fibroelastica laryngis
    m. mucosa nasi
    m. spiralis ductus
      cochlearis
    m. stapedis
    m. tympani secundaria
membrane
    buccopharyngeal m.
    hyothyroid m.
    hypoglossal m.
    mucous m.
    Reissner's m.
    Rivinus' m.
    Scarpa's m.

membrane (continued)
    Shrapnell's m.
    tectorial m.
    tympanic m.
membranous
Ménière's disease
meningioma
meningitis
mentoplasty
mesocephalic
mesoturbinal
mesoturbinate
metopantralgia
metopantritis
Metzenbaum-Lipsett scissors
Metzenbaum's
    forceps
    scissors
Meyeri sinus
Meyer's sinus
Michel's deafness
microglossia
micrognathia
microlaryngoscopy
microrhinia
microscope
    Zeiss' m.
microstomia
microsurgery
    laser m.
microtia
microtubule
Middleton's curet
migraine
Mikulicz's
    disease
    syndrome
Miller's laryngoscope
mobilization
    stapes m.
mobilizer
    Derlacki's m.
Möbius' syndrome
modiolus
Moeller's reaction
Moersch's esophagoscope
Moltz-Storz tonsillectome

Mondini's deafness
mononucleosis
Montgomery's tracheocannula
Morch's tube
Morgagni's
    sacculus
    sinus
    ventricle
Moritz-Schmidt forceps
Mosher's
    curet
    esophagoscope
    punch
    speculum
Moure's esophagoscope
mouth gag
    Davis-Crowe m.g.
    Denhardt-Dingman m.g.
    Denhardt's m.g.
    Jennings' m.g.
    Lane's m.g.
    McIvor's m.g.
    Roser's m.g.
    Sluder-Jansen m.g.
MRI – magnetic resonance
    imaging
mucocele
mucociliary
mucoid
mucoperichondrium
mucoperiosteal
mucoperiosteum
mucopurulent
mucormycosis
mucosa
mucus
multiple sclerosis
mumps
muscle
    arytenoid m.
    cricoarytenoid m.
    cricopharyngeus m.
    cricothyroid m.
    depressor septi nasi m.
    genioglossus m.
    geniohyoideus m.
    glossopalatinus m.

muscle (continued)
    glossopharyngeus m.
    helicis m.
    interarytenoid m.
    levator veli palatini m.
    longissimus m.
    palatoglossus m.
    palatopharyngeus m.
    pharyngeal constrictor m.
    pharyngopalatinus m.
    salpingopharyngeal m.
    splenius m.
    stapedius m.
    sternocleidomastoid m.
    strap m.
    stylopharyngeus m.
    temporalis m.
    tensor m. of tympanic
      membrane
    tensor m. of tympanum
    tensor veli palatini m.
    thyroarytenoid m.
    thyrohyoid m.
    vocal m.
musculoplasty
musculus
    m. temporalis
    m. tensor tympani
Museholdt's forceps
Mustarde otoplasty
myalgia
myasthenia
    m. gravis
    m. laryngis
mycosis
    m. leptothrica
Myerson's
    forceps
    saw
Myles'
    curet
    forceps
    punch
    snare
    speculum
    tonsillectome
mylohyoid

myoblastoma
myoclonus
    palatal m.
myofascitis
myositis
myringa
myringectomy
myringitis
    m. bullosa
    bullous m.
myringodectomy
myringodermatitis
myringomycosis
    m. aspergillina
myringoplasty
myringorupture
myringoscope
myringostapediopexy
myringotome
myringotomy
myrinx
myxoma
nares
naris
nasal
    n. allergy
    n. cavity
    n. congestion
    n. deformity
    n. filtration
    n. obstruction
    n. packing
    n. septum
    n. speculum
    n. tampon
    n. turbinate
    n. vestibule
    n. vestibulitis
nasalis
nasality
nasion
nasitis
nasoantral
nasoantritis
nasoantrostomy
nasobronchial
nasociliary

nasofrontal
nasograph
nasolabial
nasolacrimal
nasomanometer
nasomaxillary
nasonnement
naso-oral
nasopalatine
nasopharyngeal
    n. bursitis
nasopharyngitis
nasopharyngoscope
    Broyles' n.
    Holmes' n.
    Meltzer's n.
nasopharyngoscopy
nasopharynx
nasorostral
nasoscope
nasoseptal
nasoseptitis
nasosinusitis
nasospinale
nasotracheal
nasoturbinal
nasus
    n. externus
Nebinger-Praun operation
neck flap
    MacFee n.f.
necrosis
necrotizing
needle
    Brown's n.
    Hourin's n.
    House-Barbara n.
    House-Rosen n.
    House's n.
    McCurdy's n.
    Rosen's n.
    Shambaugh's n.
    Updegraff's n.
Neivert's retractor
neoplasm
nerve
    abducens n.

nerve (continued)
    acoustic n.
    alveolar n.
    Arnold's n.
    chorda tympani n.
    cochlear n.
    ethmoidal n.
    facial n.
    glossopharyngeal n.
    hypoglossal n.
    infraorbital n.
    infratrochlear n.
    Jacobson's n.
    laryngeal n.
    maxillary n.
    nasopalatine n.
    n. of pterygoid canal
    n. of tensor tympani
    olfactory n's
    palatine n.
    petrosal n.
    pterygopalatine n's
    trigeminal n.
    vagus n.
    vestibular n.
    vidian n.
neuralgia
    glossopharyngeal n.
    retrobulbar n.
    trigeminal n.
neurapraxia
neurilemmoma
neurofibroma
neurogenic
neuroma
    acoustic n.
nevoid
New-Lambotte osteotome
niche
nodular
nodule
noma
non-Hodgkin's lymphoma
nose
    cleft n.
    potato n.
    saddle-back n.

nose (continued)
    swayback n.
nosebleed
nostril
notch
    Carhart n.
    n. of Rivinus
    rivinian n.
Noyes' forceps
Noyes-Shambaugh scissors
NP – nasopharyngeal
    nasopharynx
NT – nasotracheal
nucha
nuchal
nucleus
    Bechterew's n.
    Deiters' n.
numatizashun. See
    pneumatization.
numo-. See words beginning
    pneumo-.
nystagmus
    aural n.
    caloric n.
    labyrinthine n.
    vestibular n.
obstruction
    airway o.
obstructive
    o. sleep apnea
occipital
occipitofrontal
occipitomastoid
occipitomental
occiput
occlusion
odynophagia
ogo
Ogston-Luc operation
olfaction
olfactory
oncocytoma
onychodystrophy
operation
    Adams' o.
    Almoor's o.

operation (continued)
    Arslan's o.
    Asch's o.
    Becker's o.
    Billroth's o.
    Caldwell-Luc o.
    Canfield's o.
    Carpue's o.
    Carter's o.
    Cassel's o.
    Cheever's o.
    Chevalier Jackson o.
    Coakley's o.
    Cody's o.
    Commando's o.
    Day's o.
    Denker's o.
    Denovilliers' o.
    Derlacki's o.
    Dott's o.
    Fergusson's o.
    Ferris-Smith o.
    Fick's o.
    Gillies' o.
    Haverhill's o.
    Heath's o.
    Heerman's o.
    Hilger's o.
    Horgan's o.
    Howorth's o.
    Indian o.
    Italian o.
    Jansen's o.
    Jarvis' o.
    Keegan's o.
    Killian's o.
    Kuhnt's o.
    Kuster's o.
    Lauren's o.
    Lempert's o.
    McGee's o.
    Nebinger-Praun o.
    Ogston-Luc o.
    radical antrum o.
    Ridell's o.
    Roberts' o.
    Rosen's o.

operation (continued)
    Rouge's o.
    Schonbein's o.
    Schuknecht's o.
    Schwartze's o.
    Shambaugh's o.
    Sistrunk's o.
    Sluder's o.
    Sonneberg's o.
    Sourdille's o.
    Stacke's o.
    Stallard's o.
    tagliacotian o.
    Vicq d'Azyr's o.
    West's o.
    Wood's o.
    Wullstein's o.
    Yankauer's o.
opisthogenia
opisthognathism
opisthotic
oral
    o. mucosa
    o. tori
orbit
orbital
    o. cellulitis
    o. floor
orbitonasal
organ
    o. of Corti
organum
    o. spirale
    o. vestibulocochleare
orifice
    tympanic o.
oroantral
oronasal
oropharynx
os
    o. epitympanicum
    o. ethmoidale
    o. frontale
    o. hyoideum
    o. interparietale
    o. lacrimale
    o. mastoideum

os (continued)
    o. nasale
    o. occipitale
    o. orbiculare
    o. palatinum
    o. parietale
    o. sphenoidale
    o. temporale
    o. unguis
    o. zygomaticum
OSA – obstructive sleep apnea
Osler-Weber-Rendu syndrome
osseosonometry
osseous
ossicle
    auditory o's
ossicula
    o. auditus
ossicular
    o. chain
    o. disarticulation
    o. system
ossiculectomy
ossiculotomy
ossiculum
osteoma
osteomyelitis
osteopetrosis
osteotome
    Cottle's o.
    Dingman's o.
    New-Lambotte o.
    Rowland's o.
    Silver's o.
ostium
    o. pharyngeum tubae
      auditivae
    o. tympanicum tubae
      auditivae
otacoustic
otagra
otalgia
    o. dentalis
    o. intermittens
    reflex o.
otalgic
otectomy

othelcosis
othematoma
othemorrhea
othygroma
otiatrics
otic capsule
oticodinia
otitic
    o. barotrauma
otitis
    o. crouposa
    o. desquamativa
    o. diphtheritica
    o. externa circumscripta
    o. externa diffusa
    o. externa furunculosa
    o. externa hemorrhagica
    o. externa mycotica
    furuncular o.
    o. haemorrhagica
    o. labyrinthica
    o. mastoidea
    o. media catarrhalis acuta
    o. media catarrhalis
      chronica
    o. media purulenta acuta
    o. media purulenta
      chronica
    o. media sclerotica
    o. media serosa
    o. media suppurativa
    o. media vasomotorica
    mucosis o.
    mucosus o.
    o. mycotica
    necrotizing external o.
    purulent o.
    o. sclerotica
Oto. – otolaryngology
    otology
otoantritis
otoblennorrhea
otocatarrh
otocephalus
otocerebritis
otocleisis
otoconia

otoconium
otocranial
otocranium
otocyst
otodynia
otoencephalitis
otoganglion
otogenic
otogenous
otography
otohemineurasthenia
Otol. – otology
Otolar. – otolaryngology
otolaryngology
otolith
otolithiasis
otologic
otologist
otology
otomassage
otomastoiditis
otomicroscope
otomicroscopy
otomucormycosis
otomyasthenia
Otomyces
otomycosis
    o. aspergillina
otomyiasis
otoncus
otonecrectomy
otoneuralgia
otoneurasthenia
otoneurology
otopathy
otopharyngeal
otophone
otopiesis
otoplasty
    Mustarde o.
otopolypus
otopyorrhea
otopyosis
otor
otorhinolaryngologist
otorhinolaryngology
otorhinology

otorrhagia
otorrhea
otosalpinx
otosclerectomy
otoscleronectomy
otosclerosis
otoscope
     Bruening's o.
     Brunton's o.
     pneumatic o.
     Siegle's o.
     Toynbee's o.
     Welch-Allyn o.
otoscopy
     pneumatic o.
otosis
otospongiosis
otosteal
otosteon
ototomy
ototoxic
ototoxicity
Owens'
     position
     view
ozena
     o. laryngis
paint
     Mandl's p.
palata
palatal
palate
     cleft p.
palateoethmoidal
palatine
palatitis
palatoglossal
palatognathous
palatograph
palatography
palatomaxillary
palatomyograph
palatonasal
palatopharyngeal
palatoplasty
palatoplegia
palatoschisis

palatostaphylinus
palatouvularis
palatum
palsy
     Bell's p.
Pang's forceps
panotitis
panseptum
pansinuitis
pansinusectomy
pansinusitis
panturbinate
Paparella's tube
papilla
     acoustic p.
     p. parotidea
papillae
     filiform p.
     p. filiformes
     foliate p.
     p. foliatae
     fungiform p.
     p. fungiformes
     lingual p.
     p. linguales
papillary
papilloma
     inverted p.
     squamous p.
paracusia
     p. acris
     p. duplicata
     p. loci
     p. willisiana
paracusis of Willis
paraglossa
paraglossia
paraglossitis
paralysis
     vocal cord p.
parapharyngeal
paries
     p. externus ductus
       cochlearis
     p. jugularis cavi tympani
     p. labyrinthicus cavi
       tympani

paries (continued)
  p. mastoideus cavi
    tympani
  p. medialis orbitae
  p. membranaceus cavi
    tympani
  p. membranaceus tracheae
  p. tegmentalis cavi
    tympani
  p. tympanicus ductus
    cochlearis
  p. vestibularis ductus
    cochlearis
parietal
parietofrontal
parietomastoid
parieto-occipital
parietosphenoid
parietosquamosal
parietotemporal
parosmia
parotid
parotidean
parotidectomy
parotitis
pars
  p. flaccida membranae
    tympani
  p. tensa membranae
    tympani
patch
  Silastic p.
Paterson's
  cannula
  forceps
pectus
  p. excavatum
peenash
pemphigoid
pemphigus
  p. vulgaris
Pendred's disease
Pennington's elevator
perforation
  Bezold's p.
  tympanic membrane p.

perforator
  Lempert's p.
  Royce's p.
  Thornwald's p.
  Wellaminski's p.
periadenitis
  p. mucosa necrotica
    recurrens
periauricular
perichondritis
perichondrium
perilabyrinth
perilabyrinthitis
perilaryngeal
perilaryngitis
perilymph
perilymphatic
periodontal
periodontitis
periorbital
periosteotome
  Dean's p.
  Fomon's p.
  Joseph's p.
periosteum
periotic
perirhinal
perisinuitis
perisinuous
perisinusitis
peritonsillar
peritonsillitis
Per-Lee tube
perpendicular plate
petiolus
  p. epiglottidis
petromastoid
petro-occipital
petropharyngeus
petrosal
petrosectomy
petrositis
petrosphenoid
petrosquamosal
petrous
pharyngalgia
pharyngeal

pharyngectasia
pharyngectomy
pharyngemphraxis
pharyngeus
pharyngism
pharyngismus
pharyngitic
pharyngitid
pharyngitis
    atrophic p.
    catarrhal p.
    croupous p.
    diphtheritic p.
    follicular p.
    gangrenous p.
    glandular p.
    granular p.
    p. herpetica
    hypertrophic p.
    p. keratosa
    membranous p.
    phlegmonous p.
    recurrent p.
    p. sicca
    p. ulcerosa
    viral p.
pharyngoamygdalitis
pharyngocele
pharyngoconjunctivitis
pharyngodynia
pharyngoepiglottic
pharyngoesophageal
pharyngoglossal
pharyngoglossus
pharyngokeratosis
pharyngolaryngeal
pharyngolaryngitis
pharyngolith
pharyngolysis
pharyngomaxillary
pharyngomycosis
pharyngonasal
pharyngo-oral
pharyngopalatine
pharyngoparalysis
pharyngopathy
pharyngoperistole

pharyngoplasty
pharyngoplegia
pharyngorhinitis
pharyngorhinoscopy
pharyngorrhagia
pharyngorrhea
pharyngosalpingitis
pharyngoscleroma
pharyngoscope
pharyngoscopy
pharyngospasm
pharyngostenosis
pharyngostomy
pharyngotherapy
pharyngotome
pharyngotomy
pharyngotonsillitis
pharyngotyphoid
pharynx
philtrum
phlebectasia
    p. laryngis
phlegm
phonation
photophore
Pierce's
    dissector
    elevator
    retractor
Pierre Robin syndrome
pillar
pinna
pinnal
piriform
plasmacytoma
platinectomy
Plaut-Vincent's angina
pledget
plegaphonia
plexus
    Kiesselbach's p.
    laryngeal p.
    pharyngeal p.
    tympanic p.
plica
    p. nervi laryngei
    p. salpingopharyngea

plica (continued)
    p. stapedis
    p. supratonsillaris
    p. triangularis
    p. vocalis
plicotomy
plug
    Mackenty's choanal p.
Plummer's bougie
Plummer-Vinson syndrome
PND – postnasal drainage
    postnasal drip
pneumatization
pneumococcal
    p. meningitis
pneumomediastinum
pneumothorax
pocket
    Rathke's p.
politzerization
Politzer's
    bag
    speculum
    test
    treatment
pollination
pollinosis
polychondritis
polycythemia
polyp
    antrochoanal p.
    Hopmann's p.
    nasal p.
polypectomy
polypoid
polyposis
polysomnography
    nocturnal p.
ponticulus
    p. auriculae
    p. promontorii
position
    Law's p.
    Mayer's p.
    Owens' p.
    Schüller's p.
    Stenver's p.

postaurale
postauricular
posturography
pouch
    Prussak's p.
    Rathke's p.
Pratt's curet
preauricular
presbycusis
Prince's scissors
probe
    Arbuckle's p.
    Jansen-Newhart p.
    Rosen's p.
    Spencer's p.
    Theobald's p.
    Welch-Allyn p.
    Yankauer's p.
procedure
    obliteration p.
    Valsalva's p.
process
    clinoid p.
    hamular p.
    mastoid p.
    styloid p.
    zygomatic p.
Proctor's
    elevator
    retractor
Proetz's treatment
prognathism
prognathous
projection
    Chausse III p.
prominentia
    p. laryngea
    p. styloidea
promontorium
    p. faciei
    p. tympani
promontory
prosthesis
    Blom-Singer p.
    House's p.
    Sheehy-House p.
    Teflon p.

prosthesis (continued)
TORP (total ossicular
replacement p.)
Prussak's
fibers
pouch
space
pseudocholesteatoma
pseudoglottis
Pseudomonas
P. aeruginosa
pterygomandibular
pterygomaxillary
pterygopalatine
ptyalectasis
ptyalism
ptyalith
ptyalize
ptyalocele
ptyalolithiasis
ptyalorrhea
punch
Adler's p.
Citelli-Meltzer p.
Gundelach's p.
Hajek-Skillern p.
Hartmann's p.
Hoffmann's p.
Lermoyez's p.
Meltzer's p.
Mosher's p.
Myles' p.
Schmeden's p.
Spencer's p.
Spies' p.
Takahashi's p.
Van Struycken's p.
Wagner's p.
Watson-Williams p.
Wilde's p.
Yankauer's p.
purulent
pyemia
otogenous p.
pyknosis
Pynchon's
applicator

Pynchon's (continued)
speculum
pyocele
pyothorax
pyramid
p. of tympanum
petrous p.
quinsy
lingual q.
Quisling's hammer
RAD – radiation absorbed dose
radiculopathy
radiography. See *Radiology and
Nuclear Medicine* section.
radiosialographic
Ramsay-Hunt disease
ramus
ranula
raphe
r. pharyngis
Rappaport's classification
rasp
Aufricht-Lipsett r.
Aufricht's r.
Berne's r.
Cottle's r.
Fomon's r.
Good's r.
Lewis' r.
Maltz-Lipsett r.
Maltz's r.
Wiener-Pierce r.
RAST – radioallergosorbent test
Rathke's
pocket
pouch
tumor
Ray-Parsons-Sunday elevator
Ray's speculum
reaction
Moeller's r.
recess
Tröltsch's r's
recessus
r. cochlearis vestibuli
r. ellipticus vestibuli
r. epitympanicus

recessus (continued)
  r. membranae tympani anterior
  r. membranae tympani posterior
  r. membranae tympani superior
  r. pharyngeus
  r. piriformis
  r. pro utriculo
  r. sphenoethmoidalis
  r. sphenoethmoidalis osseus
  r. sphericus vestibuli
Refsum disease
Reiner-Beck snare
Reiner-Knight forceps
Reissner's membrane
rem – roentgen-equivalent – man
resection
  submucous r.
respiratory
  r. mucosa
  r. tract
reticulosis
  polymorphic r.
retractor
  Allport's r.
  Aufricht's r.
  Brown's r.
  Cottle-Neivert r.
  Cottle's r.
  Davis' r.
  Dingman's r.
  Ferris-Smith-Sewall r.
  Gifford's r.
  Hajek's r.
  Haslinger's r.
  Henner's r.
  House-Urban r.
  Jansen's r.
  Latrobe's r.
  Lempert's r.
  Lothrop's r.
  Love's r.
  Luer's r.
  Luongo's r.

retractor (continued)
  Neivert's r.
  Pierce's r.
  Proctor's r.
  Schuknecht's r.
  Senn-Dingman r.
  Shambaugh's r.
  Spitman's r.
  Weitlaner's r.
  White-Proud r.
  Wullstein's r.
retroauricular
retrolabyrinthine
retromandibular
retromastoid
retronasal
retropharyngeal
retropharyngitis
retropharynx
Reuter's tube
rhabdomyosarcoma
rhinal
rhinalgia
rhinallergosis
rhinedema
rhinenchysis
rhinesthesia
rhineurynter
rhinion
rhinism
rhinitis
  allergic r.
  anaphylactic r.
  atrophic r.
  r. caseosa
  catarrhal r.
  croupous r.
  dyscrinic r.
  fibrinous r.
  gangrenous r.
  hypertrophic r.
  infectious r.
  influenzal r.
  membranous r.
  nonairflow r.
  perennial r.
  pseudomembranous r.

rhinitis (continued)
    purulent r.
    scrofulous r.
    r. sicca
    suppurative r.
    syphilitic r.
    tuberculous r.
    vasomotor r.
rhinoanemometer
rhinoantritis
rhinobyon
rhinocephalia
rhinocephalus
rhinocheiloplasty
rhinocleisis
rhinocoele
rhinodacryolith
rhinodynia
rhinogenous
rhinokyphectomy
rhinokyphosis
rhinolalia
    r. aperta
    r. clausa
rhinolaryngitis
rhinolaryngology
rhinolith
rhinolithiasis
rhinologist
rhinology
rhinomanometer
rhinometer
rhinomiosis
rhinomycosis
rhinonecrosis
rhinonemmeter
rhinoneurosis
rhinopathia
    r. vasomotoria
rhinopathy
rhinopharyngeal
rhinopharyngitis
    r. mutilans
rhinopharyngocele
rhinopharyngolith
rhinopharynx
rhinophonia

rhinophore
rhinophycomycosis
rhinophyma
rhinoplastic
rhinoplasty
    Carpue's r.
    dactylocostal r.
    English r.
    Indian r.
    Italian r.
    tagliacotian r.
rhinopneumonitis
rhinopolypus
rhinoreaction
rhinorrhagia
rhinorrhaphy
rhinorrhea
    cerebrospinal r.
rhinosalpingitis
rhinoscleroma
rhinoscope
rhinoscopic
rhinoscopy
rhinosinusitis
rhinosporidiosis
rhinostegnosis
rhinostenosis
rhinotomy
rhinotracheitis
rhinovaccination
rhinovirus
rhomboid
rhonchal
rhonchial
rhonchus
Richards' curet
Richards-Rundle syndrome
Ridell's operation
Ridley's sinus
Ridpath's curet
rima
    r. glottidis
    r. glottidis cartilaginea
    r. glottidis membranacea
    intercartilaginous r.
    intermembranous r.
    r. oris

rima (continued)
    r. vestibuli
    r. vocalis
ring
    Waldeyer's r.
Ringer's solution
Rinne's test
Rivinus'
    ducts
    gland
    incisure
    membrane
    notch
Robb's forceps
Roberts'
    applicator
    esophagoscope
    laryngoscope
    operation
Robertson's
    forceps
    knife
rod
    Corti's r's
    House's r.
Roeder's treatment
Rogers' dissector
rongeur
    Beyer's r.
    Converse's r.
    duckbill r.
    Dufourmentel's r.
    Hartmann-Herzfeld r.
    Hartmann's r.
    Hoffmann's r.
    Husks' r.
    Ivy's r.
    Kerrison's r.
    Lombard-Boies r.
    Rowland's r.
    Ruskin's r.
    Tobey's r.
    Whiting's r.
Rosenmüller's
    curet
    fossa

Rosen's
    explorer
    fenestrater
    knife
    needle
    operation
    probe
    separator
    tube
Roser's mouth gag
Rouge's operation
Rowland's
    forceps
    osteotome
    rongeur
Royce's perforator
rubella
ruga
    r. palatina
Rusch's laryngoscope
Ruskin's
    forceps
    rongeur
Ruysch's tube
sacculation
saccule
    laryngeal s.
    s. of larynx
sacculi

sacculocochlear
sacculus
    s. communis
    s. lacrimalis
    s. laryngis
    s. morgagnii
    s. proprius
    s. rotundus
    s. sphaericus
    s. ventricularis
    s. vestibularis
sagittal
St. Clair-Thompson curet
saliva
salivant
salivary
salivation

salpingitis
    eustachian s.
salpingocatheterism
salpingopharyngeal
salpingoscope
salpingoscopy
salpingostaphyline
Salvatore-Maloney tracheotome
Sanders' laryngoscope
Santorini's
    cartilage
    incisura
sarcoid
sarcoidosis
sarcoma
Sauer-Sluder tonsillectome
Sauer's tonsillectome
saw
    Clerf's s.
    Cottle's s.
    Gottschalk's s.
    Joseph-Maltz s.
    Joseph's s.
    Lamont's s.
    Maltz's s.
    Myerson's s.
    Slaughter's s.
    Woakes' s.
Sawtell's forceps
scala
    s. media
    s. tympani
    s. vestibuli
scanning
    radiosialographic s.
scapha
scarlet fever
Scarpa's
    foramen
    membrane
Schaffer's curet
Schall's tube
Scheibe's deafness
Scheinmann's forceps
Schindler's esophagoscope
Schmeden's punch

Schmincke's tumor
Schonbein's operation
Schuknecht's
    excavator
    hook
    knife
    operation
    retractor
    speculum
    stapedectomy
Schüller's
    position
    view
Schwabach's test
schwannoma
Schwartze's
    operation
    sign
scissors
    Bellucci's s.
    Boettcher's s.
    Cottle's s.
    Dean's s.
    Fomon's s.
    House's s.
    Jackson's s.
    Joseph's s.
    Knapp's s.
    Knight's s.
    Lejeune's s.
    Lillie's s.
    Lynch's s.
    Maclay's s.
    Metzenbaum-Lipsett s.
    Metzenbaum's s.
    Noyes-Shambaugh s.
    Prince's s.
    Seiler's s.
    Steven's s.
sclerosis
Scott's
    cannula
    speculum
scute
    tympanic s.
SD – septal defect

searcher
Allport's s.
Searcy's tonsillectome
SEE – Seeing Essential English
Seiffert's forceps
Seiler's
formula
knife
scissors
sella
s. turcica
sellar
semicanal
s. of auditory tube
s. of tensor tympani
muscle
semicanales
semicanalis
s. musculi tensoris
tympani
s. tubae auditivae
Semken's forceps
Sengstaken-Blakemore tube
Sengstaken's tube
Senn-Dingman retractor
sensitization
sensitized
sensorineural
Senturia's speculum
separator
House's s.
Rosen's s.
septal
septectomy
septonasal
septoplasty
septotome
septotomy
septum
s. canalis musculoturbarii
s. cartilagineum nasi
s. mobile nasi
s. nasi osseum
s. of sphenoidal sinuses
s. sinuum frontalium
s. sinuum sphenoidalium

Sewall's chisel
Sexton's knife
sfeno-. See words beginning
spheno-.
shadow
s. curve
Shambaugh-Derlacki
chisel
elevator
Shambaugh-Lempert knife
Shambaugh's
adenotome
elevator
headrest
hook
irrigator
needle
operation
retractor
Shapleigh's curet
Shearer's forceps
Shea's
curet
drill
hook
irrigator
knife
stapedectomy
tube
Sheehan's chisel
Sheehy-House prosthesis
Sheehy's
knife
tube
Shepard's tube
Shiley's tube
Shrapnell's membrane
siagantritis
siagonagra
siagonantritis
sialaden
sialadenitis
sialadenography
sialadenoncus
sialagogic
sialagogue

sialaporia
sialectasia
sialectasis
sialitis
sialoadenectomy
sialoadenitis
sialoadenotomy
sialocele
sialodochiectasis
sialodochitis
sialodochoplasty
sialogram
sialography
sialolith
sialolithiasis
sialolithotomy
sialoma
sialorrhea
sialosis
sialostenosis
sialosyrinx
sialozemia
Siegle's otoscope
Sierra-Sheldon tracheotome
sign
    Bespaloff's s.
    Biederman's s.
    Bieg's s.
    Demarquay's s.
    Ewing's s.
    Schwartze's s.
    Wreden's s.
    Zaufal's s.
Siker's laryngoscope
Silastic patch
Silver's osteotome
sinistraural
sinobronchitis
sinodural
sinography
sinus
    s. cochleae
    ethmoidal s.
    s. ethmoidalis
    frontal s.
    s. frontalis osseus
    Huguier's s.

sinus (continued)
    laryngeal s.
    mastoid s.
    s. maxillaris highmori
    s. maxillaris osseus
    maxillary s.
    s. meyeri
    Meyer's s.
    occipital s.
    s. occipitalis
    s. of Morgagni
    paranasal s's
    s. paranasales
    piriform s.
    s. posterior cavi tympani
    Ridley's s.
    sigmoid s.
    sphenoidal s.
    s. sphenoidalis
    s. sphenoidalis osseus
    s. tympani
    tympanic s.
sinusitis
    ethmoid s.
    frontal s.
    fungal s.
    hyperplastic s.
    intracranial s.
    maxillary s.
    orbital s.
    sphenoid s.
    viral s.
sinusotomy
SISI – short increment sensitivity
    index
Sistrunk's operation
situs
    s. inversus
Sjögren's syndrome
Slaughter's saw
sleep apnea
Sluder-Demarest tonsillectome
Sluder-Jansen mouth gag
Sluder's
    adenotome
    guillotine
    operation

Sluder's (continued)
    tonsillectome
Sluder-Sauer
    guillotine
    tonsillectome
SMR – submucous resection
SMRR – submucous resection
   and rhinoplasty
SMR speculum
snare
    Bosworth's s.
    Brown's s.
    Bruening's s.
    Eves' s.
    Krause's s.
    Lewis' s.
    Myles' s.
    Reiner-Beck s.
    Storz-Beck s.
    Stutsman's s.
    Tydings' s.
    Wilde-Bruening s.
    Wright's s.
Snitman's retractor
snoring
solution
    Ringer's s.
SOM – secretory otitis media
   serous otitis media
Sonneberg's operation
Sonnenschein's speculum
Sourdille's operation
space
    poststyloid s.
    prestyloid s.
    Prussack's s.
    retropharyngeal s.
speculum
    Aufricht's s.
    aural s.
    Beckman-Colver s.
    Boucheron's s.
    Chevalier Jackson s.
    Coakley's s.
    Converse's s.
    Cottle's s.
    Duplay-Lynch s.

speculum (continued)
    Duplay's s.
    Eaton's s.
    Erhardt's s.
    Farrior's s.
    Flannery's s.
    Gerzog's s.
    Gruber's s.
    Halle's s.
    Halle-Tieck s.
    Hartmann-Dewaxer s.
    Hartmann's s.
    Heffernan's s.
    Ingals' s.
    Killian's s.
    Kramer's s.
    Kyle's s.
    Lempert-Colver s.
    Lillie's s.
    Mahoney's s.
    McHugh's s.
    Mosher's s.
    Myles' s.
    nasal s.
    Politzer's s.
    Pynchon's s.
    Ray's s.
    Schuknecht's s.
    Scott's s.
    Senturia's s.
    SMR s.
    Sonnenschein's s.
    Toynbee's s.
    Tröltsch's s.
    Vienna s.
    Welch-Allyn s.
    Yankauer's s.
speechreading
Spencer's
    probe
    punch
sphenoethmoid
sphenofrontal
sphenoid
sphenoidal
sphenoidectomy
    frontoethmoid s.

sphenoiditis
sphenoidostomy
sphenoidotomy
sphenomaxillary
sphenopalatine
sphenoparietal
sphenosquamous
sphenozygomatic
Spies' punch
spine
    s. of Henle
    suprameatal s.
splint
    Asch's s.
    Carter's s.
    Erich's s.
    Jones' s.
    Kazanjian's s.
    Love's s.
    Mayer's s.
spondylosis
spoon
    Gross' s.
spot
    Koplik's s's
Spratt's curet
spud
    Gross' s.
squama
squamomastoid
SRT – speech reception test
    speech reception threshold
Stacke's operation
Stallard's operation
stapedectomy
    Guilford's s.
    Hough's s.
    House's s.
    Schuknecht's s.
    Shea's s.
stapedial
stapediolysis
stapedioplasty
stapediotenotomy
stapediovestibular
stapes

staphylagra
staphylectomy
staphyledema
staphylematoma
staphyline
staphylinus
staphylion
staphylitis
staphyloangina
staphyloncus
staphylopharyngorrhaphy
staphyloplasty
staphyloptosia
staphyloptosis
staphylorrhaphy
staphyloschisis
staphylotome
staphylotomy
Stenger's test
stenosis
Stensen's
    duct
    foramen
stent
Stenver's position
sternohyoid
sternomastoid
sternothyroid
sternotracheal
Stevens' scissors
Stoerk's blennorrhea
stomatitides
stomatitis
    aphthous s.
stomatomycosis
stomatoplasty
Storz-Beck snare
Straight's tenaculum
stria
    s. vascularis ductus
        cochlearis
stricture
stridor
Struempel's forceps
struma
Struyken's forceps

Stubbs' curet
stump
    tracheal s.
Stutsman's snare
stuttering
stylohyal
stylohyoid
styloid
stylomandibular
stylomastoid
subarachnoid
subglossitis
subglottic
sublingual
submandibular
submaxillary
submental
submucous
suctioning
sudo-. See words beginning
    pseudo-.
sudokolesteatoma. See
    pseudocholesteatoma.
sulcus
    tympanic s.
summit
    s. of nose
Sunday's elevator
suppuration
suppurative
supraclavicular
supraglottic
supraglottitis
suprahyoid
supramandibular
supramastoid
supramaxillary
supramental
supranasal
supraorbital
suprastapedial
suprasternal
supratemporal
surgical procedures. See
    operation.
Sutton's disease

suture. See *General Surgical
    Terms* section.
swimmer's ear
symptom
    Bárány's s.
    esophagosalivary s.
    Fröschel's s.
    labyrinthine s's
synchondrosis
syncytial
syndrome
    Apert's s.
    Avellis' s.
    Baelz's s.
    Bárány's s.
    Costen's s.
    Crouzon's s.
    Gradenigo's s.
    Heerfordt's s.
    Horner's s.
    Hurler's s.
    Kartagener's s.
    Klippel-Feil s.
    Lermoyez's s.
    Mikulicz's s.
    Möbius' s.
    Osler-Weber-Rendu s.
    Pierre Robin s.
    Plummer-Vinson s.
    Richards-Rundle s.
    Sjögren's s.
    toxic shock s.
    Treacher Collins s.
synechia
syringe
    irrigating s.
Tabb's curet
Takahashi's
    forceps
    punch
tampon
    nasal t.
tantalum
technique
    guillotine t.

Teflon
        prosthesis
        tube
tegmen
        t. antri
        t. cellulae
        t. mastoideotympanicum
        t. mastoideum
        t. tympani
tegmental
tegmentum
        t. auris
temple
tempora
temporal
temporalis
temporoauricular
temporofacial
temporofrontal
temporohyoid
temporomandibular
temporomaxillary
temporo-occipital
temporoparietal
temporosphenoid
temporozygomatic
tenaculum
        Cottle's t.
        Straight's t.
tendon
        stapedius t.
tentorial
tentorium
terigo-. See words beginning
        pterygo-.
test
        Bárány's t.
        Bing's t.
        caloric t.
        clivogram t.
        Doerfler-Stewart t.
        Erhard's t.
        fistula t.
        Gault's t.
        Gellé's t.
        impedance audiometry t.
        Lombard's t.

test (continued)
        Politzer's t.
        radioallergosorbent t.
        Rinne's t.
        rotation t.
        Schwabach's t.
        short increment
                sensitivity index (SISI) t.
        Stenger's t.
        Tobey-Ayer t.
        torsion t.
        tuning fork t.
        watch t.
        Weber's t.
        whisper t.
        whistle t.
Theobald's probe
Thornwald's perforator
Thornwaldt's disease
thrombophlebitis
thrombosis
        cavernous sinus t.
thrush
thyrochondrotomy
thyrocricotomy
thyroglossal
thyrohyoid
thyroid
        t. cartilage
        t. gland
thyroiditis
thyromegaly
thyrotomy
thyrotoxicosis
tia-. See words beginning
        ptya-.
tialektasis. See *ptyalectasis*.
tializm. See *ptyalism*.
tic
        t. douloureux (doo-loo-
                roo)
tinnitus
Tivnen's forceps
TM – tympanic membrane
TMJ – temporomandibular joint
Tobey-Ayer test
Tobey's rongeur

Tobold's
> forceps
> knife

tongue
> black hairy t.
> geographic t.
> scrotal t.
> t.-tie

tongue-tie

tonsil
> buried t.
> eustachian t.
> faucial t.
> hypertrophied t.
> lingual t.
> Luschka's t.
> palatine t.
> pharyngeal t.
> submerged t.

tonsilla
> t. lingualis
> t. palatina
> t. pharyngea
> t. tubaria

tonsillar

tonsillectome
> Ballenger-Sluder t.
> Beck-Mueller t.
> Beck-Schenck t.
> Brown's t.
> Daniels' t.
> Laforce's t.
> Mack's t.
> Moltz-Storz t.
> Myles' t.
> Sauer's t.
> Sauer-Sluder t.
> Searcy's t.
> Sluder-Demarest t.
> Sluder's t.
> Sluder-Sauer t.
> Tydings' t.
> Van Osdel's t.
> Whiting's t.

tonsillectomy

tonsillitis
> caseous t.

tonsillitis (continued)
> catarrhal t.
> diphtherial t.
> erythematous t.
> follicular t.
> herpetic t.
> lacunar t.
> t. lenta
> lingual t.
> mycotic t.
> parenchymatous t.
> preglottic t.
> pustular t.
> streptococcal t.
> Vincent's t.

tonsilloadenoidectomy

tonsillolith

tonsilloscope

tonsilloscopy

tonsillotome

tonsillotomy

tophi
> gouty t.

Topinard's
> angle
> line

Tornwaldt's bursitis

TORP – total ossicular
> replacement prosthesis

torticollis

torus
> t. frontalis
> t. levatorius
> t. mandibularis
> t. occipitalis
> t. palatinus
> t. tubarius

Towne's view

Toynbee's
> otoscope
> speculum

trachea

tracheal
> t. atresia
> t. cannula

tracheitis

tracheobronchial

tracheobronchitis
tracheobronchoscopy
tracheocannula
    Montgomery's t.
tracheocele
tracheoesophageal
tracheofissure
tracheofistulization
tracheolaryngeal
tracheolaryngotomy
tracheomalacia
tracheopharyngeal
tracheoplasty
tracheorrhaphy
tracheoscopy
    peroral t.
tracheostenosis
tracheostomy
tracheotome
    Salvatore-Maloney t.
    Sierra-Sheldon t.
tracheotomy
tragus
transillumination
transnasal
Trautmann's triangle
Treacher Collins syndrome
treatment
    Politzer's t.
    Proetz's t.
    Roeder's t.
trench mouth
trephination
trephine
triad
    Kartagener's t.
triangle
    Trautmann's t.
trigeminal
trismus
trisomy
    13–15 D
    18 E
trocar
    Coakley's t.
Tröltsch's
    recesses

Tröltsch's (continued)
    speculum
Troutman's
    chisel
    gouge
tube
    Anthony's t.
    auditory t.
    Blakemore's t.
    Bouchut's t.
    Castelli's t.
    Chevalier Jackson t.
    Communitrach t.
    Donaldson's t.
    endotracheal t.
    eustachian t.
    Frazier's t.
    House's t.
    intubation t.
    Jackson's t.
    Lanz' t.
    LaRocca's t.
    Lewis' t.
    Lindeman-Silverstein t.
    Mackenty's t.
    Morch's t.
    nasopharyngeal t.
    otopharyngeal t.
    Paparella's t.
    Per-Lee t.
    Reuter's t.
    Rosen's t.
    Ruysch's t.
    Schall's t.
    Sengstaken-Blakemore t.
    Sengstaken's t.
    Shea's t.
    Sheehy's t.
    Shepard's t.
    Shiley's t.
    Teflon t.
    ventilation t.
    Voltolini's t.
    Welch-Allyn t.
    Yankauer's t.
tubercle
    darwinian t.

tuberculosis
    t. of larynx
    tracheobronchial t.
tuborrhea
tubotorsion
tubotympanal
tubotympanic
    t. recess
Tucker's
    esophagoscope
    laryngoscope
tumefaction
tumor
    acoustic t.
    hypopharyngeal t.
    neuroectodermal t.
    neurogenic t.
    odontogenic t.
    Rathke's t.
    Schmincke t.
    Warthin's t.
tuning fork
    Hartmann's t.f.
tunnel
    t. of Corti
turbinate
    sphenoid t.
turbinectomy
turbinotome
turbinotomy
Tydings'
    forceps
    knife
    snare
    tonsillectome
Tydings-Lakeside forceps
tympanal
tympanectomy
tympanic
tympanichord
tympanichordal
tympanicity
tympanion
tympanitic
tympanitis
tympanoacryloplasty
tympanocentesis

tympanoeustachian
tympanogram
tympanolabyrinthopexy
tympanomalleal
tympanomandibular
tympanomastoiditis
tympanomeatal
tympanometry
tympano-ossicular system
tympanophonia
tympanoplasty
tympanosclerosis
tympanosquamosal
tympanostapedial
tympanosympathectomy
tympanotemporal
tympanotomy
tympanum
tympany
ulcer
    contact u.
uloglossitis
uloncus
ultrasonogram
ultrasonography
ultrasound
umbo
    u. of tympanic membrane
uniaural
unit
    Hertz u.
Updegraff's needle
UPP – uvulopalato-
    pharyngoplasty
uraniscochasma
uraniscolalia
uranisconitis
uranoplasty
Usher's disease
utricle
uvula
    u. palatina
    palatine u.
uvulectomy
uvulitis
uvulopalatopharyngoplasty
uvuloptosis

uvulotome
uvulotomy
vallecula
    v. epiglottica
Valsalva's procedure
valve
    Huschke's v.
Van Osdel's tonsillectome
Van Struycken
    forceps
    punch
varix
vas
vasa
    v. auris internae
vasoconstrictor
vasomotor
vault
    cartilaginous v.
velum
    v. palatinum
ventilation
ventricle
    Morgagni's v.
ventricular
ventriculocordectomy
Verga's lacrimal groove
vermilion border
vermilionectomy
vertiginous
vertigo
    paroxysmal positional v.
vestibular
    v. nerve
    v. neuronitis
    v. reflex
    v. system
vestibule
vestibulo-ocular reflex
vestibulotomy
vestibulum
    v. auris
    v. glottidis
    v. laryngis
    v. nasi
    v. oris

vibrissa
vibrissae
vibromasseur
vibrometer
Vicq d'Azyr's operation
Vienna speculum
Vieussens' annulus
view
    Law's v.
    Owens' v.
    Schüller's v.
    Towne's v.
    Waters' v.
Vincent's
    infection
    tonsillitis
virus
    Epstein-Barr v.
vocal
Vogel's curet
Voltolini's tube
vomer
vomeronasal
von Recklinghausen's disease
Waardenburg's disease
Wagner's punch
Waldeyer's ring
Walker's dissector
Walsham's forceps
Walther's ducts
Warthin's tumor
Waters' view
Watson-Williams
    forceps
    punch
web
Weber's test
Wegener's granulomatosis
Weil's forceps
Weingartner's forceps
Weisman's curet
Weitlaner's retractor
Welch-Allyn
    laryngoscope
    otoscope
    probe

Welch-Allyn (continued)
   speculum
   tube
Wellaminski's perforator
West's operation
Wharton's duct
wheezing
White-Lillie forceps
White-Proud retractor
White's forceps
Whiting's
   curet
   rongeur
   tonsillectome
whooping cough
Wiener-Pierce rasp
Wilde-Bruening snare
Wilde's
   forceps
   punch
Willis' paracusis
window
   oval w.
   round w.
windowing
Wis-Foregger's laryngoscope
Wis-Hipple's laryngoscope
Woake's saw
Wood's operation
Wreden's sign
Wright's snare
Wrisberg's cartilage

Wullstein-House forceps
Wullstein's
   bur
   forceps
   knife
   operation
   retractor
xanthosis
   x. of septum nasi
xeromycteria
xerostomia
Yankauer-Little forceps
Yankauer's
   catheter
   curet
   esophagoscope
   forceps
   laryngoscope
   operation
   probe
   punch
   speculum
   tube
Zaufal's sign
Zeiss' microscope
Zenker's diverticulum
zygoma
zygomatic
zygomaticofacial
zygomaticofrontal
zygomaticomaxillary
zygomaxillary

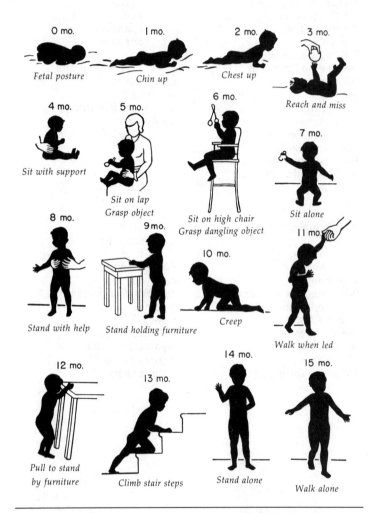

0 mo. **Fetal posture**

1 mo. **Chin up**

2 mo. **Chest up**

3 mo. **Reach and miss**

4 mo. **Sit with support**

5 mo. **Sit on lap Grasp object**

6 mo. **Sit on high chair Grasp dangling object**

7 mo. **Sit alone**

8 mo. **Stand with help**

9 mo. **Stand holding furniture**

10 mo. **Creep**

11 mo. **Walk when led**

12 mo. **Pull to stand by furniture**

13 mo. **Climb stair steps**

14 mo. **Stand alone**

15 mo. **Walk alone**

Pediatrics

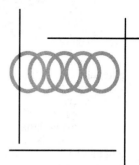

Abderhalden-Fanconi
    syndrome
abetalipoproteinemia
ABO incompatibility
abscess
    amebic a.
    Bezold's a.
    perinephric a.
    pyogenic a.
    retroesophageal a.
    retropharyngeal a.
    retrotonsillar a.
    subphrenic a.
Absidia
Abt-Letterer-Siwe
    syndrome
acanthocytosis
acantholysis
    a. bullosa
acanthosis
    a. nigricans
acatalasia
achalasia
acheiria
acholic
achondrogenesis
achondroplasia
acidosis
    diabetic a.
    hyperchloremic renal a.
    metabolic a.
aciduria
    β-aminoisobutyric a.
aclasis
    diaphyseal a.
acne
    a. conglobata
    halogen a.
    a. neonatorum

acne (continued)
    a. vulgaris
acoustic
    a. reflex
    a. trauma
acrania
acrobrachycephaly
acrocephalosyndactyly
acrocyanosis
acrodermatitis
    a. enteropathica
    papular a.
acrodynia
acromegaly
acropustulosis
Actinomyces
actinomycosis
Addison's disease
adenitis
    cervical a.
    mesenteric a.
adenocarcinoma
adenoidectomy
adenoiditis
adenoma
    islet cell a.
    a. sebaceum
adenomatosis
adenopathy
    cervical a.
adenosarcoma
adenovirus
adhesions
Adie's syndrome
adiponecrosis
    a. subcutanea neonatorum
adipsia
adnexa
adolescence

adrenal
    a. cortex
    a. crisis
    a. gland
    a. hyperplasia
    a. medulla
adrenarche
adrenocortical
adrenogenital
adynamia
    a. episodica hereditaria
aerophore
aftha. See *aphtha.*
agammaglobulinemia
aganglionosis
agenesia
    a. corticalis
agenesis
    callosal a.
    gonadal a.
    nuclear a.
    ovarian a.
    renal a.
agglutinin
agranulocytosis
AIDS – acquired immuno-
    deficiency syndrome. See
    Immunology and AIDS
    section.
akalazea. See *achalasia.*
akinesia
    a. algera
akondroplazea. See
    achondroplasia.
akrobrakesefale. See
    acrobrachycephaly.
alacrima
Albers-Schönberg syndrome
albinism
Albright's syndrome
albuminuria
Alder's anomaly
aldosteronism
    juvenile a.
Aldrich's syndrome
aleukia
    congenital a.

Alexander's disease
"Alice in Wonderland"
    syndrome
alkalosis
allergen
allergic
allergy
alopecia
    a. areata
Alper's disease
Alport's syndrome
alveolitis
alveolus
alymphocytosis
alymphoplasia
amaurosis
amaurotic familial idiocy
ambient
amebiasis
amelia
amenorrhea
aminoacidemia
aminoacidopathy
aminoaciduria
aminoaciduriasis
amnesia
    retrograde a.
amnionitis
amyloidosis
amylopectinosis
amyoplasia
    a. congenita
amyotonia
    a. congenita
anaerobic
anaphylaxis
anasarca
Ancylostoma
    A. braziliense
    A. duodenale
ancylostomiasis
Andersen's disease
Andogsky's syndrome
androgen
anemia
    aplastic a.
    breast a.

anemia (continued)
    congenital a. of newborn
    congenital nonspherocytic
      hemolytic a.
    Cooley's a.
    Czerny's a.
    erythroblastic a. of
      childhood
    familial erythroblastic a.
    Fanconi's a.
    globe cell a.
    glucose-6-phosphate
      dehydrogenase
      deficiency a.
    hemolytic a.
    a. hypochromica
      siderochrestica
      hereditaria
    hypoplastic a., congenital
    Jaksch's a.
    Larzel's a.
    Mediterranean a.
    megaloblastic a.
    microcytic a.
    a. neonatorum
    ovalocytary a.
    pernicious a., juvenile
    physiologic a.
    a. pseudoleukemica
      infantum
    pyridoxine-responsive a.
    sickle cell a.
    sideroblastic a.
    von Jaksch's a.
anemic
anencephaly
aneurysm
    aortic a.
angiitis
angiocardiography
angioedema
angiokeratoma
    a. circumscriptum
    a. of Mibelli
angioma
    spider a.
aniridia

anomaly
    Alder's a.
    May-Hegglin a.
    Pelger-Huët a.
    Peters' a.
    Poland's a.
    Undritz a.
anorchia
anorchism
anorexia
    a. nervosa
anosmia
anoxia
ansilostomiasis. See
    ancylostomiasis.
antigen
    Australia a.
antrum
anuria
anus
    imperforate a.
aorta
aortitis
Apert's disease
Apgar
    rating
    score
aphasia
    global a.
    Wernicke's a.
aphtha
    Bednar's a.
aphthous
aplasia
    a. axialis extracorticalis
      congenita
    a. cutis congenita
    gonadal a.
    Leydig cell a.
    nuclear a.
    retinal a.
    thymic a.
    thymic-parathyroid a.
aplastic
    a. anemia
    a. crisis
    a. pancytopenia

apnea
    initial a.
    late a.
    a. neonatorum
appendicitis
aqueductal
arachnidism
arachnodactyly
arachnoiditis
arak-. See words beginning
    arach-.
Aran-Duchenne disease
arbovirus
archenteronoma
areflexia
arginosuccinicaciduria
Arnold-Chiari syndrome
arrhenoblastoma
arrhinencephaly
arrhythmia
    sinus a.
arteriosclerosis
    infantile a.
arteritis
    a. umbilicalis
arthritis
    juvenile rheumatoid a.
    psoriatic a.
    septic a.
arthrogryposis
    a. multiplex congenita
ascariasis
Ascaris
    A. lumbricoides
ascites
    chylous a.
ASD–atrial septal defect
aspergillosis
asphyxia
    a. neonatorum
aspiration
asplenia
astasia
    a.-abasia
asthma
    thymic a.
astigmatism

astrocytoma
ataxia
    cerebellar a.
    Friedreich's a.
atelectasis
    congenital a.
    primary a.
athetoid
athetosis
    congenital a.
athlete's foot
atonic
atopic
atopy
atresia
    biliary a.
    esophageal a.
    ileal a.
    pyloric a.
    tricuspid a.
atrial
    a. contraction
    a. enlargement
    a. fibrillation
    a. flutter
    a. septal defect
    a. septostomy
    a. tachycardia
atrium
atrophia bulborum hereditaria
atrophy
    Déjérine-Sottas a.
    Fazio-Londe a.
    infantile a.
    Parrot's a. of the new-
        born
audiogram
audiometry
aura
Australia antigen
autism
autistic
autoprothrombin I
autosomal
Babinski's sign
bacteremia
bacteroidosis

Ballantyne-Runge syndrome
Banti's syndrome
Barlow's disease
Bartter's syndrome
Bassen-Kornzweig syndrome
Batten-Mayou disease
Beau's line
Beck's disease
Beckwith's syndrome
Bednar's aphtha
Berger's paresthesia
beriberi
Best's disease
bezoar
Bezold's abscess
Bielschowsky syndrome
biliary
    b. atresia
    b. hypoplasia
bilirubin
Blalock-Hanlon operation
Blalock-Taussig operation
blastomycosis
blefaritis. See *blepharitis.*
blefarospasm. See
    blepharospasm.
blennorrhea
blepharitis
blepharospasm
Bloch-Sulzberger syndrome
blood
    cord b.
Bloom's syndrome
Bochdalek
    foramen of B. hernia
    B. hernia
Bodian-Schwachman syndrome
Bonnevie-Ullrich syndrome
Bordetella
    B. pertussis
Bornholm's disease
botulism
Bouchut's respiration
Bourneville's syndrome
bowleg
Brachmann-de Lange syndrome
brachycephalic

brachydactyly
bradyarrhythmia
bradycardia
Brandt's syndrome
brash
    weaning b.
bronchial
bronchiectasis
bronchiolectasia
bronchiolitis
bronchitis
    acute laryngotracheal b.
    arachidic b.
    asthmatic a.
    chronic obstructive b.
    epidemic capillary b.
bronchobiliary
bronchogenic
bronchogram
bronchopneumonia
bronchopulmonary
    b. aspergillosis
    b. dysplasia
    b. lavage
bronchoscopy
bronchospasm
bronchus
    esophageal b.
Brown-Symmers disease
Brucella
brucellosis
Brudzinski's sign
bruit
    aortic b.
    carotid b.
Brushfield's spots
Bruton's disease
bruxism
brwe. See *bruit.*
Budd-Chiari syndrome
Buhl's disease
bulimia
bullous
    b. congenital
      ichthyosiform
      erythroderma
    b. dermatosis

bullous (continued)
    b. impetigo
    b. pemphigoid
Burkitt's lymphoma
burping
butterfly rash
Byler's disease
Byrd-Dew method
Caffey-Kenny disease
Caffey's disease
Caffey-Silverman syndrome
Caffey-Smyth-Roske syndrome
calculi
calculus
    urate c.
Calvé-Legg-Perthes syndrome
Camurati-Engelmann syndrome
Canavan's disease
cancer
cancerous
Candida
    C. albicans
candidiasis
candidosis
canker
caput
    c. medusae
    c. quadratum
    c. succedaneum
carbuncle
carcinogenesis
carcinoid
carcinoma
cardiac
cardiomyopathy
cardiorespiratory
cardiospasm
carditis
Caroli's disease
Carpenter's syndrome
cataplexy
cataract
catarrhal
catheter
    arterial c.
    umbilical c.
    venous c.

catheterization
cavernous
    c. hemangioma
    c. sinus thrombosis
cavus foot
celiac
    c. disease
    c. sprue
celiaca
cellulitis
cephalhematoma
cerebellar
cerebral
cerebrospinal
cerebrovascular
Chagas' disease
chalasia
chalazion
Chapple's syndrome
Charcot-Marie-Tooth-Hoffmann
    syndrome
Cheadle's disease
Chédiak-Higashi syndrome
chemotaxis
chemotherapy
chickenpox
chigger bite
Chilaiditi's syndrome
cholangitis
cholecystectomy
cholecystitis
    acute acalculous c.
cholelithiasis
cholera
    c. infantum
cholestasis
chondrodysplasia
    c. punctata
chondrodystrophia
    c. calcificans congenita
    c. fetalis calcificans
chondrodystrophy
chondro-osteodystrophy
chondrosarcoma
chordee
chorea
    Sydenham's c.

chorioepithelioma
choriomeningitis
    lymphocytic c.
chorioretinitis
Christ-Siemens-Touraine
    syndrome
chromaffinoma
chromosomal
chromosome
Chvostek's sign
circulatory
    c. arrest
    c. failure
circumcision
cirrhonosus
cirrhosis
    biliary c.
citrullinuria
Clark-Hadfield syndrome
cleft
    c. lip
    c. palate
clinodactyly
cloaca
    congenital c.
clonus
    ankle c.
clostridia
clubfoot
clubhand
CNS – central nervous
    system
coarctation
    c. of the aorta
Coat's disease
coccidioidomycosis
Cockayne's syndrome
colic
colicky
colitis
    amoebic c.
    granulomatous c.
    infectious c.
    tuberculous c.
    ulcerative c.
collodion baby
coloboma

colonization
    stool c.
Colorado tick fever
colostration
colostrum
coma
    diabetic c.
    hyperosmolar c.
Comby's sign
communicable
complex
    Eisenmenger's c.
    Ghon c.
concussion
condylomata
    c. acuminata
    c. lata
congenital
congestive
conjunctivitis
Conradi's disease
constipation
contusion
conversion
    hysterical c.
convulsion
    febrile c.
Cooley's anemia
Coombs' test
cor
    c. biloculare
    c. triloculare biatriatum
Cori's disease
Cornelia de Lange's
    syndrome
corpora
    c. quadrigemina
Corrigan's pulse
cortex
    adrenal c.
cortical
    c. hyperostosis
    c. nephron
corticosteroid
Corynebacterium
    C. diphtheriae
coryza

coxa
  c. vara
coxsackieviral
Coxsackie virus
cradle cap
craniopharyngioma
craniostenosis
craniosynostosis
craniotabes
crease
    simian c.
    sole c.
creatinine
crepitation
cretinism
crib death
cri-du-chat syndrome
Crigler-Najjar syndrome
crisis
    adrenal c.
criteria
    Jones' c.
Crohn's disease
croup
Crouzon's disease
crusta
    c. lactea
cryoprecipitate
cryptococcosis
cryptorchidism
culture
    sputum c.
    tracheal-aspirate c.
Curling's ulcer
curse
    Ondine's c.
Cushing-Rokitansky
    ulcer
Cushing's syndrome
cutaneous
    c. anthrax
    c. larva migrans
    c. leishmaniasis
    c. mucormycosis
    c. nevi
    c. vasculitis

cutis
  c. elastica
  c. hyperelastica
  c. laxa
  c. marmorata
  c. verticis gyrata
CVP–central venous pressure
cyanosis
cyst
    choledochal c.
    colloid c.
    dermoid c.
    follicular c.
    hydatid c.
    inclusion c.
    omental c.
    popliteal c.
    porencephalic c's
    urachal c.
    vitelline duct c.
cystadenocarcinoma
cystathioninuria
cystic
  c. fibrosis
  c. hygroma
cystinosis
cystinuria
cystitis
  c. cystica
  hemorrhagic c.
cystography
cytomegalovirus
Czerny's anemia
dacroadenitis
dacrostenosis
dacryocystostenosis
dactylitis
Dalrymple's sign
dance
    St. Vitus' d.
dandruff
Dandy-Walker
    deformity
    syndrome
Darrow-Gamble syndrome
Dawson's encephalitis
Debré-Sémélaigne syndrome

defect
    atrial septal d.
    ventricular septal d.
deficiency
    disaccharidase d.
    erythrocyte glutathione
      peroxidase d.
    Factor VIII d.
    fibrinogen d.
    fructose d.
    galactokinase d.
    glucose-6-phosphate
      dehydrogenase d.
    IgA d.
    IgM d.
    immunoglobulin d.
    pyruvate-kinase d.
    riboflavin d.
deformity
    cloverleaf skull d.
    Dandy-Walker d.
    Sprengel's d.
    Vookmann's d.
degeneration
    cerebellar d.
    cerebromacular d.
    congenital macular d.
    vitelliform d.
dehydration
Déjérine's disease
Déjérine-Sottas
    atrophy
    disease
de Lange's syndrome
delinquency
delirium
dengue
Dennett's diet
Dennie-Marfan syndrome
depigmentation
dermatitis
    atopic d.
    chronic bullous d.
    diaper d.
    d. excoriativa infantum
    d. exfoliativa infantum
    d. gangrenosa infantum

dermatitis (continued)
    d. herpetiformis
    Jacquet's d.
    nickel d.
    seborrheic d.
    d. venenata
dermatofibroma
dermatomyositis
dermatophytosis
dermatosis
    juvenile plantar d.
DeSanctis-Cacchione syndrome
desensitization
determination
    sweat chloride d.
de Toni-Fanconi-Debre
    syndrome
dextrocardia
Dextrostix
diabetes
    brittle d.
    d. insipidus
    d. mellitus
diabetic
diadochokinesis
dialysis
Diamond-Blackfan
    syndrome
diarrhea
diastasis
    d. recti
diastematomyelia
diencephalic syndrome
diet
    Dennett's d.
    Moro-Heisler d.
difenilthiourea. See
    diphenylthiourea.
difilobothriasis. See
    diphyllobothriasis.
diftherea. See *diphtheria.*
DiGeorge's syndrome
dilatation
    esophageal d.
diphenylthiourea
diphtheria
diphyllobothriasis

Diphyllobothrium
    D. latum
diplegia
    atonic-astatic d.
    facial d., congenital
    infantile d.
    spastic d.
Diplococcus
    D. pneumoniae
diplopia
Dirofilaria
    D. immitis
    D. tenuis
dis-. See words beginning *dys-*.
disease
    Addison's d.
    Alexander's d.
    Alper's d.
    Andersen's d.
    antiglomerular basement
      membrane antibody d.
    Apert's d.
    Aran-Duchenne d.
    Barlow's d.
    Batten-Mayou d.
    Beck's d.
    Best's d.
    Bornholm's d.
    Brown-Symmers d.
    Bruton's d.
    Buhl's d.
    Byler's d.
    Caffey-Kenny
    Caffey's d.
    Canavan's d.
    Caroli's d.
    cat scratch d.
    celiac d.
    central nervous system d.
    Chagas' d.
    Cheadle's d.
    Coat's d.
    collagen d.
    communicable d.
    Conradi's d.
    Cori's d.
    Crohn's d.

disease (continued)
    Crouzon's d.
    cytomegalic inclusion d.
      of the newborn
    cytomegalovirus d.
    Déjérine's d.
    Déjérine-Sottas d.
    Duke's d.
    Duroziez's d.
    Fabry's d.
    Factor X deficiency d.
    Farber's d.
    Feer's d.
    fibrocystic d.
    fifth d.
    Filatov-Dukes d.
    Fölling's d.
    Fordyce's d.
    ganglioside storage d.
    Gaucher's d.
    Gee-Herter-Heubner d.
    genetotrophic d.
    glycogen storage d.
    Goldstein's d.
    Graves' d.
    Hartnup's d.
    helminthic d.
    hemoglobin C-thalassemia
      d.
    hemoglobin E-thalassemia
      d.
    hemolytic d. of the
      newborn
    hemorrhagic d. of
      newborn
    Henoch's d.
    hereditary d.
    heredoconstitutional d.
    heredodegenerative d.
    Hers' d.
    Hirschsprung's d.
    Hodgkin's d.
    Huntington's d.
    Hutinel's d.
    hyaline membrane d.
    hydatid d.
    hydrocephaloid d.

disease (continued)

    I cell d.

    infantile celiac d.

    Kashin-Beck d.

    Kawasaki d.

    kinky-hair d.

    Köhler's d.

    Krabbe's d.

    Kufs' d.

    Kugelberg-Welander d.

    Leber's d.

    Legionnaires' d.

    Leigh's d.

    Leiner's d.

    Letterer-Siwe d.

    Little's d.

    Luft's d.

    Lyme d.

    maple syrup urine d.

    Marion's d.

    McArdle's d.

    Melnick-Needles d.

    Milroy's d.

    Minot's d.

    Möller-Barlow d.

    Morquio's d.

    Niemann-Pick d.

    Norrie's d.

    Oppenheim's d.

    Osler-Weber-Rendu d.

    Owren's d.

    Paas' d.

    Paget's d.

    Pelizaeus-Merzbacher d.

    pelvic inflammatory d.

    phytanic acid storage d.

    pink d.

    Pompe's d.

    Potter's d.

    pulseless d.

    Recklinghausen's d.

    Refsum's d.

    renal cystic d.

    Ritter's d.

    Sandhoff d.

    Saunders' d.

    Scheuermann's d.

disease (continued)

    Schilder's d.

    Scholz's d.

    sickle cell d.

    sickle cell-hemoglobin C d.

    sickle cell-hemoglobin D d.

    sickle cell-thalassemia d.

    Spielmeyer-Vogt d.

    spinocerebellar degenerative d.

    Stargardt's d.

    Sticker's d.

    Still's d.

    Stuart-Prower factor deficiency d.

    Swift's d.

    Tangier d.

    Tay-Sachs d.

    Thiemann's d.

    Thomsen's d.

    Thomson's d.

    Trevor's d.

    Underwood's d.

    Unverricht's d.

    van Buchem's d.

    Vogt-Spielmeyer d.

    Volkmann's d.

    von Gierke's d.

    von Hippel-Lindau d.

    von Recklinghausen's d.

    von Willebrand's d.

    Weil's d.

    Wilkins' d.

    Wilson's d.

    Winckel's d.

    Wolman's d.

    wooly hair d.

disfagia. See *dysphagia.*

disjenisis. See *dysgenesis.*

dislocation

distress

    idiopathic respiratory d. of newborn

diuresis

diverticula

diverticulosis
diverticulum
    Meckel's d.
    pharyngeal d.
doll's head maneuver
Donohue's syndrome
Down's syndrome
drooling
drugs. See *Drugs and Chemistry*
    section.
Duane's syndrome
Dubin-Johnson syndrome
Dubovitz's syndrome
Duchenne's dystrophy
duct
    müllerian d.
    omphalomesenteric d.
    Stensen's d.
    vitelline d.
ductus
    d. arteriosus
Duke's disease
duodenal
    d. ileus
    d. obstruction
duplication
    d. cysts
    d. of colon
    d. of duodenum
    d. of esophagus
    d. of ileum
    d. of rectum
    d. of stomach
Duroziez's disease
dwarfism
    pituitary d.
Dyggve-Melchior-Clausen
    syndrome
dysautonomia
    familial d.
dysbetalipoproteinemia
dyschondroplasia
dysdiadochokinesis
dysentery
    amebic d.
    bacillary d.
dysfibrinogenemia

dysfunction
    placental d.
dysgammaglobulinemia
dysgenesis
    gonadal d.
dysgerminoma
dyshepatia
    lipogenic d.
dyshidrosis
dyskeratosis
    d. congenita
dyslexia
dysmaturity
dysmenorrhea
dysmorphology
dysnomia
dysostosis
    cleidocranial d.
    craniofacial d.
    mandibulofacial d.
    metaphyseal d.
    d. multiplex
    orodigitofacial d.
dysphagia
dysplasia
    anhidrotic ectodermal d.
    arteriohepatic d.
    bronchopulmonary d.
    camptomelic d.
    chondroectodermal d.
    cleidocranial d.
    congenital alveolar d.
    craniodiaphyseal d.
    craniometaphyseal d.
    cretinoid d.
    diaphyseal d.
    diastrophic d.
    ectodermal d.
    d. epiphysealis hemimelica
    d. epiphysealis punctata
    frontometaphyseal d.
    hereditary bone d.
    hidrotic ectodermal d.
    Kniest's d.
    metaphyseal d.
    metatropic d.
    oculoauriculovertebral

dysplasia (continued)
    (OAV) d.
    oculodentodigital (ODD)
      d.
    ophthalmomandi-
      bulomelic d.
    polyostotic fibrous d.
    punctate epiphyseal d.
    Robinow's mesomelic d.
    spondyloepiphyseal d.
    spondylometaphyseal d.
    thanatophoric d.
    thymic d.
    trichorhinophalangeal d.
dyspnea
dyspraxia
dysrhythmia
dystaxia
    d. cerebralis infantilis
dysthymic
dystonia
    d. musculorum deformans
    torsion d.
dystrophy
    Duchenne's d.
    limb-girdle d.
    Meesmann's d.
    muscular d.
    oculocerebrorenal d.
    twenty-nail d.
Eagle-Barrett syndrome
EBV – Epstein-Barr virus
eccentrochondroplasia
eccentro-osteochondrodysplasia
ecchymosis
Echinococcus
    E. granulosus
    E. multilocularis
ECHO – enteric cytopathogenic
   human orphan (virus)
echocardiography
echoencephalography
echovirus
ecthyma
ectopia
    e. cordis
    e. lentis

eczema
    dyshidrotic e.
    e. herpeticum
    infantile e.
    e. marginatum
    e. neonatorum
    nummular e.
    e. vaccinatum
eczematoid
edema
    angioneurotic e.,
      hereditary
    e. neonatorum
eelworm
efeb-. See words beginning
   epheb-.
efelidez. See *ephelides.*
efelis. See *ephelis.*
effusion
Ehlers-Danlos syndrome
Eisenmenger's complex
ekimosis. See *ecchymosis.*
ekinokokus. See *Echinococcus.*
eksanthen. See *exanthen.*
ekthima. See *ecthyma.*
ekzema. See *eczema.*
elastosis
    e. performans serpiginosa
electrocardiography
electrodesiccation
electroencephalogram
electroencephalography
electrolyte
electromyography
electrophoresis
elephantiasis
    congenital e.
elliptocytosis
Ellis-van Creveld syndrome
embolism
embolus
embryo
embryoma
embryonic
emesis
emphysema
    lobar e., infantile

empyema
emulsion
    Pusey's e.
encephalitis
    Dawson's e.
    e. neonatorum
    St. Louis e.
    Schilder's e.
    viral e.
encephalocele
encephalomyelitis
encephalopathy
    demyelinating e.
    spongiform e.
encephalotrigeminal
    e. angiomatosis
enchondroma
enchondromatosis
encopresis
endocarditis
    subacute bacterial e.
endocrinopathy
endoscopy
endotracheal
    e. intubation
Entamoeba
    E. histolytica
enteritis
    bacterial e.
    regional e.
enterobiasis
Enterobius
    E. vermicularis
enterocolitis
    necrotizing e.
enteropathy
enteroviral
enuresis
eosinophilia
ependymoma
ephebiatrics
ephebic
ephebogenesis
ephebogenic
ephebology
ephelides
ephelis

EPI – Expanded Programme on
    Immunization
epicanthal
epicanthus
epidermal
epidermis
epidermolysis
    e. bullosa
epidermophytosis
epididymis
epididymitis
epidural
    e. abscess
    e. empyema
    e. hemorrhage
epifisis. See *epiphysis.*
epigastric
epilepsia
    e. partialis continua
epilepsy
    abdominal e.
    focal e.
    grand mal e.
    jacksonian e.
    myoclonus e.
    nocturnal e.
    petit mal e.
    photosensitive e.
    psychomotor e.
    rolandic e.
    temporal lobe e.
epileptic
epileptiform
epiloia
epiphyseal
epiphysis
epispadias
epistaxis
epithelioma
    e. adenoides cysticum
    basal cell e.
epituberculosis
Epstein-Barr virus
Epstein's
    pearls
    symptom
Erb-Duchenne paralysis

erithema. See *erythema.*
erithro-. See words beginning
  erythro-.
Erlacher-Blount syndrome
eruption
  Kaposi's varicelliform e.
erysipelas
Erysipelothrix
erythema
  e. chronicum migrans
  e. infectiosum
  Jacquet's e.
  e. marginatum
  e. multiforme exudativum
  e. neonatorum toxicum
  e. nodosum leprosum
  e. streptogenes
  e. toxicum
erythredema polyneuropathy
erythroblastosis
  e. fetalis
  e. neonatorum
erythroderma
  atopic e.
  e. desquamativum
erythroleukoblastosis
Escherichia
  E. coli
esophageal
  e. atresia
  e. sphincter
  e. varices
esophagitis
  infectious e.
  monilia e.
  reflux e.
esophagus
esthesioneuroblastoma
eustachian
  e. tube
eventration
Ewing's
  sarcoma
  tumor
exanthem
  e. subitum
exomphalos

exostosis
Expanded Programme on
  Immunization
exstrophy
extragonadal
extrahepatic
extrapulmonary
extrapyramidal
extrasystole
Fabry's disease
Factor D, H, I, V, VIII, IX, XI,
  XII, XIII
  deficiency
  Hageman f.
  inhibitor
Factor X deficiency disease
Fallot's tetralogy
familial
  f. osteochondrodystrophy
Fanconi-Albertini-Zellweger
  syndrome
Fanconi-Petrassi syndrome
Fanconi's
  anemia
  syndrome
Farber's
  disease
  test
farinjitis. See *pharyngitis.*
fasciculation
fascioscapulohumeral
fasciitis
  diffuse f.
  eosinophilic f.
Fazio-Londe atrophy
febrile
fecalith
  appendiceal f.
feces
Feer's disease
fenilketonurea. See
  phenylketonuria.
feochromocytoma. See
  pheochromocytoma.
fetal
  f. circulation
  f. crowding

fetal (continued)
    f. distress
    f. hydrops
    f. scalp blood sampling
fetoscopy
fetus
    acardiac f.
    harlequin f.
    viable f.
FEV – familial exudative vitro-
   retinopathy
fever
    cat scratch f.
    Colorado tick f.
    Haverhill f.
    hay f.
    paratyphoid f.
    Q f.
    rat-bite f.
    relapsing f.
    rheumatic f.
    Rocky Mountain spotted
      f.
    scarlet f.
    South African tick f.
    spotted f.
    tick f.
    typhoid f.
    typhus f.
    undulant f.
    valley f.
    West Nile f.
    yellow f.
fibrillation
    atrial f.
    ventricular f.
fibroadenoma
fibroelastosis
    endocardial f.
fibroma
    histiocytic f.
fibromatosis
fibroplasia
    retrolental f.
fibrosis
    cystic f.
    hepatic f.

fibroxanthoma
Filatov-Dukes disease
fissure
fistula
    arteriovenous f.
    bronchobiliary f.
    tracheoesophageal f.
fitobezor. See *phytobezoar.*
FJN – familial juvenile
   nephrophthisis
flaccid
flaring
    alar f.
    nasal f.
flukes
fluoridation
fluoride
fluorine
fluoroscopy
fobia. See *phobia.*
fokomelea. See *phocomelia.*
folliculitis
Fölling's disease
fontanelle
fonticulus
foramen
    f. of Bochdalek hernia
    f. of Morgagni hernia
    f. ovale
    pleuroperitoneal f.
    f. primum
    f. secundum
Fordyce's
    disease
    granule
    spots
formiminoglutamicaciduria
formula
    Hardy-Weinberg f.
fragilitas
    f. ossium
Franceschetti's syndrome
freckle
Freiberg's infraction
Frei test
frenulum
Friedreich's ataxia

frostbite
fructokinase
fructose
fructosuria
fugue state
fulminant
fungal
fungi
fungus balls
funnel chest
furuncle
furunculosis
galactose
galactosemia
gallbladder
gallstones
gamma globulin
gangliocytoma
ganglioneuroma
ganglioneuromatosis
gangliosides
gangrene
Gardnerella
    G. vaginalis
Gardner's syndrome
gargoylism
gas gangrene
Gasser's syndrome
gastritis
gastroenteritis
    eosinophilic g.
gastroesophageal
gastrointestinal
Gaucher's disease
gavage
    g. feeding
Gee-Herter-Heubner
    disease
genitalia
genu
    g. valgum
geophagia
German measles
germinoma
Gerstmann's syndrome
gestation
gestational

Ghon
    complex
    tubercle
Gianotti-Crosti syndrome
Giardia
    G. lamblia
giardiasis
    intestinal g.
gigantism
    cerebral g.
    eunuchoid g.
    fetal g.
    hyperpituitary g.
    pituitary g.
gigantoblast
Gilbert-Dreyfus syndrome
Gilbert-Lereboullet syndrome
Gilles de la Tourette's syndrome
gingivitis
    herpetic g.
gingivostomatitis
    herpetic g.
gland
    parotid g.
    Philip's g's
    salivary g.
    sublingual g.
    submaxillary g.
glanders
Glanzmann's syndrome
glaucoma
glioblastoma
glioma
    pontine g.
globulin
globus
    g. hystericus
glomerular
    g. filtration rate
    g. insufficiency
    g. proteinuria
    g. sclerosis
glomerulonephritis
glomerulotubular
glomerulus
glossitis
glucoglycinuria

glucose
glucosuria
glutathione
glutathionemia
glycinuria
glycogen
glycosuria
goiter
Goldstein's disease
Goltz-Gorlin syndrome
Goltz's syndrome
gonad
gonadarche
gonadoblastoma
gonadotropin
gonococcal
gonorrhea
Goodpasture's syndrome
Gowers' sign
G6PD – glucose-6-phosphate
    dehydrogenase
Gradenigo's syndrome
Graham Steell murmur
grand mal
Granger's sign
granule
    Fordyce's g.
granuloma
    g. annulare
    telangiectatic g.
granulomatosis
    Wegener's g.
granulomatous
graphesthesia
Graves' disease
Grünfelder's reflex
grunting
Guillain-Barré syndrome
Guthrie test
guttate
    g. parapsoriasis
    g. psoriasis
gynecomastia
habituation
Haemophilus
    H. aphrophilus
    H. influenzae

Haemophilus (continued)
    H. vaginalis
Hageman factor
hairball
Hall-Pallister syndrome
hallux
    h. valgus
hamartoma
Hamman-Rich syndrome
hammer toe
Hand-Schüller-Christian
    syndrome
Hanhart's syndrome
haptoglobin
Hardy-Weinberg formula
harlequin fetus
Hartnup's
    disease
    syndrome
Hart's syndrome
Haverhill fever
HDN – hemolytic disease of the
    newborn
Head's reflex
heart block
    Wenckebach h.b.
hebetic
Hecht's pneumonia
helminth
hemangioblastoma
hemangioma
    cavernous h.
    macular h.
hemangiomatosis
hemarthrosis
hematemesis
hematochezia
hematoma
    extradural h.
    subdural h.
    sublingual h.
    submental h.
hematopoiesis
hematuria
hemiatrophy
hemiplegia
hemivertebra

hemochromatosis
hemodialysis
hemoglobinopathy
hemolysis
hemolytic
hemophilia
hemophiliac
hemophilus
hemopneumomothorax
hemorrhage
    sternocleidomastoid h.
    subarachnoid h.
hemorrhagic
    h. cystitis
    h. fever
    h. shock
    h. telangiectasia
hemosiderosis
Henoch's disease
hepatic
hepatitis
    h. A
    h. B
    fulminant h.
    "giant cell" h.
    neonatal h.
    h. non-A
    h. non-B
hepatobiliary
hepatoblastoma
hepatocellular
hepatolenticular
hepatoma
hepatomegaly
hepatorenal
hepatosplenomegaly
hereditary
heredity
    autosomal h.
    sex-linked h.
heredoataxia
heredobiologic
heredodegeneration
heredodiathesis
heredofamilial
heredoimmunity
heredolues

heredopathia
    h. atactica
        polyneuritiformis
heredosyphilis
Hering-Breuer reflex
heritability
heritable
Hermansky-Pudlak syndrome
hermaphroditism
hernia
    Bochdalek h.
    congenital h.
    diaphragmatic h.
    hiatus h.
    incarcerated h.
    incisional h.
    inguinal h.
    Morgagni h.
    paraduodenal h.
    peritoneopericardial h.
    pleuroperitoneal h.
    retrocecal h.
    retrosternal h.
    Richter's h.
    transmesenteric h.
    umbilical h.
herniation
herniorrhaphy
herpangina
herpes
    h. labialis
    h. simplex
    h. zoster
herpesvirus
Hers' disease
heterosexual
hipsarithmea. See
    hypsarrhythmia.
Hirschsprung's disease
histidinemia
histidinuria
histiocytoma
histiocytosis
    h. X
Histoplasma
    H. capsulatum
histoplasmoma

histoplasmosis
Hodgkin's
    disease
    lymphoma
holoprosencephaly
Holt-Oram syndrome
homocystinemia
homocystinuria
homosexuality
hookworm
hordeolum
Hunter's syndrome
Huntington's disease
Hurler's syndrome
Hutchinson-Gilford syndrome
Hutchinson's syndrome
Hutinel's disease
hydranencephaly
hydroa
    h. aestivale
    h. puerorum
    h. vacciniforme
hydrocele
hydrocelectomy
hydrocephalic
hydrocephalocele
hydrocephaloid
hydrocephalus
hydrocolpos
hydrometrocolpos
hydronephrosis
hydrophobia
hydrops
    h. fetalis
hydroxyprolinemia
hygroma
hymen
    imperforate h.
hyperacidity
hyperactivity
hyperaldosteronism
hyperalphalipoproteinemia
hyperammonemia
hyperbilirubinemia
hyperbilirubinemic
hypercalcemia
    idiopathic h.

hypercalciuria
hypercapnia
hyperdibasicaminoaciduria
hyperemesis
    h. lactentium
hyperglycemia
hyperglycinemia
hyperimmunoglobulin E
hyperinsulinism
hyperkalemia
hyperkeratosis
hyperlacticacidemia
hyperlipidemia
hyperlipoproteinemia
hypermagnesemia
hypernatremia
hyperopia
hyperosmolar
    h. coma
hyperostosis
    infantile cortical h.
hyperparathyroidism
hyperplasia
    Leydig cell h.
    lymphoid h.
hyperprolinemia
hyperpyrexia
hypersegmentation
hypersensitization
hypersplenism
hypertelorism
hypertension
hyperthermia
hyperthyroidism
hyperthyroxinemia
hypertrophy
    septal h.
hyperuricemia
hyperuricosuria
hypervalinemia
hyperventilation
hyperviscosity
hypervitaminosis
hyphema
hypoadrenalism
hypoalbuminemia
hypoallergenic

hypocalcemia
hypocalcemic
hypocapnia
hypochloremia
hypochondriasis
hypochondroplasia
hypodermoclysis
hypogammaglobulinemia
    acquired h.
    congenital h.
    physiologic h.
    transient h.
hypogenesis
hypoglycemia
hypoglycemic
hypogonadism
hypokalemia
hypomagnesemia
hypomelanosis
hyponatremia
hyponatremic
hypoparathyroidism
hypopharynx
hypophosphatasia
hypophosphatemia
hypopituitarism
hypopotassemia
hypoproteinemia
hyposegmentation
hyposensitization
hypospadias
hyposplenism
hypotelorism
hypotension
hypothalamus
hypothermia
hypothyroidism
hypotonia
hypotrichosis
hypouricemia
hypoventilation
hypovitaminosis
hypovolemia
hypovolemic
hypoxemic
hypoxia
hypsarrhythmia

hysteria
I-cell disease
ichthyosiform
    i. erythroderma
ichthyosis
    lamellar i.
    i. linearis circumflexa
    i. vulgaris
    X-linked i.
icterus
    i. gravis neonatorum
    Liouville's i.
    i. melas
    i. neonatorum
idiocy
    amaurotic familial i.
    mongolian i.
idiopathic
IDM – infant of diabetic mother
IgA deficiency
IgM deficiency
iktheosis. See *ichthyosis.*
ileitis
    terminal i.
ileum
ileus
    adynamic i.
    meconium i.
    paralytic i.
imbecile
Imerslund's syndrome
iminoglycinuria
immunity
immunization
immunodeficiency
immunoelectrophoresis
immunofluorescence
immunoglobulin A, D, E, G, M
immunosuppression
immunotherapy
impaction
    fecal i.
impetigo
    bullous i.
    i. contagiosa
    i. neonatorum
incarceration

incompatibility
    ABO i.
    Rh i.
incompetence
    gastroesophageal i.
incontinence
incontinentia
    i. pigmenti achromians
incubation
incubator
infancy
infant
infantile
infarct
    bilirubin i.'s
    uric acid i.
infectious
influenza
infraction
    Freiberg's i.
inhibitor
    Factor VIII i.
insomnia
insufficiency
    adrenocortical i.
    aortic i.
intersexuality
interstitial
intertriginous
    i. candidosis
intertrigo
intestinal
in-toeing
intracellular
intracranial
intrahepatic
intrauterine
intussusception
    cecocolic i.
    colocolic i.
    ileocolic i.
    ileoileal i.
IRDS–idiopathic respiratory
  distress syndrome
iridocyclitis
iritis
irritability

ischemia
isohemagglutinin
isoimmunization
Isolette
Isospora
isovalericacidemia
Ito's nevus
Ivemark's syndrome
jacksonian epilepsy
Jacquet's
    dermatitis
    erythema
Jaksch's anemia
jamais vu
Janeway's lesion
Jansen's syndrome
Jansky-Bielschowsky
  syndrome
Jarisch-Herxheimer reaction
jaundice
    cholestatic j.
    physiologic j.
jejunum
jitteriness
jittery
Job syndrome
Johanson-Blizzard syndrome
Jones' criteria
Joseph's syndrome
Juliusberg's pustulosis
    vacciniformis acuta
juxtaglomerular
juxtamedullary
kala-azar
kalazea. See *chalasia.*
Kallmann's syndrome
Kaposi's varicelliform
    eruption
    sarcoma
karnikterus. See *kernicterus.*
Kartagener's syndrome
Kasabach-Merritt syndrome
Kashin-Beck disease
Kaufman's pneumonia
Kawasaki disease
Kayser-Fleischer ring
Kearns-Sayre syndrome
Kenny-Caffey syndrome

keratitis
  interstitial k.
keratoconjunctivitis
keratoconus
keratoderma
keratolysis
  k. neonatorum
keratoma
  k. hereditarium
  mutilans
keratopathy
  band k.
keratosis
  k. follicularis
  k. palmaris et plantaris
  k. pilaris
kerion
kernicterus
Kernig's sign
ketoacidosis
  diabetic k.
ketosis
ketotic
Kinsbourne syndrome
Klebsiella
  K. pneumoniae
Klinefelter's syndrome
Klippel-Feil syndrome
Klippel-Trenaunay-Weber
  syndrome
Kloepfer's syndrome
Klumpke's paralysis
Kniest's dysplasia
knock knees
Kocher-Debré-Sémélaigne
  syndrome
Koerber-Salus-Elschnig
  syndrome
Köhler's disease
koilonychia
kolanjitis. See cholangitis.
kolera. See cholera.
kondro-. See words beginning
  chondro-.
Koplik's spots
korea. See chorea.
korio-. See words beginning
  chorio-.

koriza. See coryza.
Krabbe's disease
Kufs' disease
Kugelberg-Welander disease
Kussmaul's respiration
Kveim test
kwashiorkor
kyphoscoliosis
kyphosis
  k. dorsalis juvenilis
labia
labyrinthitis
lacrimal
lactobezoar
lactose
  l. intolerance
lagophthalmos
Landau's
  reflex
  test
Landry-Guillain-Barré syndrome
Langer-Giedion syndrome
Langer-Saldino syndrome
lanugo
laringoskope. See laryngoscope.
larinks. See larynx.
Laron's syndrome
Larsen's syndrome
larva
  l. currens
  l. migrans
laryngeal
  l. stridor
  l. web
laryngitis
laryngoscope
laryngoscopy
laryngospasm
laryngotracheobronchitis
laryngotracheoesophageal
larynx
Larzel's anemia
Launois' syndrome
Laurence-Moon-Biedl syndrome
Laurence-Moon syndrome
lavage
  gastric l.
LBW – low birth weight

LBWI – low birth weight
    infant
LE – lupus erythematosus
Leber's disease
Legionella
    L. micdadei
    L. pneumophilia
Legionnaires' disease
Leigh's disease
Leiner's disease
leiomyoma
leishmaniasis
Lennox-Gastaut syndrome
Lennox's syndrome
lentigine(s)
leptomeningitis
leptospira
    L. icterohaemorrhagiae
    L. interrogans
leptospirosis
Leptothrix
leptotrichosis
Léri-Weill syndrome
Lesch-Nyhan syndrome
lesion
    Janeway's l.
lethargic
lethargy
Letterer-Siwe disease
leukemia
    aplastic l.
    basophilic l.
    eosinophilic l.
    granulocytic l.
    hemoblastic l.
    leukopenic l.
    lymphocytic l.
    lymphosarcoma cell l.
    mast cell l.
    megakaryocytic l.
    micromyeloblastic l.
    myeloblastic l.
    myelogenous l.
leukocoria
leukocytosis
leukodystrophy
    globoid cell l.
    sudanophilic l.

leukoencephalopathy
LeVeen shunt
lichen
    l. nitidus
    l. planus
    l. sclerosus et atrophicus
    l. scrofulosorum
    l. simplex chronicus
    l. spinulosus
    l. striatus
Lightwood-Albright syndrome
line
    Beau's l.
lingua
    l. nigra
Liouville's icterus
lipidosis
lipochondrodystrophy
lipodystrophy
lipogranulomatosis
    l. subcutanea
lipoid
lipoma
lipoprotein
Listeria
    L. monocytogenes
listeriosis
lithiasis
Little's disease
Löffler's syndrome
Louis-Bar syndrome
Lowe syndrome
L/S ratio
Luft's disease
lupus
    l. erythematosus
        disseminatus
    l. nephritis
    l. vulgaris
Lutembacher's syndrome
luteoma
Lyme disease
lymphadenitis
    mesenteric l.
lymphadenopathy
lymphangiectasis
    congenital pulmonary l.

lymphangioma
   l. circumscriptum
   l. cysticum
lymphangitis
lymphocytosis
lymphogranuloma
   l. inguinale
   l. venereum
lymphoma
      Burkitt's l.
      Hodgkin's l.
      non-Hodgkin's l.
lymphoreticulosis
lymphosarcoma
lysosomal
Macewen's sign
macrocephaly
macrogenitosomia
   m. praecox
macroglobulinemia
      Waldenström's m.
macular
Maffucci's syndrome
Magnus and de Kleijn neck
   reflexes
Majewski's syndrome
malabsorption
malaise
malaria
malformation
      bronchopulmonary
         foregut m.
      vascular m.
malignancy
Mallory-Weiss syndrome
malnutrition
malrotation
maneuver
      doll's head m.
marasmus
Marfan's syndrome
Marie's syndrome
Marinesco-Sjögren
   syndrome
Marion's disease
Marmo's method
Maroteaux-Lamy syndrome
masculinization

mastitis
   m. neonatorum
mastocytosis
mastoiditis
masturbation
Mauriac syndrome
May-Hegglin anomaly
McArdle's disease
McCune-Albright syndrome
measles
      German m.
Meckel's diverticulum
meconium
   m. ileus
   m. peritonitis
   m. plug
   m. staining
mediastinal
   m. collagenosis
   m. lymphadenitis
   m. teratoma
mediastinitis
medications. See *Drugs and*
   Chemistry section.
Mediterranean anemia
medulloblastoma
Meesmann's dystrophy
megacolon
      congenital m.
megalencephaly
melanoma
melanosis
melena
   m. neonatorum
Melkersson-Rosenthal syndrome
Melnick-Needles disease
melorheostosis
menarche
meningioma
meningismus
meningitis
      aseptic m.
      cryptococcal m.
      tuberculous m.
meningocele
meningococcemia
meningococcus
meningoencephalitis

meningoencephalomyelitis
meningoencephalo-
  myeloradiculitis
meningomyelocele
Menkes' syndrome
menometrorrhagia
menstrual
menstruation
M/E ratio
mesenteric
mesoblastic
mesoblastoma
    m. ovarii
    m. vitellinum
mesothelioma
metabolic
metabolism
metastasis
metatarsus
    m. varus
methemoglobinemia
methemoglobinuria
method
    Byrd-Dew m.
    Marmo's m.
Metopirone test
Mibelli's angiokeratoma
micrencephaly
microangiopathy
    thrombotic m.
microcephaly
microcytosis
microgastria
microlithiasis
microphallus
Microsporum
    M. audouini
    M. furfur
    M. lanosum
micturition
mielitis. See *myelitis.*
mielo-. See words beginning
    myelo-.
migraine
miksedema. See *myxedema.*
milia
miliaria

milium
Milroy's disease
Minkowski-Chauffard syndrome
Minot's disease
mio-. See words beginning *myo-.*
mitral
    m. insufficiency
    m. stenosis
    m. valve
Möbius' syndrome
Möller-Barlow disease
molluscum
    m. contagiosum
    m. fibrosum
mongolian
mongolism
    double-trisomy m.
    translocation m .
mongoloid
moniliasis
mononeuropathy
mononucleosis
    infectious m.
monoplegia
monosomy
morbilliform
Morgagni hernia
Moro embrace reflex
Moro-Heisler diet
Moro's reflex
morphea
Morquio's
    disease
    syndrome
Morquio-Ullrich syndrome
mosaicism
mucocutaneous
    m. candidosis
    m. leishmaniasis
mucoid
mucolipidosis
mucopolysaccharidosis
    m. I; m. II; m. III; m. IV;
    m. V; m. VI, m. VII,
    m. VIII
Mucor
mucormycosis

mucosal
mucoviscidosis
multiple sclerosis
mumps
murmur
    continuous m.
    diastolic m.
    functional m.
    Graham Steell's m.
    holosystolic m.
    pansystolic m.
    Still's m.
    systolic ejection m.
myalgia
myasthenia
    m. gravis
mycobacterial
Mycobacterium
    M. avium-intracellulare
    M. fortuitum-chelonei
    M. kansasii
    M. leprae
    M. marinum
    M. tuberculosis
    M. ulcerans
Mycoplasma
    M. pneumoniae
mycoplasmal
mycosis
mycotic
myelitis
    transverse m.
myelodysplasia
myelofibrosis
myelomeningocele
myelophthisis
myeloproliferative
myiasis
myocardial
myocarditis
myocardium
myoclonic
myoclonus
    jaw m.
myoglobinuria
myopathy
    mitochondrial m.

myopia
myositis
    m. ossificans
        circumscripta
    m. ossificans progressiva
myotonia
    m. congenita
    m. neonatorum
myringitis
    bullous m.
myxedema
    infantile m.
myxoma
narcolepsy
narcosis
nares
naris
nasal
    n. flaring
    n. mastocytosis
    n. polyposis
    n. septal defect
nasogastric
nasojejunal
nasopharyngeal
nasopharyngitis
nasotracheal
nausea
nefritis. See *nephritis.*
nefrosis. See *nephrosis.*
neogaster. See *pneogaster.*
neonatal
neonate
neoplasm
nephritis
nephroblastomatosis
nephrocalcinosis
nephrolithiasis
nephroma
nephropathy
nephrophthisis
nephrosis
nepiology
nesidioblastosis
Netherton's syndrome
Nettleship's syndrome

neuritis
    retrobulbar n.
neuroblastoma
neurodermatitis
neurofibromatosis
neurogenic
    n. bladder
    n. tumor
neurologic
neuromuscular
neuronal
neurosis
neurotransmitter
neutropenia
nevi
nevoxanthoendothelioma
nevus
    n. anemicus
    n. comedonicus
    n. depigmentosus
    n. flammeus
    halo n.
    n. of Ito
    n. of Ota
    n. pilosus
    n. sebaceus
    n. simplex
    n. spilus
    Spitz' n.
    strawberry n.
    n. verrucosus
Nezelof's syndrome
Niemann-Pick disease
Nocardia
nocardiosis
noma
    n. pudendi
    n. vulvae
noncalculous
non-Hodgkin's lymphoma
Noonan's syndrome
normocephalic
Norrie's disease
nosocomial
numo-. See words beginning
    pneumo-.
nyctalopia

nystagmus
obesity
obstipation
ocular
    o. aspergillosis
    o. hypertelorism
    o. hypotony
    o. myopathy
ofthalmea. See *ophthalmia.*
oksesefale. See *oxycephaly.*
okseuriasis. See *oxyuriasis.*
oliguria
Ollier's syndrome
omphalocele
Ondine's curse
onychia
oophoritis
operation. See *General Surgical*
    Terms section.
ophthalmia
    o. neonatorum
opisthotonos
    o. fetalis
Oppenheim's disease
opsoclonus
opsomyoclonus
orchidoblastoma
orchitis
organomegaly
orkitis. See *orchitis.*
oropharynx
orthomyxovirus
Ortolani's test
Osgood-Schlatter syndrome
Osler-Weber-Rendu disease
ossicular
ossification
osteitis
    o. condensans
        generalisata
    o. fibrosa
osteoarthropathy
osteoblastoma
osteochondritis
    o. deformans juvenilis
    o. dissecans
    o. ischiopubica

osteochondrodystrophia
    o. deformans
osteochondrodystrophy
osteochondroma
osteochondrosis
    o. deformans tibiae
osteodysplasty
osteodystrophia
    o. juvenilis
osteodystrophy
osteogenesis
    o. imperfecta
    o. imperfecta cystica
osteogenic
osteoid
osteoma
    osteoid o.
osteomalacia
    juvenile o.
osteomyelitis
osteopathia
    o. striata
osteopenia
osteopetrosis
    o. tarda
osteopoikilosis
osteoporosis
osteopsathyrosis
osteosarcoma
osteotabes
ostium
    o. primum defect
    o. secundum defect
otalgia
otitis
    o. externa
    o. media
otomycosis
otorrhea
otosclerosis
Oto's nevus
out-toeing
ovary
    polycystic o's
Owren's disease
oxycephaly
oxygen

oxyuriasis
Paas' disease
pachyonychia
    p. congenita
Paget's disease
palate
    cleft p.
palatopharyngeal
    p. incompetence
pallor
palsy
    brachial plexus p.
    cerebral p.
pancreas
    annular p.
pancreatitis
pancreatoblastoma
pancytopenia
panencephalitis
panniculitis
panniculus
papilledema
Papillon-Lèfevre syndrome
papilloma
papular
    p. acrodermatitis
    p. urticaria
paracentesis
parainfluenza
paralysis
    congenital abducens-
        facial p.
    congenital oculofacial p.
    Erb-Duchenne p.
    hysterical p.
    Klumpke's p.
    spastic p.
    Werdnig-Hoffmann p.
parapertussis
paraphimosis
paraplegia
parapsoriasis
parasympathetic
paratesticular
parathyroid
parathyromatosis
parenchyma

parenteral
Parenti-Fraccaro syndrome
paresis
paresthesia
    Berger's p.
paroksizmal. See *paroxysmal.*
paronychia
parotitis
paroxysmal
Parrot's atrophy of the newborn
Pasteurella
    P. tularensis
Pastia's sign
Patau's syndrome
patch
    Peyer's p's
patent ductus arteriosus
Paul-Bunnell-Davidsohn test
pavor
    p. diurnus
    p. nocturnus
PDA – patent ductus arteriosus
pearl
    Epstein's p's
pectus
    p. excavatum
pedarthrocace
pediatric
pediatrician
pedicterus
pediculosis
    p. capitis
    p. corporis
    p. pubis
pedobaromacrometer
pedobarometer
pedologist
pedometer
Pelger-Huët anomaly
Pelizaeus-Merzbacher disease
pellagra
pellagrous
Pellizzi's syndrome
pemphigoid
    bullous p.
pemphigus
    p. vulgaris

Pendred's syndrome
pentosuria
Perez's sign
periarteritis
    p. nodosa
pericardial
    p. tamponade
pericarditis
pericardium
perinatal
perineal
    p. pearls
perinephritis
peritoneal
    p. dialysis
peritoneum
peritonitis
    meconium p.
pernio
peroneal
pertussis
pes
    p. cavus
petechia
Peters' anomaly
petit mal
petrositis
Peutz-Jeghers syndrome
Peyer's patches
phagocytic
phagocytosis
phakomata
pharyngeal
pharyngitis
    lymphonodular p.
    purulent p.
    streptococcal p.
    viral p.
phenomenon
    dawn p.
    Rumpel-Leede p.
    Somogyi p.
phenylketonuria
pheochromocytoma
Philip's glands
phimosis
phlebectasia

phobia
phocomelia
phonocardiography
phycomycosis
phytobezoar
pica
Pierre Robin syndrome
pigeon
    p. breast
    p. toe
piknocytosis. See *pyknocytosis.*
pili
    p. annulati
    p. torti
pilitis. See *pyelitis.*
pilonephritis. See *pyelonephritis.*
pilonidal
    p. cyst
    p. dimple
    p. sinus
pinealoma
pingueculum
pink disease
pink-eye
pinna
pinworm
pituitary
pityriasis
    p. alba
    p. lichenoides chronica
    p. lichenoides et
       varioliformis acuta
    p. rosea
    p. rubra pilaris
PKU – phenylketonuria
placentitis
plague
plantar
    p. dermatosis, juvenile
    p. reflex
    p. wart
plethysmograph
pleurisy
pleurodynia
pleuropulmonic
plumbism
pneogaster

pneumatocele
pneumatosis cystoides intestinalis
pneumococcal
pneumococcus
Pneumocystis
    P. carinii
pneumomediastinum
pneumonia
    adenoviral p.
    p. alba
    aspiration p.
    bacterial p.
    chemical p.
    chlamydial p.
    congenital p.
    eosinophilic p.
    giant cell p.
    gram-negative p.
    Hecht's p.
    hypostatic p.
    Kaufman's p.
    lipoid p.
    lobar p.
    plasma cell p.
    pneumococcal p.
    rheumatic p.
    staphylococcal p.
    streptococcal p.
    thrush p.
    viral p.
pneumonitis
pneumopericardium
pneumoperitoneum
pneumothorax
poison
    p. ivy
    p. oak
Poison Control Centers
poisoning
    barbiturate p.
    lead p.
    petroleum distillate p.
    phenothiazine p.
    salicylate p.
    scopolamine p.
    strychnine p.
    thallium p.

Poland's
    anomaly
    syndrome
poliodystrophy
polioencephalitis
    bulbar p.
poliomyelitis
poliovirus
polyarteritis
    p. nodosa
polyarthritis
polychondritis
polycystic
polycythemia
    p. rubra vera
polydactylia
polydactyly
polydipsia
polydysplasia
    hereditary ectodermal p.
polydysspondylism
polydystrophic
polydystrophy
    pseudo-Hurler p.
polymicrogyria
polyneuritis
polyneuropathy
polyp
    inflammatory p.
    intestinal p.
    pedunculated juvenile p.
polyposis
    colonic p.
polyserositis
    idiopathic p.
polysplenia
Pompe's disease
porencephaly
porokeratosis
porphyria
    p. cutanea tarda
    p. variegata
port wine mark
potbelly
Potter's disease
PPTT – prepubertal testicular
    tumor

Prader-Willi syndrome
precocity
premature
prematurity
premenstrual
prenatal
prepubertal
prickly heat
progeria
prognathism
projectile
prolactinoma
pronate
prostration
proteinosis
proteinuria
    orthostatic p.
    postural p.
prothrombokinase
protoporphyria
prurigo
pruritus
    p. ani
pseudoachondroplasia
pseudocyst
pseudohermaphroditism
pseudohypertrophic
pseudohypoparathyroidism
pseudoleukemia
pseudomenstruation
Pseudomonas
    P. aeruginosa
    P. cepacia
pseudoparalysis
pseudotumor
    p. cerebri
psittacosis
psoriasis
psychosis
    symbiotic p.
psychosocial
psychosomatic
psychotherapy
PTA – plasma thromboplastin
    antecedent
pterygium
    p. coli

ptosis
pubarche
pubertas
    p. praecox
puberty
pubescent
Pudenz's
    reservor
    shunt
pulmonary
    p. agenesis
    p. alveolus
    p. anthrax
    p. arborization
    p. ascariasis
    p. aspergillosis
    p. atresia
    p. blastomycosis
    p. candidiasis
    p. cryptococcosis
    p. diffusion
    p. edema
    p. ejection clicks
    p. embolism
    p. eosinophilia
    p. fibrosis
    p. gangrene
    p. hemosiderosis
    p. histoplasmosis
    p. hypertension
    p. infarction
    p. lymphangiectasia
    p. mucormycosis
    p. neoplasm
    p. sequestration
    p. suppuration
    p. surfactant
    p. valve
pulmonic
    p. murmur
    p. plaque
pulse
    Corrigan's p.
puncture
    bone marrow p.
    cisternal p.
    lumbar p.

puncture (continued)
    pericardial p.
    subdural p.
purpura
    anaphylactoid p.
    p. fulminans
    p. hemorrhagica
    Schönlein-Henoch p.
    thrombocytopenic p.
    thrombotic p.
Pusey's emulsion
pustulosis
    p. vacciniformis acuta
pyelitis
pyelonephritis
pyknocytosis
pyloric
pylorospasm
pyropoikilocytosis
pyuria
Q fever
quadriplegia
quarantine
rabies
rachischisis
rachitic
    r. metaphysis
    r. rosary
radiology. See *Radiology and*
    Nuclear Medicine section.
ragadez. See *rhagades.*
rales
Ramsey-Hunt syndrome
rating
    Apgar r.
ratio
    L/S r.
    M/E r.
reaction
    Jarisch-Herxheimer r.
Recklinghausen's disease
reflex
    gagging r.
    grasp r.
    Grünfelder's r.
    Head's r.
    Hering-Breuer r.

reflex (continued)
    Landau's r.
    Magnus and de Kleijn
        neck r's
    Moro embrace r.
    Moro's r.
    rooting r.
    sucking r.
reflux
    gastroesophageal r.
    intrarenal r.
    r. nephropathy
    vesicoureteral r.
Refsum's disease
regurgitation
Reifenstein's syndrome
renal
    r. cell carcinoma
    r. cortex
    r. dysgenesis
    r. dysplasia
    r. medulla
    r. osteodystrophy
    r. parenchyma
    r. tubular acidosis
    r. tubular necrosis
    r. vein thrombosis
Rendu-Osler-Weber syndrome
reservoir
    Pudenz's r.
respiration
    Bouchut's r.
    Kussmaul's r.
respirator
    negative pressure r.
respiratory
    r. arrest
    r. distress
    r. insufficiency
    r. paralysis
    r. scoring system
resuscitation
retardation
    mental r.
reticuloendotheliosis
retinitis
    r. pigmentosa

retinoblastoma
retinopathy
retinoschisis
retrovirus
Reye's syndrome
rhabdomyosarcoma
rhagades
rheumatic
    r. fever
    r. heart disease
    r. pneumonia
rheumaticosis
rheumatism
rheumatoid
    r. arthritis
    r. factor
    r. nodules
Rh incompatibility
rhinitis
    r. medicamentosa
rhinovirus
rhizomelic
Rhus
    R. diversiloba
    R. toxicodendron
    R. venenata
Richner-Hanhart syndrome
Richter's hernia
rickets
Rickettsia
rickettsiae
rickettsial
rickettsialpox
rigidity
Riley-Day syndrome
Riley-Shwachman syndrome
ring
    Kayser-Fleischer r.
ringworm
Ritter's disease
rocker-bottom foot
Rocky Mountain spotted fever
Romaña's sign
roomatikosis. See *rheumaticosis.*
roseola
    r. infantum
rotavirus

Rothmann-Makai syndrome
Rothmund's syndrome
Rothmund-Thomson syndrome
Rotor's syndrome
roundworm
Roussy-Lévy syndrome
RS virus
RTA – renal tubular acidosis
rubella
    r. scarlatinosa
rubeola
    r. scarlatinosa
Rubinstein-Taybi syndrome
rubor
Rud's syndrome
Rumpel-Leede phenomenon
rumination
rus. See *Rhus.*
Russell's syndrome
Sabin-Feldman dye test
St. Louis encephalitis
St. Vitus' dance
Saldino-Noonan syndrome
salicylism
salmonella
salmonellosis
salmon patch
Sandhoff disease
Sanfilippo's syndrome
Sarcocystis
sarcoidosis
sarcoma
    s. botryoides
    embryonal s.
    Ewing's s.
sarcosinemia
Saunders' disease
scabies
scale
    Tanner's s.
scaphocephaly
scarlatina
scarlet fever
Scheie's syndrome
Scheuermann's disease
Scheuthauer-Marie-Sainton
    syndrome

Schick
    sign
    test
Schilder's
    disease
    encephalitis
Schiller's tumor
Schilling test
Schistosoma
    S. haematobium
    S. japonicum
    S. mansoni
schistosomiasis
schizophrenia
Scholz's disease
Schönlein-Henoch purpura
scintigraphy
scissoring
scleredema
    s. neonatorum
sclerema
    s. neonatorum
scleroderma
sclerosis
    tuberous s.
sclerosteosis
scoliosis
score
    Apgar s.
    Silverman's s.
scrofula
scrofuloderma
scrotum
"sculptured nose"
scurvy
    hemorrhagic s.
    infantile s.
sebaceous
    s. hyperplasia
seborrhea
sefalhematoma. See
    cephalhematoma.
Seip-Lawrence syndrome
seizure
    atonic s.
    autonomic s.
    hysterical s.

seizure (continued)
    infantile myoclonic s.
    jackknife s.
    lightning s.
    myoclonic s.
    neonatal s.
    sylvian s.
    tonic-clonic s.
    versive s.
    vertiginous s.
seminoma
sensory
    s. deficit
    s. loss
    s. neuropathy
    s. stimulation
sepsis
septal
septic
    s. arthritis
    s. shock
septicemia
Sertoli's tumor
serum prothrombin conversion
    accelerator
sferositosis. See *spherocytosis.*
Shigella
shigellosis
shock
    anaphylactic s.
    bacteremic s.
    cardiogenic s.
    endotoxic s.
    hypovolemic s.
    insulin s.
shunt
    LeVeen s.
    parietal s.
    Pudenz' s.
    ventricular atrial s.
    ventriculoperitoneal s.
shunting
    left-to-right ductus s.
Shwachman's syndrome
sialidosis
sickle cell
    s.c. anemia

sickle cell (continued)
    s.c. dactylitis
    s.c. hemoglobulinopathy
    s.c. nephropathy
    s.c. thalassemia
    s.c. trait
SID – sudden infant death
SIDS – sudden infant death
    syndrome
sifilis. See *syphilis.*
sign
    Babinski's s.
    Brudzinski's s.
    Chvostek's s.
    Comby's s.
    Dalrymple's s.
    Gowers' s.
    Granger's s.
    Kernig's s.
    Macewen's s.
    Pastia's s.
    Perez's s.
    peroneal s.
    Romaña's s.
    Schick s.
    Stellwag's s.
    Trousseau's s.
    von Graefe's s.
    Wreden's s.
sikosis. See *psychosis.*
silicosis
Silverman's score
silver nitrate
    s.n. conjunctivitis
Silver-Russell syndrome
Silver's syndrome
Similac
sinobronchitis
sinus
    s. arrest
    s. arrhythmia
    s. bradycardia
    s. histiocytosis
    s. of Valsalva
    paranasal s.
    pilonidal s.
    s. venosus defect

sinusitis
Sipple's syndrome
sirronosus. See *cirrhonosus.*
sirrosis. See *cirrhosis.*
sitakosis. See *psittacosis.*
situs inversus
Sjögren-Larsson syndrome
skafosefale. See *scaphocephaly.*
skeletal
    s. dysplasia
skizofrenea. See *schizophrenia.*
SLE – systemic lupus
    erythematosus
sleep apnea
smallpox
snuffles
somnambulism
Somogyi phenomenon
soriasis. See *psoriasis.*
Sotos' syndrome
South African tick fever
spasm
spasmus
    s. nutans
spastic
spasticity
SPCA – serum prothrombin
    conversion accelerator
spherocytosis
sphingolipidosis
Spielmeyer-Vogt disease
spina
    s. bifida
    s. bifida occulta
Spirillum
    S. minus
spirochetal
spirochete
Spitz nevus
spleen
    accessory s.
splenectomy
splenic flexure
splenomegaly
spondylitis
    ankylosing s.
spondylolisthesis

spondylolysis
spongioblastoma
sporotrichosis
spot
    Brushfield's s's
    Fordyce's s's
    Koplik's s's
Sprengel's deformity
sprue
squint
SRP – short rib-polydactyly
stafilokokkis. See *Staphylococcus.*
stammering
Staphylococcus
    S. aureus
    S. epidermidis
Stargardt's disease
starvation
status
    s. asthmaticus
    s. dysmyelinatus
    s. dysmyelinisatus
    s. epilepticus
steatorrhea
    idiopathic s.
Steinert's myotonic dystrophy
    syndrome
Stein-Leventhal syndrome
Stellwag's sign
stenosis
    anorectal s.
    antral s.
    aortic s.
    aqueductal s.
    esophageal s.
    hypertrophic s.
    infundibular s.
    mitral s.
    postischemic s.
    pulmonic s.
    pyloric s.
    valvular pulmonic s.
Stensen's duct
steroidogenesis
Stevens-Johnson syndrome
Sticker's disease
stigmata

Stilling-Türk-Duane syndrome
Still's
    disease
    murmur
Stock-Spielmeyer-Vogt syndrome
stomatitis
    aphthous s.
    herpetic s.
stomatocytosis
stool
    acholic s.
    currant jelly s.
strabismus
strawberry mark
Streptobacillus
    S. moniliformis
streptococcal group A, B, G
streptococci
streptococcosis
Streptococcus
    S. mutans
    S. pneumoniae
    S. viridans
streptococcus
    beta-hemolytic s.
Streptothrix
stricture
    esophageal s.
stridor
Strongyloides
    S. stercoralis
strongyloidiasis
strophulus
Stuart-Prower factor deficiency
    disease
Sturge-Weber syndrome
stuttering
stye
subclavian
subcutaneous
subdural
subphrenic
sucking
sudo-. See words beginning
    pseudo-.
sulfhemoglobinemia
Swift's disease

Swyer-James syndrome
Swyer's syndrome
Sydenham's chorea
symptom
    Epstein's s.
syncope
syndactyly
syndrome
    Abderhalden-Fanconi s.
    Abt-Letterer-Siwe s.
    Adie's s.
    adrenogenital s.
    Albers-Schönberg s.
    Albright's s.
    Aldrich's s.
    "Alice in Wonderland" s.
    Alport's s.
    Andogsky's s.
    Arnold-Chiari s.
    asplenia s.
    Ballantyne-Runge s.
    Banti's s.
    Bartter's s.
    Bassen-Kornzweig s.
    battered child s.
    Beckwith's s.
    Bielschowsky s.
    blind loop s.
    Bloch-Sulzberger s.
    Bloom's s.
    blue diaper s.
    Bodian-Schwachman s.
    Bonnevie-Ullrich s.
    Bourneville's s.
    Brachmann-de Lange s.
    Brandt's s.
    bronze baby s.
    Budd-Chiari s.
    Caffey-Silverman s.
    Caffey-Smyth-Roske s.
    Calvé-Legg-Perthes s.
    Camurati-Engelmann s.
    carcinoid s.
    carpenter's s.
    Chapple's s.
    Charcot-Marie-Tooth-
      Hoffmann s.

syndrome (continued)
 Chédiak-Higashi s.
 Chilaiditi's s.
 Christ-Siemens-Touraine
  s.
 Clarke Hadfield s.
 Cockayne's s.
 concussion s.
 Cornelia de Lange's s.
 cri-du-chat s.
 Crigler-Najjar s.
 cryptophthalmos s.
 cushingoid s.
 Cushing's s.
 Dandy-Walker s.
 Darrow-Gamble s.
 Debré-Sémélaigne s.
 de Lange's s.
 Dennie-Marfan s.
 De Sanctis-Cacchione s.
 de Toni-Fanconi-Debre s.
 Diamond-Blackfan s.
 diencephalic s.
 DiGeorge's s.
 Donohue's s.
 Down's s.
 Duane's s.
 Dubin-Johnson s.
 Dubovitz's s.
 duplication-deficiency s.
 Dyggve-Melchior-
  Clausen s.
 Eagle-Barrett s.
 Ehlers-Danlos s.
 Ellis-van Creveld s.
 empty-sella s.
 epiphyseal s.
 Erlacher-Blount s.
 Fanconi-Albertini
  Zellweger s.
 Fanconi-Petrassi s.
 Fanconi's s.
 floppy infant s.
 focal dermal hypoplasia s.
 fragile X s.
 Franceschetti's s.
 Gardner's s.

syndrome (continued)
 Gasser's s.
 Gerstmann's s.
 Gianotti-Crosti s.
 Gilbert-Dreyfus s.
 Gilbert-Lereboullet s.
 Gilles de la Tourette's s.
 Glanzmann's s.
 Goltz-Gorlin s.
 Goltz's s.
 gonadal agenesis s.
 Goodpasture's s.
 Gradenigo's s.
 gray s.
 Guillain-Barré s.
 Hallermann-Streiff s.
 Hallervorden-Spatz s.
 Hall-Pallister s.
 Hamman-Rich s.
 hand-foot s.
 Hand-Schüller-Christian s.
 Hanhart's s.
 Hartnup's s.
 Hart's s.
 hemolytic-uremic s.
 hereditary benign
  intraepithelial
  dyskeratosis s.
 Hermansky-Pudlak s.
 Holt-Oram s.
 Hunter's s.
 Hurler's s.
 Hutchinson-Gilford s.
 Hutchinson's s.
 17-hydroxylase de-
  ficiency s.
 hypoplastic left heart s.
 idiopathic respiratory
  distress s.
 Imerslund's s.
 inspissated milk s.
 Ivemark's s.
 Jansen's s.
 Jansky-Bielschowsky s.
 Job s.
 Johanson-Blizzard s.
 Joseph's s.

syndrome (continued)
- Kallman's s.
- Kartagener's s.
- Kasabach-Merritt s.
- Kearns-Sayer s.
- Kenny-Caffey s.
- kinky-hair
- Kinsbourne s.
- Klinefelter's s.
- Klippel-Feil s.
- Klippel-Trenaunay-Weber s.
- Kloepfer's s.
- Kocher-Debre-Sémélaigne s.
- Koerber-Salus-Elschnig s.
- Landry-Guillain-Barré s.
- Langer-Giedion s.
- Langer-Saldino s.
- Laron's s.
- Larsen's s.
- Launois' s.
- Laurence-Moon s.
- Laurence-Moon-Biedl s.
- Lennox-Gastaut s.
- Lennox's s.
- leopard s.
- Léri-Weill s.
- Lesch-Nyhan s.
- Lightwood-Albright s.
- Löffler's s.
- Louis-Bar s.
- Lowe's s.
- Lutembacher's s.
- Maffucci's s.
- Majewski's s.
- malabsorption s.
- Mallory-Weiss s.
- Marfan's s.
- Marie's s.
- Marinesco-Sjögren s.
- Maroteaux-Lamy s.
- Mauriac s.
- McCune-Albright s.
- meconium plug s.
- Melkersson-Rosenthal s.
- Menkes' s.

syndrome (continued)
- methionine malabsorption s.
- Minkowski-Chauffard s.
- Möbius' s.
- Morquio's s.
- Morquio-Ullrich s.
- multiple lentigines s.
- nephrotic s.
- Netherton's s.
- Nettleship's s.
- Nezelof's s.
- Noonan's s.
- Ollier's s.
- Osgood-Schlatter s.
- pancreatic insufficiency s.
- Papillon-Lèfevre s.
- Parenti-Fraccaro s.
- Patau's s.
- Pellizzi's s.
- Pendred's s.
- Peutz-Jeghers s.
- pickwickian s.
- Pierre Robin s.
- placental dysfunction s.
- Poland's s.
- postperfusion s.
- Prader-Willi s.
- prune-belly s.
- Ramsey-Hunt s.
- Reifenstein's s.
- Rendu-Osler-Weber s.
- respiratory distress s.
- Reye's s.
- Richner-Hanhart s.
- Riley-Day s.
- Riley-Shwachman s.
- Rothmann-Makai s.
- Rothmund's s.
- Rothmund-Thomson s.
- Rotor's s.
- Roussy-Lévy s.
- Rubinstein-Taybi s.
- Rud's s.
- Russell's s.
- Saldino-Noonan s.
- Sanfilippo's s.

syndrome (continued)
    Scheie's s.
    Scheuthauer-Marie-
      Sainton s.
    sebaceous nevus s.
    Seip-Lawrence s.
    Shwachman's s.
    sicca s.
    sick cell s.
    sick sinus s.
    Silver-Russell s.
    Silver's s.
    Sipple's s.
    Sjögren-Larsson s.
    sleep apnea s.
    slick-gut s.
    small left colon s.
    Sotos' s.
    stagnant loop s.
    Steinert's myotonic
      dystrophy s.
    Stein-Leventhal s.
    Stevens-Johnson s.
    Stilling-Türk-Duane s.
    Stock-Spielmeyer-Vogt s.
    Sturge-Weber s.
    sudden infant death s.
    Swyer-James s.
    Swyer's s.
    testicular feminizing s.
    Tourette's s.
    Treacher Collins s.
    trisomy 13-15 s.
    trisomy 16-18 s.
    trisomy 18 s.
    trisomy 21 s.
    Turner's s.
    Vogt's s.
    Waardenburg's s.
    Waterhouse-Friderichsen
      s.
    Watson-Alagille s.
    Weber-Christian s.
    Weill-Marchesani s.
    Werdnig-Hoffmann s.
    West's s.
    Whipple's s.

syndrome (continued)
    Wiedemann's s.
    Willebrand-Jürgens s.
    Williams' s.
    Wilson-Mikity s.
    Wiskott-Aldrich s.
    Wolff-Parkinson-White s.
    Wolfram s.
    Young's s.
    Zellweger s.
    Zinsser-Engman-Cole s.
    Zollinger-Ellison s.
synostosis
    tribasilar s.
synovitis
syphilis
syringoma
tabes
    hereditary t.
    t. infantum
    t. mesaraica
    t. mesenterica
tachyarrhythmia
tachycardia
    paroxysmal t.
tachypnea
taeniasis
takekardea. See *tachycardia.*
takipnea. See *tachypnea.*
talipes
    t. calcaneovalgus
    t. cavus
    t. equinovarus
tamponade
    cardiac t.
Tangier disease
Tanner's scale
tapeworm
Tay-Sachs disease
Teilum's tumor
telangiectasia
teratocarcinoma
teratoma
terijeum. See *pterygium.*
test. See also *Laboratory*
    Terminology section.

test
    Coombs'
    Farber's t.
    Frei t.
    Guthrie t.
    Kveim t.
    Landau's t.
    leucine tolerance t.
    Metopirone t.
    mono spot t.
    Ortolani's t.
    Paul-Bunnell-
      Davidsohn t.
    Sabin-Feldman dye t.
    Schick t.
    Schilling t.
    sweat t.
    tine t.
testes
    undescended t.
testicle
testicular
tetanus
    t. neonatorum
tetany
tetralogy
    t. of Fallot
tetraploidy
thalassemia
    t. intermedia
    t. major
    t. minor
thelarche
therapy
    aerosol t.
    hyperbaric oxygen t.
Thiemann's disease
Thomsen's disease
Thomson's disease
thoracentesis
thoracic
thoracotomy
thorax
thrombasthenia
thrombin
thrombocythemia
thrombocytopenia
    idiopathic t.

thrombocytopenic
thrombocytosis
thrombophlebitis
thrombosis
    arterial t.
thrombotic
thrombus
thrush
thumbsucking
thymoma
thyroglossal
thyroid
    t. crisis
    t. deficiency
    t. nodule
    t. storm
thyroiditis
thyrotoxicosis
tic
tinea
    t. capitis
    t. corporis
    t. cruris
    t. nigra palmaris
    t. pedis
    t. unguium
    t. versicolor
tinnitus
tissue factor
titer
    antistreptolysin t.
toeing-in
toeing-out
toewalking
tongue
    black t.
    hairy t.
    scrotal t.
    strawberry t.
tongue-tie
tonsillectomy
tonsillitis
    white t.
tonsillopharyngitis
torticollis
torulosis
tosis. See *ptosis.*

Tourette's syndrome
Toxocara
toxocariasis
toxoid
Toxoplasma
    T. gondii
toxoplasmosis
trachea
tracheobronchial
tracheobronchitis
tracheobronchomegaly
tracheoesophageal
tracheomalacia
tracheostomy
tracheotomy
trachoma
transfusion
    exchange t.
transillumination
transplantation
    kidney t.
    orthotopic liver t.
transposition
    t. of great vessels
transsexualism
Treacher Collins syndrome
tremulous
Treponema
    T. carateum
    T. pallidum
    T. pertenue
treponemal
treponematoses
Trevor's disease
trichinosis
trichobezoar
trichoepithelioma
Trichomonas
trichomoniasis
trichorrhexis
    t. invaginata
    t. nodosa
trichoschisis
trichotillomania
trichuriasis
Trichuris
    T. trichiura

tricuspid
    t. atresia
    t. insufficiency
trigonocephaly
triploidy
trismus
    t. nascentium
    t. neonatorum
trisomy 8, 9, 9p, 13, 18, 21, 22
Trousseau's sign
truncus
    t. arteriosus
Trypanosoma
    T. brucei
    T. cruzi
trypanosomiasis
tryptophanuria
tubercle
    Ghon t.
tuberculoma
tuberculosis
    abdominal t.
    extrathoracic t.
    gastrointestinal t.
    intrathoracic t.
    miliary t.
    t. papulonecrotica
    pulmonary t.
tuberculous
    t. dactylitis
    t. keratoconjunctivitis
    t. meningitis
    t. peritonitis
    t. spondylitis
tuberous
    t. sclerosis
tubular
    t. proteinuria
    t. stenosis
tularemia
tumor
    Ewing's t.
    germ cell testicular t.
    granulosa cell t.
    islet cell t.
    Leydig cell t.
    pineal t.

tumor (continued)
    pontine t.
    Schiller's t.
    Sertoli's t.
    Teilum's t.
    theca cell t.
    vitelline t.
    Wilms' t.
    yolk sac t.
tunica
    t. albuginea
Turner's syndrome
tympanites
typhlitis
typhoid
typhus
    t. degenerativus
      amstelodamensis
tyrosinemia
tyrosinosis
ulcer
    aphthous u.
    Curling's u.
    Cushing-Rokitansky u.
    duodenal u.
    peptic u.
ulcerative
ultrasonography
umbilical
umbilicus
uncinate fits
Underwood's disease
Undritz anomaly
Unverricht's disease
urachal
urachus
    patent u.
uremia
ureter
ureterocele
ureteropelvic
urethra
urethritis
URI–upper respiratory infection
urinalysis
urinary
    u. bladder

urinary (continued)
    u. tract infection
    u. voiding
urinoma
urolithiasis
urticaria
    u. pigmentosa
uveitis
uveokeratitis
uvulitis
vaccine
vagina
vaginitis
Valsalva's sinus
valve
    mitral v.
valvotomy
van Buchem's disease
varicella
    v. bullosa
    v. gangrenosa
    v. inoculata
    pustular v.
    v. pustulosa
    vaccination v.
    v.-zoster immune
      globulin (VZIG)
varicelliform
varices
varicocele
variola
varioliform
varix
vasculitis
vas deferens
vasospasm
vasovagal
venereal
venipuncture
venous hum
ventricular
    v. fibrillation
    v. hypertrophy
    v. septal defect
ventriculogram
ventriculography

vernix
  v. caseosa
verruca
  v. plana juvenilis
verrucous
vertebra
  v. plana
vertigo
vesicobullous
vesicoureteral
vesicular
Vibrio
  V. cholerae
  V. parahaemolyticus
virus
  Coxsackie v.
  ECHO v.
  Epstein-Barr v.
  herpes simplex v.
  RS v.
visceromegaly
vitiligo
vitreoretinopathy
  familial exudative v.
vitreous
VMA – vanillylmandelic acid
Vogt-Spielmeyer disease
Vogt's syndrome
Volkmann's
  deformity
  disease
volvulus
  gastric v.
  v. neonatorum
vomiting
  projectile v.
vomitus
von Gierke's disease
von Graefe's sign
von Hippel-Lindau disease
von Jaksch's anemia
von Recklinghausen's disease
von Willebrand's disease
VSD – ventricular septal defect
vulvovaginitis
VZIG – varicella-zoster immune
  globulin

Waardenburg's syndrome
Waldenström's
  macroglobulinemia
wart
  plantar w.
Waterhouse-Friderichsen
  syndrome
Watson-Alagille syndrome
weaning
Weber-Christian syndrome
Wegener's granulomatosis
Weill-Marchesani syndrome
Weil's disease
Wenckebach heart block
Werdnig-Hoffmann
  paralysis
  syndrome
Wernicke's aphasia
West Nile fever
West's syndrome
wheal
wheezing
Whipple's syndrome
whipworm
whooping cough
Wiedemann's syndrome
Wilkins' disease
Willebrand-Jürgens
  syndrome
Williams syndrome
Wilms' tumor
Wilson-Mikity syndrome
Wilson's disease
Winckel's disease
Wiskott-Aldrich syndrome
Wolff-Parkinson-White
  syndrome
Wolfram syndrome
Wolman's disease
Wreden's sign
wryneck
X chromatin
X chromosome
xanthelasmas
xanthinuria
xanthochromia
xanthogranuloma

xanthoma
- x. striata palmaris

xanthomatosis

xanthosis
- x. cutis

xanthurenic
- x. aciduria

xeroderma
- x. pigmentosum

xerography

xerophthalmia

xerosis
- x. conjunctiva
- x. cornea

xerostomia

xylulose dehydrogenase deficiency

Y chromatin

Y chromosome

yaws

yellow fever

Yersinia
- *Y. enterocolitica*
- *Y. pestis*
- *Y. pseudotuberculosis*

yolk sac carcinoma

Young's syndrome

YST – yolk sac tumor

zanthomatosis. See *xanthomatosis.*

zerofthalmea. See *xerophthalmia.*

Zellweger syndrome

Zinsser-Engman-Cole syndrome

Zollinger-Ellison syndrome

zoster

zosteriform

zygodactyly

zygomycosis

zygote

Plastic Surgery

**Secondary Myocutaneous and Cutaneous Areas
from Which Arterialized Flaps
Can Be Derived for Plastic Surgery**

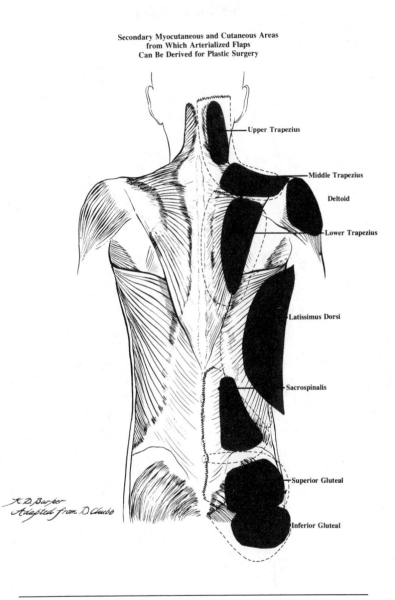

Upper Trapezius

Middle Trapezius

Deltoid

Lower Trapezius

Latissimus Dorsi

Sacrospinalis

Superior Gluteal

Inferior Gluteal

Plastic Surgery

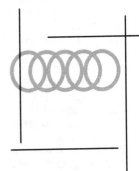

Abbé-Estlander operation
Abbe's operation
Adams' operation
akinesia
    O'Brien a.
    Van Lint a.
ala (alae)
    a. nasi
alanasi
alar
Alexander's operation
allograft
alloplasty
allotransplantation
allotriodontia
Allport's operation
Alsus-Knapp operation
alveolar
    a. arch
    a. ridge
alveololingual
alveolus
Alvis' operation
Ammon's operation
anaplasty
anaplerosis
anesthesia. See *General Surgical Terms* section.
Angelucci's operation
angkilo-. See words beginning *ankylo-*.
angle
    cheilar a.
    conchal mastoid a.
    scaphoconchal a.
ankyloblepharon
ankylochilia
anthelix

Antia-Busch chondrocutaneous flap
antitragus
aperture
    pharyngeal a.
aponeurosis
arch
    palatine a.
    zygomatic a.
area
    Kiesselbach's a.
areolar
Argamaso-Lewin composite flap
Aries-Pitanguy mammaplasty
Arlt's operation
Asch's forceps
Ashley's breast prosthesis
ATL—antitension line
atrium
auricle
auricula
auricular
Austin's knife
autocystoplasty
autograft
autografting
Bakamjian flap
Baker's velum
bandage. See *General Surgical Terms* section.
bar
    Erich's arch b.
    Passavant's b.
Bard-Parker blade
Barsky's
    elevator
    operation
Battle's operation

B-B graft
Beard-Cutler operation
Becker's operation
Bell's operation
Berke-Motais operation
Berke's operation
Bernard-Burrows operation
Biesenberger's operation
Binnie's operation
bistoury
    Brophy's b.
blade
    Bard-Parker b.
Blair-Brown
    graft
    knife
    operation
Blair's
    knife
    operation
    serrefine
Blaskovics' operation
blef-. See words beginning *bleph-.*
blepharal
blepharectomy
blepharelosis
blepharism
blepharitis
blepharoatheroma
blepharochalasis
blepharophryplasty
blepharoplasty
blepharoptosis
blepharorrhaphy
blepharostat
bone
    malar b.
    maxillary b.
    sesamoid b's
Boo-Chai craniofacial cleft
border
    mucocutaneous b.
    vermilion b.
Borges and Alexander line
bow
    Logan's b.
Brauer's operation

Braun's
    graft
    operation
Braun-Wangensteen
    graft
    operation
Brent's eyebrow reconstruction
bridge
Brophy's
    bistoury
    knife
    operation
    plate
Brown-Blair operation
Browne's needle
Brown's
    dermatome
    knife
    operation
    splint
Bruner's line
B's graft
buccal
bulla (bullae)
    b. ethmoidalis cava nasi
    b. ethmoidalis ossis
      ethmoidalis
bundle
    neurovascular b.
Bunnell's flap
Burow's operation
bursa
    pharyngeal b.
B-W graft
caliper
    Ladd's c.
Caltagirone's knife
canal
    pterygopalatine c.
canthus
    lateral c.
cartilage
    alar c.
    septal c.
    sesamoid c.
    vomeronasal c.
cartilaginous

caruncula
catheter
    Hickman c.
cauda
    c. helicis
cavum
    c. conchae
cephaloauricular angle
cephalocaudad
cervicoplasty
chalinoplasty
Charretera's flap
cheilectomy
cheilectropion
cheilitis
cheilognathoprosoposchisis
cheilognathoschisis
cheilognathouranoschisis
cheiloplasty
cheilorrhaphy
cheiloschisis
cheilostomatoplasty
cheiroplasty
chemosurgery
choana (choanae)
Chopart's operation
chordee
ciliary
clamp
    Hunt's c.
cleft
    lip
    palate
clinoid process
collagen
columella
    c. cochleae
    c. nasi
columna
comminuted
comminution
concha (conchae)
    c. auriculae
    c. sphenoidalis
conjunctiva
conjunctivoplasty
contracture

Converse's
    line
    operation
cosmesis
cosmetic
Cox's line
Crane's flap
craniofacial cleft
    Boo-Chai c.c.
    Karfik's c.c.
    Tessier's c.c.
Crawford's operation
cribriform
Crile's knife
crista
    c. galli
    c. nasalis maxillae
    c. nasalis ossis palatini
Cronin-Matthews eave flap
Cronin's operation
crus (crura)
    c. anthelicis
    c. laterale
    c. mediale
cushion
    Passavant's c.
Cutler's operation
cymba (cymbae)
    c. conchae auriculae
Davis and Kitlowski operation
Davis'
    graft
    line
debridement
deformity
    trap door d.
de Grandmont's operation
Demel and Ruttin operation
Denhardt-Dingman mouth gag
Denis-Browne needle
Denonvillier's operation
Derby's operation
dermabraded
dermabrader
    Iverson's d.
dermabrasion
dermanaplasty

dermatochalasis
dermatome
 Brown's d.
 Hall's d.
 Padgett's d.
 Reese's d.
dermatoplasty
dermolipectomy
Dieffenbach's operation
Dieffenbach-Warren operation
Dingman's
 elevator
 forceps
 osteotome
 retractor
Dorrance's operation
dorsum nasi
Dott's mouth gag
double lip
Douglas'
 graft
 operation
Dragstedt's
 graft
 operation
drain
 Penrose d.
dressing. See *General Surgical Terms* section.
drugs. See *Drugs and Chemistry* section.
duct
 lacrimal d.
 nasolacrimal d.
Duke-Elder operation
Duplay's operation
Dupuy-Dutemps operation
durum
 palatine d.
Eckstein-Kleinschmidt operation
ectropion
Edgerton's line
Eitner's operation
electrocoagulation
elevator
 Barsky's e.
 Dingman's e.

elevator (continued)
 Freer's e.
 McIndoe's e.
 Veau's e.
ellipse
elliptical
Elschnig's operation
Ely's operation
eminence
 malar e.
eminentia
 e. conchae
 e. triangularis
entropion
epicanthus
epidermatoplasty
epispadias
epithelialization
Erich's
 arch bar
 operation
eschar
Esmarch's operation
esophagoplasty
Esser's
 graft
 operation
esthetic
Estlander's
 operation
ethmofrontal
ethmoid
ethmoidal
Everbusch's operation
facial
facioplasty
faringoplasty. See *pharyngoplasty.*
farinjeal. See *pharyngeal.*
fascia
 f. lata femoris
fasciaplasty
fascioplasty
fauces
Fergus' operation
Fernandez' operation
filtrum. See *philtrum.*

fissura antitragohelicina
fissure
    antitragohelicine f.
    palpebral f.
fixation
    intermaxillary f.
flap
    Antia-Busch
      chondrocutaneous f.
    Argamaso-Lewin f.
    artery island f.
    Bakamjian f.
    bilobed f.
    bipedicle f.
    Bunnell's f.
    Charretera's f.
    compound f.
    Crane's f.
    Cronin-Matthews eave f.
    delayed f.
    double pedicle f.
    French sliding f.
    Frickle's f.
    Gillies' up-and-down f.
    Hodgson-Tuksu tumble f.
    Hueston spiral f.
    Indian rotation f.
    island leg f.
    Italian distant f.
    jump abdominal f.
    MacFee neck f.
    marsupial f.
    McGregor's forehead f.
    Millard's island f.
    Monks-Esser island f.
    Moore and Chong
      sandwich f.
    New's sickle f.
    over-and-out cheek f.
    skin f.
    Stein-Abbé lip f.
    Stein-Kazanjian lower
      lip f.
    Stenstrom foot f.
    Tagliacozzi's f.
    tumbler f.
    Wookey's neck f.

flap (continued)
    Zimany's f.
    Zovickian's f.
fold
    salpingopalatine f.
    salpingopharyngeal f.
    semilunar f.
Fomon's operation
foramen
    greater palatine f.
    Scarpa's f.
foramina
    lesser palatine f.
forceps
    Asch's f.
    Dingman's f.
    Walsham's f.
fornix
    f. conjunctivae
    superior f.
fossa
    conchal f.
    hypophyseal f.
    Rosenmüller's f.
    scaphoid f.
    f. triangularis auriculae
Fox's operation
fracture
    blow-out f.
    comminuted f.
    nasomaxillary f.
    zygomaticomaxillary f.
Freer's elevator
French
    method
    sliding flap
frenulum
frenum labiorum
Fricke's operation
Frickle's flap
Friedenwald-Guyton operation
frontal
FSR – fusiform skin revision
furrow
    palpebral f.
Gabarro's
    graft

Gabarro's (continued)
    operation
Gaillard's operation
ganglion
Gavello's operation
Gayet's operation
genioplasty
genitoplasty
genycheiloplasty
genyplasty
Gersuny's operation
Gibson-Stark and Kenedi line
Gifford's operation
Gigli's saw
Gillies-Dingman hook
Gillies'
    graft
    hook
    operation
    up-and-down flap
Gillies-Fry operation
Giralde's operation
gland
    meibomian g.
    tarsal g.
glossoplasty
gnathodynia
gnathoplasty
gnathoschisis
graft
    B-B g.
    Blair-Brown g.
    bolus tie-over g.
    Braun's g.
    Braun-Wangensteen g.
    B's g.
    B-W g.
    chessboard g.
    Davis' g.
    Douglas' g.
    Dragstedt's g.
    Esser's g.
    fascia lata g.
    free g.
    full-thickness skin g.
    Gabarro's g.
    Gillies' g.

graft (continued)
    Kebab's g.
    Konig's g.
    Ollier-Thiersch g.
    Padgett's g.
    patch g.
    pedicle g.
    pinch g.
    Reverdin's g.
    Seddon's nerve g.
    split-thickness skin g.
    stent g.
    Tanner-Vanderput g.
    Thiersch's g.
    Van Millingen's g.
    Wolfe-Krause g.
    Wolfe's g.
Grant's operation
Grimsdale's operation
groove
    sinus g.
gustatory
Guyton's operation
Hagedorn-LeMesurier
    operation
Hagedorn's operation
Hagerty's operation
Hall's dermatome
hamular
hamulus
harelip
Harman's operation
helix
hemisection
hemisphincter
    pharyngeal h.
Hess' operation
heterograft
hiatus
    h. semilunaris
Hickman catheter
Hodgson-Tuksu tumble flap
Holmes' operation
homeotransplant
homograft
homoplastic
homoplasty

hook
    Gillies-Dingman h.
    Gillies' h.
Hotchkiss' operation
Hotz' operation
Hueston spiral flap
Hughes' operation
Hunt's clamp
Hutchinson and Koop line
hyperpigmentation
hypognathous
hypospadias
Illiff's operation
immunosuppressive
implant
    Silastic i.
incision. See *General Surgical Terms* section.
incisive
incisura
    i. intertragica
Indian
    method
    rotation flap
infraorbital
infratrochlear
infundibulum
    ethmoidal i.
injection
    Silastic i.
intercartilaginous
isograft
isthmus
    i. faucium
Italian
    distant flap
    method
Iverson's dermabrader
Jaesche's operation
jenekiloplaste. See *genycheiloplasty*.
jeneplaste. See *genyplasty*.
Johnson's operation
Jones' operation
Joseph's operation
Kanavel's line
Karfik's craniofacial cleft

Kazanjian and Converse line
Kazanjian's line
Kebab's graft
Keith's needle
keloid
keloplasty
Kiesselbach's
    area
    plexus
Kilner's operation
kilo-. See *words beginning cheilo-.*
kiroplaste. See *cheiroplasty.*
Kirschner's wire
Kitlowski's operation
knife
    Austin's k.
    Blair-Brown k.
    Blair's k.
    Brophy's k.
    Brown's k.
    Caltagirone's k.
    Crile's k.
    MacKenty's k.
    Virchow's k.
koana-. See *choana.*
Kocher's line
Kolle-Lexer operation
Konig's
    graft
    operation
Kowalzig's operation
Krause-Wolfe operation
Krimer's operation
Krönlein's operation
Kuhnt-Szymanowski operation
labial
    inferior l.
    superior l.
lacus
    l. lacrimalis
Ladd's caliper
Lagleyze's operation
lamina
    posterior l.
Lancaster's operation
Landolt's eyelid reconstruction
Langenbeck's operation

Langer's line
Larsen's syndrome
Latrobe's retractor
Lauren's operation
Leahey's operation
LeMesurier's operation
leukoplakia
Lewis' line
Lexer's operation
ligament
    medial palpebral l.
line
    Borges and Alexander l.
    Bruner's l.
    cleavage l.
    contour l.
    Converse's l.
    Cox's l.
    crease l.
    crinkle l.
    Davis' l.
    dependency l.
    division l.
    dominant l.
    dynamic facial l.
    Edgerton's l.
    elastic l.
    election l.
    expression folds l.
    flexion l.
    flexure l.
    force l.
    Gibson-Stark and
      Kenedi l.
    grain l.
    gravitational l.
    Hutchinson and Koop l.
    increased tension l.
    junction l.
    Kanavel's l.
    Kazanjian and Converse l.
    Kazanjian's l.
    Kocher's l.
    Langer's l.
    Lewis' l.
    maximal tension l.
    minimal tension l.

line (continued)
    minimum extensibility l.
    natural l.
    orthostatic l.
    relaxed skin tension l.
    Stark's l.
    tension l.
    Terry's l.
    Webster's l.
    wrinkle l.
lip
    cleft l.
lipectomy
lobule
lobulus
    l. auriculae
Logan's bow
Luckett's operation
MacFee neck flap
Machek's operation
MacKenty's knife
macrocheilia
macrostomia
macrostructural
macrotia
Magnus' operation
Malbec's operation
Malbran's operation
maloplasty
mammaplasty
    Aries-Pitanguy m.
    augmentation m.
mammoplasty
    augmentation m.
mandible
Marcks' operation
margin
    orbital m.
Martin's retractor
mastoid
mastopexy
mastoplasty
mastoptosis
maxilla
maxillae
    frontal processes of m.
maxillary

maxillectomy
McCash-Randall operation
McDowell's operation
McGregor's forehead flap
McIndoe's elevator
meatus
    acoustic m.
    inferior m.
    middle m.
    superior m.
medications. See *Drugs and*
    Chemistry section.
meloncus
meloplasty
membrane
    mucous m.
mental
mentalis
mentolabial
method
    French m.
    Indian m.
    Italian m.
    triangle m.
metopoplasty
micrognathia
micrognathism
microstomia
Millard's
    island flap
    operation
Minsky's operation
Mirault-Brown-Blair operation
Mirault's operation
Mladick ear reconstruction
Monks-Esser island flap
Monks' operation
Moore and Chong sandwich flap
Morestin's operation
Motais' operation
mouth gag
    Denhardt-Dingman m.g.
    Dott's m.g.
mucomembranous
mucoperichondrium
mucoperiosteal
mucoperiosteum

mucosa
    buccal m.
Mueller's operation
Mules' operation
Müller's muscle
muscle
    frontalis m.
    glossopalatine m.
    levator m. of palatine
      velum
    Müller's m.
    pharyngopalatine m.
    platysma m.
    Riolan's m.
    superior constrictor m.
    tarsal m.
    temporalis m.
musculi
    m. levator veli palatini
    m. temporoparietalis
    m. tensor veli palatini
musculus
    m. adductor pollicis
    m. extensor pollicis brevis
    m. extensor pollicis longus
    m. flexor pollicis brevis
    m. flexor pollicis longus
    m. levator palpebrae
      superioris
    m. orbicularis oculi
    m. pectoralis major
    m. pectoralis minor
    m. salpingopharyngeus
    m. uvulae
myoplasty
nares
naris
nasal
nasion
nasoantral
nasoantritis
nasociliary
nasofrontal
nasograph
nasolabial
nasolacrimal
naso-oral

nasopalatine
nasopharyngeal
nasorostral
nasoseptal
nasoturbinal
nasus
    n. externus
natho-. See words beginning
  gnatho-.
needle
    Browne's n.
    Denis-Browne n.
    Keith's n.
    Reverdin's n.
Nelaton's operation
neoplasty
New's sickle flap
nostril
notch
    intertragic n.
O'Brien akinesia
oculi
    orbicularis o.
olfactory
Ollier-Thiersch
    graft
    operation
Ombrédanne's operation
operation
    Abbé-Estlander o.
    Abbe's o.
    Adams' o.
    Alexander's o.
    Allport's o.
    Alsus-Knapp o.
    Alvis' o.
    Ammon's o.
    Angelucci's o.
    Arlt's o.
    Barsky's o.
    Battle's o.
    Beard-Cutler o.
    Becker's o.
    Bell's o.
    Berke-Motais o.
    Berke's o.
    Bernard-Burrows o.

operation (continued)
    Biesenberger's o.
    Binnie's o.
    Blair-Brown o.
    Blair's o.
    Blaskovics' o.
    Brauer's o.
    Braun's o.
    Braun-Wangensteen o.
    Brophy's o.
    Brown-Blair o.
    Brown's o.
    Burow's o.
    Chopart's o.
    Converse's o.
    cosmetic o.
    Crawford's o.
    Cronin's o.
    Cutler's o.
    Davis and Kitlowski o.
    de Grandmont's o.
    Demel and Ruttin o.
    Denonvillier's o.
    Derby's o.
    Dieffenbach's o.
    Dieffenbach-Warren o.
    Dorrance's o.
    Douglas' o.
    Dragstedt's o.
    Duke-Elder o.
    Duplay's o.
    Dupuy-Dutemps o.
    Eckstein-Kleinschmidt o.
    Eitner's o.
    Elschnig's o.
    Ely's o.
    Erich's o.
    Esmarch's o.
    Esser's o.
    Estlander's o.
    Everbusch's o.
    Fergus' o.
    Fernandez' o.
    Fomon's o.
    Fox's o.
    Fricke's o.
    Friedenwald-Guyton o.

operation (continued)
   Gabarro's o.
   Gaillard's o.
   Gavello's o.
   Gayet's o.
   Gersuny's o.
   Gifford's o.
   Gillies' o.
   Gillies-Fry o.
   Giralde's o.
   Grant's o.
   Grimsdale's o.
   Guyton's o.
   Hagedorn-LeMesurier o.
   Hagedorn's o.
   Hagerty's o.
   Harman's o.
   Hess' o.
   Holmes' o.
   Hotchkiss' o.
   Hotz' o.
   Hughes' o.
   Illiff's o.
   Jaesche's o.
   Johnson's o.
   Jones' o.
   Joseph's o.
   Kilner's o.
   Kitlowski's o.
   Kolle-Lexer o.
   Konig's o.
   Kowalzig's o.
   Krause-Wolfe o.
   Krimer's o.
   Krönlein's o.
   Kuhnt-Szymanowski o.
   Lagleyze's o.
   Lancaster's o.
   Langenbeck's o.
   Lauren's o.
   Leahey's o.
   LeMesurier's o.
   Lexer's o.
   Luckett's o.
   Machek's o.
   Magnus' o.
   Malbec's o.

operation (continued)
   Malbran's o.
   Marcks' o.
   McCash-Randall o.
   McDowell's o.
   Millard's o.
   Minsky's o.
   Mirault-Brown-Blair o.
   Mirault's o.
   Monks' o.
   Morestin's o.
   Motais' o.
   Mueller's o.
   Mules' o.
   Nelaton's o.
   Ollier-Thiersch o.
   Ombrédanne's o.
   Owens' o.
   Pagenstecher's o.
   Panas' o.
   Parkhill's o.
   Pfeifer's o.
   Pierce-O'Connor o.
   plastic o.
   Randall's o.
   Reese's o.
   Reverdin's o.
   Rosenburg's o.
   Rose's o.
   Savin's o.
   Sayoc's o.
   Schimek's o.
   Schuchardt-Pfeifer o.
   Sédillot's o.
   Serre's o.
   Simon's o.
   Smith's o.
   Snellen's o.
   Sourdille's o.
   Spaeth's o.
   Stallard's o.
   Stein's o.
   Straith's o.
   Swenson's o.
   Szymanowski's o.
   tagliacotian o.
   Tansley's o.

operation (continued)
    Teale's o.
    Tennison's o.
    Textor's o.
    Thiersch's o.
    Thompson's o.
    Trainor-Nida o.
    Tripier's o.
    Truc's o.
    Ulloa's o.
    Van Millingen's o.
    Veau-Axhausen o.
    Veau's o.
    Verhoeff's o.
    Verweys' o.
    Vogel's o.
    von Blaskovics-Doyen o.
    von Langenbeck's o.
    V-Y o.
    Wardill-Kilner o.
    Webster's o.
    Wheeler's o.
    Wicherkiewicz' o.
    Wiener's o.
    Wies' o.
    Wolfe's o.
    Wolff's o.
    Worth's o.
    Wright's o.
    W-Y o.
    Young's o.
orbicular
orbicularis oculi
orbital
osteoplastic
osteoplasty
osteoseptum
osteotome
    Dingman's o.
osteotomy
ostium maxillare
otoplasty
Owens' operation
Padgett's
    dermatome
    graft
Pagenstecher's operation

palatal
palate
    cleft p.
palatine
palatognathous
palatomaxillary
palatonasal
palatoplasty
palatum
    p. durum
    p. durum osseum
    p. fissum
    p. molle
    p. ogivale
    p. osseum
palpebra
palpebral
palpebralis
Panas' operation
Parkhill's operation
Passavant's
    bar
    cushion
peau d'orange
pectus
    p. excavatum
pedicle
pedunculated
Penrose drain
periosteum
Pfeifer's operation
pharyngeal
pharyngoplasty
philtrum
Pierce-O'Connor operation
pillar of fauces
piriform
plate
    Brophy's p.
    perpendicular p. of
      ethmoid
    tarsal p.
plexus
    Kiesselbach's p.
plica
    p. nasi
    p. semilunaris

po dorahnj. See *peau d'orange.*
polydactylism
ponticulus
    p. auriculae
position. See *General Surgical Terms* section.
preauricular
procedure
    four-flap p.
    push-back p.
process
    hamular p.
    mastoid p.
    palatine p.
    sphenoidal p.
    uncinate p.
prognathism
prognathous
prosopoanoschisis
prosopodiplegia
prosopodysmorphia
prosoponeuralgia
prosopoplegia
prosopoplegic
prosoposchisis
prosopospasm
prosthesis
    Ashley's breast p.
pterygium
    p. colli
pterygoid
pterygomandibular
pterygomaxillary
pterygopalatine
ptosis
rafe. See *raphe.*
Randall's operation
raphe
    linear r.
    palatine r.
    palpebral r.
    pterygomandibular r.
reaction
    antigen-antibody r.
    immunity r.
reconstruction
    Brent's eyebrow r.

reconstruction (continued)
    Landolt's eyelid r.
    Mladick ear r.
    Steffanoff's ear r.
    Tagliacozzi's nasal r.
    Tanzer's auricle r.
    Wookey's pharyngoesophageal r.
Reese's
    dermatome
    operation
repair
    Rose-Thompson r.
resection
    submucous r.
retractor
    Dingman's r.
    Latrobe's r.
    Martin's r.
    Senn-Dingman r.
    Sluder's r.
retrenchment
retroauricular
retrusion
Reverdin's
    graft
    needle
    operation
revision
    W-plasty r.
    Z-plasty r.
rhinocheiloplasty
rhinokyphectomy
rhinokyphosis
rhinoplasty
rhytidectomy
rhytidoplasty
rhytidosis
rino-. See words beginning *rhino-.*
Riolan's muscle
Ritchie's tenaculum
ritidektome. See *rhytidectomy.*
ritido-. See words beginning *rhytido-.*
Rosenburg's operation
Rosenmüller's fossa
Rose's operation

Rose-Thompson repair
rostrum of sphenoid
RSTL – relaxed skin tension lines
ruga (rugae)
    r. palatina
sac
    lacrimal s.
salpingopharyngeal
Savin's operation
saw
    Gigli's s.
Sayoc's operation
scapha
scarification
Scarpa's foramen
Schimek's operation
Schuchardt-Pfeifer operation
Seddon's nerve graft
Sédillot's operation
sefalo-. See words beginning
    cephalo-.
Senn-Dingman retractor
septal
septonasal
septoplasty
septotomy
septum
    deviated nasal s.
    nasal s.
    orbital s.
    s. mobile nasi
    tarsus orbital s.
sera
    antilymphocytic s.
serrefine
    Blair's s.
Serre's operation
sfeno-. See words beginning
    spheno-.
sfenoid. See *sphenoid.*
sfenoidal. See *sphenoidal.*
shelf
    palatal s.
Silastic
    implant
    injection
Simon's operation

sinus
    paranasal s.
skafa. See *scapha.*
Sluder's retractor
Smith's operation
Snellen's operation
Sourdille's operation
Spaeth's operation
sphenoethmoid
sphenoethmoidal
sphenofrontal
sphenoid
sphenoidal
sphenopalatine
sphincter oris
splint
    Brown's s.
    volar s.
Stallard's operation
staphylectomy
staphyloplasty
staphylorrhaphy
staphylotomy
Stark's line
Steffanoff's ear reconstruction
Stein-Abbé lip flap
Stein-Kazanjian lower lip flap
Stein's operation
Stenstrom foot flap
stomatoplasty
Straith's operation
submental
sulci
    gingivolabial s.
sulcus
    s. anthelicis transversus
    s. nasolabialis
    retroauricular s.
    tympanic s.
supra-auricular
surgical procedures. See
    operation.
suture. See *General Surgical*
    Terms section.
Swenson's operation
syndrome
    Larsen's s.

syndrome (continued)
    Treacher Collins s.
Szymanowski's operation
tagliacotian operation
Tagliacozzi's
    flap
    nasal reconstruction
Tanner-Vanderput graft
Tansley's operation
Tanzer's auricle reconstruction
tarsal
tarsoplasty
tarsorrhaphy
tarsus
    t. inferior palpebrae
    t. superior palpebrae
Teale's operation
tectonic
temporal
temporomandibular
tenaculum
    Ritchie's t.
Tennison's operation
tenomyoplasty
tenoplastic
tenoplasty
terigo-. See words beginning
    pterygo-.
terigoid. See *pterygoid.*
terijeum. See *pterygium.*
Terry's line
Tessier's craniofacial cleft
Textor's operation
Thiersch's
    graft
    operation
Thompson's operation
tissue expander
tonsil
    palatine t.
    pharyngeal t.
torus
    t. frontalis
    t. levatorius
    t. mandibularis
    t. occipitalis
    t. palatinus

tosis. See *ptosis.*
tracheostomy
tragus
Trainor-Nida operation
transplant
    autogenous t.
    homogenous t.
transplantation
Treacher Collins syndrome
Tripier's operation
Truc's operation
tube
    orotracheal t.
tunica
    t. conjunctiva
        palpebrarum
turbinate
Ulloa's operation
unciform
uncinate
uraniscochasma
uraniscoplasty
uraniscorrhaphy
uranoplastic
uranoplasty
uranorrhaphy
uranoschisis
uranoschism
uranostaphyloplasty
uranostaphylorrhaphy
uranostaphyloschisis
uranosteoplasty
urethroplasty
uvula
    u. palatina
Van Lint akinesia
Van Millingen's
    graft
    operation
vault
    cartilaginous v.
Veau-Axhausen operation
Veau's
    elevator
    operation
velopharyngeal
velopharynx

velum
　　Baker's v.
　　palatine v.
Verhoeff's operation
vermilion
vermilionectomy
Verweys' operation
vestibule
Virchow's knife
Vogel's operation
vomer
vomeronasal
von Blaskovics-Doyen operation
von Langenbeck's operation
V-Y operation
Walsham's forceps
Wardill-Kilner operation
Webster's
　　line
　　operation
Wheeler's operation
Wicherkiewicz' operation
Wiener's operation
Wies' operation
wire
　　interdental w.
　　Kirschner's w.
Wolfe-Krause graft

Wolfe's
　　graft
　　operation
Wolff's operation
Wookey's
　　neck flap
　　pharyngoesophageal
　　　reconstruction
Worth's operation
W-plasty revision
Wright's operation
W-Y operation
xenograft
xenotransplantation
Young's operation
zeno-. See words beginning *xeno-*.
zigzagplasty
Zimany's flap
zoograft
zoografting
zooplasty
Zovickian's flap
Z-plasty revision
zygomatic
zygomaticofrontal
zygomaticomaxillary
zygomaticotemporal

Psychiatry, Neurology, and Neurosurgery

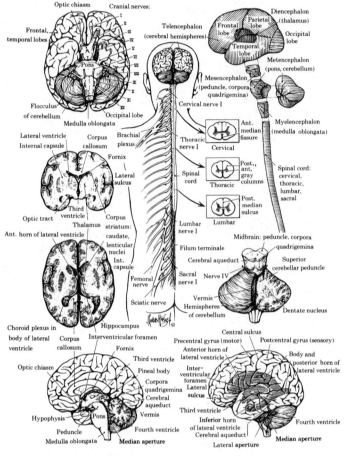

VARIOUS ASPECTS AND SECTIONS OF BRAIN AND SPINAL CORD

Psychiatry, Neurology, and Neurosurgery

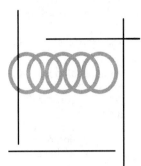

AA – achievement age
    Alcoholics Anonymous
abalienated
abalienatio
    a. mentis
abalienation
abasia
    a. atactica
    choreic a.
    paralytic a.
    paroxysmal trepidant a.
    spastic a.
    trembling a.
    a. trepidans
abasic
abducens
abducent
aberration
ablutomania
abreaction
abscess
    Dubois' a.
    epidural a.
    extradural a.
    otogenic a.
absentia
    a. epileptica
abstinence
abulia
    cyclic a.
abulic
abulomania
acalculia
acanthocytosis
acarophobia
acatamathesia

acataphasia
accident prone
acervulus
acetylcholine
ACh – acetylcholine
Achilles tendon reflex
achromatopsia
acidosis
acousma
acousmatagnosis
acousmatamnesia
acrobrachycephaly
acrocephalosyndactylia
acrodynia
acromania
acroneuropathy
acroneurosis
acroparalysis
acroparesthesia
acrophobia
acting out
adaptation
addict
addiction
    polysurgical a.
addictologist
addictology
ADE – acute disseminated
    encephalomyelitis
adenocarcinoma
adenoma
    a. sebaceum
adenovirus
adhesio
    a. interthalamica
adhesion

adiadochokinesia
adiadochokinesis
Adie's syndrome
adiposis
    a. cerebralis
    a. dolorosa
    a. orchalis
    a. orchica
    a. tuberosa simplex
adipositas
    a. cerebralis
adiposity
    cerebral a.
Adler's theory
adolescence
adolescent
adoyomanea. See *aidoiomania.*
adrenergic
adrenoleukodystrophy
Adson's
    bur
    cannula
    chisel
    clip
    conductor
    drill
    elevator
    forceps
    hook
    knife
    maneuver
    needle
    retractor
    scissors
    suction tube
adventitial
adventitious
adynamia
    a. episodica hereditaria
aero-asthenia
aerodromophobia
aeroneurosis
aerophagia
aerophagy
aerophobia
afazea. See *aphasia.*
afefobea. See *aphephobia.*

afemea. See *aphemia.*
affect
affection
affective
affectivity
affectomotor
affektepilepsie
afferent
afonea. See *aphonia.*
African meningitis
agenesia
    a. corticalis
agenesis
    callosal a.
ageusia
aggression
agitated
agitation
agitographia
agitolalia
agitophasia
agnosia
agoraphobia
agrammatica
aggrammatism
agrammatologia
agraphia
    absolute a.
    acoustic a.
    a. amnemonica
    a. atactica
    cerebral a.
    jargon a.
    literal a.
    mental a.
    motor a.
    optic a.
    verbal a.
agraphic
agromania
agyria
ahmiel-. See words beginning
    amyel-.
ahmio-. See words beginning
    amyo-.
ahservulvus. See *acervulus.*
aichmophobia

aidoiomania
AIDS-acquired
    immunodeficiency
    syndrome. See *Immunology
    with special reference to
    AIDS* section.
ailurophilia
ailurophobia
AJ-ankle jerk
akatamathesia
akatanoesis
akathisia
akinesia
akinesis
akinesthesia
akinetic
akmofobea. See *aichmophobia*.
ala
        a. cerebelli
        a. cinerea
alalia
        a. cophica
        a. organica
        a. physiologica
        a. prolongata
alalic
alcoholic
alcoholism
alcoholomania
alcoholophilia
alexanderism
Alexander's operation
alexia
alexic
alexithymia
algophilia
algophily
algophobia
algopsychalia
alienation
alienism
alienist
alkalosis
allochiria
ALS-amyotrophic lateral
    sclerosis
alteregoism

alurofilea. See *ailurophilia*.
alurofobea. See *ailurophobia*.
alveolar
Alzheimer's
    dementia
    disease
    sclerosis
    syndrome
amathophobia
amaurosis
        a. centralis
        a. cerebral
amaxophobia
ambiguous
ambivalence
ambivalent
ambiversion
ambivert
amblyopia
amenomania
ament
amentia
        a. agitata
        a. attonita
        nevoid a.
        a. occulta
        a. paranoides
        phenylpyruvic a.
        Stearn's alcoholic a.
amential
American Psychiatric Association
amerisia
ametamorphosis
amimia
        amnesic a.
        ataxic a.
amine
Ammon's horn
amnemonic
amnesia
        anterograde a.
        auditory a.
        Broca's a.
        concussion a.
        infantile a.
        Korsakoff's a.
        lacunar a.

amnesia (continued)
    localized a.
    olfactory a.
    patchy a.
    postconcussion a.
    posthypnotic a.
    psychogenic a.
    retroactive a.
    retrograde a.
    tactile a.
    transient global a.
amnesiac
amnesic
amnestic
amok
amoral
amoralia
amoralis
amphetamine
amusia
amychophobia
amyelia
amyelineuria
amyelotrophy
amygdala
    a. of cerebellum
amyloid
amyloidosis
amyostasia
amyostatic
amyosthenia
amyosthenic
amyotonia
    a. congenita
amyotrophia
    neuralgic a.
    a. spinalis progressiva
amyotrophic
amyotrophy
    diabetic a.
    neuralgic a.
anaclitic
analgesia
analysand
analysis
analysor
analytic

anamnesis
anamnestic
anancastic
anaphylaxis
anaplastic
anarithmia
anarthria
    a. literalis
Anders' disease
André-Thomas sign
anencephalia
anencephalic
anencephalohemia
anencephalous
anencephaly
anesthesia. See *General Surgical Terms* section.
aneurysm
    arterial a.
    arteriovenous a.
    berry a.
    Charcot-Bouchard a.
    cirsoid a.
    fusiform a.
    innominate a.
    intracranial a.
    miliary a.
    mycotic a.
    PICA a.
    racemose a.
aneurysmal
aneurysmectomy
angioblastoma
angiofibroma
angiography
angioma
    a. arteriale racemosum
    a. cavernosum
    cavernous a.
    encephalic a.
    a. venosum racemosum
angiomyolipoma
angioneurosis
angioneurotic
angiospasm
angophrasia
angzietas. See *anxietas*.

anhedonia
anhidrosis
anima
animus
anisocoria
anomia
anorexia
    a. nervosa
anosmia
anosmic
anosognosia
anoxia
ansa
    a. cervicalis
    a. hypoglossi
    a. lenticularis
    a. of lenticular nucleus
    a. subclavia
    a. of Vieussens
ansae
    a. nervorum spinalium
ansotomy
antecollis
antegrade
antianxiety
anticholinergic
anticoagulated
anticonvulsant
anticonvulsive
antidepressant
antihallucinatory
antiphlogistic
antisocial
antisocialism
anurizm. See aneurysm.
anxietas
    a. presenilis
    a. tibiarum
anxiety
    free floating a.
apandria
apanthropia
apanthropy
apastia
apastic
apathetic
apathic

apathism
apathy
Apert's syndrome
aphasia
    ageusic a.
    amnemonic a.
    amnesic a.
    amnestic a.
    anosmic a.
    associative a.
    Broca's a.
    global a.
aphemia
aphephobia
aphonia
    hysteric a.
    a. paranoica
apicotomy
aplasia
    a. axialis extracorticalis
        congenita
apnea
    sleep a.
apocarteresis
apophyseal
apophysis
    cerebral a.
    a. cerebri
    genial a.
apoplexy
    Broadbent's a.
    cerebellar a.
    cerebral a.
    fulminating a.
    ingravescent a.
    meningeal a.
    pituitary a.
    pontile a.
    Raymond's a.
    thrombotic a.
apperception
apperceptive
appersonification
apractic
apraxia
    akinetic a.
    a. algera

apraxia (continued)
    amnestic a.
    cortical a.
    ideational a.
    ideokinetic a.
    ideomotor a.
    innervation a.
    limb-kinetic a.
    motor a.
    oculomotor a.
    sensory a.
    transcortical a.
apraxic
aprophoria
aprosexia
apselaphesia
apsithyria
apsychia
apsychosis
aqueduct
    cerebral a.
    a. of midbrain
    a. of Sylvius
    a. of vestibule
aqueductus
    a. cerebri
arachnitis
arachnoid
arachnoidea
    a. encephali
    a. spinalis
arachnoideae
arachnoiditis
arachnophobia
Aran-Duchenne
    disease
    muscular atrophy
Arantius
    ventricle of A.
ARAS—ascending reticular
    activating system
arbor
    a. medullaris vermis
    a. vitae cerebelli
archipallial
archipallium

area
    Broca's a.
    Brodmann's a.
    Flechsig's a.
    Obersteiner-Redlich a.
    postcentral a.
    a. postpterygoidea
    a. postrema
    prefrontal a.
    premotor a.
    a. pterygoidea
    silent a.
    somatosensory a.
    vagus a.
    Wernicke's a.
areflexia
arenavirus
arhinencephalia
arithmomania
Arnold-Chiari
    deformity
    syndrome
arteriogram
arteriography
arteriosclerosis
arteritis
    cranial a.
    temporal a.
artery
    basilar a.
    callosomarginal a.
    carotid a.
    cerebellar a.
    cerebral a.
    choroidal a.
    communicating a.
    a. of Heubner
    lenticulostriate a.
    pericallosal a.
    thalamostriate a.
    vertebral a.
arthritis
    rheumatoid a.
arthropathy
asaphia
asemasia

asemia
  a. graphica
  a. mimica
  a. verbalis
assaultive
association
astasia
  a. abasia
astatic
astereocognosy
astereognosia
astereognosis
astereopsis
asterixis
asthenia
asthenic
asthenophobia
astrapophobia
astrocyte
astrocytoma
astroglia
astroid
asynchronism
asynergia
asynergy
    appendicular a.
    axial a.
    axioappendicular a.
    truncal a.
ataractic
ataraxia
ataraxic
ataraxy
ataxia
    adult onset a.
    autonomic a.
    Briquet's a.
    Broca's a.
    central a.
    cerebellar a.
    cerebral a.
    Fergusson and Critchley's
      a.
    Friedreich's a.
    frontal a.
    hereditary cerebellar a.
    hysteric a.

ataxia (continued)
    intermittent a.
    intrapsychic a.
    kinetic a.
    labyrinthic a.
    Leyden's a.
    locomotor a.
    Marie's a.
    motor a.
    noothymopsychic a.
    optic a.
    periodic a.
    progressive a.
    proprioceptive a.
    Sanger-Brown a.
    sensory a.
    spastic a.
    spinal a.
    spinocerebellar a.
    static a.
    a. telangiectasia
    thermal a.
    vasomotor a.
    vestibular a.
ataxiagram
ataxiagraph
ataxiamnesic
ataxiaphasia
atelencephalia
atelomyelia
atherothrombosis
athetoid
athetosis
atonia
atremia
atrophy
    alcoholic cerebral a.
    Aran-Duchenne muscular
      a.
    Charcot-Marie-Tooth a.
    circumscribed a. of
      brain
    convolutional a.
    Cruveilhier's a.
    degenerative a.
    Dejerine-Sottas a.
    denervated muscle a.

atrophy (continued)

    Duchenne-Aran muscular a.

    Erb's a.

    facioscapulohumeral a.

    Fazio-Londe a.

    Hoffmann's a.

    Hunt's a.

    idiopathic muscular a.

    Landouzy-Dejerine a.

    lobar a.

    multisystem a.

    myelopathic muscular a.

    neural a.

    neuritic muscular a.

    neuropathic a.

    neurotic a.

    neurotrophic a.

    olivopontocerebellar a.

    Parrot's a. of the newborn

    peroneal a.

    Pick's convolutional a.

    pseudohypertrophic muscular a.

    spinoneural a.

    Sudeck's a.

    trophoneurotic a.

    Vulpian's a.

    Werdnig-Hoffmann a.

ATS – anxiety tension state

attack

    vasovagal a.

atypical

auditory

    a. nerve

    a. nuclei

aula

aulatela

aulic

auliplexus

aura

autism

autistic

autocerebrospinal

autoerotic

autoeroticism

autoerotism

autognosis

autognostic

autokinesis

autokinetic

automatism

autonomic

autonomy

autopunition

autosomal

    a. dominant

    a. recessive

autotopagnosia

aversive

AVM – arteriovenous malformation

awla. See *aula.*

awlatela. See *aulatela.*

awlepleksus. See *auliplexus.*

awlik. See *aulic.*

axon

axonopathy

Aztec idiocy

Baastrup's syndrome

Babcock's needle

Babès' tubercles

Babinski-Nageotte syndrome

Babinski's

    law

    phenomenon

    reflex

    sign

    syndrome

Bacon's forceps

BAEP – brain-stem auditory evoked potential

Bailey's

    conductor

    leukotome

Balint's syndrome

Ballet's

    disease

    sign

ballism

ballismus

band

    Meckel's b.

Bane's forceps

Bárány's
    pointing test
    syndrome
barbiturate
Barré-Liéou syndrome
Barré's pyramidal sign
Barrett-Adson retractor
Barton-Cone tongs
Bärtschi-Rochain syndrome
basicranial
basilar
basilaris
    b. cranii
basioccipital
basion
basophobia
basophobiac
Batten-Mayou disease
Battle's sign
BEAM – brain electrical activity
    map
Beard's syndrome
Becker's dystrophy
Beckman-Adson retractor
Beckman-Eaton retractor
Beckman's retractor
Beck's syndrome
behavior
behaviorism
Bell-Magendie law
Bell's
    law
    mania
    nerve
    palsy
    phenomenon
Bender-Gestalt test
Berger rhythm
Bergeron's chorea
bestiality
bifrontal
Binswanger's
    dementia
    disease
biodynamics
Biot's respiration
bipolar

Birtcher's cautery
bisexual
bisexuality
bistoury
bitemporal
biventer
    b. cervicis
bizarre
Blackfan-Diamond syndrome
Blair's saw guide
blepharoptosis
blepharospasm
block
    spinal subarachnoid b.
    stellate b.
    sympathetic b.
    ventricular b.
body
    Nissl's b's
    pacchionian b's
    pineal b.
    Schmorl's b.
Bonhoeffer's symptom
Bonnet's syndrome
boopia
Bourneville's disease
BPV – benign positional vertigo
brace
    Hudson's b.
brachial plexus
brachium
    b. cerebelli
    b. cerebri
    b. conjunctivum
    b. copulativum
    b. of colliculus
    b. of mesencephalon
    b. opticum
    b. pontis
    b. quadrigeminum
brachybasia
brachycephalic
brachycephaly
brachycranic
bradwemaw. See *bredouillement.*
bradykinesia
bradylalia

bradylexia
bradylogia
bradyphasia
bradyphrasia
bradyphrenia
bradypsychia
bradyteleokinesis
Bragard's sign
Bragg peak
brain scan
Brain's reflex
Bravais-jacksonian epilepsy
bredouillement
bregma
Briquet's
    ataxia
    syndrome
Brissaud-Sicard syndrome
Brissaud's reflex
Bristowe's syndrome
Broadbent's apoplexy
Broca's
    amnesia
    aphasia
    area
    ataxia
    center
    convolution
    fissure
    gyrus
    space
Brodmann's area
Brown-Séquard syndrome
Brudzinski's sign
bruit
Bruns' syndrome
Brushfield-Wyatt disease
bruxism
BSAP – brief short-action
    potential
Bucy-Frazier cannula
Bucy's
    knife
    retractor
bulbonuclear
bulbopontine
bulimia

bundle
    Helweg's b.
    Meynert's b.
bunyavirus
bur
    Adson's b.
    D'Errico's b.
    Hudson's b.
    McKenzie's b.
Burdach's tract
CA – chronological age
cacergasia
cacesthenic
cacesthesia
cachinnation
cacodemonomania
cafard
café-au-lait spots
Cairns' forceps
calcarine
California encephalitis
callomania
callosal
calvaria
calvarium
Campbell's elevator
camptocormia
camptocormy
canalicular
canaliculus
canalization
cannabis
cannabism
cannula
    Adson's c.
    Bucy-Frazier c.
    Cone's c.
    Cooper's c.
    Frazier's c.
    Haynes' c.
    Kanavel's c.
    Sachs' c.
    Scott's c.
    Seletz's c.
cannulation
Capgras' syndrome
captation

carcinomatosis
    meningeal c.
carcinophobia
cardiac. See *Cardiovascular System* section.
carfol-. See words beginning *carphol-*.
carnal
carnophobia
carotid
    c. endarterectomy
    c. ischemia
carotidynia
carphologia
carphology
castration
CAT—computed axial tomography
catalepsy
cataleptic
cataleptiform
cataleptoid
cataphasia
cataphora
cataphoric
cataphrenia
cataplectic
cataplexie
    c. du reveil
cataplexis
cataplexy
catapophysis
catathymic
catatonia
catatonic
catatony
catecholamine
catharsis
cathectic
catheter
    red Robinson c.
cathexis
cathisophobia
CAT scan
cauda
    c. cerebelli
    c. equina

caudate
causalgia
cautery
    bipolar c.
    Birtcher's c.
    Mils' c.
cautionary
cavity
    Meckel's c.
cavum
    c. epidurale
    c. septi pellucidi
    c. subarachnoideale
    c. subdurale
    c. vergae
cell
    glitter c.
    Golgi c's
    Hortega's c.
    microglial c.
cella
    c. lateralis ventriculi lateralis
    c. media ventriculi lateralis
cell body
censor
    freudian c.
    psychic c.
center
    Broca's c.
    Setchenow's c's
centrencephalic
centriciput
centripetal
cephalagia
cephalhematocele
    Stromeyer's c.
cephalhematoma
    c. deformans
cephalhydrocele
cephalic
cephalocentesis
cephalogyric
cephalomeningitis
cephalometry
cephalomotor

cephaloplegia
cephalorhachidian
cerebellar
cerebellifugal
cerebellipetal
cerebellitis
cerebellofugal
cerebello-olivary
cerebellopontile
cerebellopontine
cerebellorubral
cerebellorubrospinal
cerebellospinal
cerebellum
cerebral
cerebralgia
cerebrasthenia
cerebration
     unconscious c.
cerebriform
cerebrifugal
cerebripetal
cerebritis
     saturnine c.
cerebrocardiac
cerebrocentric
cerebrogalactose
cerebrohyphoid
cerebroid
cerebrol
cerebrolein
cerebrology
cerebroma
cerebromalacia
cerebromedullary
cerebromeningeal
cerebromeningitis
cerebrometer
cerebron
cerebro-ocular
cerebropathia
     c. psychica toxemica
cerebropathy
cerebrophysiology
cerebropontile
cerebropsychosis
cerebrorachidian

cerebrosclerosis
cerebroscope
cerebroscopy
cerebrose
cerebroside
cerebrosis
cerebrospinal
cerebrospinant
cerebrospinase
cerebrostimulin
cerebrostomy
cerebrotomy
cerebrotonia
cerebrovascular
cerebrum
ceroid
cervical plexus
cervicomedullary
Céstan-Chenais syndrome
Chaddock's
     reflex
     sign
Chandler's
     forceps
     retractor
Charcot-Bouchard aneurysm
Charcot-Marie-Tooth
     atrophy
     disease
Charcot's
     disease
     gait
chemopallidectomy
chemopallidothalamectomy
cheromania
Cherry-Kerrison forceps
Cherry's
     osteotome
     retractor
     tongs
Cheyne-Stokes psychosis
Chiari-type malformation
chiasma
chiasmatic
Chinese restaurant syndrome
chisel
     Adson's c.

cholesteatoma
cholinergic
chondroma
chordoma
chordotomy
chorea
    automatic c.
    Bergeron's c.
    button-makers' c.
    chronic c.
    c. cordis
    dancing c.
    diaphragmatic c.
    c. dimidiata
    Dubini's c.
    electric c.
    epidemic c.
    c. festinans
    fibrillary c.
    c. gravidarum
    habit c.
    hemilateral c.
    Henoch's c.
    hereditary c.
    Huntington's c.
    hyoscine c.
    hysterical c.
    imitative c.
    c. insaniens
    juvenile c.
    laryngeal c.
    limp c.
    local c.
    c. major
    malleatory c.
    maniacal c.
    methodic c.
    mimetic c.
    c. minor
    c. mollis
    Morvan's c.
    c. nocturna
    c. nutans
    one-sided c.
    paralytic c.
    posthemiplegic c.
    prehemiplegic c.

chorea (continued)
    procursive c.
    rhythmic c.
    rotary c.
    saltatory c.
    school-made c.
    Schrötter's c.
    c. scriptorum
    senile c.
    simple c.
    Sydenham's c.
    tetanoid c.
    tic c.
choreal
choreic
choreiform
choreoathetoid
choreoathetosis
choreoid
choreomania
choreophrasia
choriomeningitis
    lymphocytic c.
    pseudolymphocytic c.
choroid
choroidectomy
chromosomes
Churg-Strauss syndrome
Chvostek's sign
cinerea
cingula
cingulate
cingulectomy
cingulum
cingulumotomy
circadian
    c. rhythm
circle
    c. of Willis
circumstantiality
cistern
    cerebellomedullary c.
    c. of fossa of Sylvius
    c. of lateral fossa of
      cerebrum
    c. of Pecquet
    c. of Sylvius

cistern (continued)
    subarachnoidal c's
cisterna
    c. ambiens
    c. basalis
    c. cerebellomedullaris
    c. chiasmatica
    c. chiasmatis
    c. fossae lateralis cerebri
    c. fossae Sylvii
    c. intercruralis profunda
    c. interpeduncularis
    c. magna
    c. sulci lateralis
    c. Sylvii
    c. venae magnae cerebri
cisternae
    c. subarachnoidales
    c. subarachnoideales
cisternal
cisternography
    metrizamide c.
CJD–Creutzfeldt-Jakob disease
clairaudience
clairsentience
clairvoyance
clamp
    bulldog c.
    Crutchfield's c.
    Gandy's c.
    Salibi's c.
    Wertheim's c.
classification
    Kraepelin's c.
Claude's
    hyperkinesis sign
    syndrome
claudication
    intermittent c.
    venous c.
claustra
claustrophilia
claustrophobia
claustrum
clava
climacteric
clinoid

clip
    Adson's c.
    Cushing's c.
    Heifitzs' c.
    Mayfield's c.
    McKenzie's c.
    Michel's c.
    Olivecrona's c.
    Raney's c.
    Schutz's c.
    Schwartz's c.
    Scoville-Lewis c.
    Scoville's c.
    Smith's c.
    Sugar's c.
    tantalum c.
    Weck's c.
    Yasargil's c.
clivus
clonic
clonism
clonus
    ankle c.
Cloward-Hoen retractor
Cloward's
    drill
    operation
CNS–central nervous system
coagulator
    Malis' c.
cobalt-60
cocaine
coccyx
coconscious
coconsciousness
cognition
cognitive
cognizant
colliculus
    facial c.
    inferior c.
collimator
Colorado tick fever
column
    Gowers' c.
coma
comatose

commissura
    c. alba medulae spinalis
    c. anterior cerebri
    c. cerebelli
    c. habenularum
commissure
    Meynert's c.
commitment
commotio
    c. cerebri
    c. spinalis
compensation
complex
    castration c.
    Electra c.
    inferiority c.
    Oedipus c.
compression
compulsion
compulsive
computed tomography
conamen
conarium
conation
conative
concept
conception
conconscious
concretism
concussion
condensation
conditioning
conduction
    bone c.
    c. velocity
conductor
    Adson's c.
    Bailey's c.
    Davis' c.
    Kanavel's c.
Cone's
    cannula
    needle
    retractor
confabulation
confidentiality
configuration

conflict
confluens
    c. sinuum
confusion
congenital
connector
    Rochester's c.
Conolly's system
conscience
conscious
consciousness
constellation
constitution
    ideo-obsessional c.
    psychopathic c.
content
    latent c.
Contour's retractor
contraction
    Gowers' c.
contraversion
    ocular c.
contrecoup
conus
    c. medullaris
conversion
    c. disorder
    c. reaction
convexobasia
convolution
    Broca's c.
    Heschl's c.
    occipitotemporal c.
    c's of cerebrum
    Zuckerkandl's c.
convulsant
convulsibility
convulsion
    choreic c.
    clonic c.
    coordinate c.
    epileptiform c.
    febrile c.
    hysteroid c.
    mimetic c.
    mimic c.
    myoclonic c.

convulsion (continued)
    puerperal c.
    salaam c.
    static c.
    tetanic c.
    tonic-clonic c.
    uremic c.
convulsive
Cooper's cannula
coprolagnia
coprolalomania
coprophagia
coprophagy
coprophilia
coprophiliac
coprophobia
Corning's puncture
cornu
    c. anterius ventriculi
      lateralis
    c. inferius ventriculi
      lateralis
    c. medullae spinalis
corona
    c. radiata
coronal
corpora
    c. amylacea
    c. arenacea
    c. bigemina
    c. flava
    c. quadrigemina
    c. restiformis
corporeal
corpus
    c. amygdaloideum
    c. callosum
    c. fornicis
    c. medullare cerebelli
    c. medullare vermis
    c. nuclei caudati
    c. ossis sphenoidalis
    c. pineale
    c. pyramidale medullae
    c. rhomboidale
    c. striatum
    c. trapezoideum

correlation
cortex (cortices)
    cerebral c.
    limbic c.
    precentral c.
    premotor c.
cortical
corticectomy
cortices
corticoafferent
corticoautonomic
corticobulbar
corticocerebral
corticodiencephalic
corticoefferent
corticomesencephalic
corticopeduncular
corticopontine
corticospinal
corticothalamic
costotransversectomy
costovertebral
Cotard's syndrome
Cotte's operation
counterphobia
countertransference
coxsackievirus groups A and B
CPM – central pontine
    myelinolysis
Craig's scissors
Crane's mallet
cranial
cranialis
craniamphitomy
craniectomy
cranioacromial
cranioaural
craniocele
craniocerebral
craniomalacia
craniomeningocele
craniopharyngioma
cranioplasty
craniopuncture
craniorachischisis
cranioschisis
craniosclerosis

cranioscopy
craniospinal
craniostenosis
craniostosis
craniosynostosis
craniotabes
craniotome
craniotomy
craniotonoscopy
craniotopography
craniotympanic
craniovertebral
cranitis
cranium
crescent
crescentic
cretin
cretinism
cretinistic
cretinoid
cretinous
Creutzfeldt-Jakob disease
cribriform
Crile's
    forceps
    knife
criminaloid
criminosis
crisis
    Lundvall's blood c.
crista
    c. galli
cross-tolerance
Crouzon's disease
crura
crus
    c. cerebelli ad pontem
    c. cerebri
crusta
Crutchfield-Raney tongs
Crutchfield's
    clamp
    drill
    tongs
Cruveilhier's atrophy
cryptococcosis

cryptogenic
    c. drop attacks
cryptomnesia
cryptomnesic
cryptoneurous
cryptopsychic
cryptopsychism
CSF–cerebrospinal fluid
CSM–cerebrospinal meningitis
CST–convulsive shock therapy
CT–computed tomography
CT scan
culmen monticuli
cuneate
cuneus
cunnilingus
curet
    Govons' c.
    Hibbs' c.
    Meyerding's c.
    Pratt's c.
    Raney's c.
    Volkman's c.
cushingoid
Cushing's
    clip
    depressor
    disease
    drill
    forceps
    law
    medulloblastoma
    reaction
    retractor
    spatula
    spoon
    syndrome
    tumor
CVA–cerebrovascular accident
CVOD–cerebrovascular
    obstructive disease
cyanosis
cybernetics
cycloplegic
cyclothymia
cyclothymiac
cyclothymic

cyclothymosis
cysticercosis
cytomegalovirus
cytoskeletal
daler. See *délire.*
Dana's operation
dance
    St. Vitus' d.
Dandy's
    hemostat
    hook
    scissors
Dandy-Walker syndrome
Darkschewitsch's
    fibers
    nucleus
Davidoff's retractor
Davidson's retractor
Davis'
    conductor
    forceps
    retractor
    spatula
dazhah aproova. See *déjà
    éprouvé.*
dazhah fa. See *déjà fait.*
dazhah ontondoo. See *déjà
    entendu.*
dazhah ponsa. See *déjà pensé.*
dazhah rakonta. See *déjà raconté.*
dazhah vakoo. See *déjà vécu.*
dazhah voo. See *déjà vu.*
dazhah vooloo. See *déjà voulu.*
dazhanara. See *degéneré.*
decerebellation
decerebrate
decerebration
decerebrize
decision
    Durham's d.
declinator
declive
    d. monticuli cerebelli
decompression
    cerebral d.
    subtemporal d.
decortication

decursus
    d. fibrarum cerebralium
decussation
    Forel's d.
    fountain d. of Meynert
defecalgesiophobia
defense mechanism
deflection
deformity
    Arnold-Chiari d.
degeneration
    alcoholic cerebellar d.
    axonal d.
    Holmes' d.
    spongiform d.
    striatonigral d.
    wallerian d.
degenerative
degéneré
degenitalize
dehumanization
déjà entendu
déjà éprouvé
déjà fait
déjà pensé
déjà raconté
déjà vécu
déjà voulu
déjà vu
dejection
Dejerine-Roussy syndrome
Dejerine's
    sign
    syndrome
Dejerine-Sottas atrophy
de la Camp's sign
delinquent
deliquium
    d. animi
délire
    d. de toucher
deliria
deliriant
delirifacient
delirious
delirium
    d. mussitans

delirium (continued)
    d. schizophrenoides
    d. sine delirio
    d. tremens
de lunatico inquirendo
delusion
delusional
dement
demented
dementia
    Alzheimer's d.
    Binswanger's d.
    epileptic d.
    hydrocephalic d.
    d. myoclonica
    paralytic d.
    d. paralytica
    d. paranoides
    paretic d.
    d. praecox
    d. praesenilis
    presenile d.
    progressive d.
    d. pugilistica
    semantic d.
    senile d.
    static d.
    terminal d.
    toxic d.
demonomania
demyelinate
demyelination
dendrite
denervation
Dennie-Marfan syndrome
dependence
dependency
depersonalization
depraved
deprementia
depressant
depressed
depression
    agitated d.
    involutional d.
    pacchionian d's
    postdormital d.

depressive
depressor
    Cushing's d.
deprivation
deranencephalia
Dercum's disease
derealization
dereism
dereistic
derencephalocele
dermatomyositis
dermoid
D'Errico-Adson retractor
D'Errico's
    bur
    drill
    forceps
    retractor
De Sanctis-Cacchione syndrome
desensitization
deterioration
determinism
    psychic d.
Devic's syndrome
DeVilbiss'
    forceps
    rongeur
    trephine
diachesis
diadochokinesia
diadochokinesis
diadochokinetic
diakesis. See *diachesis.*
diaphoresis
diaphragma
    d. sellae
diastematocrania
diastematomyelia
diatela
diaterma
dichotomy
diencephalic
diencephalohypophysial
diencephalon
dilemma
Dimitri's disease
dinomania

diocoele
diplegia
    atonic-astatic d.
    spastic d.
diploë
diplopia
diplopiaphobia
dipsomania
dipsopathy
dipsosis
dis-. See also words beginning
   dys-.
disc
    herniated d.
    intervertebral d.
disciplinary
discography
disease
    Alzheimer's d.
    Anders' d.
    Aran-Duchenne d.
    Ballet's d.
    Batten-Mayou d.
    Binswanger's d.
    Bourneville's d.
    Brushfield-Wyatt d.
    Charcot-Marie-Tooth d.
    Charcot's d.
    Creutzfeldt-Jakob d.
    Crouzon's d.
    Cushing's d.
    Dercum's d.
    Dimitri's d.
    Down's d.
    Dubini's d.
    Dubois' d.
    Duchenne-Aran d.
    Duchenne's d.
    Economo's d.
    Erb-Charcot d.
    Erb-Goldflam d.
    Erb-Landouzy d.
    Erb's d.
    Frankl-Hochwart's d.
    Friedreich's d.
    Fürstner's d.
    Gerlier's d.

disease (continued)
    Gilles de la Tourette's d.
    glycogen storage d.
    Goldflam's d.
    Gowers' d.
    Huntington's d.
    Hunt's d.
    Janet's d.
    Kalischer's d.
    Koshevnikoff's d.
    Krabbe's d.
    Laségue's d.
    Leigh's d.
    Little's d.
    Machado-Joseph d.
    Marchiafava-Bignami d.
    Menkes' d.
    Merzbacher-Pelizaeus d.
    Mills' d.
    Morel-Kraepelin d.
    multicore d.
    Niemann-Pick d.
    Parkinson's d.
    Pelizaeus-Merzbacher d.
    Pick's d.
    Rendu-Osler-Weber d.
    Romberg's d.
    Roth-Bernhardt d.
    Roth's d.
    Schilder's d.
    Schmorl's d.
    Scholz's d.
    Simmonds' d.
    Spielmeyer-Vogt d.
    Steiner's d.
    Strümpell's d.
    Sturge's d.
    Sturge-Weber-Dimitri d.
    Tay-Sachs d.
    Thomsen's d.
    Tourette's d.
    Unverricht's d.
    Vogt's d.
    von Hippel-Lindau d.
    von Recklinghausen's d.
    Weber's d.
    Werdnig-Hoffmann d.

disease (continued)
>Wernicke's d.
>white matter d.
>Wilson's d.
>Winkelman's d.
>Ziehen-Oppenheim d.

disfajea. See *dysphagia.*
disfazea. See *dysphasia.*
disfemia. See *dysphemia.*
disfonia. See *dysphonia.*
disfor-. See words beginning
>*dysphor-.*
disfrasia. See *dysphrasia.*
disfrenia. See *dysphrenia.*
disk. See *disc.*
diskectomy
diskogram
disorder
>affective d.
>anxiety d.
>bipolar d.
>conversion d.
>cyclothymic d.
>dissociative d.
>dysthymic d.
>obsessive-compulsive d.
>panic d.
>paranoid d.
>personality d.
>psychosexual d.
>schizophrenic d.
>somatoform d.
disorientation
displacement
dissector
>Hurd's d.
>Oldberg's d.
>Sheldon-Pudenz d.
dissociation
distaxia
>cerebral d.
distortion
distractibility
disvolution
divagation
DNA – deoxyribonucleic
>acid

dolichocephalic
dolichocephalism
domatophobia
dominance
Down's
>disease
>syndrome
dramatism
dramatization
drapetomania
dream
>clairvoyant d.
>d. interpretation
>veridical d.
dressing. See *General Surgical
>Terms* section.
drill
>Adson's d.
>Cloward's d.
>Crutchfield's d.
>Cushing's d.
>D'Errico's d.
>Hall's d.
>Hudson's d.
>McKenzie's d.
>Raney's d.
>Stille's d.
dromomania
dromophobia
drop spells
drugs. See *Drugs and Chemistry*
>section.
DSA – digital subtraction
>angiography
DST – dexamethasone
>suppression test
DT – delirium tremens
DTP – distal tingling on
>percussion
DTR – deep tendon reflex
Dubini's
>chorea
>disease
Dubois'
>abscess
>disease
>method

Duchenne-Aran
    disease
    muscular atrophy
Duchenne-Erb paralysis
Duchenne's
    disease
    dystrophy
ductus
    d. perilymphatici
Duncan's ventricle
dura
dural
dura mater
    d. m. encephali
    d. m. of brain
    d. m. of spinal cord
    d. m. spinalis
duramatral
duraplasty
durematoma
Durham's decision
duroarachnitis
durosarcoma
dysarthria
    d. literalis
    d. syllabaris spasmodica
dysarthric
dysautonomia
dysbasia
    d. angiosclerotica
    d. angiospastica
    d. intermittens
       angiosclerotica
    d. lordotica progressiva
    d. neurasthenica
       intermittens
dysbulia
dysbulic
dyscalculia
dyscephaly
dyschiria
dysdiadochokinesia
dysergasia
dysergastic
dysergia
dysesthesia
dysgeusia

dysgraphia
dyskinesia
    d. algera
dyskinetic
dyslalia
dyslexia
dyslogia
dysmetria
dysnomia
dysosmia
dyspareunia
dysphagia
dysphasia
dysphemia
dysphonia
dysphoretic
dysphoria
dysphoriant
dysphoric
dysphrasia
dysphrenia
dysplasia
dyspnea
dyspraxia
dysproteinemia
dysrhythmia
dyssocial
dyssymbolia
dyssymboly
dyssynergia
    d. cerebellaris myoclonica
    d. cerebellaris progressiva
dystaxia
    d. agitans
dystectia
dysthymia
dysthymic
dystonia
    cranial d.
    d. musculorum deformans
    segmental d.
    torsion d.
dystrophia
    d. myotonica
dystrophoneurosis
dystrophy
    autosomal-dominant

dystrophy (continued)
    distal d.
    Becker's d.
    Duchenne's d.
    Emery-Dreifuss d.
    Erb's d.
    facioscapulohumeral d.
    Landouzy-Dejerine d.
    limb-girdle d.
    muscular d.
    myotonic d.
    oculopharyngeal d.
    reflex sympathetic d.
    scapulohumeral d.
    scapuloperoneal d.
    thyroneural d.
dystropic
dystropy
Eaton-Lambert syndrome
Ebbinghaus' test
EBV – Epstein-Barr virus
eccentric
ecchordosis physaliphora
ecdemomania
echoencephalography
echogram
echographia
echokinesis
echolalia
echolalus
echomimia
echomotism
echopathy
echophrasia
echopraxia
echopraxis
echovirus
eclampsia
eclysis
ecmnesia
ecomania
Economo's disease
ecophobia
ecphoria
ecphorize
ecphory
ECT – electroconvulsive therapy

ectocinerea
ectopia
edema
    Huguenin's e.
edipism
edipus. See *Oedipus.*
EEE – eastern equine
    encephalomyelitis
EEG – electroencephalogram
efferent
ego
egocentric
egodystonic
egomania
egosyntonic
egotistical
egotropic
eidetic
ejaculation
    premature e.
eko-. See words beginning *echo-.*
elaboration
elation
Electra complex
electroconvulsive
electrocorticography
electroencephalogram
electroencephalograph
electroencephalography
electroencephaloscope
electrolyte
    e. imbalance
electromyogram
electromyography
electronarcosis
electroneuromyography
electrophysiologic
electroplexy
electroshock
electrospectrography
electrospinogram
electrostimulation
elevator
    Adson's e.
    Campbell's e.
    Frazier's c.
    Freer's e.

elevator (continued)
    Hajek-Ballenger e.
    Hibbs' e.
    Killian's e.
    Langenbeck's e.
    Love-Adson e.
    Rochester's e.
    Woodson's e.
ellipsis
emasculate
emasculation
embolism
    cerebral e.
embolalia
embolus
Emery-Dreifuss dystrophy
EMG – electromyogram
EMI – Electric and Musical
    Industries (brain scanner)
EMI scan
emotion
emotional
empathize
empathy
emprosthotonos
empyema
    subdural e.
encephalalgia
encephalatrophy
encephalemia
encephalic
encephalitis
    acute demyelinating e.
    California e.
    eastern e.
    herpes simplex e.
    e. lethargica
    Venezuelan equine e.
    von Economo's e.
    western e.
encephaloarteriography
encephalocele
encephalocoele
encephalocystocele
encephalogram
encephalolith
encephaloma

encephalomalacia
encephalomeningitis
encephalomeningocele
encephalomeningopathy
encephalomyelitis
    parainfectious e.
encephalomyelocele
encephalomyeloneuropathy
encephalomyelopathy
encephalomyeloradiculitis
encephalomyeloradiculoneuritis
encephalomyeloradiculopathy
encephalomyocarditis
encephalon
encephalonarcosis
encephalopathia
    e. alcoholica
encephalopathy
    metabolic e.
    postanoxic e.
    Wernicke's e.
encephalophyma
encephalopsy
encephalopsychosis
encephalopuncture
encephalopyosis
encephaloradiculitis
encephalorrhagia
encephalosclerosis
encephaloscope
encephaloscopy
encephalosepsis
encephalosis
encephalospinal
encephalothlipsis
encephalotome
encephalotomy
encopresis
endarterectomy
endarteritis
endocarditis
    bacterial e.
endocrinasthenia
endocrinotropic
endogenous
endomorph
endomorphic

endomorphy
endothelioma
    dural e.
ENG – electronystagmography
engram
enomania
enosimania
ensef-. See words beginning
    enceph-.
enterovirus
entropy
enuresis
environment
EOM – extraocular movements
epencephalic
epencephalon
ependopathy
ependyma
ependymal
ependymitis
ependymoblast
ependymoblastoma
ependymocyte
ependymocytoma
ependymoma
ependymopathy
epicoele
epicritic
epidemiology
epidermoid
epidermoidoma
epidural
epilepsia
    e. gravior
    e. major
    e. minor
    e. mitior
    e. nutans
    e. partialis continua
    e. procursiva
    e. rotatoria
    e. tarda
epilepsy
    abdominal e.
    Bravais-jacksonian e.
    catamenial e.
    cortical e.

epilepsy (continued)
    corticoreticular e.
    cryptogenic e.
    diurnal e.
    focal e.
    grand mal e.
    hysterical e.
    idiopathic e.
    jacksonian e.
    juvenile myoclonic e.
    Lafora's type of e.
    larval e.
    latent e.
    limbic e.
    matutinal e.
    menstrual e.
    musicogenic e.
    myoclonus e.
    nocturnal e.
    petit mal e.
    photosensitive e.
    physiologic e.
    primary e.
    procursive e.
    psychic e.
    psychomotor e.
    reflex e.
    rolandic e.
    secondary e.
    sensory e.
    serial e.
    sylvian e.
    symptomatic e.
    tardy e.
    temporal lobe e.
    tonic e.
    traumatic e.
    uncinate e.
    Unverricht-Lundborg
        type of e.
epileptic
    e. equivalent
    e. seizure
epileptiform
epileptogenic
epileptogenous
epileptoid

epileptologist
epileptology
epileptosis
epiloia
episode
    psycholeptic e.
episthotonos
epithalamus
epithelioma
    e. myxomatodes
      psammosum
epithelium
    mesenchymal e.
EPP – end plate potential
Epstein-Barr virus
equilibrium
Erb-Charcot disease
Erb-Goldflam disease
Erb-Landouzy disease
Erb's
    atrophy
    disease
    dystrophy
    sclerosis
    syndrome
erectile
eremophobia
erethism
erethisophrenia
erethistic
erethitic
ergasia
ergasiatrics
ergasiatry
ergasiology
ergasiomania
ergasiophobia
ergasthenia
ergomania
ergomaniac
ergometer
erithredema. See *erythredema.*
erithro-. See words beginning
    erythro-.
erogenous
erotic
eroticism

eroticomania
erotism
    anal e.
    muscle e.
    oral e.
erotogeneis
erotogenic
erotographomania
erotomania
erotomaniac
erotopath
erotopathy
erotophobia
erotopsychic
erotosexual
erratic
erythredema polyneuropathy
erythromelalgia
erythrophobia
eschar
    neuropathic e.
ESP – extrasensory perception
EST – electroshock therapy
estheticokinetic
eunoia
euphoretic
euphoria
euphoriant
euphoric
euphorigenic
eupnea
eupneic
excitability
excitable
excitation
excitomotor
exencephalia
exhibitionism
exhilarant
existential
existentialism
exogenous
exteroceptive
exterofection
exterofective
extracranial
extradural

extramedullary
extrapsychic
extrapyramidal
extraversion
extrovert
facetectomy
facies
    Parkinson's f.
facioscapulohumeral
factitous
Fajersztajn's sign
falik. See *phallic.*
falx
    f. cerebelli
    f. cerebri
familial
fan-. See words beginning *phan-.*
Fañana
    glia of F.
fantasy
fascia
    dentate f.
fasciculation
fasciculus
    f. aberrans of Monokow
    f. cuneatus
    f. gracilis
    f. lenticularis
    f. of Foville
    f. of Gowers
    f. of Rolando
fastigium
Fazio-Londe atrophy
feeblemindedness
fellatio
felo-de-se
fenil-. See words beginning
    phenyl-.
fenomenon. See *phenomenon.*
fenotype. See *phenotype.*
Ferguson's forceps
Fergusson and Critchley's
    ataxia
Ferris-Smith forceps
festination
fetish
fetishism

fever
    Colorado tick f.
fiber
    Darkschewitsch's f's
fibrae
    f. arcuatae cerebri
    f. arcuatae externae
    f. arcuatae internae
    f. cerebello-olivares
    f. corticonucleares
    f. corticospinales
    f. pyramidales medullae
fibrillation
fibroblastoma
    meningeal f.
fibroma
fibrosarcoma
figure
    fortification f's
fila
    f. olfactoria
    f. radicularia nervorum
        spinalium
filum
    f. durae matris spinalis
    f. of spinal dura mater
    f. terminale
fissure
    Broca's f.
    calcarine f.
    dentate f.
    Pansch's f.
    Rolando's f.
    f. of Sylvius
fistula
fixation
    freudian f.
fizeo-. See words beginning
    physio-.
flagellantism
Flatau's law
Flechsig's area
flegmatik. See *phlegmatic.*
flexibilitas
    f. cerea
flight
    f. of ideas

floccillation
flocculus
fluid
    cerebrospinal f.
    xanthochromic f.
fobia. See *phobia.*
fobic. See *phobic.*
fobofobia. See *phobophobia.*
Foix-Alajouanine syndrome
fold
    Veraguth's f.
folee. See *folie.*
folia cerebelli
folie
    f. à deux
    f. circulaire
    f. du doute
    f. du pourquoi
    f. gemellaire
    f. musculaire
    f. raisonnante
folium
    f. cacuminis
    f. vermis
fontanel
fontanelle
foramen
    f. caecum medullae
      oblongatae
    f. cecum ossis frontalis
    interventricular f.
    Luschka's f.
    Magendie's f.
    f. magnum
    f. occipitale magnum
    f. of Monro
    f. ovale ossis sphenoidalis
    f. rotundum ossis
      sphenoidalis
    f. spinosum
foramina
foraminotomy
forceps
    Adson's f.
    Bacon's f.
    Bane's f.
    bayonet f.

forceps (continued)
    Cairns' f.
    Chandler's f.
    Cherry-Kerrison f.
    Crile's f.
    Cushing's f.
    Davis' f.
    D'Errico's f.
    DeVilbiss' f.
    Ferguson's f.
    Ferris-Smith f.
    Gerald's f.
    Gruenwald's f.
    Hudson's f.
    Hurd's f.
    Leksell's f.
    Lewin's f.
    Love-Gruenwald f.
    Love-Kerrison f.
    Luer's f.
    McKenzie's f.
    Oldberg's f.
    Raney's f.
    Ruskin's f.
    Schlesinger's f.
    Schutz's f.
    Scoville's f.
    Sewall's f.
    Smithwick's f.
    Spence-Adson f.
    Spence's f.
    Spurling's f.
    Stevenson's f.
    Stille-Liston f.
    Stille-Luer f.
    Sweet's f.
    Wilde's f.
forebrain
foreconscious
Forel's decussation
forensic
formatio
    f. alba
    f. grisea
    f. reticularis pontis
    f. vermicularis
formication

fornix
    f. cerebri
Förster-Penfield operation
fossa
    cerebellar f.
    cerebral f.
    cranial f.
    f. cranii anterior
    f. cranii media
    f. cranii posterior
    posterior f.
Fothergill's neuralgia
fovea
Foville's
    fasciculus of F.
    syndrome
    tract
frame
    Stryker's f.
Francke's striae
Frankl-Hochwart's disease
Frazier's
    cannula
    elevator
    hook
    retractor
    suction tube
Frazier-Spiller operation
free association
Freer's elevator
fren-. See words beginning *phren-*.
French S-shaped retractor
frenetic
freno-. See words beginning
    phreno-.
frenzy
freudian
Freud's
    cathartic method
    theory
Friderichsen-Waterhouse
    syndrome
Friedmann's vasomotor
    syndrome
Friedreich's
    ataxia
    disease

Friedreich's (continued)
    tabes
frigidity
Fröhlich's syndrome
Froin's syndrome
frons
    f. cranii
frontal
fronto-occipital
frontotemporal
frustration
FTA-ABS – fluorescent
    treponemal antibody
    absorption (test)
fugue
    epileptic f.
    psychogenic f.
functional
fundus
funduscope
funduscopic
funicular
funiculitis
funiculus
    f. cuneatus
    f. cuneatus medullae
        oblongatae
    f. gracilis medullae
        oblongatae
    f. medullae spinalis
    f. solitarius
    f. teres
    f. ventralis
furibund
furor
    f. epilepticus
furrow
Fürstner's disease
GABA – gamma-aminobutyric
    acid
gait
    ataxic g.
    cerebellar g.
    Charcot's g.
    double-step g.
    drag-to g.
    equine g.

gait (continued)
    festinating g.
    Oppenheim's g.
    scissor g.
    staggering g.
    steppage g.
    swing-to g.
    tabetic g.
galea
    g. aponeurotica
    tendinous g.
Galt's trephine
galvanism
galvanopalpation
gamophobia
Gandy's clamp
ganglia
    basal g.
ganglion
    gasserian g.
    Meckel's g.
    trigeminal g.
ganglionectomy
ganglioneure
ganglioneuroblastoma
ganglioneuroma
gangliosympathectomy
Ganser's
    symptom
    syndrome
Garcin's syndrome
Gardner's
    needle
    operation
gargoylism
gegenhalten
gelasmus
Gélineau's syndrome
Gelpi's retractor
gene
genetic
geniculate
geniculum
genotype
genu
    g. corporis callosi
    g. nervi facialis

geophagia
geophagist
gephyrophobia
Gerald's forceps
geriatric
geriatrics
geriopsychosis
Gerlier's disease
Gerstmann's syndrome
gestaltism
Gestalt theory
Gifford's retractor
Gigli's saw
Gilles de la Tourette's
    disease
    syndrome
Gill's operation
glabella
gland
    pituitary g.
glia
    cytoplasmic g.
    fibrillary g.
    g. of Fañana
glial
glioblast
glioblastoma
    g. multiforme
gliocytoma
gliofibrillary
gliogenous
glioma
    astrocytic g.
    ependymal g.
    ganglionic g.
    g. multiforme
    g. sarcomatosum
gliomatosis
gliomatous
gliomyoma
gliomyxoma
glioneuroma
gliophagia
gliopil
gliosa
gliosarcoma

gliosis
    basilar g.
    cerebellar g.
    diffuse g.
    hemispheric g.
    hypertrophic nodular g.
    isomorphic g.
    lobar g.
    perivascular g.
    spinal g.
    unilateral g.
gliosome
globus
    g. hystericus
    g. pallidus
glossolalia
glossopharyngeal
glycorrhachia
Goldflam's disease
Golgi cells
Goll's tract
gouge
    Hibbs' g.
    Meyerding's g.
Govons' curet
Gowers'
    column
    contraction
    disease
    fasciculus
    sign
    syndrome
    tract
Gradenigo's syndrome
Graham's hook
grandiosity
grand mal
granulomatosis
graphesthesia
gratification
"gray matter"
Gruenwald's forceps
GSR – galvanic skin response
guard
    Sachs' g.
guide
    Blair's saw g.

Guillain-Barré syndrome
gumma
gummata
gustatory
gyri
    g. annectentes
    g. breves insulae
    g. cerebri
    g. insulae
    g. occipitales
    g. operti
    g. orbitales
    g. profundi cerebri
    g. transitivi cerebri
gyrus
    g. angularis
    Broca's g.
    g. callosus
    cingulate g.
    g. cinguli
    dentate g.
    g. dentatus
    g. fasciolaris
    g. fornicatus
    fusiform g.
    g. fusiformis
    hippocampal g.
    g. hippocampi
    g. infracalcarinus
    g. limbicus
    g. lingualis
    marginal g.
    g. marginalis
    g. olfactorius
    g. parahippocampalis
    g. paraterminalis
    precentral g.
    g. precentralis
    g. rectus
    supramarginal g.
    g. temporalis
    g. uncinatus
habenula
habitual
habituation
habromania
Haenel's symptom

Hajek-Ballenger elevator
Hallervorden-Spatz syndrome
Hall's
    drill
    neurotome
hallucination
    auditory h.
    depressive h.
    gustatory h.
    haptic h.
    hypnagogic h.
    lilliputian h.
    olfactory h.
    reflex h.
    stump h.
    tactile h.
    visual h.
hallucinative
hallucinatory
hallucinogen
hallucinogenesis
hallucinogenetic
hallucinogenic
hallucinosis
hallucinotic
Halstead-Reitan test
hamartoma
Hamby's retractor
Harris' migrainous neuralgia
haut-mal
Haynes'
    cannula
    operation
headache
    cluster h.
    exertional h.
    migraine h.
    orgasmic h.
    tension h.
    vascular h.
headrest
    Light-Veley h.
hebephrenia
hebephreniac
hebetude
heboid
heboidophrenia

hedonia
hedonic
hedonism
hedonophobia
Heifitz's clip
Helweg's
    bundle
    tract
hemangioblastoma
hemangioendothelioma
hemangioma
hemangiomatosis
hemangiosarcoma
hematoma
    epidural h.
    subdural h.
hematomyelia
hemiachromatopsia
hemianencephaly
hemianesthesia
hemianopia
hemiballism
hemiballismus
hemichorea
hemicrania
hemicraniectomy
hemihypesthesia
hemihypoplasia
hemilaminectomy
hemiparesis
hemiplegia
hemisection
hemisphere
    cerebellar h.
    cerebral h.
hemispherectomy
hemispherium
    h. cerebelli
hemodialysis
hemorrhage
    cerebellar h.
    epidural h.
    intracerebral h.
    intracranial h.
    intraparenchymal h.
    intraventricular h.
    pontine h.

hemorrhage (continued)
    putaminal h.
    subarachnoid h.
    subdural h.
    thalamic h.
hemostat
    Dandy's h.
    Kolodny's h.
Henoch's chorea
hepatic
    h. coma
hereditary
heredity
heredoataxia
hermaphrodite
herniation
    h. of intervertebral disk
    h. of nucleus pulposus
    tonsillar h.
    transtentorial h.
    uncal h.
heroin
herpes
    genital h.
    h. simplex
    h. zoster
herpesvirus
hertz
Heschl's convolution
heteroerotism
heterosexual
heterosexuality
heterosuggestion
heterotonic
heterotopia
Heubner's artery
Hibbs'
    curet
    elevator
    gouge
hindbrain
hipnagojik. See *hypnagogic.*
hipno-. See words beginning
    hypno-.
hipo-. See words begining
    hypo-.
hippocampal

hippocampus
    h. leonis
    h. nudus
Hirschberg's reflex
histrionic
HIV – human immunodeficiency
    virus
hodology
Hoen's skull plate
Hoffmann's
    atrophy
    sign
holergasia
holergastic
holism
holistic
Holmes'
    sign
    degeneration
holorachischisis
Holter's shunt
Homén's syndrome
homicidal
homicidomania
homilophobia
homolateral
homonymous
homosexual
homosexuality
homunculus
hook
    Adson's h.
    Dandy's h.
    Frazier's h.
    Graham's h.
horn
    Ammon's h.
Horner's syndrome
Horsley's separator
Hortega's cell
Horton's syndrome
hostility
H-reflex
HSE – herpes simplex encephalitis
Hudson's
    brace
    bur

Hudson's (continued)
    drill
    forceps
Huguenin's edema
Huntington's
    chorea
    disease
Hunt's
    atrophy
    disease
    neuralgia
    paradoxical phenomenon
    striatal syndrome
    tremor
Hurd's
    dissector
    forceps
Hurler's syndrome
hydranencephaly
hydrargyromania
hydrencephalocele
hydrencephalomeningocele
hydrocephalic
hydrocephalocele
hydrocephaloid
hydrocephalus
    communicating h.
    h. ex vacuo
    noncommunicating h.
    obstructive h.
    otitic h.
hydrocephaly
hydromeningitis
hydromeningocele
hydromicrocephaly
hydromyelia
hydromyelocele
hydromyelomeningocele
hydrophobia
hygroma
    subdural h.
hyla
hypalgesia
hypencephalon
hyperalgesia
hypercalcemia
hypercorticism

hyperdipsia
hyperesthesia
hypergeusesthesia
hypergeusia
hyperhidrosis
hyperkinesia
hyperkinesis
hyperkinetic
hypernatremia
hypernea
hyperneic
hypernoia
hyperosmia
hyperosmolar
hyperostosis
    h. cranii
    h. frontalis interna
    Morgagni's h.
hyperpathia
hyperphrenia
hyperplasia
hyperpnea
hyperreflexia
hypersomnia
hypertarachia
hypertension
hyperthermia
hyperthymergasia
hyperthymia
hyperventilation
hypervolemia
hypesthesia
hypnagogic
hypnoanalysis
hypnoanesthesia
hypnobatia
hypnogenic
hypnolepsy
hypnonarcoanalysis
hypnonarcosis
hypnopompic
hypnosia
hypnosis
hypnotherapy
hypnotic
hypnotism
hypnotize

hypoactive
hypocalcemia
hypochondria
hypochondriac
hypochondriacal
hypochondriasis
hypodipsia
hypoesthesia
hypogeusia
hypoglycemia
hypoglycorrhachia
hypohidrosis
hypokinesia
hypomania
hypomaniac
hypomanic
hypomimia
hyponatremia
hypophonia
hypophrenosis
hypophyseal
hypophysectomy
hypophysis
    h. cerebri
hypophysitis
hypophysoma
hypoplasia
hyporeflexia
hyposmia
hypotelorism
    orbital h.
hypotension
    orthostatic h.
hypothalamic
hypothalamotomy
hypothalamus
hypothermia
hypothermic
hypotonia
hypotonic
hypoventilation
    alveolar h.
hypovolemia
hypoxemia
hypoxia
hypsarrhythmia

hysteria
    anxiety h.
    canine h.
    conversion h.
    fixation h.
    h. libidinosa
    h.-malingering
    monosymptomatic h.
hysteric
hysterical
hystericism
hystericoneuralgic
hysteriform
hysteroepilepsy
hysteroepileptogenic
hysteroerotic
hysterogenic
hysteroid
hysteromania
hysteronarcolepsy
hysteroneurasthenia
hysteroneurosis
hysteropia
hysteropsychosis
iatrogenic
ICA–internal carotid artery
ICAO–internal carotid artery
    occlusion
ICP–intracranial pressure
ICT–insulin coma therapy
ictal
ictus
    i. epilepticus
    i. paralyticus
    i. sanguinis
id
ideal
    ego i.
idealization
ideation
    incoherent i.
ideational
idée
    i. fixe
identification
ideodynamism
ideogenetic

idetik. See *eidetic.*
idiocy
    absolute i.
    amaurotic familial i.
    athetosic i.
    Aztec i.
    cretinoid i.
    developmental i.
    diplegic i.
    eclamptic i.
    epileptic i.
    erethistic i.
    genetous i.
    hemiplegic i.
    hydrocephalic i.
    intrasocial i.
    Kulmuk i.
    microcephalic i.
    mongolian i.
    paralytic i.
    paraplegic i.
    plagiocephalic i.
    profound i.
    scaphocephalic i.
    sensorial i.
    spastic amaurotic axonal i.
    torpid i.
    traumatic i.
    xerodermic i.
idioglossia
idioglottic
idiohypnotism
idioimbecile
idioneural
idioneurosis
idiopathic
idiophrenic
idiopsychologic
idiosyncrasy
idiosyncratic
idiot
    erethistic i.
    mongolian i.
    pithecoid i.
    profound i.
    i.-savant
    superficial i.

idiot (continued)
    torpid i.
idiotropic
illusion
illusional
image
imagines
imago
imbecile
imbecility
immature
impotence
impoverishment
imprinting
impulse
    irresistible i.
impulsion
    wandering i.
inadequacy
inadequate
incallosal
incest
incision. See *General Surgical*
    Terms section.
incisura
    i. cerebelli
    i. clavicularis sterni
    i. frontalis
    i. temporalis
    i. tentorii cerebelli
incoherent
incompetent
incontinence
incoordination
incorrigible
incubus
indifference
    belle i.
indifferent
Indoklon therapy
indole
indusium griseum
inebriation
ineon. See *inion.*
infantile
infantilism

infarction
    brain stem i.
    cerebral i.
    lacunar i.
    watershed i.
infection
    abortive i.
    acute productive/lytic i.
    defective i.
    latent i.
    transforming i.
influenza
infundibulum
    i. hypothalami
inhibition
iniencephaly
inion
innervated
insane
insanity
    adolescent i.
    affective i.
    alcoholic i.
    alternating i.
    anticipatory i.
    choreic i.
    circular i.
    climacteric i.
    communicated i.
    compound i.
    compulsive i.
    consecutive i.
    cyclic i.
    doubting i.
    emotional i.
    hereditary i.
    homicidal i.
    homochronous i.
    hysteric i.
    idiophrenic i.
    impulsive i.
    manic-depressive i.
    moral i.
    perceptional i.
    periodic i.
    polyneuritic i.
    primary i.

insanity (continued)
    puerperal i.
    recurrent i.
    senile i.
    simultaneous i.
    toxic i.
insanoid
insensible
insight
insolation
    hyperpyrexial i.
insomnia
insomniac
insomnic
inspectionism
instinct
    death i.
    ego i.
    herd i.
instinctive
insula
insultus
    i. hystericus
integration
intellect
intellection
intellectualization
intelligence
intercourse
interictal
interneuron
interpediculate
interpeduncular
interpretation
interstitial
interventricular
intervertebral
intoxication
    water i.
intracephalic
intracerebellar
intracerebral
intracisternal
intracranial
intralobar
intramedullary
intraosseous

intraparietal
intrapsychic
intraspinal
intrathecal
intravascular
    i. coagulation
intraventricular
introjection
introspection
introversion
introvert
inversion
    sexual i.
invert
involuntary
involutional
iodoventriculography
ipsilateral
ipsiversion
    ocular i.
IQ–intelligence quotient
irascibility
irreversible
irritability
irritation
    cerebral i.
    spinal i.
ischemia
    brain stem i.
    transient carotid i.
ischogyria
island of Reil
ismus. See *isthmus.*
isolation
IST–insulin shock therapy
isthmus
    i. of cingulate gyrus
jacksonian epilepsy
Jackson's
    law
    rule
    syndrome
Jakob-Creutzfeldt syndrome
jamais vu
Janet's
    disease
    test

Jansen's retractor
Javid's shunt
jefirofobea. See *gephyrophobia.*
Jobst stocking
Joffroy's reflex
Jolly's reaction
Jung's method
juvenile
kakergasea. See *cacergasia.*
kakesthenik. See *cacesthenic.*
kakesthezea. See *cacesthesia.*
kakinashun. See *cachinnation.*
kakodemonomanea. See
    cacodemonomania.
Kalischer's disease
Kanavel's
    cannula
    conductor
Kanner's syndrome
karnshvoont. See *kernschwund.*
Kearns-Sayer syndrome
kemo-. See words beginning
    chemo-.
kenophobia
keraunoneurosis
kernicterus
Kernig's sign
kernschwund
keromanea. See *cheromania.*
Kerrison's rongeur
Killian's elevator
Kiloh-Nevin syndrome
kinanesthesia
kinesiesthesiometer
kinesiology
kinesioneurosis
kinesis
kinesodic
kinesthesia
kinesthetic
kinetic
KJ–knee jerk
KK–knee kick
Kleine-Levin syndrome
Klemme's retractor
kleptolagnia
kleptomania

kleptomaniac
kleptophobia
Klippel-Feil syndrome
Klippel-Feldstein syndrome
Klüver-Bucy syndrome
knife
    Adson's k.
    Bucy's k.
    Crile's k.
kolesteatoma. See *cholesteatoma.*
kolinerjik. See *cholinergic.*
Kolodny's hemostat
kooroo. See *kuru.*
kor-. See words beginning *chor-.*
koro
Korsakoff's
    amnesia
    psychosis
    syndrome
Koshevnikoff's disease
Krabbe's
    disease
    sclerosis
Kraepelin's classification
Krause's
    operation
    ventricle
Kretschmer types
Kulmuk idiocy
kuru
kyphoscoliosis
labile
lability
labiochorea
labyrinthitis
lactacidemia
lacuna
Lafora's
    epilsepsy
    sign
laliophobia
laloneurosis
lalophobia
lambda
Lambert-Eaton myasthenic
    syndrome
Lambotte's osteotome

lamella
lamina
    inferior l. of sphenoid
        bone
    l. medullaris lateralis
        corporis striati
    l. medullaris medialis
        corporis striati
    l. ossium cranii
laminae
    l. albae cerebelli
    l. medullares cerebelli
    l. medullares thalami
laminagram
laminagraph
laminectomy
laminotomy
Landouzy-Dejerine
    atrophy
    dystrophy
Landry's paralysis
Langenbeck's elevator
lapsus
    l. linguae
    l. memoriae
Lasègue's
    disease
    sign
latah
latency
latent
laterality
lateropulsion
law
    Babinski's l
    Bell-Magendie l.
    Bell's l.
    Cushing's l.
    Flatau's l.
    Jackson's l.
    Magendie's l.
    wallerian l.
Leichtenstern's sign
Leigh's disease
Leksell's
    forceps
    rongeur

lemniscus
Lennox-Gastaut syndrome
Lennox's syndrome
lenticular
lenticulo-optic
lenticulostriate
lentivirus
leprosy
leptocephalia
leptomeningeal
leptomeninges
leptomeningioma
leptomeningitis
    l. interna
    sarcomatous l.
leptomeningopathy
leptomeninx
Leriche's operation
Leri's sign
lesbian
lesbianism
Lesch-Nyhan syndrome
lesion
    space-occupying
      intracranial l.
lethargy
    hysteric l.
    induced l.
    lucid l.
lethe
letheomania
lethologica
leukodystrophy
    globoid cell l.
    metachromatic l.
    sudanophilic l.
leukoencephalitis
leukoencephalopathy
    metachromatic l.
    progressive multifocal l.
    subacute sclerosing l.
leukoerythroblastosis
leukomyelitis
leukomyelopathy
leukotome
    Bailey's l.
    Love's l.

leukotomy
Lewin's forceps
Leyden's ataxia
Lhermitte's sign
libidinal
libidinous
libido
    bisexual l.
    ego l.
Lichtheim's
    plaques
    sign
ligamenta
    l. flava
ligamentum
    l. denticulatum
    l. flavum
Light-Veley headrest
likenshadel. See *lückenschädel.*
limbic
lingula
    l. cerebelli
lipohyalinosis
Lissauer's
    paralysis
    tract
lithium
Little's disease
lobe
    caudate l. of cerebrum
    crescentic l. of
      cerebellum
    flocculonodular l.
    limbic l.
    occipital l.
    parietal l.
    quadrangular l. of
      cerebellum
    quadrate l. of cerebral
      hemisphere
    temporal l.
    temporosphenoidal l. of
      cerebral hemisphere
lobectomy
lobotomy
    frontal l.
    prefrontal l.
    transorbital l.

lobule
    l. of cerebellum
    posteromedian l.
lobulus
    l. centralis cerebelli
    l. paracentralis
    l. parietalis
    l. quadrangularis cerebelli
    l. semilunaris
lobus
    l. frontalis
    l. occipitalis
    l. olfactorius
    l. parietalis
    l. temporalis
locus
    l. ceruleus
    l. ferrugineus
logagnosia
logagraphia
logamnesia
logaphasia
logasthenia
logoklony
logokophosis
logomania
logoneurosis
logopathy
logoplegia
logorrhea
logospasm
lordosis
Love-Adson elevator
Love-Gruenwald
    forceps
    rongeur
Love-Kerrison forceps
Love's
    leukotome
    retractor
LP – lumbar puncture
LSD – lysergic acid diethylamide
Lucae's mallet
lucid
lückenschädel
Luer's forceps
luko-. See words beginning
   leuko-.

lumbar puncture
lumbosacral
lunacy
lunatic
lunatism
Lundvall's blood crisis
lupus
    l. erythematosus
lura
lural
Luschka's foramen
Lust's reflex
lymphoma
lymphosarcoma
lyssavirus
MA – mental age
Machado-Joseph disease
macrencephalia
macrocrania
macrogyria
macromania
macromelia
    m. paresthetica
maculocerebral
Magendie's
    foramen
    law
    spaces
magnetic resonance imaging
maladjustment
malformation
    arteriovenous m.
    Chiari-type m.
malingerer
malingering
Malis' coagulator
malleation
mallet
    Crane's m.
    Lucae's m.
    Meyerding's m.
maneuver
    Adson's m.
    Valsalva's m.
mania
    acute hallucinatory m.
    akinetic m.

mania (continued)
    m. à potu
    Bell's m.
    dancing m.
    doubting m.
    epileptic m.
    hysterical m.
    m. mitis
    periodical m.
    puerperal m.
    Ray's m.
    reasoning m.
    religious m.
    m. secandi
    transitory m.
    unproductive m.
maniac
maniaphobia
manic
manic-depressive
manifest
mannerism
MAOI – monoamine oxidase
    inhibitor
Marchiafava-Bignami disease
Marie's
    ataxia
    sclerosis
marihuana, marijuana
marital
marrowbrain
masochism
masochist
Mayfield's clip
MBP – myelin basic protein
MCA – middle cerebral
    artery
McCarthy's reflex
McKenzie's
    bur
    clip
    drill
    forceps
MD – muscular dystrophy
measles
mechanism
    defense m.

mechanism (continued)
    neutralizing m.
Meckel's
    band
    cavity
    ganglion
mecocephalic
medications. See *Drugs and*
    Chemistry section.
medicerebellar
medicerebral
medulla
    m. oblongata
    m. spinalis
medullary
medullispinal
medullitis
medulloblast
medulloblastoma
    Cushing's m.
medulloencephalic
medulloepithelioma
megalomania
megalomaniac
melancholia
    affective m.
    m. agitata
    agitated m.
    m. attonita
    flatuous m.
    m. hypochondriaca
    involution m.
    m. religiosa
    m. simplex
    stuporous m.
    m. with delirium
melancholiac
melanin
melanoma
melanotic
melomania
melyuh. See *milieu.*
membrane
    arachnoid m.
memory
    affect m.
    anterograde m.

menarche
Mendel-Bekhterew reflex
Ménière's syndrome
meningeal
meningematoma
meningeocortical
meningeoma
meningeorrhaphy
meninges
meninghematoma
meningina
meninginitis
meningioma
 angioblastic m.
 mesodermal m.
 olfactory groove m.
meningiomatosis
meningism
meningismus
meningitic
meningitides
meningitis
 acute aseptic m.
 African m.
 aseptic m.
 benign lymphocytic m.
 cerebral m.
 cerebrospinal m.
 granulomatous m.
 gummatous m.
 lymphocytic m.
 meningococcic m.
 metastatic m.
 m. necrotoxica reactiva
 occlusive m.
 m. ossificans
 otitic m.
 parameningococcus m.
 purulent m.
 Quincke's m.
 septicemic m.
 m. serosa
 m. serosa circumscripta
 m. serosa circumscripta
  cystica
 serous m.
 m. sympathica

meningitis (continued)
 syphilitic m.
 torula m.
 torular m.
 tubercular m.
 tuberculous m.
 viral m.
meningitophobia
meningoarteritis
meningoblastoma
meningocele
meningocephalitis
meningocerebritis
meningococcemia
 acute fulminating m.
meningococci
meningococcidal
meningococcin
meningococcosis
meningococcus
meningocortical
meningocyte
meningoencephalitis
meningoencephalocele
meningoencephalomyelitis
meningoencephalomyelopathy
meningoencephalopathy
meningoexothelioma
meningofibroblastoma
meningogenic
meningoma
meningomalacia
meningomyelitis
meningomyelocele
meningomyeloencephalitis
meningomyeloradiculitis
meningomyelorrhaphy
meningo-osteophlebitis
meningopathy
meningopneumonitis
meningorachidian
meningoradicular
meningoradiculitis
meningorecurrence
meningorrhagia
meningorrhea
meningothelioma

meningotyphoid
meningovascular
meninguria
meninx
    m. fibrosa
    m. serosa
    m. tenuis
    m. vasculosa
Menkes' disease
mentalia
mentation
meralgia
    m. paresthetica
merergastic
merorachischisis
Merzbacher-Pelizaeus disease
mesencephalon
mesencephalotomy
mesmerism
mesoglia
metacoele
metaphrenia
metaplexus
metapsyche
metapsychics
metapsychology
metatela
metathalamus
metencephal
metencephalic
metencephalon
metencephalospinal
methemoglobinemia
method
    Dubois' m.
    Freud's cathartic m.
    Jung's m.
    Pavlov's m.
methomania
metonymy
Meyerding's
    curet
    gouge
    mallet
    osteotome
    retractor
Meyer's theory

Meynert's
    bundle
    commissure
    decussation
    tract
Michel's clip
microaneurysm
microcephaly
microcrania
microglia
microglial
microgliocyte
microglioma
microgliomatosis
microgyri
microgyrus
micromania
microneurosurgery
microscopy
microsurgery
micturition
midbrain
mid-pons
miel-. See words beginning *myel-*.
mielo-. See words beginning
    myelo-.
migraine
    fulgurating m.
    ophthalmic m.
    ophthalmoplegic m.
migrateur
milieu
Millard-Gubler syndrome
Mills' disease
Mils' cautery
Minnesota Multiphasic
    Personality Inventory test
mio-. See words beginning *myo-*.
miosis
misaction
misandria
misanthropia
miso-. See also words beginning
    myso-.
misocainia
misogamy
misogyn

misogyny
misologia
misoneism
misopedia
mitho-. See words beginning
    mytho-.
mitochondrial
MMPI – Minnesota Multiphasic
    Personality Inventory
M'Naghten rule
Möbius' syndrome
Mönckeberg's sclerosis
mongolian idiot
mongolism
mongoloid
Monokow
        fasciculus aberrans of M.
monomania
monomoria
mononeuropathy
        m. multiplex
monophasic
monoplegia
monorecidive
monoxyhemoglobin
Monro
        foramen of M.
monticulus
        m. cerebelli
Morel-Kraepelin disease
Morgagni's hyperostosis
moria
moron
moronity
morphinomania
Morquio's sign
Morvan's chorea
motoneuron
motor
motorium
        m. commune
MRI – magnetic resonance
    imaging
MS – multiple sclerosis
multifocal
mumps
Munchausen's syndrome

muscle
    digastric m.
    frontalis m.
    gluteus maximus m.
    intercostal m.
    latissimus dorsi m.
    occipitalis m.
    orbicularis oculi m.
    rhomboid major m.
    rhomboid minor m.
    sartorius m.
    scalenus m.
    sternocleidomastoid m.
    temporalis m.
    teres major m.
    teres minor m.
    trapezius m.
mutation
mute
mutism
    akinetic m.
    hysterical m.
myalgia
myasthenia
    m. gravis pseudoparalytica
myatonia
mydriasis
    spinal m.
myelalgia
myelanalosis
myelapoplexy
myelasthenia
myelatelia
myelatrophy
myelauxe
myelencephalitis
myelencephalon
myelencephalospinal
myelencephalous
myeleterosis
myelic
myelin
myelinated
myelinization
myelinoclasis
    acute perivascular m.
    central pontine m.

myelinoclasis (continued)
    postinfection perivenous
      m.
myelinogeny
myelinolysin
myelinolysis
    central pontine m.
myelinopathy
myelinosis
myelitis
myeloarchitecture
myelobrachium
myelocele
myelocoele
myelocone
myelocyst
myelocystic
myelocystocele
myelocystomeningocele
myelocyte
myelodysplasia
myeloencephalic
myeloencephalitis
myelofibrosis
myelogenesis
myelogeny
myelogram
myelography
myeloid
myeloma
myelomalacia
myelomeningitis
myelomeningocele
myelon
myeloneuritis
myelo-opticoneuropathy
myeloparalysis
myelopathy
myelophthisis
myeloplegia
myeloradiculitis
myeloradiculodysplasia
myeloradiculopathy
myelorrhagia
myelorrhaphy
myelosarcoma
myeloschisis

myeloscintogram
myelosclerosis
myelosis
myelospasm
myelospongium
myelosyphilis
myelosyphilosis
myelotome
myelotomy
    commissural m.
Myerson's sign
myoclonia
    m. epileptica
myoclonic
myoclonus
    ocular m.
    palatal m.
    spinal m.
myofascial
myoglobinuria
myohypertrophia
    m. kymoparalytica
myokymia
myoneural
myopathy
    alcoholic m.
    centronuclear m.
    endocrine m.
    glucocorticoid-induced m.
    hypertrophic branchial m.
    hypothyroid m.
    infiltrative m.
    mitochondrial m.
    myotubular m.
    nemaline (rod) m.
    thyrotoxic m.
myositis
    m. ossificans
myotonia
    m. congenita
mysophilia
mysophobia
mythomania
mythophobia
mythoplasty
myxovirus
Naffziger's syndrome

napex
narcism
narcissism
narcissistic
narcoanalysis
narcodiagnosis
narcohypnosis
narcolepsy
narcoleptic
narcolysis
narcomania
narcosis
narcosomania
narcosynthesis
narcotic
nasion
necrencephalus
necromania
necrophilia
necrophilism
necrophobia
necrosadism
necrosis
needle
    Adson's n.
    Babcock's n.
    Cone's n.
    Gardner's n.
    New's n.
    Sachs' n.
    Ward-French n.
neencephalon
negativism
neocerebellum
neokinetic
neolalia
neolalism
neologism
neopallium
neophilism
neophobia
neophrenia
neoplasm
neostriatum
neothalamus
nerve
    abducens n.

nerve (continued)
    accessory n.
    acoustic n.
    afferent n.
    autonomic n.
    Bell's n.
    n. conduction study
    cranial n.
    efferent n.
    facial n.
    glossopharyngeal n.
    hypoglossal n.
    intermediate n.
    mandibular n.
    maxillary n.
    oculomotor n.
    olfactory n.
    ophthalmic n.
    optic n.
    parasympathetic n.
    spinal n.
    sympathetic n.
    trigeminal n.
    trochlear n.
    vagus n.
neuradynamia
neuragmia
neural
neuralgia
    cervicobrachial n.
    cranial n.
    Fothergill's n.
    glossopharyngeal n.
    hallucinatory n.
    Harris' migrainous n.
    Hunt's n.
    migrainous n.
    postherpetic n.
    trigeminal n.
    vidian n.
neuranagenesis
neurangiosis
neurapophysis
neurapraxia
neurarchy
neurasthenia
neurastheniac

neurasthenic
neurataxia
neurataxy
neuratrophia
neuratrophic
neuratrophy
neuraxial
neuraxis
neuraxitis
neuraxon
neure
neurectasia
neurectomy
    presacral n.
neurectopia
neurenteric
neurergic
neurexeresis
neuriatry
neuridine
neurilemma
neurilemmitis
neurilemmoma
neurilemoma
    acoustic n.
    trigeminal n.
neurinoma
    acoustic n.
neuritic
neuritis
neuroactive
neuroallergy
neuroamebiasis
neuroanastomosis
neuroanatomy
neuroarthropathy
neuroastrocytoma
neurobehavioral
neuroblast
neuroblastoma
neurobrucellosis
neurocanal
neurocardiac
neurocentrum
neuroceptor
neurochemistry
neurochitin

neurocirculatory
neurocladism
neuroclonic
neurocommunications
neurocranial
neurocranium
neurocrine
neurocrinia
neurocyte
neurocytology
neurocytoma
neurodegenerative
neurodendrite
neurodiagnosis
neurodynia
neuroelectricity
neuroelectrotherapeutics
neuroencephalomyelopathy
neuroendocrine
neuroendocrinology
neuroepithelium
neurofibril
neurofibrilla
neurofibrillae
neurofibrillar
neurofibroma
neurofibromatosis
neurofilament
neurofixation
neurogangliitis
neuroganglion
neurogen
neurogenesis
neurogenic
    n. bladder
neurogenous
neuroglia
    fascicular n.
    peripheral n.
neurogliocytoma
neuroglioma
neurogliosis
neuroglycopenia
neurogram
neurography
neurohumoralism
neurohypophysis

neuroimmunology
neuroinduction
neurokeratin
neurolabyrinthitis
    viral n.
neurolemma
neuroleptic
neurolipomatosis
neurologia
neurological
neurologist
neurology
neurolymph
neurolysis
neuroma
    acoustic n.
    medullated n.
    myelinic n.
    plexiform n.
    Verneuil's n.
neuromalacia
neuromatosis
neuromere
neuromittor
neuromotor
neuromyasthenia
neuromyelitis
    n. optica
neuromyotonia
neuron
neuronal
neuronitis
neuronopathy
neuro-ophthalmology. See
    Ophthalmology section.
neuroparalysis
neuroparalytic
neuropath
neuropathic
neuropathogenesis
neuropathology
neuropathy
    alcohol-nutritional n.
    amyloid n.
    brachial plexus n.
    compression-entrapment
      n.

neuropathy (continued)
    diabetic n.
    focal n.
    granulomatous n.
    infectious n.
    ischemic n.
    multifocal n.
    peripheral n.
    selective autonomic n.
    trigeminal n.
neurophonia
neuroplasty
neuropsychiatrist
neuropsychiatry
neuropsychic
neuropsychopathy
neuropsychosis
neuropyra
neuropyretic
neuroradiology
neurorecidive
neurorecurrence
neuroregulation
neurorelapse
neuroretinopathy
    hypertensive n.
neurorrhaphy
neurorrheuma
neurosarcokleisis
neurosarcoma
neurosclerosis
neurosecretion
neurosegmental
neurosensory
neuroses
neurosis
    anxiety n.
    association n.
    cardiac n.
    compensation n.
    compulsion n.
    conversion n.
    depersonalization n.
    depressive n.
    expectation n.
    fatigue n.
    fixation n.

neurosis (continued)
  gastric n.
  homosexual n.
  hypochondriacal n.
  hysterical n.
  intestinal n.
  obsessional n .
  obsessive-compulsive n.
  occupational n.
  pension n.
  phobic n.
  professional n.
  rectal n.
  regression n.
  sexual n.
  torsion n.
  transference n.
  traumatic n.
  vegetative n.
  war n.
neurosism
neuroskeletal
neuroskeleton
neurosome
neurospasm
neurosplanchnic
neurospongioma
neurospongium
neurostatus
neurosthenia
neurosurgeon
neurosurgery
  microvascular n.
  stereotaxic n.
neurosyphilis
  congenital n.
  ectodermogenic n.
  meningeal n.
  meningovascular n.
  mesodermogenic n.
  paretic n.
  tabetic n.
neurosystemitis
  n. epidemica
neutotabes
  n. diabetica
neurotagma

neurotherapy
neurothlipsis
neurotic
neurotica
neuroticism
neurotization
neurotmesis
neurotome
  Hall's n.
neurotomography
neurotomy
  retrogasserian n.
neurotoxin
neurotransducer
neurotransmitter
neurotripsy
neurotrophasthenia
neurotubule
neurovirulence
neurovirulent
New's needle
Niemann-Pick disease
nihilism
nimfo-. See words beginning
  nympho-.
Nissl's bodies
nistagmus. See *nystagmus.*
noctiphobia
nocturnal
nodule
  Schmorl's n.
non compos mentis
nonendocrine
non sequitur
notencephalocele
Nothnagel's
  sign
  syndrome
notomyelitis
NPT – nocturnal penile
  tumescence
NREM – non-rapid eye
  movement
nuclei
  n. arcuati
nucleus
  n. accumbens

nucleus (continued)
    n. ambiguus
    n. basalis
    cuneate n.
    Darkschewitsch's n.
    n. gracilis
    hypoglossal n.
    n. lateralis medullae
      oblongatae
    n. pulposus
    red n.
    reticular n.
    vestibular n.
numo-. See words beginning
    pneumo-.
nura-. See words beginning
    neura-.
nuro-. See words begining *neuro-*.
nympholepsy
nymphomania
nymphomaniac
nystagmus
nystagmus-myoconus
OA – occipital artery
Obersteiner-Redlich area
obesity
    hypothalamic o.
obex
obliteration
    cortical o.
obnubilation
OBS – organic brain syndrome
obsession
obsessive
obsessive-compulsive
obtund
obtundation
occipital
occipitalis
occipitalization
occipito-atloid
occipito-axoid
occipitobasilar
occipitobregmatic
occipitocervical
occipitofacial
occipitofrontal

occipitomastoid
occipitomental
occipitoparietal
occipitotemporal
occipitothalamic
occiput
occlusion
oculocephalic
oculogyric
oedipism
Oedipus complex
Oehler's symptom
ofthal-. See words beginning
    ophthal-.
oksesefale. See *oxycephaly*.
Oldberg's
    dissector
    forceps
    retractor
olfactory
oligergasia
oligergastic
oligodendrocyte(s)
oligodendroglia
oligodendroglioma
oligomania
oligophrenia
    phenylpyruvic o.
    o. phenylpyruvica
oligopsychia
oligoria
oliva
olivary
olive
    inferior o.
    spurge o.
    superior o.
Olivecrona's clip
olivifugal
olivipetal
olivopontocerebellar
omahl. See *haut-mal*.
Ommaya's reservoir
onanism
oneiric
oneirism
oneiroanalysis

oneirodynia
oneirogenic
oneirophrenia
oneiroscopy
onikotilomanea. See
    onychotillomania.
oniomania
onirik. See *oneiric.*
onirizm. See *oneirism.*
oniro-. See words beginning
    oneiro-.
onomatomania
onomatopoiesis
onychotillomania
operation
    Alexander's o.
    Cloward's o.
    Cotte's o.
    Dana's o.
    Förster-Penfield o.
    Frazier-Spiller o.
    Gardner's o.
    Gill's o.
    Haynes' o.
    Krause's o.
    Leriche's o.
    Pancoast's o.
    Puusepp's o.
    Smithwick's o.
    Sonneberg's o.
    Torkildsen's o.
opercula
operculum
ophthalmencephalon
ophthalmoplegia
opiate
opioid
opisthion
opisthotonos
Oppenheim's
    gait
    sign
opsoclonus
orientation
oriented
orthopsychiatry
orthostatic

oscillopsia
osmolar
osmotherapy
osteoarthritis
osteogenic
osteoma
osteomalacia
osteoplastic
osteoplasty
osteotome
    Cherry's o.
    Lambotte's o.
    Meyerding's o.
    Stille's o.
osteotomy
otitis
    malignant external o.
otohemineurasthenia
otomastoiditis
overcompensation
overdetermination
overlay
    emotional o.
    psychogenic o.
overt
overtone
    psychic o.
oxycephaly
pacchionian
pachycephalia
pachyleptomeningitis
pachymeningitis
pakeonean. See *pacchionian.*
paleencephalon
paleocerebellar
paleocerebellum
paleocortex
paleophrenia
paleothalamus
palikinesia
palilalia
palinphrasia
pallesthesia
pallidal
pallidectomy
pallidoansection
pallidoansotomy

pallidofugal
pallidotomy
pallidum
pallium
palsy
    Bell's p.
    pseudobulbar p.
    supranuclear p.
    ulnar p.
Pancoast's operation
pandysautonomia
Pandy's test
panencephalitis
panic
panophobia
Pansch's fissure
pantaphobia
pantophobia
pantophobic
papilledema
papilloma
    p. neuroticum
papovavirus
paracoele
paraganglioma
paraganglion
paragrammatism
paragraphia
parainfluenza
paralexia
paralogia
    thematic p.
paralogism
paralysis
    p. agitans
    bulbar p.
    conjugate p.
    cortical p.
    Duchenne-Erb p.
    Landry's p.
    Lissauer's p.
    Todd's p.
    Werdnig-Hoffmann p.
paramedian
parameningeal
paramyoclonus

paramyotonia
    p. congenita
paramyxovirus
paranoia
    p. hallucinatoria
    heboid p.
    litigious p.
    p. originaria
    querulous p.
    p. simplex
paranoiac
paranoic
paranoid
paranoidism
paranomia
paranormal
paranosic
paranosis
paraparesis
parapathia
paraphasia
paraphasic
paraphasis
paraphemia
paraphia
paraphilia
paraphiliac
paraphobia
paraphora
paraphrasia
paraphrenia
    p. confabulans
    p. expansiva
    p. phantastica
    p. systematica
paraphrenic
paraphronia
paraplegia
paraplegic
parapraxia
parapsychology
parapsychosis
parareaction
parasellar
parasomnia
parasympathetic
parasympathin

parasympatholytic
parasympathomimetic
parataxic
    p. distortion
paratonia
paratonic
paratrophy
parenchymal
parergasia
parergastic
paresis
paresthesia
parietal
parietofrontal
parieto-occipital
parietotemporal
Parinaud's syndrome
parkinsonian
parkinsonism
    drug-induced p.
    postencephalitic p.
    primary p.
    secondary p.
    vascular p.
parkinsonism-plus
Parkinson's
    disease
    facies
    syndrome
paroksizmal. See
   paroxysmal.
parorexia
paroxysmal
Parrot's
    atrophy of the newborn
    sign
Parry-Romberg syndrome
pars
    p. centralis ventriculi
      lateralis cerebri
    p. cervicalis medullae
      spinalis
    p. frontalis radiationis
      corporis callosi
    p. inferior fossae
      rhomboideae

pars (continued)
    p. inferior gyri frontalis
      medii
    p. intermedia fossae
      rhomboideae
    p. lumbalis medullae
      spinalis
    p. marginalis sulci cinguli
    p. occipitalis radiationis
      corporis callosi
    p. opercularis gyri
      frontalis inferioris
    p. orbitalis gyri frontalis
      inferioris
    p. parasympathica
      systematis nervosi
      autonomici
    p. parietalis operculi
    p. parietalis radiationis
      corporis callosi
    p. petrosa ossis temporalis
    p. posterior commissurae
      anterioris cerebri
    p. posterior rhinencephali
    p. subfrontalis sulci cinguli
    p. superior fossae
      rhomboideae
    p. superior gyri frontalis
      medii
    p. sympathica systematis
      nervosi autonomici
passive-aggressive
pathergasia
pathognomonic
pathognomy
pathophobia
pathway
    dopaminergic nigrostriatal
      p.
Patrick's test
Pavlov's method
pavor
    p. diurnus
    p. nocturnus
peak
    Bragg p.

Pecquet's
    cistern
    reservoir
pederasty
pederosis
pedophilia
pedophilic
pedophobia
peduncle
    cerebellar p.
    cerebral p.
    p. of flocculus
    p. of hypophysis
    p. of pineal body
    p. of thalamus, inferior
    olfactory p.
    olivary p. of Schwalbe
    pineal p.
pedunculotomy
pedunculus
    p. cerebellaris, inferior,
        medius, superior
    p. cerebri
    p. corporis callosi
    p. corporis pinealis
    p. flocculi
    p. thalami inferior
PEG – pneumoencephalography
Pelizaeus-Merzbacher
   disease
pellagra
perception
    extrasensory p.
perceptorium
perceptual
percutaneous
Perez's sign
perfusion
pericranitis
pericranium
periosteal
periosteum
peripheral nervous system
peronarthrosis
perseveration
persona

personality
    affective p.
    alternating p.
    anankastic p.
    antisocial p.
    asthenic p.
    compulsive p.
    cycloid p.
    cyclothymic p.
    disordered p.
    double p.
    dual p.
    dyssocial p.
    explosive p.
    hysterical p.
    inadequate p.
    multiple p.
    obsessive-compulsive p.
    paranoid p.
    passive-aggressive p.
    passive-dependent p.
    psychopathic p.
    schizoid p.
    seclusive p.
    shut-in p.
    sociopathic p.
    split p.
perversion
pervert
pessimism
PET – positron emission
   tomography
petechia (petechiae)
petit mal
petroclinoid
petrosal
petrosphenoid
PETT – positron emission
   transverse tomography
phagocytosis
phakoma
phakomatosis
phallic
phaneromania
phantasm
phantasmatomoria

phantasmoscopia
phantasy. See *fantasy.*
phantom limb
pharmacomania
pharmacophilia
pharmacophobia
pharmacopsychosis
phenomenology
phenomenon
 Babinski's p.
 Bell's p.
 Hunt's paradoxical p.
 Trousseau's p.
phenothiazine
phenotype
phenylketonuria
phenylpyruvic
 p. oligophrenia
pheochromocytoma
phlebitis
phlegmatic
phobia
phobic
phobophobia
phonatory
phrenemphraxis
phrenic
phrenicectomy
phreniclasia
phrenicoexeresis
phreniconeurectomy
phrenicotomy
phrenicotripsy
phrenology
phrenopathic
phrenopathy
phrenoplegia
phthisiomania
phthisiophobia
physiopathic
physiopsychic
pia
 p. mater
pia-arachnitis
pia-arachnoid
piaglia
pial

pia mater
 p. m. encephali
 p. m. spinalis
piamatral
piarachnitis
piarachnoid
pica
PICA – posterior inferior
 cerebellar artery
PICA aneurysm
Pick's
 convolutional atrophy
 disease
picornavirus
piknic. See *pyknic.*
pikno-. See words beginning
 pykno-.
pileum
pileus
pineal
pinealectomy
pinealoma
Pinel's system
Piotrowski's sign
pira-. See words beginning *pyra-.*
piro-. See words beginning *pyro-.*
pituitary
pituitectomy
PKU – phenylketonuria
plagiocephalic
plagiocephaly
plane
 axial p.
 coronal p's
 sagittal p's
plaque
 Lichtheim's p's
 Redlich-Fisher miliary p's
 senile p's
plate
 Hoen's skull p.
platybasia
pleocytosis
plexus
 brachial p.
 carotid p.
 cervical p.

plexus (continued)
    p. cervicobrachialis
    choroid p.
    p. choroideus ventriculi
        lateralis
    p. choroideus ventriculi
        quarti
    p. choroideus ventriculi
        tertii
    lumbosacral p.
    p. vertebralis
pneumocephalon
    p. artificiale
pneumocephalus
pneumoencephalogram
pneumoencephalography
pneumoencephalomyelogram
pneumoencephalomyelography
pneumoencephalos
pneumomyelography
PNI – psychoneuroimmunology
PNS – partial nonprogressing
    stroke
peripheral nervous system
poikilothermia
poliencephalomyelitis
polioclastic
poliodystrophy
polioencephalitis
polioencephalomeningomyelitis
polioencephalomyelitis
polioencephalopathy
poliomyelencephalitis
poliomyelitis
    bulbar p.
    cerebral p.
    spinal paralytic p.
poliomyelopathy
polioneuromere
poliovirus
polyarteritis
    p. nodosa
polyclonia
polycythemia
    p. vera
polymerization
polymodal

polymyositis
polyneural
polyneuralgia
polyneuritic
polyneuritis
polyneuromyositis
polyneuropathy
    symmetrical p.
    uremic p.
polyneuroradiculitis
polynuclear
polyparesis
polyphagia
polytomography
polyvinyl
pons (pontis)
    p. cerebelli
    p. varolii
pons-oblongata
pontibrachium
ponticulus
pontile
pontine
pontobulbia
pontocerebellar
porencephalia
porencephalic
porencephalitis
porencephaly
poriomania
pornographomania
pornolagnia
porphyria
position. See *General Surgical
    Terms* section.
postanoxic
postictal
postsynaptic
potency
potential
    brain stem auditory
        evoked p.
    somatosensory evoked p.
    visual evoked p.
pouch
    Rathke's p.
Powassan virus

Pratt's curet
precocious
precocity
precognition
preconscious
preconvulsant
preconvulsive
precuneus
predilection
predisposition
prefrontal
preganglionic
pregenital
preoblongata
priapism
processus
        p. clinoideus anterior
        p. clinoideus medius
        p. clinoideus posterior
prodromal
projection
pronation
propons
proprioceptive
proprioceptor
prosencephalon
prosopagnosia
proton beam (Bragg peak)
protuberance
        occipital p.
psalis
psalterium
pseudocoele
pseudocoma
pseudodelirium
pseudodementia
pseudohypertrophy
pseudoincontinence
pseudologia
        p. fantastica
Pseudomonas
        P. aeruginosa
pseudopapilledema
pseudosclerosis
        p. spastica
pseudosyncope
pseudotabes

pseudotumor
        p. cerebri
psychalgalia
psychalgia
psychalgic
psychalia
psychanalysis
psychanopsia
psychasthene
psychasthenia
psychasthenic
psychataxia
psyche
psycheclampsia
psychedelic
psychiater
psychiatric
psychiatrist
psychiatry
psychic
psychinosis
psychlampsia
psychoalgalia
psychoallergy
psychoanaleptic
psychoanalysis
psychoanalyst
psychoanalytic
psychoanalyze
psychoasthenics
psychoauditory
psychobacillosis
psychobiological
psychobiology
psychocatharsis
psychocentric
psychochemistry
psychochrome
psychochromesthesia
psychocoma
psychocortical
psychodelic
psychodiagnosis
psychodiagnostics
psychodometer
psychodometry
psychodrama

psychodynamics
psychodysleptic
psychoepilepsy
psychogalvanometer
psychogenesis
psychogenia
psychogenic
psychogenous
psychogeriatrics
psychognosis
psychognostic
psychogogic
psychogram
psychograph
psychokinesia
psychokinesis
psychokym
psycholagny
psycholepsy
psycholeptic
psycholinguistics
psychologic
psychological
psychologist
psychology
psychomathematics
psychometer
psychometric
psychometry
psychomotor
psychoneuroses
psychoneurosis
    p. maidica
    paranoid p.
psychonomy
psychonosema
psychonosis
psychoparesis
psychopath
psychopathia
    p. martialis
    p. sexualis
psychopathic
psychopathist
psychopathology
psychopathosis
psychopathy

psychopharmacology
psychophonasthenia
psychophylaxis
psychophysical
psychophysics
psychophysiology
psychoplegia
psychoplegic
psychopneumatology
psychoprophylactic
psychoprophylaxis
psychoreaction
psychorhythmia
psychorrhagia
psychorrhea
psychorrhexis
psychosensorial
psychosensory
psychoses
psychosexual
psychosis
    bipolar p.
    Cheyne-Stokes p.
    gestational p.
    idiophrenic p.
    involutional p.
    Korsakoff's p.
    manic p.
    manic-depressive p.
    paranoiac p.
    paranoid p.
    polyneuritic p.
    p. polyneuritica
    postpartum p.
    puerperal p.
    schizoaffective p.
    senile p.
    situational p.
    toxic p.
    unipolar p.
    zoophil p.
psychosolytic
psychosomatic
psychosomaticist
psychosomimetic
psychosurgery
psychotechnics

psychotherapeutics
psychotherapy
psychotic
psychotogenic
psychotomimetic
psychotonic
psychotropic
psychrophobia
pterion
ptosis
puberty
pubescence
Pudenz'
    reservoir
    shunt
    tube
    valve
puerile
puerilism
pulvinar
puncture
    cisternal p.
    Corning's p.
    lumbar p.
    thecal p.
    ventricular p.
purpura
    thrombocytopenic p.
putamen
Puusepp's
    operation
    reflex
pyknic
pyknoepilepsy
pyknophrasia
pyramid
pyramidal
pyramidotomy
pyramis
pyrolagnia
pyromania
quadrantanopia
quadriplegia
Queckenstedt's sign
querulous
Quincke's meningitis
Quinquaud's sign

rabies
"raccoon eyes"
rachialbuminimetry
rachialgia
rachicentesis
rachidial
rachidian
rachigraph
rachilysis
rachiocampsis
rachiocentesis
rachiochysis
rachiodynia
rachiometer
rachiomyelitis
rachioscoliosis
rachiotomy
rachischisis
rachitis
rachitome
rachitomy
radicular
radiculectomy
radiculitis
radiculoganglionitis
radiculomedullary
radiculomeningomyelitis
radiculomyelopathy
radiculoneuritis
radiculoneuropathy
radiculopathy
radioactive brain scan
radioencephalogram
radioencephalography
radiography
radiology. See *Radiology and*
    Nuclear Medicine section.
radionuclide
Raeder's syndrome
rafe. See *raphe.*
rahpor. See *rapport.*
rake-. See words beginning *rachi-.*
rakeal-. See words beginning
    rachial-.
rakeo-. See words beginning
    rachio-.
rakiskisis. See *rachischisis.*

rakitis. See *rachitis.*
Ramirez's shunt
ramisection
ramitis
Ramsay-Hunt syndrome
ramus
Raney's
    clip
    curet
    drill
    forceps
raphe
rapport
Rathke's
    pouch
    tumor
rational
rationalization
Raymond's apoplexy
Ray's mania
reaction
    Cushing's r.
    r. formation
    Jolly's r.
reality testing
receptor
recess
recessus
    r. infundibuli
    r. lateralis fossae
        rhomboidei
    r. lateralis ventriculi quarti
    r. pinealis
    r. suprapinealis'
    r. triangularis
recidivism
recidivist
Redlich-Fisher miliary plaques
red Robinson catheter
reflex
    Achilles tendon r.
    axon r.
    Babinski's r.
    Brain's r.
    Brissaud's r.
    carotid sinus r.
    cerebral cortex r.

reflex (continued)
    Chaddock's r.
    ciliospinal r.
    Hirschberg's r.
    H-r.
    Joffroy's r.
    Lust's r.
    McCarthy's r.
    Mendel-Bechterew r.
    palmomental r.
    proprioceptive r.
    Puusepp's r.
    quadrupedal extensor r.
    Remak's r.
    Riddoch's mass r.
    Rossolimo's r.
    Schaefer's r.
    Strümpell's r.
    tarsophalangeal r.
    Throckmorton's r.
    wrist clonus r.
regression
    atavistic r.
Reil
    island of R.
reinnervation
Reitan-Indiana aphasic screening
    test
REM – rapid eye movement
Remak's reflex
Rendu-Osler-Weber disease
Rendu's tremor
reovirus
repertoire
repression
reservoir
    Ommaya's r.
    Pecquet's r.
    Pudenz' r.
    Rickham's r.
    Rickham-Salmon r.
resistance
respiration
    Biot's r.
restibrachium
restiform
retardate

retardation
  psychomotor r.
rete
  r. canalis hypoglossi
reticular
retractor
  Adson's r.
  Barrett-Adson r.
  Beckman-Adson r.
  Beckman-Eaton r.
  Beckman's r.
  Bucy's r.
  Chandler's r.
  Cherry's r.
  Cloward-Hoen r.
  Cone's r.
  Contour's r.
  Cushing's r.
  Davidoff's r.
  Davidson's r.
  Davis' r.
  D'Errico-Adson r.
  D'Errico's r.
  Frazier's r.
  French S-shaped r.
  Gelpi's r.
  Gifford's r.
  Hamby's r.
  Jansen's r.
  Klemme's r.
  Love's r.
  Meyerding's r.
  Oldberg's r.
  Sachs' r.
  Scoville's r.
  Senn's r.
  Sheldon's r.
  Snitman's r.
  Taylor's r.
  Tower's r.
  Tuffier-Raney r.
  Tuffier's r.
  Ullrich's r.
  Weitlaner's t.
  Yasargil's r.
retrobulbar
retrocollis

retrogasserian
retrograde
retropulsion
retrovirus
Reye's syndrome
rhabdomyoma
rhabdovirus
rhinencephalon
rhinorrhea
    cerebrospinal r.
rhizotomy
rhombencephalon
rhombocoele
rhomboid
rhythm
    alpha r.
    Berger r.
    beta r.
    gamma r.
Rickham-Salmon reservoir
Rickham's reservoir
Riddoch's mass reflex
rigidity
    cerebellar r.
    hemiplegic r.
    lead-pipe r.
    nuchal r.
rigor
    r. nervorum
    r. tremens
Riley-Day syndrome
Rimbaud-Passouant-Vallat
    syndrome
rimula
RIND – reversible ischemic
    neurologic disability
rinensefalon. See
    rhinencephalon.
rinorea. See *rhinorrhea.*
risus
    r. caninus
    r. sardonicus
rizotomee. See *rhizotomy.*
RNA – ribonucleic acid
Rochester's
    connector
    elevator

Rolandi
    substantia r.
Rolandic fissure
Rolando
    fasciculus of R.
    tubercule of R.
rolandometer
rombensefalon. See
   rhombencephalon.
rombergism
Romberg's
    disease
    sign
rombosel. See *rhombocoele.*
rongeur
    DeVilbiss' r.
    gooseneck r.
    Kerrison's r.
    Leksell's r.
    Love-Gruenwald r.
    Schlesinger's r.
    Spurling's r.
    Stille-Luer r.
Rorschach test
Roser-Braun sign
Rossolimo's reflex
rostral
rostrum
    r. corporis callosi
Roth-Bernhardt disease
Roth's disease
Roussy-Cornil syndrome
rubella
rubrospinal
rule
    Jackson's r.
    M'Naghten r.
rumination
    obsessive r.
Rumpf's sign
Ruskin's forceps
Sachs'
    cannula
    guard
    needle
    retractor
    spatula

Sachs' (continued)
    suction tube
sacroiliac
sacrospinal
sacrovertebral
sadism
sadist
sadistic
sadomasochistic
Saenger's sign
sagittal
St. Louis encephalitis virus
St. Vitus' dance
sal-. See words beginning *psal-.*
Salibi's clamp
saltation
saltereum. See *psalterium.*
Sanger-Brown's ataxia
Sarbó's sign
sarcoma
    reticulum cell s. of brain
satellitosis
satyriasis
satyromania
saw
    Gigli's s.
    Stille-Gigli s.
scan
    brain s.
    CAT s.
    CT s.
    EMI s.
scanner
scanning
    radioisotope s.
scanography
scaphocephalia
scapuloperoneal
Schaefer's reflex
Schilder's disease
schizocephalia
schizogyria
schizoid
schizoidism
schizophasia
schizophrenia
    ambulatory s.

schizophrenia (continued)
    catatonic s.
    hebephrenic s.
    latent s.
    paranoid s.
    pseudoneurotic s.
    reactive s.
    schizoaffective s.
schizophreniac
schizophrenic
schizophreniform
schizophrenosis
Schlesinger's
    forceps
    ronguer
Schmorl's
    body
    disease
    nodule
Schrötter's chorea
Schutz's
    clip
    forceps
Schwalbe
    olivary peduncle of S.
schwannoma
Schwann's
    sheath
    white substance
Schwartz-Jampel syndrome
Schwartz's clip
sciatica
scintiscanner
scissors
    Adson's s.
    Craig's s.
    craniotomy s.
    Dandy's s.
    Smellie's s.
    Stevenson's s.
    Strully's s.
    Taylor's s.
scleroderma
scleromeninx
sclerosis
    Alzheimer's s.
    amyotrophic lateral s.

sclerosis (continued)
    annular s.
    anterolateral s.
    arterial s.
    arteriolar s.
    arteriopapillary s.
    benign s.
    bone s.
    bulbar s.
    cerebellar s.
    cerebral s.
    cerebrospinal s.
    cervical s.
    s. circumscripta pericardii
    diffuse s.
    disseminated s.
    Erb's s.
    familial centrolobar s.
    hyperplastic s.
    insular s.
    Krabbe's s.
    Marie's s.
    mesial temporal s.
    miliary s.
    Mönckeberg's s.
    multiple s.
    nodular s.
    posterolateral s.
    presenile s.
    s. redux
    renal arteriolar s.
    transitional s.
    s. tuberosa
    tuberous s.
    unicellular s.
    vascular s.
    venous s.
    ventrolateral s.
scoliosis
scotoma
scotomization
scotophobia
Scott's cannula
Scoville-Lewis clip
Scoville's
    clip
    forceps

Scoville's (continued)
  retractor
scrapie
sedative
sefal-. See words beginning
  cephal-.
Seguin's signal symptom
seizure
  akinetic s.
  atonic s.
  audiogenic s.
  cerebral s.
  jackknife s.
  jacksonian s.
  myoclonic s.
  neonatal s.
  partial s.
  photogenic s.
  psychic s.
  psychomotor s.
  uncinate s.
sejunction
selenoplegia
selenoplexia
Seletz's cannula
self-suspension
sella
  s. turcica
sellar
semicoma
semicomatose
semicretinism
seminarcosis
Senn's retractor
sensorial
sensorineural
sensorium
sensory
SEP – somatosensory evoked
  potential
separator
  Horsley's s.
sepsis
septal
  s. nuclei
septum
  s. pellucidum

septum (continued)
  s. pontis
serotonin
Setchenow's centers
Sewall's forceps
sexual
  s. masochism
  s. sadism
sfeno-. See words beginning
  spheno-.
sfenoid. See *sphenoid*.
sheath
  myelin s.
  Schwann's s.
Sheldon-Pudenz dissector
Sheldon's retractor
shingles
shunt
  Holter's s.
  Javid's s.
  Pudenz's s.
  Ramirez's s.
  Silastic ventricular-
    peritoneal s.
  ventricular atrial s.
shwonnoma. See *schwannoma*.
Shy-Drager syndrome
siatika. See *sciatica*.
sibling
Siegert's sign
sifilis. See *syphilis*.
sifilo-. See words beginning
  syphilo-.
sign
  André-Thomas s.
  Babinski's s.
  Ballet's s.
  Barré's pyramidal s.
  Battle's s.
  Bragard's s.
  Brudzinski's s.
  Chaddock's s.
  Chvostek's s.
  Claude's hyperkinesis s.
  Dejerine's s.
  de la Camp's s.
  Fajersztajn's s.

sign (continued)
    Gowers' s.
    Hoffmann's s.
    Holmes' s.
    Kernig's s.
    Lafora's s.
    Laségue's s.
    Leichtenstern's s.
    Leri's s.
    Lhermitte's s.
    Lichtheim's s.
    Morquio's s.
    Myerson's s.
    Nothnagel's s.
    Oppenheim's s.
    Parrot's s.
    Perez's s.
    Piotrowski's s.
    Queckenstedt's s.
    Quinquaud's s.
    Romberg's s.
    Roser-Braun s.
    Rumpf's s.
    Saenger's s.
    Sarbo's s.
    Siegert's s.
    Signorelli's s.
    Soto-Hall s.
    Stewart-Holmes s.
    Strümpell's s.
    Thomas' s.
    Tinel's s.
    Trousseau's s.
    Turyn's s.
    Vanzetti's s.
    Wartenberg's s.
    Weber's s.
    Westphal's s.
Signorelli's sign
sika-. See words beginning
    psycha-.
sikal-. See words beginning
    psychal-.
sikan-. See words beginning
    psychan-.
sikas-. See words beginning
    psychas-.

sike-. See words beginning
    psyche-.
siki-. See words beginning
    psychi-.
siko-. See words beginning
    psycho-.
Silastic ventricular-peritoneal
    shunt
siliqua
    s. olivae
Simmonds' disease
sin-. See also words beginning
    cin- and *syn-.*
sinciput
sinerea. See *cinerea.*
singulum. See *cingulum.*
singulumotome. See
    cingulumotomy.
sinistrocerebral
sinistrosis
sinus
    carotid s.
    cavernous s.
    cerebral s.
    s. durae matris
    dural s.
    s. pericranii
    sagittal s.
    s. sagittalis inferior
    s. sagittalis superior
    subarachnoidal s.
sinusitis
siringo-. See words beginning
    syringo-.
Sjögren-Larssen syndrome
Sjögren's syndrome
skafosefalea. See *scaphocephalia.*
skizo-. See words beginning
    schizo-.
sklero-. See words beginning
    sclero-.
skull
SLE – systemic lupus
    erythematosus
SLR – straight leg raising
SMA – supplementary motor area
Smellie's scissors

Smith's clip
Smithwick's
    forceps
    operation
Snitman's retractor
SOA-MCA – superficial occipital
    artery to middle cerebral
    artery
sociology
sociopath
sodomy
soma
somatic
somatization
somatomotor
somatophrenia
somatopsychic
somatopsychosis
somatosensory
somatotopic
somnambulism
somniloquism
somnipathy
somnolence
somnolentia
somnolism
somopsychosis
Sonneberg's operation
Soto-Hall sign
space
    Broca's s.
    Magendie's s's
    subarachnoid s.
    subdural s.
spasm
spastic
spatial
spatula
    Cushing's s.
    Davis' s.
    Sachs' s.
    Woodson's s.
Spence-Adson forceps
Spence's forceps
sphenoethmoid
sphenofrontal
sphenoid

sphenoidal
sphenoidostomy
sphenoidotomy
sphenotemporal
Spielmeyer-Sjögren syndrome
Spielmeyer-Vogt disease
spina
    s. bifida
    s. bifida occulta
spinal cord
spine
spinobulbar
spinocerebellar
spinogalvanization
spinogram
spinothalamic
spinous
splanchnicectomy
splanchnicotomy
splanknekotome. See
    splanchnicotomy.
splanknesektome. See
    splanchnicectomy.
splenium
    s. corporis callosi
spondylitis
spondylodesis
spondylolisthesis
spondylolysis
spondylomalacia
spondylopathy
spondylopyosis
spondyloschisis
spondylosis
    s. chronica
       ankylopoietica
    rhizomelic s.
spondylosyndesis
spondylotomy
spongioblast
spongioblastoma
spongiocyte
spoon
    Cushing's s.
spot
    café-au-lait s's
    Trousseau's s.

spreader
 Turek's s.
 Wiltberger's s.
Spurling's
 forceps
 rongeur
stability
STA-MCA – superficial temporal artery to middle cerebral artery
stammering
Stanford-Binet test
Staphylococcus
 S. aureus
stasiphobia
status
 s. choreicus
 s. convulsivus
 s. cribalis
 s. cribrosus
 s. dysgraphicus
 s. dysmyelinatus
 s. dysmyelinisatus
 s. dysraphicus
 e. epilepticus
 s. hemicranicus
 s. lacunaris
 s. lacunosus
 s. marmoratus
 petit mal s.
 s. spongiosus
 s. verrucosus
 s. vertiginosus
Stearn's alcoholic amentia
stefaneon. See *stephanion.*
Steiner's disease
stellate
stellectomy
stenion
stephanion
stereoanesthesia
stereoencephalotomy
stereognosis
stereotactic
stereotaxis
stereotypy

Stevenson's
 forceps
 scissors
Stewart-Holmes sign
Stille-Gigli saw
Stille-Liston forceps
Stille-Luer
 forceps
 rongeur
Stille's
 drill
 osteotome
stimulate
stimuli
stimulus
stocking
 Jobst s's
stratum
 s. album profundum corporis quadrigemini
 s. gangliosum cerebelli
 s. gelatinosum
 s. granulosum cerebelli
 s. griseum centrale cerebri
 s. griseum colliculi superioris
 s. interolivare lemnisci
 s. moleculare cerebelli
 s. nucleare medullae oblongatae
 s. olfactorium
 s. opticum
 s. pyramidale
 s. reticulatum
 s. zonale corporis quadrigemini
 s. zonale thalami
strephosymbolia
stria
 s. fornicis
 habenular s.
 s. lancisii
 s. medullaris thalami
 meningitic s.
 olfactory s.
 s. pinealis
 s. terminalis

striae
    Francke's s.
    s. medullares acusticae
    s. medullares fossae
       rhomboideae
    s. medullares ventriculi
       quarti
striatum
stridor
    laryngeal s.
strikninomanea. See
    strychninomania.
stroke
    atherothrombotic s.
    cardioembolic s.
Stromeyer's cephalhematocele
strontium
    radioactive s.
Strully's scissors
Strümpell's
    disease
    reflex
    sign
strychninomania
Stryker's frame
stupor
    anergic s.
    delusion s.
    epileptic s.
    lethargic s.
    postconvulsive s.
stuporous
Sturge's disease
Sturge-Weber-Dimitri disease
Sturge-Weber syndrome
stuttering
    labiochoreic s.
subarachnoid
subarachnoiditis
subclavian
subconscious
subconsciousness
subcortical
subdural
subependymal
subgaleal
subjective

sublimate
sublimation
subpial
subpontine
substance
    white s. of Schwann
substantia
    s. alba
    s. cinerea
    s. corticalis cerebelli
    s. gelatinosa
    s. grisea
    s. innominata
    s. nigra
    s. perforata
    s. reticularis alba gyri
       fornicati
    s. reticularis alba
       medullae oblongatae
    s. reticularis grisea
       medullae oblongatae
    s. Rolandi
substitution
subthalamus
suction tube
    Adson's s.t.
    Frazier's s.t.
    Sachs' s.t.
Sudeck's atrophy
sudo-. See words beginning
    pseudo-.
Sugar's clip
suicidal
suicide
sulci
sulcus
    anterolateral s.
    s. basilaris pontis
    calcarine s.
    callosal s.
    cingulate s.
    s. circularis
    s. collateralis
    s. corporis callosi
    s. hippocampi
    s. hypothalamicus
    lateral s.

sulcus (continued)
  s. limitans
  s. lunatus
  medial frontal s.
  median s.
  oculomotor s.
  paramedial s.
superdural
superego
supination
suppression
supratentorial
surgical procedures. See
  operation.
surrogate
suture. See *General Surgical
  Terms* section.
Sweet's forceps
Sydenham's chorea
sylvian
Sylvii
  cisterna S.
  cisterna fossae S.
Sylvius
  aqueduct of S.
  cistern of fossa of S.
  cistern of S.
  fissure of S.
  ventricle of S.
symbiosis
symbol
  phallic s.
symbolism
symbolization
symbolophobia
sympathectomy
  chemical s.
  lumbar s.
  periarterial s.
sympathetic
sympatheticomimetic
sympatheticoparalytic
sympatheticotonia
sympatheticotonic
sympathicoblastoma
sympathicodiaphtheresis
sympathicogonioma

sympathicopathy
sympathicotherapy
sympathicotripsy
sympathicus
sympathin
sympatholytic
sympathomimetic
sympathy
symptom
  Bonhoeffer's s.
  Ganser's s.
  Haenel's s.
  Oehler's s.
  Seguin's signal s.
  Trendelenburg's s.
synapse
  axodendritic s.
  axodendrosomatic s.
  axosomatic s.
synclonus
syncopal
syncope
  cardiac s.
  carotid sinus s.
  micturition s.
  vasodepressor s.
  vasovagal s.
syndrome
  acquired
    immunodeficiency s.
  acute organic brain s.
  Adie's s.
  alcohol withdrawal s.
  Alzheimer's s.
  Apert's s.
  Arnold-Chiari s.
  Baastrup's s.
  Babinski-Nageotte s.
  Babinski's s.
  Balint's s.
  Bárány's s.
  Barré-Liéou s.
  Bärtschi-Rochain s.
  Beard's s.
  Beck's s.
  Blackfan-Diamond s.
  Bonnet's s.

syndrome (continued)
- Briquet's s.
- Brissaud-Sicard s.
- Bristowe's s.
- Brown-Séquard s.
- Bruns' s.
- callosal s.
- Capgras' s.
- capsular thrombosis s.
- capsulothalamic s.
- carpal tunnel s.
- Céstan-Chenais s.
- "Chinese restaurant" s.
- Churg-Strauss s.
- Claude's s.
- Cotard's s.
- Cushing's s.
- Dandy-Walker s.
- Dejerine-Roussy s.
- Dejerine's s.
- Dennie-Marfan s.
- De Sanctis-Cacchione s.
- Devic's s.
- Down's s.
- Eaton-Lambert s.
- Erb's s.
- Foix-Alajouanine s.
- Foville's s.
- Friderichsen-Waterhouse s.
- Friedmann's vasomotor s.
- Fröhlich's s.
- Froin's s.
- Ganser's s.
- Garcin's s.
- Gélineau's s.
- Gerstmann's s.
- Gilles de la Tourette's s.
- Gowers' s.
- Gradenigo's s.
- Guillain-Barré s.
- Hallervorden-Spatz s.
- Homén's s.
- Horner's s.
- Horton's s.
- Hunt's striatal s.
- Hurler's s.

syndrome (continued)
- Jackson's s.
- Jakob-Creutzfeldt s.
- Kanner's s.
- Kearns-Sayre s.
- Kiloh-Nevin s.
- Kleine-Levin s.
- Klippel-Feil s.
- Klippel-Feldstein s.
- Klüver-Bucy s.
- Korsakoff's s.
- Lambert-Eaton myasthenic s.
- Lennox-Gastaut s.
- Lennox's s.
- Lesch-Nyhan s.
- Ménière's s.
- Millard-Gubler s.
- Möbius' s.
- Munchausen's s.
- Naffziger's s.
- Nothnagel's s.
- organic brain s.
- Parinaud's s.
- Parkinson's s.
- Parry-Romberg s.
- pickwickian s.
- Raeder's s.
- Ramsay-Hunt s.
- Reye's s.
- Riley-Day s.
- Rimbaud-Passouant-Vallat s.
- Roussy-Cornil s.
- scalenus anticus s.
- Schwartz-Jampel s.
- Shy-Drager s.
- Sjögren-Larssen s.
- Sjögren's s.
- sleep apnea s.
- Spielmeyer-Sjögren s.
- Sturge-Weber s.
- subclavian steal s.
- thoracic outlet s.
- trisomy D s.
- trisomy E s.
- trisomy 13-15 s.

syndrome (continued)
    trisomy 16-18 s.
    trisomy 18 s.
    trisomy 21 s.
    Vogt-Koyanagi-Harada s.
    Vogt's s.
    Wallenberg's s.
    Waterhouse-Friderichsen
      s.
    Wernicke-Korsakoff s.
    West's s.
synesthesia
synesthesialgia
synkinesis
synreflexia
syntactic
syntaxis
synthesis
syntonic
syphilis
    meningovascular s.
syphilitic
syphilophobia
syphilopsychosis
syringobulbia
syringocele
syringocoele
syringoencephalia
syringoencephalomyelia
syringomeningocele
syringomyelia
    s. atrophica
syringomyelitis
syringomyelocele
syringomyelus
syringopontia
syrinx
system
    autonomic nervous s.
    central nervous s.
    Conolly's s.
    peripheral nervous s.
    Pinel's s.
tabes
    cerebral t.
    diabetic t.
    t. dorsalis

tabes (continued)
    t. ergotica
    Friedreich's t.
    t. spinalis
    vessel t.
tabetic
taboparesis
tache
    t. cerebrale
    t. meningeale
    t. spinale
tachycardia
tachyphrasia
tachyphrenia
taedium
    t. vitae
taenia
    t. chorioidea
    t. cinerea
    t. fimbriae
    t. fornicis
    t. hippocampi
    t. medullaris thalami
      optici
    t. pontis
    t. semicircularis corporis
      striati
    t. tectae
    t. thalami
    t. violacea
taeniae
    t. acusticae
    t. telarum
tahsh. See *tache.*
tantalum sheet
tapeinocephaly
tapetum
    t. corporis callosi
    t. ventriculi
tardive
tasikinesia
TAT—thematic apperception test
Taylor's
    retractor
    scissors
Tay-Sachs disease
tectospinal

tedeum. See *taedium.*
tegmental
tegmentum
    hypothalamic t.
    t. of pons
    t. rhombencephali
    subthalamic t.
tela
    t. choroidea
telangiectasia
telencephalon
telepathy
temp. dext. – to the right temple
tempora
temporal
temporalis
temporoauricular
temporofacial
temporofrontal
temporohyoid
temporomalar
temporomandibular
temporomaxillary
temporo-occipital
temporoparietal
temporopontile
temporosphenoid
temporozygomatic
temp. sinist. – to the left temple
tenia
    t. choroidea
    t. telae
teniola
tentorium
    t. cerebelli
    t. of hypophysis
tephromalacia
tephromyelitis
teratoma
tereon. See *pterion.*
test
    Bárány's pointing t.
    Bender-Gestalt t.
    dexamethasone
      suppression t.
    Ebbinghaus' t.
    edrophonium t.

test (continued)
    finger-nose t.
    finger-to-finger t.
    Halstead-Reitan t.
    heel-knee t.
    heel-shin t.
    Janet's t.
    Minnesota Multiphasic
      Personality Inventory t.
    Pandy's t.
    Patrick's t.
    projective human figure
      drawing t.
    Reitan-Indiana aphasic
      screening t.
    Rorschach t.
    Stanford-Binet t.
    thematic apperception t.
    Tobey-Ayer t.
    Wada's t.
    Walter's bromide t.
    Wechsler's Adult
      Intelligence Scale t.
    Wechsler's Intelligence
      Scale for Children t.
    Wittenborn Psychiatric
      Rating Scale t.
    Yerkes-Bridges t.
    Ziehen's t.
tetraplegia
TGA – transient global amnesia
thalamencephalic
thalamencephalon
thalamic
thalamocele
thalamocortical
thalamolenticular
thalamotegmental
thalamotomy
thalamus (thalami)
theory
    Adler's t.
    Freud's t.
    Gestalt t.
    Meyer's t.
therapy
    beam t.

therapy (continued)
    behavior t.
    carbon dioxide t.
    convulsive shock t.
    drug t.
    electric convulsive t.
    electroshock t.
    family t.
    group t.
    Indoklon t.
    lithium t.
    milieu t.
    play t.
    sex t.
    shock t.
Thomas' sign
Thomsen's disease
Throckmorton's reflex
thromboangiitis
    t. obliterans
thrombocytosis
thrombosis
thrombus
thymergastic
thymopathy
thyrotoxicosis
TIA – transient ischemic attack
tic
    t. de pensée
    t. de sommeil
    t. douloureux
    t. nondouloureux
tigroid
Tinel's sign
tinnitus
titubation
    lingual t.
tizeo-. See words beginning
    phthisio-.
Tobey-Ayer test
Todd's paralysis
togavirus
tolerance
tomography
    computed t.
tongs
    Barton-Cone t.

tongs (continued)
    Cherry's t.
    Crutchfield-Raney t.
    Crutchfield's t.
tonsil
    t. of cerebellum
tonsilla
    t. cerebelli
    t. of cerebellum
tonus
    neurogenic t.
topagnosis
topectomy
Torkildsen's operation
torticollis
tortipelvis
toruloma
tosis. See *ptosis*.
Tourette's disease
Tower's retractor
toxiphrenia
trabecula
    t. cerebri
    t. cinerea
    t. cranii
trabs
    t. cerebri
trachelism
trachelismus
tract
    Burdach's t.
    cerebellorubral t.
    cerebellorubrospinal t.
    cerebellospinal t.
    corticospinal t.
    extrapyramidal t.
    Foville's t.
    Goll's t.
    Gowers' t.
    Helweg's t.
    Lissauer's t.
    Meynert's t.
    neospinothalamic t.
    paleospinothalamic t.
    pyramidal t.
    spinocerebellar t.
    spinothalamic t.

tract (continued)
    sympathetic t.
    tectospinal t.
tractotomy
    mesencephalic t.
trait
trance
tranquilizer
transcortical
transection
    spinal t.
transference
transorbital
transsexual
transsexualism
transvestism
trauma
    psychic t.
traumasthenia
treatment
    Weir Michell t.
tremor
    epileptoid t.
    flapping t.
    Hunt's t.
    intention t.
    intermittent t.
    kinetic t.
    t. linguate
    motofacient t.
    t. potatorum
    Rendu's t.
    striocerebellar t.
    volitional t.
tremulous
Trendelenburg's symptom
trephination
trephine
    DeVilbiss' t.
    Galt's t.
Treponema
    T. pallidum
trichologia
trichopoliodystrophy
trichotillomania
tricyclic
trigeminal

trigone
trigonocephaly
trigonum
    t. acustici
    t. cerebrale
    t. collaterale
    t. habenulae
    t. lemnisci
    t. nervi hypoglossi
    t. olfactorium
triplegia
trismus
trisomy D, E, 13-15, 16-18,
    18, 21
Trousseau's
    phenomenon
    sign
    spot
    twitching
truncal
truncus
    t. corporis callosi
    t. lumbosacralis
    t. symphathicus
trypanosomiasis
TSH - thyroid-stimulating
    hormone
TTP - thrombotic
    thrombocytopenic purpura
tube
    Pudenz's t.
tuber
    t. annulare
    t. anterius hypothalami
    t. cinereum
    t. vermis
tubercle
    Babès' t.
    t. of Rolando
tuberculoma
    t. en plaque
tuberculum
Tuffier-Raney retractor
Tuffier's retractor
tumor
    cerebellopontine-angle t.
    Cushing's t.

tumor (continued)
    extramedullary t.
    intramedullary t.
    parasagittal t.
    parasellar t.
    paravertebral t.
    Rathke's t.
    sellar t.
    supratentorial t.
Turek's spreader
Turyn's sign
twitch
twitching
    fascicular t.
    fibrillar t.
    Trousseau's t.
type
    Kretschmer t's
ufor-. See words beginning
    euphor-.
ulegyria
Ullrich's retractor
ululation
unarousable
uncinate
unconscious
uncus
underhorn
unoia. See *eunoia*.
unresponsive
Unverricht-Lundborg type of
    epilepsy
Unverricht's disease
uremia
urolagnia
urophobia
vadum
vagabondage
vagal
vagotomy
vagotonia
vagus
vallecula
    v. cerebelli
    v. sylvii
Valsalva's maneuver

valve
    Pudenz's v.
Vanzetti's sign
varicella-zoster
varix
    aneurysmoid v.
varolian
vasculopathy
vasoactive
    v. amines
vasoconstriction
vasovagal
VDRL – Venereal Disease
    Research Laboratory
vegetative
velamenta cerebri
velum
    medullary v.
venereal
Venezuelan equine encephalitis
ventral
ventricle
    Duncan's v.
    Krause's v.
    v. of Arantius
    v's of brain
    v. of cerebrum
    v. of cord
    v. of myelon
    v. of Sylvius
    terminal v. of spinal cord
    Verga's v.
    Vieussen's v.
ventricornu
ventricornual
ventricose
ventricular
ventriculitis
ventriculoatriostomy
ventriculocisternostomy
ventriculogram
ventriculography
ventriculomegaly
ventriculometry
ventriculoperitoneal
ventriculopuncture
ventriculoscope

ventriculoscopy
ventriculostium
ventriculostomy
ventriculosubarachnoid
ventriculus
    v. dexter cerebri
    v. lateralis cerebri
    v. quartus cerebri
    v. sinister cerebri
    v. terminalis medullae
      spinalis
    v. tertius cerebri
ventromedial
VEP – visual evoked potential
Veraguth's fold
verbigeration
verbomania
Verga's ventricle
vermis
    v. cerebelli
Verneuil's neuroma
vertebra
    basilar v.
    v. dentata
    v. magnum
    odontoid v.
    v. plana
    prominent v.
    sternal v.
vertebrae
    cervical v.
    coccygeal v.
    lumbar v.
    sacral v.
    thoracic v.
vertebral
vertebrobasilar
vertex
    v. cranii
    v. cranii ossei
vertiginous
vertigo
    central v.
    encephalic v.
    epileptic v.
    hysterical v.
    neurasthenic v.

vertigo (continued)
    paralyzing v.
    vestibular v.
vesania
vestibular
vestibulo-ocular reflex
vestibulopathy
vibratory
vicious
Vieussen's
    ansa
    ventricle
virus
    Epstein-Barr v.
    human immunodeficiency
      v.
    Powassan v.
    St. Louis encephalitis v.
visna
visuopsychic
vitselzookt. See *witzelsucht.*
Vogt-Koyanagi-Harada
    syndrome
Vogt's
    disease
    syndrome
volatile
volition
volitional
Volkman's curet
von Economo's encephalitis
von Hippel-Lindau disease
von Recklinghausen's disease
voyeurism
vulnerability
vulnerable
Vulpian's atrophy
Wada's test
WAIS – Wechsler's Adult
    Intelligence Scale
Wallenberg's syndrome
wallerian
    degeneration
    law
Walter's bromide test
Ward-French needle
Wartenberg's sign

Waterhouse-Friderichsen
  syndrome
wave
    alpha w's
    beta w's
    brain w's
    delta w's
    plateau w.
    random w's
    theta w's
Weber's
    disease
    sign
Wechsler's Adult Intelligence
  Scale test
Wechsler's Intelligence Scale for
  Childen test
Weck's clip
WEE – western equine
  encephalomyelitis
Weir Mitchell treatment
Weitlaner's retractor
Werdnig-Hoffmann
    atrophy
    disease
    paralysis
Wernicke-Korsakoff syndrome
Wernicke's
    area
    disease
    encephalopathy
Wertheim's clamp
Westphal's sign
West's syndrome
white matter disease
Wilde's forceps
Willis' circle
Wilson's disease
Wiltberger's spreader
wing
    sphenoid w.
Winkelman's disease

WISC – Wechsler's Intelligence
    Scale for Children
withdrawal
Wittenborn Psychiatric Rating
    Scale test
witzelsucht
Woodson's
    elevator
    spatula
WPRS – Wittenborn Psychiatric
    Rating Scale
xanthochromia
xanthochromic
xanthocyanopsia
xanthogranulomatosis
xenophobia
Yasargil's
    clip
    retractor
Yerkes-Bridges test
zan-. See words beginning *xan-.*
zelotypia
zenophobia. See *xenophobia.*
Ziehen-Oppenheim disease
Ziehen's test
zona
    z. reticularis
    z. rolandica
    z. spongiosa
zoophobia
Zuckerkandl's convolution
zygapophyseal
zygion
zygoma
zygomatic
zygomaticofacial
zygomaticofrontal
zygomaticomaxillary
zygomatico-orbital
zygomaticosphenoid
zygomaticotemporal
zygomaxillary

Radiology and
Nuclear Medicine

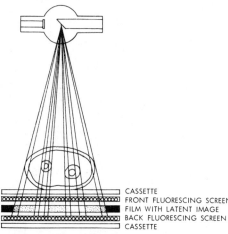

CASSETTE
FRONT FLUORESCING SCREEN
FILM WITH LATENT IMAGE
BACK FLUORESCING SCREEN
CASSETTE

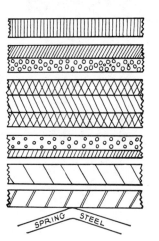

Cassette Front	Bakelite
Intensifying Screen	Cardboard Backing
	Calcium Tungstate
X-ray Film	Silver Bromide Crystals
	Cellulose Acetate Base
	Silver Bromide Crystals
Intensifying Screen	Calcium Tungstate
	Cardboard Backing
Backing	Felt Cushion Back
Cassette Back	Steel Back

SPRING STEEL

(Courtesy of Meschan, I.: Radiographic Positioning and Related Anatomy, 2nd ed. Fig. 2-9, p. 26. Philadelphia, W. B. Saunders Company, 1978).

Radiology and
Nuclear Medicine

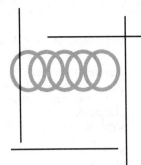

abduction
aberrant
aberration
    chromatid-type a.
    chromosome a.
    commatic a.
abnormalities
ABR – American Board of
    Radiology
Abrodil contrast medium
abscessogram
abscopal
absorbance
absorbed fraction
absorber
absorptiometer
absorption
    a. coefficient
Acacia
acanthus
accelerated
accelerator
    linear a.
acetabular rim
acetabulum
acetic anhydride
acetrizoate sodium
acetylated
acetylation
acinar-like
acquisition time
ACR – American College of
    Radiology
ACTH – adrenocorticotropic
    hormone
actinium

actinogen
actinogenesis
actinogram
actinograph
actinography
actinokymography
actinon
actinopraxis
actinoscopy
activation
ADC – analog-to-digital
    conversion
adduction
adrenocorticotropic hormone
Adrian-Crooks type cassette
AEC – Atomic Energy
    Commission
afterglow
agent
    contrast a.
aggregated
AHRA – American Hospital
    Radiology Administrators
air
    a. bronchogram
    a. crescent sign
    "a. dome" sign
    a. insufflation
    a. monitor
airflow obstruction diseases
air-space disease
AIUM – American Institute of
    Ultrasound in Medicine
Albers-Schönberg position
albumin
    iodinated I 125 serum a.

albumin (continued)
  iodinated I 131 serum a.
  macroaggregated a.
aldosterone
algebraic reconstruction
  technique
algorithm
alignment
  Cooley-Tukey a.
allowed beta transition
alpha
  a. chamber
  a. decay
  a. particle
  a. radiation
  a. ray
  a. threshold
alumina
aluminum
alveolar
alveoli
alveolobronchogram
alveologram
American Board of Radiology
American College of Radiology
American Hospital Radiology
  Administrators
American Institute of
  Ultrasound in Medicine
American Registry of Diagnostic
  Medical Sonographers
American Roentgen Ray Society
American Society of Radiologic
  Technologists
americium
Amipaque contrast medium
amniography
A-mode – amplitude modulation
   A-m. ultrasonography
ampere
amphoteric
amplification
  gas a.
amplifier
  buffer a.
  linear a.
  nuclear pulse a.

amplifier (continued)
  pulse a.
  voltage a.
amplitude modulation
ampulla
  a. of Vater
a.m.u. – atomic mass unit
analog
  a. computations
  a. photo
  a. rate meter
analog-to-digital conversion
analysis
  activation a.
  basic volume image a.
  chemical a.
  correlation a.
  least-squares a.
  neutron activation a.
  quantitative a.
  regression a.
  saturation a.
analyzers
  multichannel a.
ancillary
aneurysm
Anger camera
angioblastoma
angiocardiogram
angiocardiography
  intravenous a.
  radionuclide a.
  selective a.
  venous a.
Angioconray contrast medium
Angiografin contrast medium
angiogram
angiography
  biliary a.
  carotid a.
  cerebral a.
  digital subtraction a.
  peripheral a.
  renal a.
  vertebral a.
  visceral a.
angiology

angiolymphangioma
angioscintigraphy
Angiovist contrast medium
angle
  a. board
  cardiophrenic a.
  subcarinal a.
Angstrom unit
angular
  a. frequency
  a. momentum
angulator
anion
annihilation
  a. photons
  a. radiation
anode
  rotating a.
  stationary a.
anomalous
anteflexion
antegrade
anteroposterior view
anteversion
antibody
anticoincidence circuit
antigenic
antimony
antineutrino
antinuclear
antiparticle
antiproton
antrum
anuria
aortic
  a. arch
  a. knob
aortogram
aortography
  abdominal a.
  catheter a.
  lumbar a.
  retrograde a.
  selective visceral a.
  thoracic a.
  translumbar a.
  venous a.

aortography (continued)
  visceral a.
AP – anteroposterior
apical
aponeurosis
apophyseal
apophysis
appearance
  "applecore-like" a.
  "ball-in-hand" a.
  "beaded" a.
  "beaked" a.
  "beaten brass" a.
  "bone within bone" a.
  "bubble-like" a.
  "candle dripping" a.
  "cobblestone" a.
  "coiled-spring" a.
  "cotton ball" a.
  "cotton-wool" a.
  double-bubble a.
  drumstick a.
  "frayed string" a.
  "ground glass" a.
  "hair-standing-on-end" a.
  "hammered brass" a.
  "hot-cross-bun" a.
  "inverse comma" a.
  "jail bars" a.
  "kernel of popcorn" a.
  "lacelike" a.
  "leafless tree" a.
  "light bulb" a.
  "moth-eaten" a.
  "onion skin" a.
  "pancake" a.
  "panda" a.
  "picture frame" a.
  "popcorn-like" a.
  "pruned-tree" a.
  "punched out" a.
  "railroad track" a.
  "rugger jersey" a.
  "saber shin" a.
  "sandwich" a.
  "scottie dog" a.
  "shell of bone" a.

appearance (continued)
"soap bubble" a.
"spadelike" a.
"sunburst" a.
"sun-ray" a.
"Swiss Alps" a.
"trefoil" a.
"weblike" a.
"wineglass" a.
"wormy" a.
applecore-like
apposition
arachnodactyly
arachnoid
arachnoiditis
ARDMS – American Registry of
Diagnostic Medical
Sonographers
areae gastricae
argon
ARRS – American Roentgen Ray
Society
ARRT – American Registry of
Radiologic Technologists
arsenic
ART – algebraic reconstruction
technique
arteriogram
coronary a.
"pruned-tree" a.
wedge a.
arteriography
brachiocephalic a.
carotid a.
celiac a.
cerebral a.
coronary a.
digital subtraction a.
femoral a.
mesenteric a.
peripheral a.
pulmonary a.
renal a.
selective a.
vertebral a.
visceral a.
arterioles

arteriosclerosis
arteriosus
patent ductus a.
arteriovenous
arteritis (arteritides)
arthritis
arthrogram
double-contrast a.
arthrography
air a.
double-contrast a.
opaque a.
articulare
articulation
artifact
ascites
aspergillosis
asplenia
ASRT – American Society of
Radiologic Technologists
assay
erythropoietin a.
astatine
astrocytoma
asymmetry
atelectasis
atlas (C-1) (vertebra)
atom
Na a's
a. smasher
tagged a.
atomic
a. energy
a. mass unit
a. number
a. spectrum
a. weight
atomization
atony
atresia
atrophy
attenuation
a. coefficient
attenuator
Auger
effect
electron

auscultation
autocorrelation function
autofluoroscope
    digital a.
autogenous
autoradiograph
autoradiography
    contact a.
    dip-coating a.
    film-stripping a.
    thick-layer a.
    two-emulsion a.
autotomogram
autotomography
autotransformer formula
avalanche
    Townsend's a.
average life
Avogadro's number
axial
axis (C-2) (vertebra)
axis
    celiac a.
    longitudinal a.
    vertical a.
    X a.
    Y a.
azygography
azygos vein
B–Bucky (film in cassette in
    Potter-Bucky diaphragm)
    tomogram with oscillating
    Bucky
BA–barium
background
    b. activity
    b. count
    b. erase
    b. radiation
backscatter
    b. peak
balloon
    b. catheterization
    b. dilatation
    image data intra-aortic
        counter-pulsation b.
    b. tamponade

Ball's method
balsa wood block
barium
    b. enema
    b. meal
    b. sulfate
    b. swallow
    b. vaginography
barn
"barrel chest"
barreling distortion
basilar
basket cells
Bayes' theorem
BBB–blood-brain barrier
BE–barium enema
bead chain cystography
beam
    b. barrier
    b. CT scanner
    electron b.
    b. flattening filter
    b. monitor
    b. quality comparison
    b. therapy
    useful b.
    x-ray b.
beamsplitter
Béclére's position
BEI–butanol-extractable iodine
Benassi's position
berkelium
beryllium
beta
    b. decay
    b. emitter
    b. particle
    b. radiation
    b.-ray
    b. transition
betatron
BEV–billion electron volts
bevatron
bezoar
biliary
Biligrafin contrast medium
Biligram contrast medium

Biliodyl contrast medium
Bilivistan contrast medium
Bilopaque contrast medium
Biloptin contract medium
bimolecular
binding energy
bioassay
    erythropoietin b.
biological half life
biopsy
biosynthesis
bisacodyl tannex
bismuth
Blackett-Healy position
Bloch's scale
block
    alveolar-capillary b.
    balsa wood b.
blood flow study
    cerebral b.f.s.
    pulmonary b.f.s.
blood pool
    b.p. imaging
    b.p. scan
blood volume measurements
blurring
B-mode – brightness modulation
BOBA – beta-oxybutyric acids
Bohr
    B. equation
    B. radius
bolus
bombardment
bone
    b. marrow scanning
    b. scan
    b. seeker
boron
bosselated
bosselation
Bracco contrast medium
brachytherapy
Bragg
    curve
    peak
brain scan
brain stem

"braking" radiation
branch
branching
    b. decay
    b. fraction
    b. ratio
breeder reactor
bregma
bremsstrahlung
BRH – Bureau of Radiological
    Health
broad-beam scattering
Broden's position
bromine
bronchogram
bronchography
    Cope-method b.
    percutaneous
      transtracheal b.
bronchopulmonary
bronchoradiography
bronchoscopy
    fiberoptic b.
    nonfiberoptic b.
bronchus
    lower lobe b.
    main stem b.
    middle lobe b.
    upper lobe b.
BSP – Bromsulphalein
bubble-like
Bucky grid
bunamiodyl
Bureau of Radiological
    Health
c. – curie
cadmium
calcific
    c. shadows
calcification
calcium (with scandium 47)
calculogram
calculography
calculus
    ureteral c.
Caldwell-Moloy method
Caldwell's position

calibration
    E-dial c.
calibrator
    digital isotope c.
    radioisotope c.
calices
caliectasis
californium
calorie
camera
    Anger c.
    cine c.
    gamma c.
    Isocon c.
    Medx c.
    Multicrystal c.
    Orthicon c.
    pinhole c.
    positron scintillation c.
    radioisotope c.
    scintillation c.
    video display c.
Camp-Coventry position
Camp-Gianturco method
Camp's grid cassette
Cannon's ring
cannulation
Cantor's tube
capacitance
capacitive reactance
capture
    cross section c.
    gamma ray c.
carbon
    c. dioxide
cardiac
    c. output
    c. shunt detection
cardioangiography
    retrograde c.
Cardio-Conray contrast medium
Cardiografin contrast medium
cardiography
    M-mode c.
cardiophrenic
cardiopulmonary
cardioscan

carina
carrier
    c. -free radioisotope
cartilaginous
cassette
    Adrian-Crooks type of c.
    Camp's grid c.
    multisection c.
    c. tunnel
    c. unloader
    Wisconsin kV p test c.
CAT – chlormerodrin
        accumulation test
    computed axial
        tomography
    computer assisted
        tomography
catabolism
cataphoresis
catenary system
catheter
    aortic flush pigtail c.
    c. aortography
    c. arteriography
    central venous pressure c.
    French polyethylene c.
    Grollman pigtail c.
    Grüntzig balloon-tip c.
    headhunter c.
    c. induced thrombosis
    Ingram's trocar c.
    intraluminal c.
    intraperitoneal c.
    nasogastric c.
    pigtail angiographic c.
    radiopaque c.
    retrograde c.
    Ring-McLean c.
    sheathed c.
    sidewinder c.
    Simmons' c.
    subclavian c.
    Swan-Ganz c.
    trocar c.
    umbilical c.
    Von Sonnenberg's c.

catheterization
    balloon c.
    cardiac c.
    Seldinger's c.
cathode
caudad
caudal
cavogram
cavography
cb – cardboard or plastic film
    holder without intensifying
    screens
CBG – corticosteroid-binding
    globulin
CCK – cholecystokinin
CCT – cranial computed
    tomography
cecum
cell
    polygonal c.
    reticuloendothelial c.
cellulitis
cephalad
cephalic
cephalometry
    ultrasonic c.
Cerenkov radiation production
cerium
ceruloplasmin
cesium (with barium 137m)
chamber
    ionization c.
    multiwire proportional c.
    spark c.
    Wilson c.
charcoal
Chassard-Lapiné projection
Chausse's view
chemotherapeutic
chemotherapy
chemotoxic
Cherenkov counter
chlorine
chlormerodrin
    c.-cysteine
    c. Hg 197
    c. Hg 203

cholangiogram
    endoscopic retrograde c.
    intraoperative c.
    intravenous c.
    operative c.
    percutaneous transhepatic
    c.
    retrograde c.
    transhepatic c.
    T-tube c.
cholangiographic
cholangiography
    delayed operative c.
    direct percutaneous
      transhepatic c.
    intraoperative c.
    intravenous c.
    operative c.
    percutaneous
      hepatobiliary c.
    percutaneous transhepatic
    c.
    postoperative c.
    transabdominal c.
    transhepatic c.
    T-tube c.
cholangiopancreatography
    endoscopic retrograde c.
cholangiotomogram
Cholebrine contrast medium
cholecystocholangiography
cholecystogram
cholecystographic
cholecystography
    intravenous c.
    oral c.
cholecystokinin-pancreozymin
cholecystosonography
choledochogram
choledochograph
choledochography
cholegraphy
cholescintigram
cholescintigraphy
    radionuclide c.
Cholografin contrast medium
    C. methylglucamine

Cholovue contrast medium
chromatid-type aberration
chromatoelectrophoretic
chromatogram
chromatographic
chromatography
chromic phosphate P 32
chromium
    c. Cr 51 serum albumin
chromosome
    c.-type aberration
Ci–curie
cicatricial
cicatrix (cicatrices)
cine
    c. camera
    c. CT scan
    c. study
cineangiocardiography
cineangiograph
cineangiography
cinebronchography
cinedensigraphy
cinefluorography
cinefluoroscopy
cinematography
cinematoradiography
cinemicrography
cinephlebography
cineradiography
cineroentgeno-
   fluorography
cineroentgenography
cineurography
circle of confusion
circuit
    anticoincidence c.
    coincidence c.
    magnetic c.
    phototube output c.
circuitry
cistern
    basal c.
    cerebellomedullary c.
    chiasmatic c.
    interpeduncular c.
    c. of Sylvius

cistern (continued)
    subarachnoidal c.
    terminal c's
cisternal puncture
cisternogram
cisternography
    radionuclide c.
cisternomyelography
clavicle
Cleaves' position
clinodactyly
    factitious c.
    traumatic c.
clinoids
cloud chamber
Clysodrast contrast medium
coarsening
cobalt
Cobb's method
Code and Carlson radiograph
coded-aperture imaging
Codman's triangle
coefficient
    linear absorption c.
    mass absorption c.
    partition c.
coeur en sabot
coffin
coincidence
    c. circuit
    c. counting
    c. detection
    c. loss
    c. sum peak
coinlike
Colcher-Sussman method
cold
    c. lesion
    c. spot
collecting system
collimate
collimation
collimator
    automatic c.
    converging c.
    diverging c.
    focusing c.

collimator (continued)
    multihole c.
    parallel-hole c.
    pin-hole c.
    single-hole c.
    thick-septa c.
    thin-septa c.
colloid
colloidal gold
colon
    ascending c.
    descending c.
    transverse c.
colonoscopy
colorimetric
colorimetrically
combined transmission-emission
   scintiphoto
comparison view
compartmental analysis
complex
    chlormerodrin-cysteine c.
compression
Compton's
    C. edge
    C. effect
    C. electron
    C. photon
    C. scatter
    C. scattering
    C. wavelength
computed
    c. myelogram
    c. myelography
    c. tomography
computer
computerized
    c. axial tomography
    c. radiography
    c. tomography
concept
    "ring of bone" c.
condenser
conductivity
    thermal c.
conductor
cone

coned-down view
configuration
confluent
conical
Conray contrast medium
constant
    permeability c.
    Planck's c.
constriction
contamination
contour
contrast
    c. radiography
    c. studies
contrast media
    Abrodil
    acetrizoate
    acetrizoic acid
    amidotrizoic acid
    Amipaque
    Angioconray
    Angiografin
    Angiovist
    barium sulfate
    benzoic acid
    Biligrafin
    Biligram
    Biliodyl
    Bilivistan
    Bilopaque
    Biloptin
    bismuth
    Bracco
    brominized oil
    bunamiodyl
    calcium
    Cardio-Conray
    Cardiografin
    cerium
    Cholebrine
    Cholografin
    Cholovue
    Clysodrast
    Conray
    Cystografin
    Cystokon
    diaginol

contrast media (continued)
diatrizoate
diatrizoic acid
diodine
diodone
Diodrast
Dionosil
diprotrizoate
Duografin
Duroliopaque
dysprosium
Endobile
Endografin
Ethiodane
ethiodized oil
Ethiodol
ethyliodophenylundecyl
gadolinium
Gastrografin
glucagon
Hexabrix
Hippuran
Hypaque
Hytrast
Intropaque
iobenzamic acid
iobutoic acid
iocarmate meglumine
iocarmic acid
iocetamate
iocetamic acid
iodamic acid
iodamide
iodatol
iodecol
iodide
iodipamide
iodized oil
iodoalphionic acid
iodohippurate
iodomethamate
iodophendylate
iodophthalein
iodopyracet
iodoxamate
iodoxamic acid
iodoxyl

contrast media (continued)
ioglicate
ioglicic acid
ioglucol
ioglucomide
ioglunide
ioglycamic acid
ioglycamide
iogulamide
iohexol
iomide
Iopamidol
iopanoate
iopanoic acid
iophendylate
iophenoxic acid
ioprocemic acid
iopromide
iopronic acid
iopydol
iopydone
iosefamate
iosefamic acid
ioseric acid
iosulamide
iosumetic acid
iotasul
ioteric acid
iothalamate
iothalamic acid
iotrol
iotroxamide
iotroxic acid
ioxaglate
ioxaglic acid
ioxithalamate
ioxithalamic acid
iozomic acid
ipodate
ipodic acid
Isopaque
Isovue
Kinevac
Lipiodol
Liquipake
magnesium
Magnevist

contrast media (continued)
    manganese chloride
    meglumine
    methiodal
    methylglucamine
    metrizamide
    metrizoate
    metrizoic acid
    Micropaque
    Microtrast
    Monophen
    Myodil
    Neo-Iopax
    Niopam
    Novopaque
    Nyegaard
    Omnipaque
    Orabilex
    Oragrafin
    Oravue
    Osbil
    Pantopaque
    phenobutiodyl
    phentetiothalein
    potassium bromide
    Praestholm
    Priodax
    propyliodone
    Raybar 75
    Rayvist
    Renografin
    Reno-M-30
    Reno-M-60
    Reno-M-Dip
    Renovist
    Renovue
    Retro-Conray
    Salpix
    sincalide
    Sinografin
    Skiodan
    Skiodan Acacia
    sodium
    Solu-Biloptin
    Solutrast
    Steripaque-BR
    Steripaque-V

contrast media (continued)
    tantalum-178
    Telebrix
    Telepaque
    Teridax
    tetrabromophen-
        olphthalein
    tetraiodophenolphthalein
    Thixokon
    thorium dioxide
    thorium tartrate
    Thorotrast
    triiodobenzoic acid
    Triosil
    tyropanoate
    tyropanoic acid
    Umbradil
    Urografin
    Uromiro
    Uropac
    Urovision
    Vasiodone
conversion coefficient
converter
    digital to analog c.
convolutional
coolant
Cooley-Tukey algorithm
Cope-method bronchography
copper
coprecipitation
coprolith
Corbin technique
coronal
corresponding ray
cortex
corticosteroids
cosmotron
costophrenic
costotransverse
costovertebral
cotton-wool appearance
coulomb force
count density
count rate
counter
    boron c.

counter (continued)
    Cherenkov c.
    Geiger-Müller c.
    proportional c.
    radiation c.
    scintillation c.
    whole-body c.
counting rate meter
craniad
cranial computed tomography
craniograph
craniography
crater
    ulcer c.
^{51}Cr-heated RBC's
critical mass
cross-fire treatment
cruciform
crus (crura)
    c. commune
    diaphragmatic c.
cryomagnet
cryptoscope
    Satvioni's c.
cryptoscopy
CT–computed tomography
CT body scanner
curie
curium
current
    alternating c.
    direct c.
    eddy c.
    pulsating c.
    saturation c.
    single-phase c.
    three-phase c.
    unidirectional c.
curve
    Bragg c.
cut
    tomographic c.
Cutie Pie
CXR–chest x-ray
cyanocobalamin Co 57, Co 58,
    Co 60
Cyber 170/720

Cybex ergometer
cycle
    Krebs' c.
    pentose c.
cycle-length window
cyclotron
cysteine
Cystografin contrast medium
cystogram
    triple-voiding c.
cystography
    bead chain c.
    radionuclide c.
    retrograde c.
    triple-voiding c.
Cystokon contrast medium
cystoscopy
cystoureterogram
cystoureterography
cystourethrogram
    micturition c.
    retrograde c.
    voiding c.
cystourethrography
    "chain" c.
    expression c.
    isotope voiding c.
    micturition c.
    radionuclide voiding c.
    retrograde c.
    voiding c.
D–mean dose
dacryocystography
data
    ferrokinetic d.
datacamera
daughter nuclide
DDC–direct display console
dead time
de Broglie's wavelength
decade scaler
decay
    alpha d.
    beta d.
    branching d.
    d. constant
    exponential d.

decay (continued)
    isometric d.
    d. mode
    nuclear d.
    positron d.
    d. product
    radioactive d.
    d. scheme
decompression
decontamination
decubitus
decussation
dee
de-excitation
defecography
defect
    filling d.
    napkin-ring d.
defibrillation
defibrillator
deflation
deflection
deformity
    cloverleaf d.
    valgus d.
    varus d.
delimitation
delineation
delta ray
demarcation
    no line of d.
    "shell-like" d.
demineralization
demyelinization
denatured
densitometer
densitometry
    quantitative CT d.
density
    background d.
    calcific d.
    inherent d.
    ionization d.
densography
6-deoxy-1-galactose
deoxyribonucleic acid
DES – diffuse esophageal spasm

descending
detection
    beta d.
detector
    collimation scintillation d.
    crystalline phosphor d.
    dielectric track d.
    quadrature d.
    radiation d.
    semiconductor d.
    tissue-equivalent d.
    x-ray d.
deuterium
deuteron
dextrogram
DI – diagnostic imaging
diagrammatic radiography
diaphragm
    Potter-Bucky d.
diaphragmatic
diapositive
diatrizoate meglumine
diatrizoate sodium
diethyltriamine-penta-acetic acid
differentiation
diffusion
digital
    d. subtraction angiography
    d. subtraction
        arteriography
diisofluorophosphate
dimer
    ionic d's
    nonionic d's
dimerization
Dimer X
Diodrast contrast medium
Dionosil contrast medum
dioxide
diphenyloxazole
diphosphonate
diploë
diplogram
dipolar
dipole
diprotrizoate
discography

discoid
discriminator
disintegration rate
diskogram
diskography
distal
distended
distortion
    pin-cushion d.
distribution
    depth dose d.
    gaussian d.
    maxwellian d.
    Poisson d.
    spatial dose d.
diverticulitis
diverticulosis
diverticulum (diverticula)
DNA–deoxyribonucleic acid
Doerner-Hoskins distribution law
dominance
Dooley, Caldwell and Glass
    method
Doppler
    D. echocardiography
    D. effect
    D. ultrasonography
    D. ultrasound
dorsal
dose
    absorbed d.
    cumulative d.
    depth d.
    doubling d.
    erythema d.
    d. estimate
    exit d.
    genetically significant d.
    integral d.
    lethal d.
    maximum permissible d.
    mean d.
    nominal single d.
    organ tolerance d.
    d. reciprocity theorem
    threshold erythema d.
    tissue tolerance d.

dose (continued)
    tumor lethal d.
dosimeter
    pencil d.
    pocket d.
    thermoluminescent d.
    ultraviolet fluorescent d.
    Victoreen d.
dosimetric
dosimetry
    pion d.
dot scan
Dotter's tube
"double-bubble"
double-contrast
"doughnut" sign
DPTA–diethylenetriamine
    penta-acetic acid
drip-infusion
    d.-i. pyelography
    d.-i. urography
drugs. See *Drugs and Chemistry*
    section.
DSA–digital subtraction
    angiography
DTPA–diethyltramine penta-
    acetic acid
duct
    common bile d.
    cystic d.
    hepatic d.
    pancreatic d.
ductography
    peroral retrograde
        pancreaticobiliary d.
dumping syndrome
duodenal
    d. bulb
    d. loop
    d. papilla
duodenogram
duodenography
    hypotonic d.
duodenum
Duografin contrast medium
dural
dura mater

Duroliopaque contrast medium
D-xylose
dye
      halogenated
          phenolphthalein d.
      rose bengal d.
Dynapix
Dyne
dynode
dysphagia
dysprosium
echo
      e. planar imaging
      e. ranging
      e. texture
      e. time
echocardiogram
echocardiography
      two-dimensional e.
echoencephalography
echogram
echoic
echolaminography
ECT – emission computed
    tomography
edge
      Compton e.
      e. packing
E-dial calibration
EDR – effective direct radiation
    electrodermal response
EEG – electroencephalogram
effect
      Auger e.
      Compton e.
      Doppler e.
      isotope e.
effective
      e. half-life
      e. renal plasma flow
Eindhoven's magnet
einsteinium
ejection fraction
elastic collision
electrocardiogram
electrocardiography
electrodynamometer

electroencephalogram
electrokymogram
electrokymograph
electrokymography
electrolyte
electromagnetic
      e. induction
      e. radiation
electromagnetism
electrometer
      dynamic-condenser e.
      vibrating-reed e.
electron
      Auger e.
      bound e.
      e. capture
      Compton e.
      e. multiplier tube
      secondary e.
      e. volt(s)
electronneutrino
electrophoresis
electrophoretically
electroscope
electrostatic
element
      daughter e.
      parent e.
ellipsoid
elliptical
Elon
elutriation
Embden-Meyerhof glycolytic
    pathway
EMI – Electric and Musical
    Industries (scanner)
emission
      beta e.
      e. computed tomography
      filament e.
      photoelectric e.
      thermonic e.
      e. tomography
emitter
emulsion
      nuclear e.
encephalo-arteriography

encephalogram
encephalography
encephalometry
Endobile contrast medium
endodiascope
endodiascopy
endoergic reaction
Endografin contrast medium
endoscopy
enema
     barium e.
     cleansing e.
     opaque e.
energy
     atomic e.
     binding e.
     chemical potential e.
     electrical potential e.
     electromagnetic e.
     e. frequency
     kinetic e.
     mechanical potential e.
     nuclear e.
     photon e.
     potential e.
     quadrant e.
     radiant e.
     e. resolution
     e. spectrum
     thermal e.
     e. wavelength
     x-ray e.
enteropathy
     exudative e.
enzyme
epididymography
epididymovesiculography
epidurography
epigastrium
equation
     Bohr e.
equilibrium
     radioactive e.
     secular e.
     transient e.
equivalence
     mass energy e.

erbium
ERCP – endoscopic retrograde
     cholangiopancreatography
ergometer
     Cybex e.
Erlenmeyer flask-like
ERPF – effective renal plasma
     flow
erythropoietin
esofa-. See words beginning
     esopha-.
esophagogram
esophagography
esophagoscopy
esophagospasm
esophagram
esophagraphy
ESU – electrostatic unit
Ethiodane contrast medium
ethiodized oil
Ethiodol contrast medium
EU – excretory urography
Euler's number
europium
eV – electron volt
eversion
examination
     double-contrast e.
excitation
excretory urography
expiration
exponential
extension
extrapolate
E-zero offset
faceted
faceting
factor
     intrinsic f.
     geometry f.
fasciagram
fasciagraphy
fascicle
fasciculation
fast Fourier transformation
fatty meal
feather analysis

fecalith
Feist-Mankin position
femoral
    f. head
    f. neck
    f. shaft
Ferguson's method
fermium
ferrokinetics
ferromagnetic relaxation
ferrous citrate Fe 59
fetogram
fetography
FEV—forced expiratory volume
fibercolonoscope
fibergastroscope
fiberoptic
fiberscope
fiberscopic
fibronuclear
fibrosis
Fick's
    law
    position
    principle
FID—free induction decay
filling defect
film
    f. badge
    comparison f.
    f. density calibration
    lateral decubitus f.
    plain f.
    prone f.
    rapid processing f.
    sequential f.
    serial f.
filter
    inherent f.
    Thoreau's f.
filtration
fission
fistulogram
fistulography
fixer
fixing time
flail chest

"flank stripe"
flask-like
    Erlenmeyer f.-l.
fleb-. See words beginning *phleb-*.
Fleischner's position
flexion
flexure
flocculent
flood source
floppy disk
fluorescence
fluorescent
    f. phosphor
    f. ray
    f. scan
    f. screen
fluorine F 18
fluorography
fluorometer
fluorometry
fluoronephelometer
fluororoentgenography
fluoroscope
fluoroscopic
fluoroscopy
    computerized f.
    digital f.
    image-amplified f.
flurescence. See *fluorescence*.
fluroskope. See *fluoroscope*.
fluroskopic. See *fluoroscopic*.
fluoroskopy. See *fluoroscopy*.
flux
fluxes
focal
    f. spot
    f. zone
foramen
    f. lacerum
    f. magnum
    obturator f.
    f. ovale
    f. spinosum
foreign body
formatter
formula
    autotransformer f.

formula (continued)
  projection f.
fossa
Fourier
  direct transformation
    imaging
  discrete transformation
  multislice modified KWE
    direct imaging
  transformation
    reconstruction
  transformation
    zeugmatography
  two-dimensional imaging
  two-dimensional
    projection
    reconstruction
four-valve-tube rectification
four-vessel angiography
fraction
  penetration f.
  scatter f.
fractional
fractionation
frames
francium
free peritoneal air
French polyethylene catheter
Fresnel zone plate
Friedman's position
fucose
fulcrum
full-width at half-maximum
fundus
fusion
FWHM – full width at half
  maximum
FZ – focal zone
Ga – gallium
^{57}Ga citrate
gadolinium
  g.-159 hydroxycitrate
galactography
galactose
gallium
  g. citrate Ga 67
  radioactive g. Ga 67

gallium (continued)
  g. scanning
  g. uptake
galvanometer
gamma
  g.-aminobutyrate
  g. camera
  g. cascade
  g. emitter
  g. film
  g. heating
  g. radiation
  g. radiography
  g. ray(s)
  g.-ray counter
  g.-ray level indicator
  g.-ray scanner
  g.-ray spectra
  g.-ray spectrometer
  g. scanning
  g. well counter
gammopathy
  monoclonal g.
gantry
gastrocamera
Gastrografin contrast medium
gastrointestinal
gastropathy
gated
  g. blood pool imaging
  g. CT scanner
  g. imaging
gating
gaussian distribution
Gaynor-Hart position
Geiger-Müller counter
General Electric CT/T7 scanner
generator
  direct current g.
  electric g.
  electrostatic g.
  molybdenum-technetium
    g.
  polyphase g.
  6-pulse 3-phase g.
  12-pulse 3-phase g.
  radionuclide g.

generator (continued)
    resonance g.
    supervoltage g.
    three-phase g.
    Triphasix g.
    Van de Graaff's g.
    x-ray g.
genetic
geographic
geometrical efficiency
geometry factor
germanium
GE scan – gastroesophageal scan
GFR – glomerular filtration rate
GI – gastrointestinal
Girout's method
glabella
glandulography
glow modular tube
glucagon
gluconeogenesis
glucose
glutamate
goitrogen
gold Au 198
gonion
gradient
    g. coil
    g. magnetic field
graininess
granuloma
Grashey's position
grid
    Bucky g.
    g. cassette (or oscillating g.)
    focused g.
    Potter-Bucky g.
Grollman pigtail catheter
ground state
Grüntzig balloon-tip catheter
GSD – genetically significant dose
gynecography
gynogram
gynography
gyromagnetic
Haas position

hafnium
"hair-on-end"
"hairpin" loop
half-life
    biological h.
    effective h.
    physical h.
half-thickness
half-time of exchange
half-value layer
"Hampton's hump"
Hampton's view
haustration
haustrum (haustra)
heavy particle therapy
helium
hematocrit
    mean circulatory h.
"hemi-diaphragms"
hemithorax
hepatic flexure
hepatogram
hepatography
hepatolienography
hepatophlebography
hepatosplenography
Heublein's method
Hexabrix contrast medium
Hg meralluride
Hickey's position
hilum
Hippuran contrast medium
histogram mode
histography
historadiography
holmium
holography
homogeneity
homogeneous
homogeneously
honeycomb
    h. lung
hot lesion
Hounsfield unit
hourglass chest
HSA – human serum albumin

HVL – half-value layer
hyaline
  h. arteriosclerosis
  h. cartilage
  h. membrane disease
hybrid
hydrogen
  h. atom
hydronephrosis
hydroquinone
hydrothorax
hydroxycitrate
Hypaque contrast media
  H.-Cysto
  H. M.
  H. Meglumine
  H. Sodium
hyperlucency
hypertrophy
hypoaeration
hysterography
hysterosalpingogram
hysterosalpingography
Hytrast contrast medium
I – iodine
ICRP – International
    Commission on
    Radiological Protection
ICRU – International
    Commission on Radiation
    Units and Measures
ilium
ill-defined
image
  i. aliasing
  i. amplifier
  i. analysis
  calculated i.
  i. chains
  i. contrast
  i. converter
  fluoroscopic i.
  i.-forming system
  gated i.
  i. intensification
  i. intensifier system
  i. intensifier tube

image (continued)
  inversion recovery i.
  i. noise
  nuclear magnetic
    resonance i's
  i. orthicon tube
  parametric i.
  phantom i.
  i. quality
  radiographic i.
  i. reconstruction
  i. reformation
  renal i.
  i. resolution
  saturation recovery i.
  scout i.
  i. sharpness
  i. slice thickness
  spin echo i.
  static renal i.
  x-ray i.
imaging
  acoustic i.
  adrenal i.
  blood pool i.
  cardiac blood pool i.
  coded-aperture i.
  diagnostic i.
  digital vascular i.
  direct Fourier
    transformation i.
  dynamic volume i.
  echo-planar i.
  electrostatic i.
  flow i.
  gated blood pool i.
  gray-scale i.
  heavy ion i.
  infarct-avid i.
  iosotope colloid i.
  isotope hepatobiliary i.
  longitudinal section i.
  lymph node i.
  magnetic resonance i.
  microwave i.
  multigated i.
  multiplanar i.

imaging (continued)
  multiple-gated blood pool
    i.
  multiple line scan i.
  multiple spin echo total
    volume i.
  multislice modified KWE
    direct Fourier i.
  myocardial infarct i.
  myocardial perfusion i.
  nuclear i.
  nuclear magnetic
    resonance i.
  perfusion i.
  planar i.
  planar spin i.
  projection reconstruction
    i.
  pyrophosphate i.
  quantitative brain i.
  radionuclide i.
  reconstructive i.
  reticuloendothelial i.
  rotating frame i.
  selective excitation
    projection
    reconstruction i.
  sensitive plane projection
    reconstruction i.
  sequential first pass i.
  sequential plane i.
  single slice modified
    KWE direct Fourier i.
  spin-echo i.
  spin-warp i.
  thallium-201 i.
  three-dimensional i.
  three-dimensional echo
    planar i.
  three-dimensional Fourier
    i.
  three-dimensional KWE
    direct Fourier i.
  three-dimensional
    projection
    reconstruction i.
  transverse section i.

imaging (continued)
  two-dimensional Fourier i.
  two-dimensional Fourier
    transformation i.
  two-dimensional KWE
    direct Fourier i.
  two-dimensional modified
    KWE direct Fourier i.
  ultrasound i.
  ventilation perfusion i.
  volume i.
IMPH – 1-iodomercuri-2-
    hydroxypropane
immobilization device
    Pigg-O-Stat i.d.
immunoadsorbent
immunoassay
immunoelectrophoresis
immunofiltration
immunofluorescence
immunogenetics
immunoglobulin
I_n chelate
^{111}In chloride
indium-111
inductance
induction
industrial monitoring
inferior ramus
inflation
Ingram's trocar catheter
inherent
inhibition
inion
injection
    perinephric air i.
    transduodenal fiberscopic
      duct i.
^{111}In-labeled IgG
insoluble
inspiration
insufflation
    perirenal i.
    retroperitoneal gas i.
insulinase
insulin-iodine
intensification factor

intensity
interaction
intercartilaginous rim
interface
internal conversion
International Commission on
    Radiation Units and
    Measures
International Commission on
    Radiological Protection
interspace
interstitial disease
interstitium
intertrochanteric
intracavitary
^{113m}In-transferrin
intraperitoneal
intrinsic
Intropaque contrast medium
intubation
intussusception
inverse square law
inversion
in vitro
in vivo
iodinated
      i. I 131 aggregated
        albumin (human)
      i. contrast media
      i. I 125 fibrinogen
      i. I 125 serum albumin
      i. I 131 serum albumin
        (human)
iodination
iodine
      i. PVP bond
      radioactive i.
iodipamide
iodoalphionic acid
iodohippurate sodium
iodomethamate
iodophthalein sodium
iodopyracet
ion
      amphoteric dipolar i.
ionic
ionization

ionizing
ionograph
ionography
Iopamidol contrast medium
iopanoic acid
iophendylate
iophenoxic acid
iopydol
iopydone
iothalamate
ipodate calcium
IRA-400 resin
iridium
iron
      i. hydroxide
      radioactive i.
irradiated
irradiation
ischium
Isherwood's position
isobar
isobaric transition
Isocon camera
isoelectric
isomer
isomeric
      i. decay
      i. transition
Isopaque contrast medium
isotone
isotope
      i. bone scan
      i. colloid imaging
      i. effect
      i. hepatobiliary imaging
      radioactive i.
      i. study
      i. voiding cystourethrog-
        raphy
isotopic
Isovue contrast medium
IVC–intravenous cholangiogram
IVCU–isotope voiding
      cystourethrography
IVP–intravenous pyelogram
jejunum
Johnson's position

joint mice
junction
      myoneural j.
      rectosigmoid j.
K-capture
Kerley's
      A line
      B line
ker-on-sa-bo. See *coeur en sabot*.
ketone bodies
kev. – kilo electron volts
kHz – kilohertz
kidney washout
kilocalorie
kilocurie
kilohertz
kilomegacycle
kilovolt
kilovoltage
kineradiography
kinescope
kinetic energy
kinetics
Kinevac contrast medium
kol. See words beginning *chol-*.
kolangi-. See words beginning
    cholangi-.
kole-. See words beginning *chole-*.
kolo-. See words beginning *cholo-*.
K radiation
Krebs cycle
krypton-81M
K-shell
KUB – plain view of abdomen
    (kidneys, ureters, bladder)
Kurzbauer's position
kymograph
kymography
      roentgen k.
kymoscope
kymoscopy
lacelike
lactose-barium
lambda
lambdoidal suture
laminagram
laminagraph

laminagraphy
laminated
lamination
laminogram
laminography
lamp
      Wood's l.
lanthanum
LAO – left anterior oblique
Laquerrière-Pierquin position
Larkin's position
laryngogram
laryngography
      contrast l.
laryngopharyngography
laser beam
laterality
latitude
Lauenstein and Hickey
    projection
law
      Doerner-Hoskins
        distribution l.
      Fick's l.
      inverse-square l.
      l. of inertia
      l. of reciprocity
      l. of thermodynamics
      Ohm's l.
Lawrence's position
lawrencium
Law's
      position
      view
LD_{50} – median lethal dose
lead
lens
      Thorpe plastic l.
Leonard-George position
lepton
lesion
      annular l.
      "apple core" l.
      "butterfly" l.
      cold l.
      "doughnut" l.
      "dumbbell" l.

lesion (continued)
    ellipsoid l.
    hot l.
    "napkin ring" l.
    "ring-like" l.
    sessile l.
    space occupying l.
    wedge-shaped l.
LET – linear energy transfer
levoangiocardiogram
levocardiogram
levogram
Lewis' position
licorice powder
lienography
ligament of Treitz
Lilienfeld's position
Lindblom's position
line
    acanthomeatal l.
    auricular l.
    canthomeatal l.
    glabelloalveolar l.
    glabellomeatal l.
    infraorbital l.
    infraorbitomeatal l.
    interorbital l.
    interpupillary l.
    Kerley's A l.
    Kerley's B l.
    McGregor's l.
    pubococcygeal l.
    Reid's base l.
linear
    l. accelerator
    l. attenuation
    l. compartmental system
    l. energy transfer
    l. focus
Lipiodol contrast medium
lipogenesis
lipping
Liquipake contrast medium
list mode
lithium
LMR – localized magnetic
    resonance

localization
loopogram
loose bodies
lopamidol
lordotic
    anteroposterior l.
      projection
    apical l. projection
Lorenz's position
Löw-Beer position
LPO – left posterior oblique
lucent
lumen
lung
    l. markings
    l. root
lutetium
lymphadenogram
lymphadenography
lymphangiogram
lymphangiography
lymphography
MAA – macroaggregated albumin
macroaggregated
    m. albumin
macroangiography
macromolecules
macroradiography
macroscopic
magenblase
magic numbers
magnesium
magnet
    beam-bending m.
    cryostable m.
    Eindhoven's m.
    permanent m.
    resistive m.
    superconductive m.
    Walker's m.
magnetic
    artifical permanent m.
    m. circuit
    m. dipole
    m. disc
    m. domain
    m. field

magnetic (continued)
  m. field strength
  m. flux
  m. focal plane
  m. force
  m. gradient
  m. induction
  m. lines of force
  m. material
  m. moment
  m. nuclei
  m. permeability
  m. pole
  m. recording
  m. resonance imaging
  m. retentivity
  superconducting m.
magnetization
Magnevist contrast medium
magnification
malum coxae senilis
mamillary system
mammogram
mammography
mandible
manganese
mannitol
maplike
mask node subtraction
mass
  atomic m.
  intraluminal m.
  relativistic m.
Massiot polytome
mastogram
mastography
matrix mode
maxicamera
maxwellian distribution
Mayer's
  position
  view
mc., mCi–millicurie
μc., μCi–microcurie
McGregor's line
mean
  m. deviation

mean (continued)
  m. free path
  m. gonad dose
  m. life
media
  contrast m.
medial
mediastinal
"mediastinal crunch"
mediastinoscopy
mediastinum
medium
  contrast m.
Medx
  M. camera
  M. scanner
Meese's position
megavoltage
meglumine
  m. diatrizoate
  m. iodipamide
  m. iothalamate
mendelevium
Mercuhydrin
mercurihydroxypropane
mercury
mesenteric
  m. arteriography
mesentery
meson
metallic
metastable state
method
  Ball's m.
  Caldwell-Moloy m.
  Camp-Gianturco m.
  Cobb's m.
  Colcher-Sussman m.
  Dooley, Caldwell, and
    Glass m.
  Ferguson's m.
  Girout's m.
  Heublein's m.
  Monte Carlo m.
  Ottonello's m.
  parallax m.
  Parama's m.

method (continued)
    Pfeiffer-Comberg m.
    Sommer-Foegella m.
    Sweet's m.
    Thoms' m.
    Wolf's m.
    Zimmer's m.
methylcellulose gel
metoclopramide
metric
    m. system
metrizamide
    m.-assisted computed
        tomography
metrizoate sodium
metrizoic acid
metrosalpingography
metrotubography
Mev. – million electron volts
MHP – 1-mercuri-2-
    hydroxypropane
microangiogram
microcurie
microdosimetry
microembolism
microembolization
microfarad
micron
Micropaque contrast medium
microparticle
microradiogram
microradiography
microscopy
microsphere
Microtrast contrast medium
microtron
Miller-Abbott tube
Miller's position
milliamperage
milliampere-minute
milliampere-second
millicurie
    m.-hour
milliequivalent
milligamma
milliliter
millimicrocurie

millimicrogram
milliroentgen
millisecond
milliunit
millivolt
minification
minometer
MLD – median lethal dose
MLSI – multiple line scan
    imaging
MMFR – maximum
    midexpiratory flow rate
M-mode scanning
modulation
    amplitude m.
    brightness m.
    image m.
    object m.
    m. transfer function
molar volume
molecular
    m. vibrations
molecule
molybdenum
monitor
    beam m.
    radiation m.
monitoring
Monophen contrast medium
Monte Carlo method
mosaic
Mossbauer's spectrometer
mottled
MPD – maximum permissible
    dose
MRI – magnetic resonance
    imaging
MTF – modulation transfer
    function
mucosa
multicrystal camera
multigated
    m. angiography
    m. imaging
multilanigraph
multiplaner
    m. imaging

multiplaner (continued)
    m. scanning
multiple-nuclide
multiscaler
mutation
myelocisternoencephalography
myelogram
myelography
    opaque m.
Myodil contrast medium
Na atoms
nanocurie
nanogram
"napkin ring"
    "n.r." defect
    "n.r." lesion
narrow-beam half-thickness
nasion
nasopharyngography
National Council on Radiation
    Protection and
    Measurements
National Radiological
    Commission
National Radiological Protection
    Board
nc., nCi–nanocurie
NCRPM–National Council on
    Radiation Protection and
    Measurements
negatron
    n. emission
neodymium
Neo-Iopax contrast medium
neon
neostigmine
nephrogram
nephrography
nephropyelography
nephrosonography
nephrostogram
nephrotomogram
nephrotomography
    infusion n.
nephrourography
neptunium
neuroangiographic

neuroradiology
neuroroentgenography
neutrino
neutron
    epithermal n.
    fast n.
    intermediate n.
    n. number
    slow n.
    thermal n.
niche
nickel
niobium
Niopam contrast medium
nitrogen
nitrous oxide
NMR–nuclear magnetic
    resonance
nobelium
node
    lymph n's
    mesenteric n.
nodular
Nölke's position
nomogram
nonhomogeneous
nonlinearity
normalized plateau slope
Novopaque contrast medium
NRC–National Radiological
    Commission
    Nuclear Regulatory
    Commission
NRPB–National Radiological
    Protection Board
NSD–nominal single dose
nuchal
nuchofrontal
nuclear
    n. angiography
    n. cardiology
    n. decay
    n. disintegration
    n. emulsion
    n. energy
    n. fission
    n. force

nuclear (continued)
    n. fusion
    n. magnetic moments
    n. medicine
    n. imaging
    n. particle
    n. probe
    n. radiation
    n. reaction
    n. reactor
    n. relaxation
    n. scanner
    n. scanning
    n. scintigraphy
    n. signal
    n. spin
    n. structure
nuclear magnetic resonance
    n. m. r. images
    n. m. r. imaging
    n. m. r. Fourier
      transformation
    n. m. r. phantoms
    pulsed n. m. r.
    n. m. r. relaxation rate
      enhancement
    n. m. r. scanning
      sequences
    n. m. r. signal intensity
    n. m. r. spectra
    n. m. r. spectral
      parameters
    n. m. r. spectrometer
    n. m. r. spectroscopy
    n. m. r. spin warp method
    n. m. r. tomography
Nuclear Regulatory Commission
nuclease
nuclei
nucleide
nucleiform
nucleography
nucleoid
nucleoliform
nucleon
    n. number
nucleonics

nucleoprotein
nucleoreticulum
nucleoside
nucleotherapy
nucleotide
nucleus
nuclide
number
    atomic n.
    Avogadro's n.
    body atomic n.
    effective atomic n.
    Euler's n.
    mass n.
    nucleon n.
    n. profile
numo-. See words beginning
    pneumo-.
Nyegaard contrast medium
oblique
obliquity
obturator foramen
OCG–oral cholecystogram
OCR–optical character
    recognition
odontoid
Ohm's law
OIH–orthoidohippurate
oleic acid I 125
omentoportography
Omnipaque contrast medium
oncology
    radiation o.
opacification
opacified
opaque
operating voltage
Orabilex contrast medium
Oragrafin contrast medium
Oravue contrast medium
orbit
orbitography
ordography
orientation
Orthicon camera
orthodiagram
orthodiagraph

orthodiagraphy
orthodiascope
orthodiascopy
orthoiodohippurate
orthopantomography
orthoroentgenography
orthoskiagraph
orthovoltage
Osbil contrast medium
oscilloscope
osmium
osteoporosis
osteoscope
ostium
OTD – organ tolerance dose
Ottonello's method
overexposure
"overlap shadow"
overvoltage
oxidation
oxygen
^{32}P – radioactive phosphorus
PA – posteroanterior
packing fraction
PAH – para-aminohippurate
pair production
palatograph
palatography
palatomyograph
palladium
palliative
palmitate
palmitic acid
panagraphy
"pancake"
    "p." appearance
    "p." compression
pancreatogram
pancreatography
pangynecography
panography
Panorex
pantomographic
pantomography
    concentric p.
    eccentric p.

Pantopaque contrast medium
para-aminohippuric acid
parallax method
paramagnetic
Parama's method
parameter
parametric image
parenchyma
"parentheses-like" calcification
parent nuclide
parietography
particle
    viral p.
parturition
pastille radiometer
pathway
    Embden-Meyerhof
      glycolytic p.
pattern
    alveolar p.
    "broken bough" p.
    "butterfly" p.
    convolutional p.
    corkscrew p.
    cystic p.
    "fingerprint" p.
    "hair brush" p.
    "hanging fruit" p.
    haustral p.
    "herring-bone" p.
    honeycomb p.
    "mimosa" p.
    rugal p.
    solid p.
    start test p.
    three-dimensional
      physiologic flow p.
patulous
Pauli's exclusion principle
Pawlow's position
PC – pentose cycle
pc., pCi – picocurie
peak
    Bragg p.
Pearson's position
pectus excavatum

pedicle
PEEP – positive end-expiratory
  pressure
PEG – pneumoencephalography
peizoelectric
pelves
pelvicephalography
pelvicephatometry
pelvimetry
pelviography
pelvioradiography
pelvioscopy
pelviradiography
pelviroentgenography
pelvis (pelves)
pemphigus
penetration
    radiographic p.
penetrology
penetrometer
pentose cycle
penumbra
percussion
percutaneous
perfusion study
perinephric
peripheral
periphery
peristalsis
peristaltic
peritoneal fluid
peritoneography
permeability constant
perpendicular
pertechnetate
PET – positron emission
  tomography
petrous tips
PETT – positron emission
  transverse tomography
Pfeiffer-Comberg method
pharmacoradiology
pharyngoesophagraphy
pharyngography
phenolphthalein
phenolsulfonphthalein

phenoltetrachlorophthalein
phenomenon
    interference p.
    vacuum p.
phentetiothalein
phenylalanine
phenyldiphenyloxadiazole
phenyloxazolyl
phlebogram
phlebography
phlebolith
phonation
phosphate
phosphor
phosphorated
phosphorescence
phosphorus
phosphorus 32 diiso-
  fluorophosphate
Phospho-soda
photocathode
photodisintegration
photodisplay unit
photoelectric
    p. absorption
    p. effect
    p. interaction
photoelectron
photoflow
photofluorographic
photomicrograph
photomultiplier tube
photon
    Compton p.
    degraded p.
photoneutron
photonuclear
    p. effect
    p. reaction
photopeak
photorecording
photoroentgenography
photoscanner
photosensitivity
photosensitization
phototimer

phototube output circuit
picocurie
picture-frame-like
piezoelectric crystal
pig
Pigg-O-Stat immobilization
     device
pile
pinhole collimator
pion beam
Pirie transoral projection
piriform
pisiform
PIT – plasma iron turnover
pitchblende
Pitressin
pixel – picture element
placentography
Planck's
     constant
     quantum theory
plane
     coronal p.
     cross-sectional p.
     median-sagittal p.
planigram
planigraphy
plasma
plasmapheresis
plateau
platelets
platelike
platinum
plethysmography
     electrical impedance p.
pleura
pleural
     p. effusion
pleurography
pluridirectional tomography
plutonium
pneumarthrogram
pneumarthrography
pneumatogram
pneumatograph
pneumencephalography
pneumoalveolography

pneumoangiogram
pneumoangiography
pneumoarthrogram
pneumoarthrography
pneumocardiograph
pneumocardiography
pneumocystography
pneumocystotomography
pneumoencephalogram
pneumoencephalography
     cerebral p.
pneumoencephalomyelogram
pneumoencephalomyelography
pneumofasciogram
pneumogastrography
pneumogastroscopy
pneumogram
pneumography
     cerebral p.
     retroperitoneal p.
pneumogynogram
pneumomediastinogram
pneumomediastinography
pneumomyelography
pneumonograph
pneumonography
pneumoperitoneography
pneumoperitoneum
     diagnostic p.
pneumopyelogram
pneumopyelography
pneumoradiography
     retroperitoneal p.
pneumoretroperitoneum
pneumoroentgenogram
pneumoroentgenography
pneumothorax
     diagnostic p.
pneumotomography
pneumoventriculogram
pneumoventriculography
pocket chamber
Poisson distribution
"poker" spine
polarity
polonium
polycycloidal tomography

polymer
polyp
polytome
    Massiot p.
polytomogram
polytomography
polyvinylpyrrolidone
popcorn-like
POPOP – 1,4-bis-2-(5-
    phenyloxazolyl)-benzene
pork insulin
porous
portacamera
portography
portophlebography
portosplenography
portovenography
portwine marks
position
    abduction p.
    adduction p.
    Albers-Schönberg p.
    AP (anteroposterior) p.
    Béclére's p.
    Benassi's p.
    Blackett-Healy p.
    Broden's p.
    brow-down p.
    brow-up p.
    Caldwell's p.
    Camp-Coventry p.
    Cleaves' p.
    cross-table lateral p.
    decubitus p.
    erect p.
    eversion p.
    extension p.
    Feist-Mankin p.
    Fick's p.
    Fleischner's p.
    flexion p.
    Friedman's p.
    frog-leg p.
    Gaynor-Hart p.
    Grashey's p.
    Haas' p.
    Hickey's p.

position (continued)
    inlet p.
    inversion p.
    Isherwood's p.
    Johnson's p.
    Kurzbauer's p.
    Laquerrière-Pierquin p.
    Larkin's p.
    lateral p.
    Lawrence's p.
    Law's p.
    Leonard-George p.
    Lewis' p.
    Lilienfeld's p.
    Lindblom's p.
    Lorenz' p.
    Löw-Beer p.
    Mayer's p.
    Meese's p.
    Miller's p.
    Nölke's p.
    oblique p.
    PA (posteroanterior) p.
    Pawlow's p.
    Pearson's p.
    prone p.
    recumbent p.
    Schüller's p.
    semierect p.
    semirecumbent p.
    Settegast's p.
    Staunig's p.
    Stecher's p.
    Stenver's p.
    supine p.
    Tarrant's p.
    Taylor's p.
    Titterington's p.
    Towne's p.
    Trendelenburg's p.
    Twining's p.
    Wigby-Taylor p.
    Zanelli's p.
positrocephalogram
positron
    p.-coincidence
    p. decay

positronium
posteroanterior view
postirradiation
post release radiography
postvoid radiography
potassium
    p. perchlorate
potential
    p. difference
    p. gradient
Potter-Bucky
    diaphragm
    grid
PPD–phenyldiphenyloxadiazole
PPO–2,5-diphenyloxazole
Praestholm contrast medium
praseodymium
preamplifier
predetector
principle
    Fick's p.
    Pauli's exclusion p.
Priodax contrast medium
Pro-Banthine
probe
    fiberoptic p.
    scintillation p.
process
    bremsstrahlung p.
    neutron absorption p.
    spinous p.
    superior articulating p.
    transverse p.
processor
    array p.
projection
    anteroposterior lordotic p.
    apical lordotic p.
    axial p.
    axillary p.
    ball-catcher's p.
    basilar p.
    basovertical p.
    biplane p.
    blowout view p.
    Chassard-Lapiné p.
    cone-down p.

projection (continued)
    craniocaudad p.
    cross-sectional transverse p.
    dorsoplantar p.
    erect fluoro spot p.
    flexion, extension p.
    p. formula
    frontal p.
    half-axial p.
    inferior-superior p.
    inferior-superior tangential p.
    inferosuperior axial p.
    intraoral p.
    lateral oblique axial p.
    lateral transcranial p.
    lateral transfacial p.
    lateromedial oblique p.
    Lauenstein and Hickey p.
    L-5, S-1 p.
    lumbosacral p.
    medial oblique axial p.
    mediolateral p.
    navicular p.
    nuchofrontal p.
    oblique lateral p.
    parieto-orbital p.
    pillar p.
    Pirie transoral p.
    plantodorsal p.
    posteroanterior lordotic p.
    recumbent lateral p.
    Runström p.
    scaphoid p.
    semiaxial p.
    semiaxial anteroposterior p.
    semiaxial transcranial p.
    skyline p.
    stereo right lateral p.
    submentovertical axial p.
    "sunrise" p.
    superoinferior p.
    tangential p.
    Templeton and Zim carpal tunnel p.

projection (continued)
    transtabular AP (PA) p.
    transthoracic p.
    tunnel p.
    verticosubmental p.
    Waters' p.
promethium
pronate
pronation
prone
propagation
propantheline bromide
proportional counter
propyliodone
prostatography
Prostigmin
protactinium
protein
proton
protuberance
    external occipital p.
proximal
"pruned hilum"
psoas
PSP–phenolsulfonphthalein
ptosis
PTRA–percutaneous
    transluminal renal
    angioplasty
pubic rami
pubis (pubes)
pulmonary pedicle
pulse-height analyzer
punctate
PVP–polyvinylpyrrolidone
pyelofluoroscopy
pyelogram
    hydrated p.
    retrograde p.
pyelography
    drip infusion p.
    intravenous p.
    percutaneous antegrade p.
    retrograde p.
    washout p.
pyeloscopy
pyloric stenosis

pylorus
pyrogen
pyrogenic
quantification
quantitative
quantum (quanta)
    q. theory
quenching
R–roentgen
rabbit
racemose
rachitic
rad–radiation adsorbed dose
radian
radiant energy
radiation
    r. absorbed dose
    alpha r.
    annihilation r.
    background r.
    beta r.
    "braking" r.
    bremsstrahlung r.
    r. burn
    characteristic r.
    r. colitis
    corpuscular r.
    cosmic r.
    r. counter
    cyclotron r.
    r. dermatitis
    r. detector
    direct r.
    dose equivalent r.
    electromagnetic r.
    r. energy
    r. enteropathy
    r. equivalent man
    r. exposure
    gamma r.
    r. gastritis
    r. hepatitis
    infrared r.
    r. injury
    r. intensity
    interstitial r.
    ionization r.

radiation (continued)
    r. leakage
    man-made environmental
       r.
    Maxwell's theory of r.
    r. monitor
    monochromatic r.
    monoenergetic r.
    natural r.
    r. necrosis
    nuclear r.
    occupational r.
    optic r.
    r. osteitis
    photon theory of r.
    r. physics
    r. pneumonia
    r. pneumonitis
    primary r.
    r. protection
    recoil r.
    remnant r.
    scattered r.
    r. sickness
    specific r.
    spontaneous r.
    r. syndrome
    terrestrial r.
    r. therapy
    thermal r.
    ultraviolet r.
    r. warning symbol
    white r.
    r. window
radiation production
    Cerenkov r.p.
radiculopathy
radioactive
    r. decay
    r. disintegration
    r. effluents
    r. element
    r. equilibrium
    r. fallout
    r. gallium
    r. gases
    r. half-life

radioactive (continued)
    r. isotope
    r. nuclide
    r. series
    r. source
    r. thorium
radioactivity
radioactor
radioanaphylaxis
radioassay
radioautograph
radiobe
radiobioassay
radiobiological
radiobiologist
radiobiology
radiocalcium
radiocarbon
radiocardiogram
radiocardiography
radiochemical purity
radiochemistry
radiochemotherapy
radiochemy
radiocholecystography
radiochroism
radiochromatography
radiocinematograph
radiocolloid
radiocurable
radiode
radiodensity
radiodermatography
radiodiagnosis
radiodiagnostics
radiodiaphane
radioelectrocardiogram
radioelectrocardiograph
radioelectrocardiography
radioelement
radioencephalogram
radioencephalography
radiofluorine
radiofrequency
radiogallium
radiogenic
radiogold

radiogram
radiograph
    Code and Carlson r.
radiographic
    r. density
    r. effect
radiography
    biomedical r.
    body section r.
    pan-oral r.
    stereoscopic r.
radiohepatographic
radioimmunity
radioimmunoassay
radioimmunodiffusion
radioimmunoelectrophoresis
radioimmunoprecipitation
radioinduction
radioiodine
radioiron
radioisotope
radiokymography
radiolead
radiologic
radiological
radiologist
radiology
radiolucency
radiolucent
radiometallography
radiometer
    pastille r.
    photographic r.
radiometric
    r. analysis
radiomicrometer
radiomimetic
radion
radionitrogen
radionuclides. See also *Drugs
    and Chemistry* section.
    gamma emitting r's
    r. imaging
    r. kinetics
    r. purity
    r. scanning
radiopacity

radiopaque
radioparency
radioparent
radiopathology
radiopelvimetry
radiopharmaceutical
radiophosphorus
radiophotography
radiophylaxis
radiopotassium
radiopotentiation
radiopulmonography
radioreceptor
radioresistant
radioscope
radioscopy
radiosensitive
radiosensitivity
radiosodium
radiospirometry
radiostereoscopy
radiostrontium
radiosulfur
radiotellurium
radiotherapeutics
radiotherapy
    computerized r.
    interstitial r.
    intracavitary r.
radiothorium
radiotracer
radiotransparency
radiotransparent
radium
radius
    Bohr r.
radon
range
RAO – right anterior oblique
rate meter
ratio
    gyromagnetic r.
    target-to-nontarget r.
ray
    alpha r.
    beta r.
    cathode r.

ray (continued)
    central r.
    cosmic r.
    delta r.
    fluorescent r.
    gamma r.
    grenz r.
    infrared r.
    parallel r.
    roentgen r.
    secondary r.
    vertical r.
Raybar 75 contrast medium
Rayopak
Rayvist contrast medium
RBC's – red blood cells
RBL – Reid's base line
rd. – rutherford
reaction
    biomolecular r.
    thermonuclear r.
reactor
    nuclear r.
recanalization
recess
    azygoesophageal r.
    epitympanic r.
recovery time
recumbency
recumbent
redundancy
redundant
reformat
refractory
region of interest
Reid's base line
relativistic mass
REM – roentgen equivalent – man
REMP – roentgen equivalent –
    man period
renocystogram
Renografin contrast medium
renogram
renography
Reno-M-30 contrast medium
Reno-M-60 contrast medium
Reno-M-dip contrast medium

Renovist contrast medium
Renovue contrast medium
rentgen. See roentgen.
rentgenogram. See
    roentgenogram.
rentgenologe. See roentgenology.
rentgenologic. See roentgenologic.
REP – roentgen equivalent –
    physical
resin
resistive magnet
resolution
    spatial r.
resonance
    r. capture
    nuclear magnetic r.
resonant
reticular
reticulation
retrococcygeal
Retro-Conray contrast medium
retrograde
retroperitoneal
RF – radiofrequency
rhenium
rhodium
RIA – radioimmunoassay
ribose
ribosome
ribosyl
ribothymidine
ribulose
ring
    Cannon's r.
    "r. of bone"
Ring-McLean catheter
ripple voltage
R-meter
RNA – ribonucleic acid
roentgen
roentgenogram
roentgenography
roentgenologic
roentgenologist
roentgenology
rotography
roto-tomography

RP – retrograde pyelogram
RPM – rapid processing mode
    (par speed screens)
RPO – right posterior oblique
rubidium
ruga (rugae)
rugal pattern
Runström's
    projection
    view
RUQ – right upper quadrant
ruthenium
rutherford
s – screen containing cassette
sacrum
sagittal
saline solution
salpingography
Salpix contrast medium
Salyrgan
samarium
sarcoidosis
saturation current
Satvioni's cryptoscope
SBFT – small bowel follow-
    through
scale
    Bloch's s.
scaler
scalloped
scalloping
scan
    adrenal s.
    blood pool s.
    bone s.
    brain s.
    capillary blockade
      perfusion s.
    CT s.
    dynamic CT s.
    fluorescent s.
    hepatobiliary s.
    isotope bone s.
    liver/spleen s.
    multiple gated blood
      pool s.
    multislice full line s.

scan (continued)
    nongated CT s.
    perfusion lung s.
    renal s.
    salivary gland s.
    selective excitation line s.
scandium
scanner
    CT body s.
    General Electric CT/T7
      800 s.
    Medx s.
    neurodiagnostic s.
    nuclear s.
    radioisotope s.
    rectilinear s.
    supercam scintillation s.
    tomographic multiplane s.
    whole body s.
scanning
    A-mode (amplitude
      modulation) s.
    B-mode (brightness
      modulation) s.
    bone marrow s.
    brain s.
    cine CT s.
    compound s.
    contiguous s.
    full line s.
    gallium s.
    gamma s.
    infarct s.
    lacrimal s.
    line s.
    linear s.
    M-mode (time-motion) s.
    multiplanar s.
    nuclear s.
    perfusion s.
    point s.
    radioisotope s.
    radionuclide s.
    real-time s.
    renal s.
    rotate-rotate s.
    rotate-stationary s.

scanning (continued)
    sector s.
    sensitive point s.
    s. sequence
    single pass s.
    s. spot
    three-phase bone s.
    transverse s.
    water path s.
    whole body s.
scanography
    slit s.
    spot s.
scatter
    Compton s.
scattering
    Compton s.
    ultrasound s.
Schüller's position
scimitar
    s. shadow
    "s. sign"
    s. syndrome
scintiangiography
scintigram
scintigraphic
scintigraphy
    perfusion s.
    ventilation s.
scintillation
    s. camera
    s. probe
    s. scan
scintiphotograph
scintiphotography
scintiphotosplenoportography
scintiscan
scintiscanner
scintiview
scoliosis
Seidlitz powder test
Seldinger's catheterization
selenium
selenomethionine Se 75
self
    s.-absorption
    s.-quenched counter tube

self (continued)
    s.-scattering
sella turcica
senograph
senography
sensitivity
    plane s.
    point s.
sensitometer
    electroluminescent s.
sensitometry
Sephadex
sequential
sequestration
serialoangiocardiography
serialogram
serialograph
series
    gastrointestinal s.
    small bowel s.
seronegative
seropositive
serpiginous
Settegast's position
shadow
    psoas s.
shadowgram
shadowgraph
shadowgraphy
shaggy
shape
    "baseball bat" s.
    "cricket bat" s.
shield
    lead gonad s.
shielding
sialadenitis
sialadenography
sialoangiography
sialogram
sialography
sigmoidoscopy
sign
    air bronchogram s.
    air crescent s.
    air dome s.
    doughnut s.

sign (continued)
>   fat pad s.
>   meniscus s.
>   rim s.
>   silhouette s.
>   string s.
>   Westmark's s.

silhouette
silicon
silver
>   s. iodide

Simmons' catheter
Sinografin contrast medium
sinogram
sinography
sinti-. See words beginning
>   *scinti-*.

sinus
>   costophrenic s.
>   frontal s.
>   sphenoid s.

sinusography
>   cerebral s.

skeletal
skiagram
skiagraph
skiagraphy
Skiodan contrast medium
>   S. Acacia

"skip areas"
slice
>   CT s.
>   s. geometry
>   s. selection

slug
SNR – signal-to-noise ratio
sodium
>   s. bromide
>   s. chromate Cr 51
>   s. diatrizoate
>   s. iodide I 123, I 125, I 131
>   s. iodipamide
>   s. iodohippurate I 131
>   s. iodomethamate
>   s. iothalamate I 125
>   s. ipodate
>   s. methiodal

sodium (continued)
>   s. pertechnetate Tc 99m
>   s. phosphate P 32
>   s. radioiodide
>   s. rose bengal I 131
>   s. thorium tartrate
>   s. tyropanoate

solarization
solenoid
solid-state
>   s.-s. physics

solubilize
Solu-Biloptin contrast medium
soluble
solution
>   hundredth-normal s.
>   hypertonic s.
>   molal s.

Solutrast contrast medium
Sommer-Foegella method
sonar
sonarography
sonofluoroscope
sonofluoroscopy
sonogram
sonography
space
>   retroperitoneal s.
>   subarachnoid s.

spadelike
spallation
spatial
specific activity
speckled
SPECT – single photon emission
>   computed tomography

spectrometer
>   beta-ray s.
>   gamma-ray s.
>   mass s.
>   Mossbauer's s.
>   scintillation s.

spectrometry
>   pulse height s.

spectrophotofluorometer
spectrophotometer
>   absorption s.

spectrophotometry
spectroscope
spectroscopic
spectroscopy
spectrum
     chromatic s.
     electromagnetic s.
     thermal s.
     x-ray s.
sphere
spherical
spiculated
spindling
spine
     lumbar s.
     sacral s.
spin-echo imaging
spin-lattice relaxation time
spinogram
spinthariscope
spintherometer
spintometer
splenic flexure
splenography
splenoportogram
splenoportography
spot film
     s. f. device
     s. f. radiography
     s. f. study
star test pattern
Staunig's position
Stecher's position
Stenver's
     position
     view
stereocinefluorography
stereofluoroscopy
stereogram
stereograph
stereography
stereometry
stereomicroradiography
stereoradiogram
stereoradiograph
stereoradiography
stereoroentgenography
stereoroentgenometry

stereosalpingography
stereoscope
stereoscopic
stereoscopy
stereoskiagraphy
Steripaque-BR contrast
     medium
Steripaque-V contrast medium
straggling
stratigraphy
stress films
stridor
strontium (with yttrium 90)
     s. nitrate Sr 85
     s. Sr 87m
study
     air contrast s.
     barium meal s.
     blood flow s.
     cine s.
     double-contrast s.
     dual-contrast s.
     horizontal beam s.
     iodized oil s.
     lumbar, flexion, and
       extension s.
     motility s.
     perfusion s.
     perirenal air s.
     phonation s.
     quantitative regional
       lung
       function s.
     retrococcygeal air s.
     retroperitoneal air s.
     single-contrast s.
     spot film s.
     tracer s.
     ventilation s.
     videotape s.
     washout s.
subluxation
subpleural
subtraction
     s. angiography
     second order s.
     s. venography
succinic semialdehyde

sulcus
  s. for optic chiasm
  sigmoid s.
sulfur
superimposed
superimposition
superior
  s. ramus
supernumerary
supinate
supination
supine
suppuration
swallow
  barium s.
Swan-Ganz catheter
Sweet's method
Swiss Alps appearance
Sylvius' cistern
symmetrical
symphysis
  s. pubis
synchrotron
synthesis
system
  catenary s.
  linear s.
  mamillary s.
  metric s.
  three-compartment s.
  three-phase s.
  two-compartment s.
T – tesla
T_3 – triiodothyronine
tagged atom
tagging
tamponade
tannic acid
tantalum-178
target
Tarrant's position
tautography
Taylor's position
Tc – technetium
^{99m}Tc
  ^{99m}Tc-labeled 2,6-
    dimethylacetanilide
    iminodiacetic acid

^{99m}Tc (continued)
  ^{99m}Tc-labeled
    pyridoxylideneglutamate
    (PYG)
  ^{99m}Tc lidofenin
technetium
  t. 99m acetanili-
    doiminodiacetic acid
  t. 99m aggregated
    albumin kit
  t. 99m albumin
  t. 99m albumin
    microspheres kit
  t. 99m antimony
  t. 99m blood pool study
  t. 99m colloid
  t. 99m diethylenetriamine
    penta-acetic acid
  t. 99m 2,3-
    dimercaptosuccinic acid
  t. 99m etidronate sodium
    kit
  t. 99m ferric hydroxide
  t. 99m generator
  t. 99m glucoheptonate
  t. 99m HAM perfusion
    scan
  t. 99m imidodiphos-
    phonate
  t. 99m iminodiacetic acid
  t. 99m macroaggregates
  t. 99m medronate sodium
    kit
  t. 99m methylene
    diphosphonate
  t. 99m microspheres
  t. 99m pentetate sodium
    kit
  t. 99m pertechnetate
  t. 99m phosphate uptake
  t. 99m phytate
  t. 99m pyridoxy-
    lideneglutamate
  t. 99m pyrophosphate
  t. 99m radiopharma-
    ceutical
  t. 99m serum albumin
    kit

technetium (continued)
    t. 99m stannous
        pyrophosphate/
        polyphosphate kit
    t. 99m sulfur colloid
technique
    autoradiographic t.
    chromatographic-
        fluorometric t.
    Corbin t.
    drip infusion t.
    supervoltage t.
    Welin's t.
TED–threshold erythema dose
Telebrix contrast medium
telecardiogram
telecardiography
telecobolt
telefluoroscopy
telemetry
teleoroentgenogram
teleoroentgenography
Telepaque contrast medium
teleradiography
teleroentgenogram
teleroentgenography
teleroentgentherapy
teletherapy
tellurium
Templeton and Zim carpal
    tunnel projection
terbium
Teridax contrast medium
tesla
test
    chlormerodrin
        accumulation t.
    fat absorption t.
    gastrointestinal blood
        loss t.
    gastrointestinal protein
        loss t.
    positive washout t.
    radioimmunoprecipita-
        tion t.
    radioiodine t.
    Seidlitz powder t.

test (continued)
    string t.
    triiodothyronine red cell
        uptake t.
    triiodothyronine resin t.
    washout t.
testosterone
thallium
    t. 201 imaging
    t. myocardial scan
    t. perfusion scintigraphy
    t. 201 stress testing
thallous chloride Tl 201
theorem
    Bayes' t.
theory
    Planck's quantum t.
therapy
    beam t.
    deep roentgen ray t.
    megavolt t.
thermal neutrons
thermogram
thermograph
thermography
thermoluminescent
thermonuclear
thermovision
thiosemicarbazide
thiosemicarbazone
Thixokon contrast medium
Thoms' method
Thoreau's filter
thorium
    t. dioxide
Thorotrast contrast
    medium
Thorpe plastic lens
three-phase system
thulium
thumb-printing
thymidine
thyratron
thyroxine
Thyrx timer
Ti–titanium
time-activity curve

timer
    Thyrx t.
tin (with indium-113m)
titanium
Titterington's position
Tl – thallium
TLD – thermoluminescent
    dosimeter
    tumor lethal dose
TM – time motion
tomogram
tomograph
tomography
    axial transverse t.
    circular t.
    computed t.
    computer assisted t.
    computerized axial t.
    emission computed t.
    focal plane t.
    hypercycloidal t.
    linear t.
    longitudinal section t.
    metrizamide-assisted
      computed t.
    panoramic t.
    plesiosectional t.
    pluridirectional t.
    polycycloidal t.
    positron emission t.
    positron emission
      transverse t.
    quantitative computed t.
    radionuclide emission t.
    rotational t.
    simultaneous multifilm t.
    single photon emission
      computed t.
    skip t.
    transmission, computer-
      assisted t.
    transversal t.
    wide angle t.
tomolaryngography
tomoscopy
tortuous
tourniquet

Towne's
    position
    view
Townsend's avalanche
tracer
trachea
tracheobronchoscopy
transducer
    sector t.
transferrin
transformation
    fast-Fourier f.
transformer
    filament t.
    high-voltage t.
    ratio t.
    step-down t.
    step-up t.
transillumination
transmission electron microscopy
transmutation
transverse
    t. colon
    t. magnetization
tree
    tracheobronchial t.
Treitz
    ligament of T.
Trendelenburg's position
triangle
    Codman's t.
triangular
triangulation
trichloroacetic acid
triiodothyronine
triolein (glyceral trioleate) I 131
Triosil contrast medium
Triphasix generator
tritium
triton
trochanter
    greater t.
    lesser t.
TSC – technetium sulfur colloid
TTD – tissue tolerance dose
T-tube
    T-t. cholangiogram

T-tube (continued)
 T-t. cholangiography
tube
 Cantor's t.
 Dotter's t.
 Miller-Abbott t.
 photomultiplier t.
tungsten
Twining's position
tympanography
UGI–upper gastrointestinal
UIBC–unsaturated iron-binding
 capacity
ulceration
ultrasonogram
ultrasonograph
ultrasonographic
ultrasonography
 A-mode u.
ultrasonoscope
ultrasound
 Doppler u.
 real-time u.
ultraviolet
Umbradil contrast medium
undulating
unit
 Angstrom u.
 Hounsfield u.
unsaturated
 u. compounds
upper GI series
uptake
uranium
ureterocystography
ureterogram
ureterography
ureteropyelography
urethrocystogram
urethrocystography
urethrogram
 excretory u.
urethrography
Urografin contrast medium
urogram
 drip-infusion u.

urography
 excretory u.
 intravenous u.
 percutaneous antegrade u.
 retrograde u.
urokymography
Uromiro contrast medium
Uropac contrast medium
uroradiology
Uroselectan
Urovision contrast medium
uterography
uterosalpingogram
uterosalpingography
uterotubography
vaginogram
vaginography
vanadium
Van de Graeff generator
vascular
 v. groove
Vasidone contrast medium
vasography
Vasopressin
Vater
 ampulla of V.
VCG–vectocardiogram
 vectocardiography
VCUG–voiding
 cystourethrogram
vectocardiogram
vectocardiography
vector
velocity
Velpeau's axillary view
venacavogram
venacavography
venogram
venography
 limb v.
 peripheral v.
 selective v.
 splenoportal v.
ventriculogram
ventriculography
 cardiac v.
 cerebral v.

ventriculography (continued)
    contrast v.
    radionuclide v.
vermiform
vermography
vertebra
vesiculogram
    seminal v.
vesiculography
Victoreen dosimeter
videodensitometric
videodensitometry
videometry
view
    "ball catcher's" v.
    Chaussé's v.
    comparison v.
    coned-down v.
    decubitus v.
    dorsal v.
    frog-leg v.
    Hampton's v.
    kyphotic v.
    lateral v.
    lateral decubitus v.
    Law's v.
    lordotic v.
    Mayer's v.
    normal anteroposterior v.
    oblique v.
    overcouch v.
    panoramic v.
    pantomographic v.
    plantar v.
    posterior v.
    profile ray v.
    recumbent v.
    Runström's v.
    "scottie dog" v.
    scout v.
    skyline v.
    Stenver's v.
    stereoscopic v.
    stress v.
    submentovertical v.
    superoinferior v.
    "swimmer's v.

view (continued)
    tangential v.
    Towne's v.
    Velpeau's axillary v.
    Waters' v.
viscerography
viscus
visualization
    double-contrast v.
voltage
volume
    atomic v.
    v. imaging
    molar v.
volvulus
Von Sonnenberg's catheter
voxel – volume element
Walker's magnet
Waters'
    projection
    view
wave
    electromagnetic w.
wavelength
    Compton's w.
    de Broglie's w.
weight
    atomic w.
    w.-bearing
Welin's technique
Westmark's sign
whole-body counting
wide angle tomography
Wigby-Taylor position
Wilson chamber
Wisconsin kV p test cassette
wolfram
Wolf's method
Wood's lamp
X axis
Xe – xenon
xenon
    x. Xe 133
xerogram
xerography
xeromammography
xeroradiogram

xeroradiograph
xeroradiography
xerosialography
xerotomography
x-ray
Xu–X-unit
xylose
Y–yttrium
Y axis
Yb–ytterbium
ytterbium
      y. Yb pentetate sodium
yttrium

Zanelli's position
zero. See words beginning *xero-*.
zeugmatography
Zimmer's method
zinc
zirconium (with niobium-95)
zone plate
      Fresnel z.p.
zonogram
zonography
      stereoscopic z.
zwitterion

Respiratory System

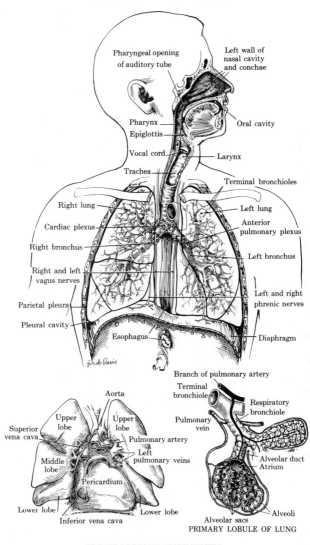

ORGANS OF RESPIRATORY SYSTEM

Pharyngeal opening of auditory tube

Left wall of nasal cavity and conchae

Pharynx

Oral cavity

Epiglottis

Vocal cord

Larynx

Trachea

Terminal bronchioles

Right lung

Left lung

Cardiac plexus

Anterior pulmonary plexus

Right bronchus

Left bronchus

Right and left vagus nerves

Parietal pleura

Left and right phrenic nerves

Pleural cavity

Esophagus

Diaphragm

Branch of pulmonary artery

Aorta

Terminal bronchiole

Upper lobe

Upper lobe

Respiratory bronchiole

Superior vena cava

Pulmonary vein

Pulmonary artery

Middle lobe

Left pulmonary veins

Alveolar duct Atrium

Pericardium

Lower lobe

Inferior vena cava

Lower lobe

Alveoli

Alveolar sacs

PRIMARY LOBULE OF LUNG

(Courtesy of Dorland's Illustrated Medical Dictionary, 27th ed. Plate 46. Philadelphia, W. B. Saunders Company, 1988).

Respiratory System

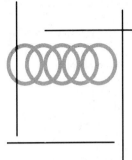

aasmus
Abelson's cannula
ABPA – allergic
    bronchopulmonary
    aspergillosis
Abraham's
    cannula
    sign
Abrams' needle
abscess
ACMI bronchoscope
acoustic reflection method
acquired immunodeficiency
    syndrome
acromegaly
Actinomyces
    A. bovis
actinomycosis
    pulmonary a.
Adair's forceps
adenocarcinoma
adenoma
    bronchial a.
    chondromatous a.
adenomatosis
    pulmonary a.
adenopathy
    hilar a.
adenosquamous
adenovirus
adhesions
    a. of pleura
adjuvant
Adson's test
aeration
aerobic capacity
aerodermectasia
aeroemphysema

aeroionotherapy
aeroporotomy
aerosol
AFB – acid-fast bacillus
agenesis
AIDS – acquired
    immunodeficiency
    syndrome. See *Immunology*
    section.
airway
    a. closure
    a. conductance
    a. epithelium
    a. heat loss
    a. hyperactivity
    a. narrowing
    a. osmolarity
    a. permeability
    a. reactivity
    a. receptors
    a. resistance
    a. tone
Albert's bronchoscope
alkalosis
    respiratory a.
Allen's test
allergic
allergy
Allis' forceps
alpha
    a. chain disease
alveobronchiolitis
alveolar
alveoli
    a. pulmonis
alveolitis
    diffuse sclerosing a.
alveolobronchogram

alveolocapillary
alveolus
Ambu bag
amebiasis
    pulmonary a.
American Thoracic Society
amyloidosis
anaerobiosis
anapnoic
anapnotherapy
Andrews-Pynchon tube
Andrews' retractor
anesthesia. See *General Surgical Terms* section.
aneurysm
    mycotic a.
angiogram
angiography
    pulmonary a.
angioimmunoblastic
    a. lymphadenopathy
angiokeratoma
    a. corporis diffusum
angiotensin
anomaly
    Freund's a.
antagonist(s)
anthracosilicosis
anthracosis
anthropotoxin
antiasthma
antibody
    monoclonal a's
antigen(s)
aorta
    retroesophageal a.
A&P – auscultation and percussion
apex
apical
apices
apicolysis
apnea
    deglutition a.
    obstructive sleep a.
    traumatic a.
apneic

apneumatosis
apneumia
apneusis
apparatus
    Fell-O'Dwyer a.
applicator
    Plummer-Vinson radium a.
arch
    aortic a.
arcus
    a. costarum
ARD – acute respiratory disease
area
    Krönig's a.
argon
Argyle chest tube
Arloing-Courmont test
Arneth's syndrome
artery
    pulmonary a.
    subclavian a.
arytenoid
asbestos
asbestosis
aspergillosis
    pulmonary a.
Aspergillus
asphyxia
aspiration
aspirator
    Broyles' a.
Assmann's
    focus
    infiltrate
asthma
    allergic a.
    alveolar a.
    bronchial a.
    cotton dust a.
    emphysematous a.
    essential a.
    grinders' a.
    intrinsic a.
    millers' a.
    miners' a.
    occupational a.

asthma (continued)
    potters' a.
    steam-fitters' a.
    stone-strippers' a.
asthmatic
atelectasis
    absorption a.
    compression a.
    lobar a.
    lobular a.
    obstructive a.
    relaxation a.
    resorption a.
    rounded a.
    secondary a.
    segmental a.
atelectatic
Atkins-Cannard tube
Atlee's clamp
atmograph
atmotherapy
atresia
atrial
atrium
    pulmonary a.
atrophy
    senile a. of lung
auscultation
Ayerza's
    disease
    syndrome
azoospermia
azygography
azygos
Babcock's forceps
BAC–bronchioloalveolar
    adenocarcinoma
Baccelli's sign
bacilli
bacillus
    Friedländer's b.
    rhinoscleroma b.
Bacillus
    B. pneumoniae
    B. subtilis
bacterial
Bacteroides

bag
    Ambu b.
bagassosis
Bailey's catheter
Balme's cough
Bard's syndrome
baritosis
Bársony-Polgár syndrome
Beatty-Bright friction sound
Behçet's syndrome
Belsey's repair
Benedict-Roth spirometer
Benedict's
    gastroscope
    retractor
berylliosis
Bethea's sign
Bethune's tourniquet
Biermer's change
bifurcatio
    b. tracheae
bifurcation
bilharziasis
bimodal therapy
biomarker
biopsy
    scalene lymph node b.
Biot's
    breathing
    respiration
bistoury
    Jackson's b.
Blakemore's tube
Blalock-Taussig operation
blastomycosis
bleb
    subpleural b.
blennothorax
"blue bloaters"
Blumenau's test
Bohr isopleth method
Boies' forceps
bolus
BOOP–bronchiolitis obliterans
    organizing pneumonia
Bornholm's disease
Boros' esophagoscope

botulism
bougie
    Hurst's b.
    Jackson's b.
    Trousseau b.
BP—bronchopleural
brachytherapy
bradykinin
Bragg-Paul pulsator
breathing
    Biot's b.
    bronchial b.
    frog b.
    glossopharyngeal b.
    intermittent positive-
      pressure b.
Brewster's retractor
Broch's syndrome
bronchadenitis
bronchi
    hyparterial b.
    lobar b.
    b. lobares
    segmental b.
    b. segmentales
bronchia
bronchial
    b. adenoma
    b. brushing
    b. challenge test
    b. circulation
    b. lavage
    b. obstruction
    b. reactivity
    b. stenosis
bronchiectasis
    capillary b.
    chemical b.
    cylindrical b.
    cystic b.
    follicular b.
    pseudocylindrical b.
    saccular b.
bronchiectatic
bronchiloquy
bronchiocele
bronchiocrisis

bronchiolalveolar
bronchiolar
    b. lavage
    b. stenoses
bronchiole
    alveolar b.
    lobular b.
    respiratory b's
    terminal b's
bronchiolectasis
bronchioli respiratorii
bronchiolitis
    acute obliterating b.
    b. exudativa
    b. fibrosa obliterans
    vesicular b.
    viral b.
bronchiolus
bronchiospasm
bronchitic
bronchitis
    arachidic b.
    Castellani's b.
    catarrhal b.
    cheesy b.
    chronic b.
    croupous b.
    epidemic capillary b.
    ether b.
    exudative b.
    fibrinous b.
    hemorrhagic b.
    infectious asthmatic b.
    mechanic b.
    membranous b.
    b. obliterans
    phthinoid b.
    plastic b.
    polypoid b.
    productive b.
    pseudomembranous b.
    putrid b.
    secondary b.
    staphylococcal b.
    streptococcal b.
    suffocative b.
    verminous b.

bronchitis (continued)
    vesicular b.
bronchium
bronchoadenitis
bronchoalveolar
bronchoalveolitis
bronchoaspergillosis
bronchobiliary
bronchoblastomycosis
bronchoblennorrhea
bronchocandidiasis
bronchocavernous
bronchocele
bronchocentric
    b. granulomatosis
bronchocephalitis
bronchoclysis
bronchoconstrictor
bronchodilatation
bronchodilation
bronchodilator
bronchoesophageal
bronchoesophagology
bronchoesophagoscopy
bronchogenic
bronchogram
bronchography
broncholith
broncholithiasis
bronchologic
bronchology
bronchomalacia
bronchomotor
bronchomycosis
bronchonocardiosis
broncho-oidiosis
bronchopathy
bronchophony
    pectoriloquous b.
    sniffling b.
    whispered b.
bronchoplasty
bronchoplegia
bronchopleural
bronchopleuropneumonia
bronchopneumonia
bronchopneumonitis

bronchopneumopathy
bronchopulmonary
bronchoradiography
bronchorrhagia
bronchorraphy
bronchorrhea
bronchoscope
    ACMI b.
    Albert's b.
    Broyles' b.
    Bruening's b.
    Chevalier Jackson b.
    coagulation b.
    costophrenic b.
    Davis' b.
    double-channel irrigating
      b.
    Emerson's b.
    fiberoptic b.
    Foregger's b.
    Haslinger's b.
    Holinger-Jackson b.
    Holinger's b.
    hook-on b.
    Jackson's b.
    Jesberg's b.
    Kernan-Jackson b.
    Michelson's b.
    Moersch's b.
    Negus' b.
    Overholt-Jackson b.
    Pilling's b.
    Riecker's b.
    Safar's b.
    Staple's b.
    Storz's b.
    telescope b.
    Tucker's b.
    ventilation b.
    Waterman's b.
    Yankauer's b.
bronchoscopic
bronchoscopy
bronchosinusitis
bronchospasm
bronchospirochetosis
bronchospirography

bronchospirometer
bronchospirometry
bronchostaxis
bronchostenosis
bronchostomy
bronchotetany
bronchotome
bronchotomy
bronchotracheal
bronchotyphoid
bronchotyphus
bronchovesicular
bronchus
    apical b.
    cardiac b.
    eparterial b.
    lingular b.
    lobar b.
    main stem b.
    b. principalis dexter
    b. principalis sinister
    stem b.
    tracheal b.
brong-. See words beginning
    bronch-.
Broyles'
    aspirator
    bronchoscope
    dilator
    esophagoscope
    forceps
    telescope
    tube
brucella
Bruening's
    bronchoscope
    esophagoscope
    forceps
bruit
    b. d'airain (brwe da ra)
    b. de bois (brwe duh bwah)
    b. de craquement (brwe
      duh krak maw)
    b. de cuir neuf (brwe duh
      kwer nuf)
    b. de frolement (brwe
      duh frol maw)

bruit (continued)
    b. de grelot (brwe duh
      gruh lo)
    b. de pot fêlé (brwe duh
      po fe la)
brwe. See *bruit*.
Buhl's desquamative pneumonia
bulbospinal tract
bulla (bullae)
    emphysematous b.
Burghart's symptom
button
    Moore's tracheostomy b's
byssinosis
calcicosilicosis
calcicosis
calcification
cancrocirrhosis
Candida
    C. albicans
candidiasis
cannula
    Abelson's c.
    Abraham's c.
    Pritchard's c.
    Rockey's c.
cannulation
capillary
Caplan's syndrome
Carabelli's tube
carcinoembryonic
carcinogen
carcinoid
carcinoma
    alveolar cell c.
    anaplastic c.
    bronchiolar c.
    bronchogenic c.
    epidermoid c.
    squamous cell c.
carcinomatosis
carcinomatous
cardia
    incompetent c.
cardiopulmonary
carina
    c. of trachea

Carlens'
    catheter
    mediastinoscope
carotid
Carswell's grapes
cartilage
    cricoid c.
caseation
Casoni's test
Castellani's bronchitis
catheter
    Bailey's c.
    Carlens' c.
    Lloyd's c.
    Metras' c.
    Thompson's c.
    Zavod's c.
caval
cavernoscopy
cavernostomy
cavernous
cavitary
cavitation
cavum
CEA – carcinoembryonic antigen
Cegka's sign
Celestin's tube
cell
    ciliated c.
    clonogenic c.
    dust c.
    endocrine c.
    Langhans' c.
    metaplastic c.
    mucous c.
    stem c.
chalicosis
change
    Biermer's c.
    Gerhardt's c. of sound
Chaussier's tube
chemotherapy
Chevalier Jackson
    bronchoscope
    esophagoscope
    tube
Cheyne-Stokes respiration

cholesterohydrothorax
chondroadenoma
chondroma
chylomediastinum
chylopleura
chylopneumothorax
chylorrhea
chylothorax
cinebronchogram
cineradiography
circadian rhythm
circumscribed
clamp
    Atlee's c.
    Davidson's c.
    Hudson's c.
    Kantrowicz's c.
    Kapp-Beck c.
    Kinsella-Buie c.
    Lees' c.
    Mueller's c.
    Price-Thomas c.
    Ralks' c.
    Rockey's c.
    Rubin's c.
    Sarot's c.
    Thomson's c.
classification
clavicle
clavicular
clavipectoral
coagulopathy
coalescence
coarctation
Coccidioides
    C. immitis
coccidioidomycosis
coin lesion
collagen
collapse
    c. of the lung
collapsotherapy
Collins' respirometer-spirometer
colloid
congestion
    pleuropulmonary c.
coniosporosis

coniotoxicosis
COPD – chronic obstructive
    pulmonary disease
Cope's needle
cor
       c. pulmonale
Cordes' forceps
core vesicles
Corrigan's
       pneumonia
       respiration
corticosteroid
Corynebacterium
costa
costal
costectomy
costophrenic
costopleural
costopneumopexy
costovertebral
cough
       Balme's c.
       barking c.
       compression c.
       extrapulmonary c.
       mechanical c.
       minute gun c.
       Morton's c.
       productive c.
       reflex c.
       c. response
       Sydenham's c.
       tea taster's c.
       c. threshold
       trigeminal c.
       whooping c.
       winter c.
Coxsackie virus
CPAP – continuous positive
    airway pressure
CPR – cardiopulmonary
    resuscitation
Crafoord's
       forceps
       scissors
Craig's test
creatine kinase

crepitant
cricoid
cricopharyngeus
cricotracheotomy
croup
croupette
croupy
crus (crura)
cryoglobulinemia
cryptococcosis
Cryptococcus
       C. neoformans
cryptogenic
CT – computed tomography
cupula
       c. of pleura
curse
       Ondine's c.
cutaneous
CVA – costovertebral angle
cyanosis
       pulmonary c.
cyst
       bronchogenic c.
       dermoid c.
       enteric c.
       neurenteric c.
       pericardial c.
       thymic c.
cystic
       c. firbrosis
cytogenic
cytology
cytomegalovirus
cytoskeletal
D'Amato's sign
Daniel's operation
Darling's disease
Davidson's clamp
Davis' bronchoscope
Debove's membrane
decannulation
decarbonization
décollement
decompression sickness
decortication
       d. of lung

deficiency
  alpha-1-antitrypsin d.
degeneration
  cerebellar d.
  trabecular d.
Delmege's sign
Delorme's operation
density
  conglomerate d.
Depaul's tube
dermatomyositis
Desnos'
  disease
  pneumonia
desquamative
DeVilbiss nebulizer
dextrocardia
diaphragm
diaphragmatic
  d. excursion
  d. pacing
  d. paralysis
diffusion
  d. components
  d. limitation
dilator
  Broyles' d.
  Einhorn's d.
  Jackson-Trousseau d.
  Jackson's d.
  Laborde's d.
  Patton's d.
  Plummer's d.
  Plummer-Vinson d.
  Sippy's d.
  Steele's d.
  Trousseau-Jackson d.
  Trousseau's d.
diminution
DIP–desquamative interstitial
  pneumonitis
diphtheria
Diplococcus
  D. pneumoniae
discission
  d. of pleura

disease
  alpha-chain d.
  Ayerza's d.
  black lung d.
  Bornholm's d.
  brown lung d.
  Darling's d.
  Desnos' d.
  Fabry's d.
  farmer's lung d.
  Gaucher's d.
  grinder's d.
  Hamman's d.
  Hodgkin's d.
  hyaline membrane d.
  Kartagener's d.
  Löffler's d.
  Lucas-Championnière's d.
  pigeon breeder's d.
  Pompe's d.
  pulmonary embolic d.
  Shaver's d.
  silo filler's d.
  Takayasu's d.
  Thomsen's d.
  Whipple's d.
  Woillez's d.
dissector
  Lynch's d.
diuretic
diverticulum
  pharyngoesophageal d.
  Rokitansky's d.
  supradiaphragmatic d.
  Zenker's d.
Douglas' bag spirometer
drainage system(s)
  closed water seal d.s.
  continuous suction d.s.
  Glover's d.s.
  Monaldi's d.s.
  postural d.s.
  redivac d.s.
  Snyder's surgivac d.s.
  sump d.s.
  surgivac suction d.s.
  three-bottle d.s.

drainage system(s) (continued)
    tidal d.s.
    two-bottle d.s.
    underwater seal d.s.
    vacuum d.s.
    waterseal d.s.
Drinker's respirator
drugs. See *Drugs and Chemistry*
    section.
Duchenne's muscular dystrophy
Duguet's siphon
Durham's tube
Duval-Crile forceps
dysphagia
dyspnea
    expiratory d.
    inspiratory d.
    nocturnal d.
    nonexpansional d.
    orthostatic d.
    Traube's d.
dyspneic
dystrophy
    Duchenne's muscular d.
dysynapsis
Eaton agent pneumonia
Eaton-Lambert syndrome
echocardiography
ECHO virus
edema
    pulmonary e.
    vernal e
Eder-Hufford esophagoscope
effect
    "horse-race" e.
effusion
    pleural e.
EGF – epidermal growth factor
EGL – eosinophilic granuloma of
    the lung
egophony
EIAL – exercise induced airflow
    limitation
Einhorn's dilator
Eisenmenger's syndrome
electrocardiogram
electrodiagnostic

electrophrenic
elevator
    Jackson's e.
Ellis' sign
Eloesser's
    flap
    operation
EM – electron microscopy
embolism (emboli)
    pulmonary e.
Emerson's bronchoscope
emphysema
    alveolar e.
    atrophic e.
    bullous e.
    centrilobular e.
    compensatory e.
    cystic e.
    diffuse e.
    false e.
    focal-dust e.
    gangrenous e.
    generalized e.
    glass blower's e.
    hypertrophic e.
    hypoplastic e.
    idiopathic unilobar e.
    interlobular e.
    interstitial e.
    Jenner's e.
    lobar e.
    loculated e.
    mediastinal e.
    obstructive e.
    panacinar e.
    panlobular e.
    paracicatricial e.
    paraseptal e.
    pulmonary e.
    senile e.
    small-lunged e.
    subcutaneous e.
    subfascial e.
    surgical e.
    traumatic e.
    unilateral e.
    vesicular e.

emphysematous
empyema
    e. benignum
    interlobar e.
    metapneumonic e.
    pneumococcal e.
    putrid e.
    sacculated e.
    streptococcal e.
    synpneumonic e.
    thoracic e.
    tuberculous e.
empyemic
encephalitis
endobronchial
endobronchitis
endorphin
endoscopic
endoscopy
endothelial
endotracheal
endotracheitis
enzyme
eosinophilia
eosinophilic
eparterial
epicardia
epidermal
epidermoid
epiglottis
epithelial
equation
    Henderson-Hasselbalch e.
Equen's magnet
Erich's forceps
ERV – expiratory reserve volume
Escherichia
    E. coli
Escherich's test
esofa-. See words beginning
    esopha-.
esophagalgia
esophageal
esophagectasia
esophagectomy
esophagism
    hiatal e.

esophagitis
    reflux e.
esophagocele
esophagocologastrostomy
esophagoduodenostomy
esophagodynia
esophagoenterostomy
esophagofundopexy
esophagogastrectomy
esophagogastroanastomosis
esophagogastroplasty
esophagogastroscopy
esophagogastrostomy
esophagogram
esophagography
esophagojejunogastrostomosis
esophagojejunostomy
esophagolaryngectomy
esophagomalacia
esophagometer
esophagomycosis
esophagomyotomy
esophagopharynx
esophagoplasty
esophagoplication
esophagoptosis
esophagosalivation
esophagoscope
    Boros' e.
    Broyles' e.
    Bruening's e.
    Chevalier Jackson e.
    Eder-Hufford e.
    Haslinger's tracheo-
      broncho e.
    Holinger's e.
    Jackson's e.
    Jesberg's e.
    Lell's e.
    Moersch's e.
    Mosher's e.
    Moure's e.
    Roberts' e.
    Schindler's e.
    Tucker's e.
    Yankauer's e.
esophagoscopy

esophagospasm
esophagostenosis
esophagostoma
esophagostomy
esophagotome
esophagotomy
esophagus
Estlander's operation
eupnea
evagination
eventration
    diaphragmatic e.
EVLW – extravascular lung water
Ewart's sign
expansion
expectorant
expectoration
expiration
expiratory
exsufflation
exsufflator
extracellular
extrapulmonary
extrathoracic
extratracheal
extravascular
Fabry's disease
faringo-. See words beginning
   pharyngo-.
farinjeal. See *pharyngeal.*
farinks. See *pharynx.*
Fauvel's granules
FEF – forced expiratory flow
Fell-O'Dwyer apparatus
FET – forced expiratory time
FEV – forced expiratory
   volume
fever
    Q f. (Q. for query)
    zinc fume f.
fiberoptic
fiberscope
    Hirschowitz's
      gastroduodenal f.
fibrocystic
fibrogastroscopy
fibroleiomyomatosis

fibroma
    f. of lung
fibroplasia
    retrolental f.
fibrosarcoma
fibrosing
fibrosis
    cystic f.
    diffuse interstitial
      pulmonary f.
    idiopathic f.
    interstitial f.
    mediastinal f.
    pulmonary f.
fibrothorax
fibrotic
fibrous
field
    Krönig's f.
FIF – forced inspiratory flow
Finochietto's forceps
Fischer's needle
fissure
    f. of lung
fistula
    bronchocutaneous f.
    bronchopleural f.
    esophagobronchial f.
    pulmonary arteriovenous
      f.
    tracheal f.
    tracheoesophageal f.
flap
    Eloesser's f.
flem. See *phlegm.*
Floyd's needle
fluoroscopy
flutter
    mediastinal f.
focus
    Assmann's f.
foramen
    f. ovale basis cranii
    f. ovale ossis sphenoidalis
forceps
    Adair's f.
    Allis' f.

forceps (continued)
    Babcock's f.
    Boies' f.
    Broyles' f.
    Bruening's f.
    Cordes' f.
    Crafoord's f.
    Duval-Crile f.
    Erich's f.
    Finochietto's f.
    Fraenkel's f.
    Harrington-Mayo f.
    Holinger's f.
    Jackson's f.
    Johnson's f.
    Julian's f.
    Kahler's f.
    Killian's f.
    Kocher's f.
    Kolb's f.
    Krause's f.
    Leyro-Diaz f.
    Lovelace's f.
    Lynch's f.
    Mayo-Russian f.
    Moersch's f.
    Myerson's f.
    Nelson's f.
    New's f.
    Patterson's f.
    Pennington's f.
    Price-Thomas f.
    Roberts' f.
    Rockey's f.
    Russian f.
    Sam Roberts f.
    Sarot's f.
    Scheinmann's f.
    Seiffert's f.
    Tobold-Fauvel f.
    Tuttle's f.
    Yankauer-Little f.
Foregger's bronchoscope
Forlanini's treatment
fossa
    supraclavicular f.
Fowler's operation

Fraenkel's forceps
FRC–functional residual
    capacity
Frederick's needle
fremitus
    bronchial f.
    pleural f.
    rhonchal f.
    tactile f.
    tussive f.
fren-. See words beginning *phren-.*
Freund's anomaly
Friedländer's
    bacillus pneumonia
    pneumobacillus
    pneumonia
Friedreich's sign
Friedrich's operation
furrow
    Schmorl's f.
FVC–forced vital capacity
Gabriel Tucker tube
gallium scan
gamma camera
gangrene
    g. of lung
gastrocamera
    Olympus model GTF-A g.
gastroesophageal
    g. reflux
gastroscope
    Benedict's g.
Gaucher's disease
geotrichosis
Gerhardt's change of sound
Ghon tubercle
Gibson's rule
glanders
    g. of lung
glass blower's emphysema
Glenn's operation
glomectomy
glomus
glossopharyngeal
    g. breathing
    g. nerve
glottis

Glover's drainage system
goiter
Goldstein's hemoptysis
Goodpasture's syndrome
granule
    Fauvel's g's
granuloma
    eosinophilic g.
granulomatosis
    lymphomatoid g.
    pulmonary g.
    sarcoid g.
    Wegener's g.
granulomatous
grape
    Carswell's g's
graphite
Guillain-Barré syndrome
Guisez's tube
Haemophilus
    H. influenzae
    H. pertussis
Haight's retractor
hamartoma
    intrapulmonary h.
    h. of lung
Hamburger's test
Hamman-Rich syndrome
Hamman's
    disease
    sign
Harrington-Mayo forceps
Haslinger's
    bronchoscope
    tracheo-
        bronchoesophagoscope
hay fever
Heaf test
heaves
Hccht's pneumonia
Heimlich's maneuver
helium
    h. dilution method
    h. equilibration time
    h. washout
hemangioendothelioma
hemangioma

hemangiomatosis
hemibody
hemidiaphragm
hemiplegia
hemithorax
hemodynamic
hemophilia
Hemophilus. See *Haemophilus.*
hemopneumothorax
hemoptysis
    endemic h.
    Goldstein's h.
    Manson's h.
    parasitic h.
hemorrhage
hemosiderosis
    idiopathic pulmonary h.
hemothorax
Henderson-Hasselbalch
    equation
hepatic
hepatitis B
Hering-Breuer reflex
Hermansky-Pudlak syndrome
hernia
    diaphragmatic h.
    hiatal h.
    hiatus h.
    h. of lung
hernial
herpes
    h. zoster
hiatus
    esophageal h.
hibernoma
hiccup
hilar
hilum
hilus
    h. pulmonis
Himmelstein's valvulotome
Hirschowitz's gastroduodenal
    fiberscope
Hirtz's rale
histamine
    h. challenge
histiocytoma

histiocytosis
  h. X
Histoplasma
  H. capsulatum
histoplasmosis
Hitzenberg's test
Hodgkin's disease
Holinger-Jackson bronchoscope
Holinger's
  bronchoscope
  esophagoscope
  forceps
  laryngoscope
  telescope
  tube
hook
  New's h.
Hoover's sign
Hopp's laryngoscope
Horner's syndrome
"horse-race" effect
Hudson's clamp
Hurst's bougie
Hurwitz's trocar
hyalinization
hydropneumothorax
hydrops
  h. of pleura
hydrothorax
  chylous h.
hygroma
hyparterial
hyperaldosteronism
hyperbaric chamber
hypercalcemia
hypercapnia
hyperinflation
hyperlipidemia
hyperlucency
hyperlucent
hyperplasia
hyperresonance
hypersecretion
hypertension
  pulmonary h.
hypertrophy
hyperventilation

hypogammaglobulinemia
hypophosphatemia
hypoventiliation
hypoxemia
hypoxia
hypoxic
IC – inspiratory capacity
idiopathic
I/E – inspiratory-expiratory ratio
immotile cilia syndrome
immunity
immunoglobulin
  A (IgA)
  D (IgD)
  E (IgE)
  G (IgG)
  M (IgM)
immunohistochemistry
immunotherapy
impaction
  mucoid i.
impedance
impressio
  i. cardiaca pulmonis
IMV – intermittent mandatory
  ventilation
incarcerated
incision. See *General Surgical
  Terms* section.
infarction
  pulmonary i.
infectious
  i. mononucleosis
infiltrate
  Assmann's i.
infiltration
inflammation
inflation
influenza
infrapulmonic
INH – isoniazid
inhalant
  antifoaming i.
inhalation
inhaler
inspiration
inspiratory

inspissated
insufficiency
    pulmonary i.
insufflation
    endotracheal i.
intercostal
interlobar
intermedius
interstitial
intrabronchial
intracardiac
intracavitary
intracellular
intractable
intrapleural
intrapulmonary
intrathoracic
intratracheal
intubation
    endotracheal i.
invasive
ionizing
ions
IPPB – intermittent positive
    pressure breathing
IPPO – intermittent positive
    pressure inflation with
    oxygen
irradiation
isotope
    radioactive i.
isovolume
    i. pressure
isthmus
    Krönig's i.
IT – inhalation test
    inhalation therapy
    intratracheal tube
Jackson's
    bistoury
    bougie
    bronchoscope
    dilator
    elevator
    esophagoscope
    forceps
    laryngoscope

Jackson's (continued)
    operation
    retractor
    scalpel
    scissors
    tenaculum
    tube
Jackson-Trousseau dilator
Jacobaeus' operation
jade workers
Jenner's emphysema
Jesberg's
    bronchoscope
    esophagoscope
Johnson's forceps
jugular
Julian's forceps
Jürgensen's sign
jute workers
Kahler's forceps
Kantrowicz's clamp
Kaplan's needle
Kapp-Beck clamp
Kartagener's
    disease
    syndrome
    triad
Kaufman's pneumonia
kemotherapy. See chemotherapy.
Kernan-Jackson bronchoscope
Killian's
    forceps
    tubes
kilo-. See words beginning chylo-.
Kinsella-Buie clamp
Kistner's tube
Klebsiella
    K. pneumoniae
knife
    Lynch's k.
Kocher's forceps
Kohn's pore
Kolb's forceps
kondro-. See words beginning
    chondro-.
Krause's forceps
krico. See words beginning crico-.

Krogh's apparatus spirometer
Krönig's
    area
    field
    isthmus
    percussion
Kussmaul-Kien respiration
Kussmaul's
    respiration
    sign
Kveim test
kyphoscoliosis
Laborde's dilator
Laennec's
    pearls
    sign
Langhans' cells
Lanz's tube
laparothoracoscopy
Laplace's law
laringo-. See words beginning
    laryngo-.
larinjeal. See *laryngeal.*
larinks. See *larynx.*
laryngeal
laryngitis
laryngopharyngitis
laryngopharynx
laryngoscope
    Holinger's l.
    Hopp's l.
    Jackson's l.
    Lewy's l.
    Welch-Allyn l.
laryngoscopy
laryngospasm
laryngotomy
laryngotracheal
laryngotracheitis
laryngotracheobronchitis
laryngotracheobronchoscopy
laryngotracheoscopy
laryngotracheotomy
larynx
laser
Lautier's test
lavage

law
    Laplace's l.
Lee's clamp
Legionnaire's pneumonia
Legroux's remission
leiomyoma
Leitner's syndrome
Lell's esophagoscope
Lennarson's tube
Lepley-Ernst tube
leptomeningeal
leptospirosis
Leredde's syndrome
lesion
    coin l.
leukemia
leukopenia
Lewis' tube
Lewy-Rubin needle
Lewy's laryngoscope
Leyro-Diaz forceps
Lignières' test
Linguatula
lingula
    l. pulmonis sinistri
lingulectomy
Linton's tube
LIP – lymphocytic interstitial
    pneumonitis
lipoma
LL – left lung
    lower lobe
LLL – left lower lobe
Lloyd's catheter
lobar
lobectomy
lobitis
lobostomy
loculated
Löffler's
    disease
    pneumonia
    syndrome
Lore-Lawrence tube
Louisiana pneumonia
Lovelace's forceps
Lowenstein's medium

LTB–laryngotracheobronchitis
Lucas-Championnière disease
Luer's tube
Lukens' retractor
LUL–left upper lobe
lung
    arc-welder l.
    artificial l.
    bird-breeder's l.
    black l.
    brown l.
    cardiac l.
    coalminer's l.
    drowned l.
    eosinophilic l.
    farmer's l.
    fibroid l.
    harvester's l.
    honeycomb l.
    hyperlucent l.
    iron l.
    masons' l.
    miners' l.
    pigeon-breeder's l.
    polycystic l.
    silo filler's l.
    thresher's l.
    l. transplantation
    trench l.
    vanishing l.
    wet l.
    white l.
lungmotor
lungworm
lupus
    l. erythematosus
lymphadenectomy
lymphadenitis
lymphadenopathy
    subcarinal l.
lymphangiectasis
    congenital pulmonary l.
lymphangiography
lymphangiomyomatosis
    pulmonary l.
lymphangitic
lymphoblastoma

lymphoid
lymphoma
lymphomatoid
lymphosarcoma
Lynch's
    dissector
    forceps
    knife
    scissors
macroglobulinemia
    Waldenström's m.
macrophage
    alveolar m.
magnet
    Equen's m.
magnetic resonance imaging
main stem bronchus
malformation
Malm-Himmelstein
    valvulotome
maneuver
    Heimlich's m.
    Müller's m.
    Valsalva's m.
Manson's hemoptysis
Mantoux test
manubrium
Marfan's syndrome
Martin's tube
Maugeri's syndrome
Mayo-Russian forceps
Mayo's scissors
mechanism
    wave speed m.
mediastinal
mediastinitis
mediastinography
mediastinopericarditis
mediastinoscope
    Carlens' m.
mediastonoscopy
mediastinotomy
mediastinum
medications. See *Drugs and*
    Chemistry section.
medicolegal
medicothorax

  Lowenstein's m.
MEFV—maximum expiratory
  flow volume
Meigs' syndrome
melioidosis
  pulmonary m.
membrane
  Debove's m.
Mendelson's syndrome
mesothelioma
metabolic
metaplasia
metastases
  hematogenous m.
  lymphangitic m.
  mediastinal m.
  miliary m.
  nodular m.
  pleural m.
metastasis (metastases)
metastatic
method
  acoustic reflection m.
  Bohr isopleth m.
Metras' catheter
Metzenbaum's scissors
mica
Michelson's bronchoscope
microlithiasis
  pulmonary alveolar m.
Micropolyspora
  M. faeni
microscopy
  electron m.
  light m.
midthorax
migratory
miliary
mist
  ultrasonic m.
Moersch's
  bronchoscope
  esophagoscope
  forceps
Monaldi's
  drainage system

Monaldi's (continued)
  operation
Monilia
  M. albicans
monoclonal
mononucleosis
Moore's tracheostomy buttons
Morch's tube
Morton's cough
Mosher's
  esophagoscope
  tube
Mounier-Kuhn syndrome
Moure's esophagoscope
MRI—magnetic resonance
  imaging
MSVC—maximal sustained
  ventilatory capacity
mucin
mucociliary
mucoid
mucopurulent
Mucor
mucormycosis
mucous
  m. hypersecretion
  m. plugging
  m. plugs
mucoviscidosis
mucus
Mueller's clamp
Müller's
  maneuver
  test
multinucleated
multiple sclerosis
murmur
  cardiopulmonary m.
  cardiorespiratory m.
  respiratory m.
muscle
  scalenus m.
  serratus m.
  strap m.
myasthenia
  m. gravis
myasthenic

Mycobacterium
    M. tuberculosis
Mycoplasma
    M. pneumoniae
Myerson's
    forceps
    saw
Nachlas' tube
Naffziger's syndrome
Nathan's test
nebulizer
    DeVilbiss n.
needle
    Abrams' n.
    Cope's n.
    Fischer's n.
    Floyd's n.
    Frederick's n.
    Kaplan's n.
    Lewy-Rubin n.
Negus' bronchoscope
Nelson's
    forceps
    scissors
neuroendocrine
neurofibroma
neurofilament
neuron-specific enolase
neurophysin
neurosecretory
New's
    forceps
    hook
    tube
Nocardia
    N. asteroides
nocardial
nocardiosis
nodal
node
    bronchopulmonary
      lymph n.
    mediastinal lymph n.
    pulmonary lymph n.
    tracheobronchial
      lymph n.
nodular
nodularity

noninvasive
NSCLS – non small cell lung
    carcinoma
NSE – neuron-specific enolase
nucleus
numektome. See *pneumectomy.*
numo-. See words beginning
    pneumo-.
obesity
obstruction
obstructive
obturator
occlusion
Octomyces
    O. etiennei
oculocutaneous
    o. albinism
oleothorax
Olympus model GTF-A
    gastrocamera
oncogene
oncology
Ondine's curse
operation
    Blalock-Taussig o.
    Daniel's o.
    Delorme's o.
    Eloesser's o.
    Estlander's o.
    Fowler's o.
    Friedrich's o.
    Glenn's o.
    Jacobaeus' o.
    Monaldi's o.
    Overholt's o.
    Potts-Smith-Gibson o.
    Ransohoff's o.
    Schede's o.
    Semb's o.
    Tuffier's o.
    Wilms' o.
ornithosis
oropharynx
orthodeoxia
orthopnea
orthopneic
OSA – obstructive sleep
    apnea

osteoarthropathy
  pulmonary o.
osteoblastic
Overholt-Jackson bronchoscope
Overholt's operation
oxyetherotherapy
ozone
P & A – percussion and
  auscultation
palate
palliative
panbronchiolitis
Pancoast's
    syndrome
    tumor
PAP – positive airway pressure
    primary atypical
      pneumonia
papilloma
paracentesis
    p. pulmonis
    p. thoracis
paragonimiasis
Paragonimus
    P. westermani
para-influenza
paraneoplastic
paraplegic
parasternal
parenchyma
paries
    p. membranaceus bronchi
    p. membranaceus tracheae
parietal
paroksizm. See paroxysm.
paroksizmal. See paroxysmal.
paroxysm
paroxysmal
pars
    p. thoracalis esophagi
Patterson's
    forceps
    trocar
Patton's dilator
patulous
pCO$_2$ – carbon dioxide pressure
PCP – *Pneumocystis carinii*
    pneumonia

PE – pharyngoesophageal
    pleural effusion
    pulmonary edema
    pulmonary embolism
peak
    p. expiratory flow rate
    p. flow gauge
    p. flow meter
pearl
    Laennec's p's
pectoral
pectoralis
pectoriloquy
pectorophony
pectus
    p. carinatum
    p. excavatum
    p. gallinatum
    p. recurvatum
pedunculated
PEEP – positive end-expiratory
    pressure
PEFR – peak expiratory flow
    rate
penicilliosis
Penicillium
Pennington's forceps
percussion
    Krönig's p.
    respiratory p.
percutaneous
Perez's sign
perfusion
peribronchial
peribronchiolar
peribronchiolitis
peribronchitis
pericardial
pericarditis
    tuberculous p.
pericardium
periesophageal
periesophagitis
perihilar
peripheral
    p. airway resistance
    p. edema

peripneumonia
    p. notha
pertussis
Peyrot's thorax
PFT – pulmonary function test
Pfuhl-Jaffe sign
Pfuhl's sign
phagocyte
    alveolar p.
pharyngeal
pharyngitis
pharyngoesophageal
pharyngospasm
pharyngostenosis
pharyngotomy
pharynx
phenomenon
    Raynaud's p.
phlegm
phonation
photofluorogram
photofluorography
phrenic nerve
phrenicectomy
phreniclasia
phrenicoexeresis
phrenicotomy
phrenicotripsy
phrenitis
phthisis
    bacillary p.
    colliers' p.
    diabetic p.
    fibroid p.
    flax dressers' p.
    grinders' p.
    miner's p.
    nodosa p.
    potters' p.
    pulmonary p.
    stone cutters' p.
PI – pulmonary incompetence
    pulmonary infarction
PIE – pulmonary infiltration
    and eosinophilia
    pulmonary interstitial
    emphysema

Pilling's
    bronchoscope
    tube
"pink puffer"
piriform
pituitary
    p. fossa
    p. snuff
planigram
planimetric
plaque
plasmacytoma
platypnea
platysma
plethysmograph
    body p.
plethysmography
    impedance p.
    inductive p.
pleura
    cervical p.
    costal p.
    diaphragmatic p.
    mediastinal p.
    parietal p.
    pericardial p.
    pulmonary p.
    visceral p.
pleuracentesis
pleuracotomy
pleural
    p. cavity
    p. effusion
    p. mesothelioma
    p. pressure
    p. shock
    p. space
pleuralgia
pleurectomy
pleurisy
    adhesive p.
    blocked p.
    circumscribed p.
    costal p.
    diaphragmatic p.
    diffuse p.

pleurisy (continued)
    encysted p.
    exudative p.
    fibrinous p.
    hemorrhagic p.
    ichorous p.
    indurative p.
    interlobular p.
    mediastinal p.
    metapneumonic p.
    plastic p.
    pulmonary p.
    pulsating p.
    purulent p.
    sacculated p.
    serofibrinous p.
    serous p.
    suppurative p.
    visceral p.
    wet p.
pleuritic
pleuritis
pleurobronchitis
pleurocele
pleurocentesis
pleuroclysis
pleurodynia
    epidemic p.
pleurogenous
pleurography
pleurohepatitis
pleurolith
pleurolysis
pleuroparietopexy
pleuropericardial
pleuropericarditis
pleuroperitoneal
pleuroperitoneum
pleuropneumonia
pleuropneumonia-like
pleuropneumonolysis
pleuropulmonary
pleurorrhea
pleuroscopy
pleurothoracopleurectomy
pleurotome

pleurotomy
pleurotyphoid
pleurovisceral
plexus
    p. aorticus thoracicus
    brachial p.
    esophageal p.
    mediastinal p.
    p. pulmonalis
    subpleural mediastinal p.
plication
    fundal p.
plombage
    extraperiosteal p.
Plummer's dilator
Plummer-Vinson
    dilator
    radium applicator
PND–paroxysmal nocturnal
    dyspnea
pneogram
pneograph
pneometer
pneoscope
pneumal
pneumatic
pneumatocele
pneumatodyspnea
pneumatometer
pneumatometry
pneumatophore
pneumatosis
    p. pulmonum
pneumectomy
pneumoalveolography
pneumoangiography
pneumobacillus
    Friedländer's p.
pneumobronchotomy
pneumobulbar
pneumocardial
pneumocentesis
pneumochirurgia
pneumocholecystitis
pneumochysis
pneumococcal
pneumococcic

pneumococcus
pneumoconiosis
 bauxite p.
 coal workers' p.
 collagenous p.
 hard metal p.
 mica p.
 noncollagenous p.
 rheumatoid p.
 p. siderotica
 talc p.
pneumocystic
Pneumocystis
 P. carinii
pneumoenteritis
pneumoerysipelas
pneumogastric
pneumogram
pneumography
pneumohemothorax
pneumohydrothorax
pneumolithiasis
pneumomalacia
pneumomediastinography
pneumomediastinum
pneumomelanosis
pneumomycosis
pneumonectasis
pneumonectomy
pneumonedema
pneumonemia
pneumonere
pneumonia
 abortive p.
 acute p.
 p. alba
 amebic p.
 anthrax p.
 p. apostematosa
 aspiration p.
 atypical p.
 bacterial p.
 bilious p.
 bronchial p.
 Buhl's desquamative p.
 caseous p.
 catarrhal p.

pneumonia (continued)
 cheesy p.
 cold agglutinin p.
 Corrigan's p.
 croupous p.
 deglutition p.
 Desnos' p.
 desquamative p.
 desquamative interstitial p.
 diffuse lymphoid interstitial p.
 p. dissecans
 double p.
 Eaton agent p.
 embolic p.
 ephemeral p.
 fibrinous p.
 Friedländer's bacillus p.
 Friedländer's p.
 gangrenous p.
 giant cell p.
 Hecht's p.
 hypostatic p.
 indurative p.
 influenzal p.
 p. interlobularis purulenta
 interstitial plasma cell p.
 Kaufman's p.
 Klebsiella p.
 Legionnaire's p.
 lingular p.
 lipoid p.
 lobar p.
 lobular p.
 Löffler's p.
 Louisiana p.
 metastatic p.
 migratory p.
 mycoplasmal p.
 obstructive p.
 parenchymatous p.
 pleurogenetic p.
 pneumococcal p.
 Pneumocystis carinii p.
 purulent p.
 rheumatic p.

pneumonia (continued)
    Riesman's p.
    septic p.
    staphylococcal p.
    Stoll's p.
    streptococcal p.
    suppurative p.
    toxemic p.
    transplantation p.
    tuberculous p.
    tularemic p.
    typhoid p.
    unresolved p.
    vagus p.
    varicella p.
    viral p.
    wandering p.
    woolsorter's p.
pneumonic
pneumonitis
    aspiration p.
    cholesterol p.
    desquamative interstitial
      p.
    eosinophilic p.
    granulomatous p.
    hypersensitivity p.
    kerosene p.
    lymphocytic interstitial p.
    malarial p.
    pneumocystis p.
    uremic p.
pneumonocentesis
pneumonochirurgia
pneumonocirrhosis
pneumonocyte
    granular p.
    membranous p.
pneumonograph
pneumonography
pneumonolipoidosis
pneumonolysis
pneumonomelanosis
pneumonomoniliasis
pneumonopathy
    eosinophilic p.
pneumonopexy

pneumonophthisis
pneumonoresection
pneumonorrhaphy
pneumonosis
pneumonotherapy
pneumonotomy
pneumoparesis
pneumopericardium
pneumoperitoneum
pneumopexy
pneumopleuritis
pneumopleuroparietopexy
pneumopyothorax
pneumoresection
pneumorrhagia
pneumosepticemia
pneumoserothorax
pneumosilicosis
pneumotachograph
pneumotachometer
pneumotachygraph
pneumotaxic center
pneumotherapy
pneumothorax
    artifical p.
    clicking p.
    closed p.
    diagnostic p.
    extrapleural p.
    spontaneous p.
    tension p.
    valvular p.
pneumotoxin
pneumotropic
pneumotropism
pneumotyphoid
pneumotyphus
PO_2–oxygen pressure
Polisar-Lyons tube
polyarteritis
    p. nodosa
polychondritis
polycythemia
polymyositis
polypeptide
polysomnography
Pompe's disease

pore
> Kohn's p.

portacaval

position. See *General Surgical Terms* section.

postpneumonic

post-tussis

Pottenger's sign

Potts-Smith-Gibson operation

poudrage
> pleural p.

PP – pink puffers (emphysema)

PPB – positive pressure breathing

PPD – purified protein derivative

PPLO – pleuropneumonia-like organism

pretracheal

Price-Thomas
> clamp
> forceps

Pritchard's cannula

profundoplasty

proteinosis
> pulmonary alveolar p.

Proteus

pseudobronchiectasis

pseudocoarctation

Pseudomonas
> *P. aeruginosa*

psittacosis

pulmogram

pulmolith

pulmometer

pulmometry

pulmonary
> p. abscess
> p. amyloidosis
> p. congestion
> p. edema
> p. embolism
> p. eosinophilia
> p. fibrosis
> p. function
> p. hemosiderosis
> p. hypertension
> p. perfusion
> p. sulcus

pulmonary (continued)
> p. telangiectasia
> p. thromboembolism
> p. thromboses
> p. valve
> p. vasculature
> p. veno-occlusive disease
> p. venules

pulmonic

pulmonitis

pulmonohepatic

pulmonology

pulmonoperitoneal

pulmotor

pulsator
> Bragg-Paul p.

purpura
> thrombocytopenic p.
> thrombotic thrombocytopenic p.

purulent

PX – pneumothorax

pyopneumothorax

pyothorax

Q fever (Q for query)

quadriplegia

radiation
> r. dermatitis
> r. esophagus
> r. fibrosis
> r. myelitis
> r. oncology
> r. pericarditis
> r. pneumonitis

radiocurability

radiogram

radiography

radioisotope

radiology

radiolucent

radionuclide

radiopaque

radiosensitivity

radiotherapy

radon

rale
> amphoric r.

rale (continued)
    atelectatic r.
    bronchial r.
    bubbling r.
    cavernous r.
    cellophane r.
    clicking r.
    collapse r.
    consonating r.
    crackling r.
    crepitant r.
    r. de retour
    extrathoracic r.
    gurgling r.
    guttural r.
    Hirtz's r.
    r. indux
    inspiratory r's
    moist r.
    r. muqueux
    pleural r.
    r. redux
    sibilant r.
    Skoda's r.
    sonorous r.
    subcrepitant r.
    tracheal r.
    "Velcro" r's
    vesicular r.
    whistling r.
Ralk's clamp
Ramond's sign
Ransohoff's operation
Raynaud's phenomenon
RDS – respiratory distress
    syndrome
receptors
    H_1
    H_2
reflex
    Hering-Breuer r.
    inspiratory-inhibitory r.
reflux
regurgitation
    esophageal r.
Reid index

remission
    Legroux's r.
rentgenograhfe. See
    roentgenography.
reoxygenation
repair
    Belsey's r.
resonance
    bandbox r.
    bell-metal r.
    cracked-pot r.
    shoulder-strap r.
    skodaic r.
resonant
respiration
    amphoric r.
    anaerobic r.
    asthmoid r.
    Biot's r.
    bronchial r.
    bronchocavernous r.
    bronchovesicular r.
    cavernous r.
    Cheyne-Stokes r.
    cogwheel r.
    Corrigan's r.
    electrophrenic r.
    external r.
    internal r.
    Kussmaul-Kien r.
    Kussmaul's r.
    paradoxical r.
    puerile r.
    Seitz's metamorphosing r.
    stertorous r.
    tubular r.
    vesicular r.
    vesiculocavernous r.
    vicarious r.
respirator
    cabinet r.
    cuirass r.
    Drinker r.
respiratory
    r. acidosis
    r. bronchiolitis
    r. center drive

respiratory (continued)
    r. distress syndrome
    r. rate
    r. syncytial virus
respirometer
    Wright r.
retractor
    Andrews' r.
    Bernay's r.
    Brewster's r.
    flexible shaft r.
    Haight's r.
    Jackson's r.
    Lukens' r.
    Robinson's r.
    Shurly's r.
retrolental
retrosternal
rhinitis
rhinovirus
rhonchal
rhonchial
rhonchus
RI – respiratory illness
rib spreader
    Tuffier's r.s.
rickettsial
Riecker's bronchoscope
Riesman's pneumonia
ring
    Schatzki's r.
    vascular r's
Riviere's sign
RL – right lung
RLC – residual lung capacity
RLL – right lower lobe
RM – respiratory movement
RML – right middle lobe
Roberts'
    esophagoscope
    forceps
Robinson's retractor
Rockey's
    cannula
    clamp
    forceps
    scope

roentgenography
Rokitansky's diverticulum
rong-. See words beginning
    rhonc-.
Roussel's sign
RSV – respiratory syncytial virus
RTF – respiratory tract fluid
Rubin's clamp
RUL – right upper lobe
rule
    Gibson's r.
Russian forceps
RV – respiratory volume
Safar's bronchoscope
Salvatore-Maloney tracheotome
Sam Roberts forceps
sarcoid
sarcoidosis
sarcoma
Sarot's
    clamp
    forceps
saw
    Myerson's s.
scalene
scalenectomy
scalenotomy
scalpel
    Jackson's s.
scan
    CAT (computerized axial
      tomography) s.
    gallium s.
    ^{99m}Tc-labeled MAA s.
scanning
    radionuclide s.
Schatzki's ring
Schede's operation
Scheinmann's forceps
Schindler's esophagoscope
schistosomiasis
    pulmonary s.
Schmorl's furrow
scintigraphy
scissors
    Crafoord's s.
    Jackson's s.

scissors (continued)
    Lynch's s.
    Mayo's s.
    Metzenbaum's s.
    Nelson's s.
    Sweet's s.
SCLC – small cell lung cancer
        squamous cell, large cell
        (carcinoma)
scleroderma
    pulmonary s.
sclerosis
    diffuse systemic s.
    multiple s.
scoliosis
scope
    Rockey's s.
segment
    bronchopulmonary s.
segmenta
    s. bronchopulmonalia
segmental
Seiffert's forceps
Seitz's metamorphosing
        respiration
Semb's operation
Sengstaken-Blakemore tube
septicemia
septum
    s. bronchiale
    s. mediastinale
sequestration
    pulmonary s.
sequoiosis
serosanguineous
serpiginous
Shaver's disease
Shenstone's tourniquet
Shibley's sign
shunt
    portacaval s.
Shurly's retractor
siderosilicosis
siderosis
Sierra-Sheldon tracheotome
sign
    Abraham's s.

sign (continued)
    Baccelli's s.
    Bethea's s.
    Cegka's s.
    D'Amato's s.
    Delmege's s.
    Ellis' s.
    Ewart's s.
    Friedreich's s.
    Hamman's s.
    Hoover's s.
    Jürgensen's s.
    Kussmaul's s.
    Laennec's s.
    Perez's s.
    Pfuhl-Jaffe s.
    Pfuhl's s.
    Pottenger's s.
    Ramond's s.
    Riviere's s.
    Roussel's s.
    Shibley's s.
    Skoda's s.
    Sternberg's s.
    Westermark's s.
    Williams' s.
    Williamson's s.
silica
silicatosis
silicosiderosis
silicosis
    infective s.
silicotuberculosis
SIMV – synchronized
        intermittent mandatory
        ventilation
singultus
sinobronchitis
sinus
    s. trunci pulmonalis
sinusitis
siphon
    Duguet's s.
Sippy's dilator
sitakosis. See *psittacosis.*
situs
    s. inversus viscerum

Skoda's
    rale
    sign
    tympany
snoring
Snyder's surgivac drainage
  system
solitary nodule
sonorous
sound
    Beatty-Bright friction s.
    cracked-pot s.
    esophageal s.
    hippocratic s.
    respiratory s.
    to-and-fro s.
Souttar's tube
space
    Traube's s.
sphingolipid
Spinhaler
spirochetosis
    bronchopulmonary s.
spirogram
spirograph
spirography
spirometer
    Benedict-Roth s.
    Collins' respirometer-s.
    Douglas' bag s.
    Krogh's apparatus s.
    Tissot's s.
    Venturi's meter s.
    Wright's respirometer-s.
spirometry
    bronchoscopic s.
spirophore
splenization
    hypostatic s.
splenopneumonia
sputum
    s. aeroginosum
    albuminoid s.
    s. coctum
    s. crudum
    s. cruentum
    egg yolk s.
    globular s.

sputum (continued)
    green s.
    icteric s.
    moss-agate s.
    nummular s.
    prune juice s.
    rusty s.
squama
    s. alveolaris
squamous cell
stannosis
Staphylococcus
    S. aureus
Staple's bronchoscope
status
    s. asthmaticus
Steele's dilator
stenosis
stereoscopy
sternal
Sternberg's sign
sternoclavicular
sternocostal
sternomastoid
sternotomy
stenotracheal
sternum
steroid
stethoscope
Stevens-Johnson syndrome
Stoll's pneumonia
Storz's bronchoscope
stricture
stridor
    s. serraticus
study
    cytological s.
    enzyme s.
subcutaneous
submucosa
subpleural
substernal
succussion
    hippocratic s.
suctioning
    endotracheal-bronchial s.
sudo-. See words beginning
    pseudo-.

suffocation
sulcate
sulcus
    s. pulmonalis thoracis
    subclavian s. of lung
    s. subclavius
      pulmonis
supraclavicular
surgical procedures. See
    operation.
suture. See *General Surgical
    Terms.*
SVC–superior vena cava
Sweet's scissors
Sydenham's cough
symptom
    Burghart's s.
syncytial
syndrome
    acquired
      immunodeficiency s.
    Arneth's s.
    Ayerza's s.
    Bard's s.
    Bársony-Polgár s.
    Behçet's s.
    Brock's s.
    Caplan's s.
    Eaton-Lambert s.
    Eisenmenger's s.
    Goodpasture's s.
    Guillain-Barré s.
    Hamman-Rich s.
    Hermansky-Pudlak s.
    Horner's s.
    hyperlucent lung s.
    immotile cilia s.
    Kartagener's s.
    Leitner's s.
    Leredde's s.
    Löffler's s.
    Marfan's s.
    Maugeri's s.
    Meigs' s.
    Mendelson's s.
    middle lobe s.
    Mounier-Kuhn s.

syndrome (continued)
    Naffziger's s.
    Pancoast's s.
    Stevens-Johnson s.
    Trousseau's s.
    Williams-Campbell s.
    Wilson-Mikity s.
    Young's s.
system
    respiratory s.
systemic
Takayasu's disease
talcosis
TB–tuberculosis
telangiectasia
    pulmonary t.
telescope
    Broyles' t.
    Holinger's t.
    right-angle t.
tenaculum
    Jackson's t.
teratodermoid
teratoma
test
    Adson's t.
    Allen's t.
    Arloing-Courmont t.
    Blumenau's t.
    Casoni's t.
    coccidioidin t.
    Craig's t.
    Escherich's t.
    Hamburger's t.
    Heaf t.
    histoplasmin skin t.
    Hitzenberg's t.
    Kveim t.
    Lautier's t.
    Lignières' t.
    Mantoux t.
    Müller's t.
    Nathan's t.
    patch t.
    pulmonary function t.
    sweat t.
    tine tuberculin t.

test (continued)
    tuberculin t.
    Valsalva's t.
    V_{isov} t.
    Vollmer's t.
    Weinberg's t.
    Youman-Parlett t.
Thompson's catheter
Thomsen's disease
Thomson's clamp
thoracentesis
thoracic
thoracicoabdominal
thoracobronchotomy
thoracocautery
thoracocentesis
thoracocyllosis
thoracocyrtosis
thoracodynia
thoracogastroschisis
thoracograph
thoracolaparotomy
thoracolysis
    t. praecordiaca
thoracometer
thoracometry
thoracoplasty
    costoversion t.
thoracopneumograph
thoracopneumoplasty
thoracoschisis
thoracoscope
thoracoscopy
thoracostenosis
thoracostomy
thoracotomy
thorax
    barrel-shaped t.
    cholesterol t.
    Peyrot's t.
    pyriform t.
thrombosis
thymectomy
thymoma
thymus
thymusectomy
thyrotoxicosis

tine test
tisis. See *phthisis.*
Tissot's spirometer
TLC–total lung capacity
    total lung compliance
Tobold-Fauvel forceps
tomography
tonsilar
torulosis
tourniquet
    Bethune's t.
    Shenstone's t.
toxoplasmosis
trachea
tracheaectasy
tracheal
    t. length
    t. mucus
    t. mucus velocity
    t. stenosis
trachealgia
tracheitis
tracheobronchial
tracheobronchitis
tracheobronchomegaly
tracheobronchoscopy
tracheocele
tracheoesophageal
tracheofissure
tracheofistulization
tracheogenic
tracheolaryngeal
tracheomalacia
tracheopathia
    t. osteoplastica
tracheopharyngeal
tracheophony
tracheoplasty
tracheopyosis
tracheorrhagia
tracheorrhaphy
tracheoschisis
tracheoscopy
tracheostenosis
tracheostoma
tracheostomize
tracheostomy

tracheotome
 Salvatore-Maloney t.
 Sierra-Sheldon t.
tracheotomize
tracheotomy
transbronchial
transdiaphragmatic
transillumination
transplantation
transpulmonary
transthoracic
transthoracotomy
transtracheal
Traube's
 dyspnea
 space
treatment
 Forlanini's t.
tree
 bronchial t.
 tracheobronchial t.
triad
 Kartagener's t.
trichinosis
Trichomonas
 T. pulmonalis
Trichosporon
 T. cutaneum
trocar
 Hurwitz's t.
 Patterson's t.
Trousseau-Jackson dilator
Trousseau's
 bougie
 dilator
 syndrome
truncus
 t. bronchomediastinalis
  dexter
 t. pulmonalis
tube
 Andrews-Pynchon t.
 Argyle chest t.
 Atkins-Cannard t.
 Blakemore's t.
 Broyles' t.
 Carabelli's t.

tube (continued)
 Celestin's t.
 Chaussier's t.
 Chevalier Jackson t.
 Depaul's t.
 Durham's t.
 fiberoptic t.
 Gabriel Tucker t.
 Guisez's t.
 Holinger's t.
 intubation t.
 Jackson's t.
 Killian's t's
 Kistner's t.
 Lanz's t.
 Lennarson's t.
 Lepley-Ernst t.
 Lewis' t.
 Linton's t.
 Lore-Lawrence t.
 Luer's t.
 Martin's t.
 Morch's t.
 Mosher's t.
 Nachlas' t.
 New's t.
 Pilling's t.
 Polisar-Lyons t.
 Sengstaken-Blakemore t.
 Souttar's t.
 thoracostomy t.
 tracheostomy t.
 Tucker's t.
tubercle
 Ghon t.
 scalene t.
tubercular
tuberculin
tuberculoid
tuberculoma
tuberculomyces
tuberculosilicosis
tuberculosis
 acute miliary t.
 anthracotic t.
 cestodic t.
 exudative t.

tuberculosis (continued)
    hilus t.
    miliary t.
    pulmonary t.
    tracheobronchial t.
tuberculous
tuberous
    t. sclerosis
Tucker's
    bronchoscope
    esophagoscope
    tube
Tuffier's
    operation
    rib spreader
tumor
    alveolar cell t.
    amyloid t.
    epidermoid t.
    oat cell t.
    Pancoast's t.
    sulcus t.
    teratoid t.
    thymic t.
tunica
    t. adventitia esophagi
    t. mucosa bronchiorum
    t. mucosa esophagi
    t. mucosa laryngis
    t. mucosa tracheae
    t. muscularis esophagi
    t. muscularis tracheae
Tuttle's forceps
tympanic
tympany
    bell t.
    skodaic t.
    Skoda's t.
ulceration
ulcerative
    u. colitis
underwater seal drainage
UPP – uvulopalatopharyngo-
    plasty
URI – upper respiratory
    infection

uvulopalatopharyngo-
    plasty
Valsalva's
    maneuver
    test
valvulotome
    Himmelstein's v.
    Malm-Himmelstein v.
varices
varix
VC – vital capacity
vectorcardiography
vein
    azygos v.
    brachial v.
    cephalic v.
    innominate v.
    thymic v.
Velcro rale
vena
    v. cava
venesection
venogram
veno-occlusive
venous
ventilation
    alveolar v.
    intermittent mandatory v.
    synchronized intermittent
        mandatory v.
ventilatory
Venti-mask
ventral
ventricular
Venturi's meter spirometer
viral
virus
    v. bronchopneumonia
    Coxsackie v.
    ECHO (enteric
        cytopathogenic human
        orphan) v.
    parinfluenza v.
    respiratory syncytial v.
visceropleural
Visov test

visualization
    laryngoscopic v.
V_{max}
    25%
    50%
    75%
    O_2
Vollmer's test
vomiting
V/Q
    distribution
    imbalance
    nonuniformity
    ratio
Waldenström's
    macroglobulinemia
Waterman's bronchoscope
wave-speed mechanism
wedge
    w. angiogram
    w. pressure
Wegener's granulomatosis
Weinberg's test
Welch-Allyn laryngoscope
welders
Westermark's sign
wheeze

Whipple's disease
whooping cough
Williams-Campbell syndrome
Williams' sign
Williamson's sign
Wilms' operation
Wilson-Mikity syndrome
windpipe
Woillez's disease
wool workers
Wright's respirometer-spirometer
xenon
xerotrachea
X histiocytosis
xiphocostal
xiphoid
YAG laser therapy
Yankauer-Little forceps
Yankauer's
    bronchoscope
    esophagoscope
Youman-Parlett test
Young's syndrome
Zavod's catheter
Zenker's diverticulum
zifo-. See words beginning *xipho-.*
zinc fume fever

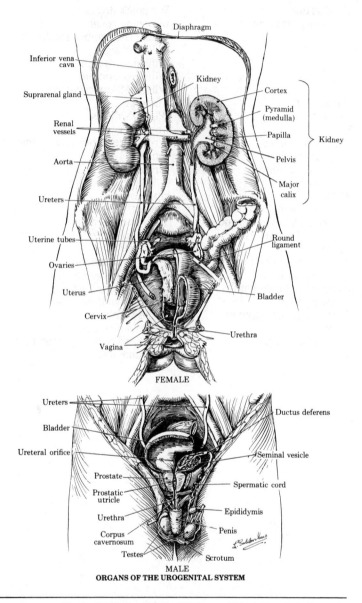

ORGANS OF THE UROGENITAL SYSTEM

(Courtesy of Dorland's Illustrated Medical Dictionary, 27th ed. Plate 47. Philadelphia, W. B. Saunders Company, 1988.)

Urology

aberrant
ablation
abscess
acetone
acetonuria
achromaturia
acidosis
    renal tubular a.
acinar
Acmistat catheter
Acmi-Valentine tube
aconuresis
acquired immunodeficiency
  syndrome
acraturesis
actinomycosis
acuminata
    condylomata a.
    verruca a.
adapter
    Ralks' a.
Addis' method
Addison's disease
adenitis
adenoacanthoma
adenocarcinoma
    acinar a.
    ductal a.
    urachal a.
adenoma
    cortical a's
    feminizing a.
adenomatosis
adenomyosarcoma
adenosarcoma
    embryonal a.
ADH – antidiuretic
  hormone

adiposis
    a. orchalis
    a. orchica
adrenal
    Marchand's a's
adrenalectomy
adrenalinuria
adrenalism
adrenalitis
adrenalopathy
adrenic
adrenin
adrenitis
adrenocortical
adrenocorticotropic
adrenogenital
adrenogenous
adrenokinetic
adrenomedullotropic
adrenomegaly
adrenopathy
adrenopause
adrenoprival
adrenostatic
adrenotoxin
adrenotropic
adrenotropin
adrenotropism
adventitia
aerocystography
aerocystoscope
aerocystoscopy
afferent
agenesis
agenitalism
agenosomia
aglomerular
aidoiitis

AIDS – acquired
    immunodeficiency
    syndrome
Albarran's
    gland
    test
    tubules
albiduria
albuginea
    a. penis
albugineotomy
albumin
albuminaturia
albuminuria
    adventitious a.
    globular a.
    nephrogenous a.
    postrenal a.
    renal a.
    residual a.
albuminuric
Alcock-Hendrickson lithotrite
Alcock's
    catheter
    lithotrite
Alcock-Timberlake obturator
alcoholuria
aldosterone
    a. adenoma
    a. suppression test
aldosteronism
alginuresis
alkaline
Allemann's syndrome
Allis' forceps
allograft
Alyea's clamp
amebiasis
    a. of bladder
aminoglutethimide
ampulla
    a. ductus deferentis
    Henle's a.
    a. of vas deferens
amyloidosis
anaplasia
anaplastic

anastomosis
    pyeloileocutaneous a.
    transuretero-ureteral a.
Andrews' operation
androblastoma
androgen
    a. ablation
    a. deprivation
    a. precursors
    a. suppression
anesthesia. See *General Surgical Terms* section.
aneurysm
aneurysmal
aneurysmatic
angiogram
    renal a.
angiography
angioma
angiomyolipoma
angle
    costovertebral a.
angulation
anischuria
ankylurethria
annulus
    a. urethralis
anorchia
anorchid
anorchidic
anorchidism
anorchis
anorchism
anovesical
antiandrogen
antibody
    cytophilic a's
    cytotoxic a's
    monoclonal a's
anticoagulation
antigen
    A a.
    B a.
    cryptic T a.
    Factor VIII a.
    O a.
    P54 a.

antigen (continued)
    T a.
    Thomsen-Friedenreich a's
antigenic
    a. modulation
anuresis
anuretic
anuria
    angioneurotic a.
    calculous a.
    obstructive a.
    postrenal a.
    prerenal a.
    renal a.
    suppressive a.
anuric
aorta
aorticorenal
aortography
apex
    a. of bladder
    a. prostatae
    a. vesicae urinariae
aponeurosis
    Denonvilliers' a.
arcuate
ardor
    a. urinae
areolar
argon laser
Arnold and Gunning's method
arteriography
arteriole
    glomerular a.
    glomerular a., afferent
    glomerular a., efferent
    Isaacs-Ludwig a.
    postglomerular a.
    preglomerular a.
    renal a.
arteriorenal
arteriosclerotic
arteriovenous
artery
    arcuate a.
    cremasteric a.
    dorsal a.

artery (continued)
    gluteal a.
    helcine a.
    hypogastric a.
    iliac a.
    interlobar a.
    interlobular a.
    perineal a.
    pudendal a.
    renal a.
    spermatic a.
    vesical a.
asbestos
ascites
aspermatism
aspermatogenesis
aspermia
aspiration
asthenospermia
atonic
atony
atresia
atrophic
atrophy
atypia
azoospermatism
azoospermia
azotemia
    extrarenal a.
    prerenal a.
azotemic
    a. osteodystrophy
azoturia
azoturic
Babcock's clamp
bacille Calmette-Guérin vaccine
backflow
    pyelovenous b.
bacteriuria
bah-fon. See *bas-fond.*
balanic
balanitis
    b. circinata
    b. circumscripta
        plasmacellularis
    b. diabetica
    Follmann's b.

balanitis (continued)
    b. gangraenosa
    gangrenous b.
    b. xerotica obliterans
balanoblennorrhea
balanocele
balanoplasty
balanoposthitis
balanoposthomycosis
balanopreputial
balanorrhagia
balanus
Balkan
    B. nephritis
    B. nephropathy
bar
    Mercier's b.
Bardex's catheter
Bard's catheter
Bartter's syndrome
basement membrane
bas-fond
basket
    Browne's b.
    Councill's b.
    Dormia's b.
    Ferguson's b.
    Howard's b.
    Johnson's b.
    Mitchell's b.
Bates' operation
Baumrucker's resectoscope
BCG – bacille Calmette-Guérin
    (vaccine)
Belfield's operation
Bellini's
    ducts
    tubules
Bell's
    law
    muscle
Bence Jones
    cylinders
    protein method
    proteinuria
    urine
Benedict and Franke's method

Benedict and Osterberg's method
Bengt-Johanson repair
benign
Bennett's operation
Bergenhem's operation
Bergman's sign
Bertin's column
Bertrand's method
Bethune's rib cutter
Bevan-Rochet operation
Bevan's operation
bifid
bifurcation
Bigelow's
    lithotrite
    operation
bilabe
bilharzial
bilirubin
bilirubinuria
biomodulation
biopsy
    brush b.
    fine-needle aspiration b.
    renal b.
    transperineal b.
    transrectal b.
    transurethral b.
Bittorf's reaction
bladder
    atonic b.
    autonomic b.
    dome of b.
    fasciculated b.
    ileocecal b.
    irritable b.
    nervous b.
    neurogenic b.
    sacculated b.
    stammering b.
    urinary b.
Blake's forceps
blastema
Blasucci's catheter
blennorrhagia
blennorrhea
blennuria

Boari's operation
body
    b. of Highmore
    wolffian b.
boggy
boo-zhe. See *bougie.*
Bottini's operation
bougie
    b. à boule
    acorn-tipped b.
    b. coudé
    LeFort's b.
    olive tip b.
    Otis' b.
    Philips' b.
    Ruschelit's b.
boutonnière
Bowen's disease
Bowman's capsule
Bozeman's forceps
BPH – benign prostatic
    hypertrophy
Braasch's
    catheter
    cystoscope
    forceps
Brenner's tumor
Brewer's infarcts
Bricker's operation
brightism
Bright's disease
Brodny's clamp
Brödel's line
Brown-Buerger cystoscope
Browne's basket
Brunn's nest
bubo
    chancroidal b.
    gonorrheal b.
    venereal b.
bubonulus
Buck's fascia
Buerger-McCarthy forceps
Bugbee's electrode
bulbitis
bulbocavernosus
bulbourethral

bulbous
bulbus
    b. penis
    b. urethrae
bullous
Bumpus'
    forceps
    resectoscope
BUN – blood urea nitrogen
Bunim's forceps
Burkitt's lymphoma
Buschke-Loewenstein tumor
Butterfield's cystoscope
Bywaters' syndrome
Cacchi-Ricci syndrome
cachexia
    urinary c.
caffeine
calcification
calculi
calculus
    alternating c.
    coral c.
    cystine c.
    decubitus c.
    dendritic c.
    encysted c.
    fibrin c.
    gonecystic c.
    hemp seed c.
    indigo c.
    matrix c.
    mulberry c.
    nephritic c.
    oxalate c.
    prostatic c.
    renal c.
    spermatic c.
    stag-horn c.
    struvite c.
    ureteral c.
    urethral c.
    uric acid c.
    urinary c.
    urostealith c.
    vesical c.
    vesicoprostatic c.

calculus (continued)
    xanthic c.
caliber
calibrated
calibration
calibrator
caliceal
calicectasis
calicectomy
calices
calices renales
    c.r. majores
    c.r. minores
calicine
caliectasis
caliectomy
calix
calyceal
calycectasis
calycectomy
calyces
calyces renales
    c.r. majores
    c.r. minores
calyx
Campbell's
    catheter
    forceps
    procedure
    retractor
    sound
    trocar
Camper's fascia
cannulation
CAPD—continued ambulatory
   peritoneal dialysis
capillaries
capistration
capsula
    c. adiposa renis
    c. fibrosa renis
    c. glomeruli
capsulae renis
capsular
capsule
    adipose c.
    Bowman's c.

capsule (continued)
    fibrous c. of corpora
      cavernosa penis
    Gerota's c.
    glomerular c.
    müllerian c.
    c. of glomerulus
    pelvioprostatic c.
    perinephric c.
    suprarenal c.
capsulectomy
capsuloma
capsuloplasty
capsulorrhaphy
capsulotomy
caput
    c. gallinaginis
carcinoma
    embryonal c.
    epibulbar c.
    granular cell c.
    c. in situ
    renal cell c.
    c. scroti
    squamous cell c.
    transitional cell c.
    verrucous c.
carcinosarcoma
Carson's catheter
caruncle
    morgagnian c.
cast
    blood c.
    epithelial c.
    fat c.
    wax c.
castrate
castration
catecholamine(s)
Cathclin's segregator
catheter
    Acmistat c.
    acorn tip c.
    Alcock's c.
    Bardex's c.
    Bard's c.
    Blasucci's c.

catheter (continued)
    Braasch's c.
    Campbell's c.
    Carson's c.
    cathematic c.
    c. coudé
    Councill's c.
    Coxeter's c.
    de Pezzer c.
    Emmett-Foley c.
    filiform c.
    Foley c.
    Foley-Alcock c.
    French-Robinson c.
    Furniss' c.
    indwelling c.
    latex c.
    LeFort's c.
    Malecot's c.
    McIver's c.
    Nélaton's c.
    olive tip c.
    Owen's c.
    Pezzer's c.
    Philips' c.
    polyethylene c.
    red Robinson c.
    retention c.
    return flow hemostatic c.
    Silastic mushroom c.
    spiral tip c.
    Tiemann's c.
    ureteral c.
    whistle tip c.
    Winer's c.
    Wishard's c.
catheterization
    retrourethral c.
catheterize
cauda
    c. epididymidis
cavernous
cavography
cavum
    c. retzii
C-clamp

Cecil's
    operation
    repair
cell
    Leydig's c's
    natural killer c's
    renal c's
    Sertoli's c.
    signet c's
    suppressor c's
cellule
cervix
chancre
    Nisbet's c.
chancroid
chemolysis
chemotherapy
cholesteatoma
chondrosarcoma
chorda
    c. gubernaculum
    c. spermatica
chordae
chordee
chorditis
choriocarcinoma
chorioepithelioma
chromaffinoma
chromosomal
    c. markers
chylocele
    parasitic c.
chyloderma
chyluria
cinefluorography
cineurography
circumcise
circumcision
circumferential
Civale's operation
Cl—chloride
clamp
    Alyea's c.
    Babcock's c.
    Brodny's c.
    C-c.
    Cunningham's c.

clamp (continued)
    Goldblatt's c.
    Gomco's c.
    Guyon-Pean c.
    Guyon's c.
    Halsted's c.
    Herrick's c.
    Hyams' c.
    Kantor's c.
    Mayo's c.
    Ockerblad's c.
    pedicle c.
    penile c.
    rubber-shod c.
    Stille's c.
    Stockman's c.
    Tatum's c.
    Walther-Crenshaw c.
    Walther's c.
    Wertheim-Cullen c.
    Wertheim-Reverdin c.
    Wertheim's c.
    Young's c.
    Zipser's c.
Clark's operation
classification
    Marshall-Jewett-Strong c.
clean catch urine specimen
cloaca
    congenital c.
    persistent c.
CMV – cytomegalovirus
cocarcinogen
Cock's operation
colic
    renal c.
collagen
collagenase
collecting system
Colles' fascia
colliculectomy
colliculi
colliculitis
colliculus
    bulbar c.
    seminal c.
    c. seminalis

Collings' electrode
colloid
collum
    c. glandis penis
colony count
column
    Bertin's c.
    c. of Sertoli
concentric
concrement
concretion
condyloma
    c. acuminatum
    c. latum
congenital
Conn's syndrome
continence
continent
contracture
convoluted
Cooke-Apert-Gallais syndrome
cooler
    Eissner's prostatic c.
Coombs' test
Cooper's irritable testis
Coppridge's forceps
copulation
copulatory
Corbus' disease
cord
    genital c.
    gubernacular c.
    nephrogenic c.
    spermatic c.
corditis
corona
    c. glandis penis
    c. of glans penis
coronal
corpora
    c. amylacea
    c. cavernosa
corpus
    c. cavernosum penis
    c. cavernosum urethrae
        virilis
    c. epididymidis

corpus (continued)
    c. glandulae
      bulbourethralis
    c. glandulare prostatae
    c. Highmori
    c. highmorianum
    c. penis
    c. spongiosum penis
    c. vesicae urinariae
    c. vesiculae seminalis
    c. Wolffi
cortex
    adrenal c.
    c. glandulae suprarenalis
    renal c.
    c. renis
cortiadrenal
cortical
corticosteroid
Corynebacterium
    C. parvum
costovertebral angle
coudé
    bougie c.
    catheter c.
Councill's
    basket
    catheter
    stone dislodger
counterimmunoelectrophoresis
counterirritation
Cowper's gland
Coxeter's catheter
creatinine
Creevy's evacuator
cremaster
    internal c. of Henle
cremasteric
Crenshaw's forceps
CRF–chronic renal failure
crisis
    Dietl's c.
crista
    c. urethralis masculinae
    c. urethralis virilis
crus (crura)
    c. penis

cryogenic
cryopreservation
cryptorchid
cryptorchidectomy
cryptorchidism
cryptorchidopexy
cryptorchidy
cryptorchism
crystalloid
crystalluria
crystalluridrosis
C & S–culture and sensitivity
Culp's ureteropelvioplasty
cuneiform
Cunningham's clamp
Cushing's syndrome
cutaneous
CVA–costovertebral angle
cyclamate
cylinders
    Bence Jones c's
cylindruria
cyst
    adrenal c.
    dermoid c.
    epidermoid c.
    medullary c.
    pyelogenic c.
    renal c.
    retroperitoneal c.
    testicular c.
    wolffian c.
cystalgia
cystathioninuria
cystatrophia
cystauchenitis
cystauchenotomy
cystauxe
cystectasia
cystectasy
cystectomy
cysteine
cystelcosis
cystendesis
cysterethism
cysthypersarcosis
cystic

cystidolaparotomy
cystidotrachelotomy
cystine
cystinosis
cystinuria
cystistaxis
cystitis
    allergic c.
    amicrobic c.
    bacterial c.
    catarrhal c.
    chemical c.
    c. colli
    croupous c.
    cystic c.
    c. cystica
    diphtheritic c.
    c. emphysematosa
    eosinophilic c.
    exfoliative c.
    c. follicularis
    gangrenous c.
    glandular c.
    c. glandularis
    hemorrhagic c.
    incrusted c.
    interstitial c.
    mechanical c.
    panmural c.
    papillary c.
    c. papillomatosa
    c. senilis feminarum
    subacute c.
    submucous c.
cysto–cystoscopic examination
cystocele
cystochrome
cystochromoscopy
cystocolostomy
cystodynia
cystoenterocele
cystoepiplocele
cystogram
    air c.
    excretory c.
    gravity c.
    postvoiding c.

cystogram (continued)
    voiding c.
cystography
cystolith
cystolithectomy
cystolithiasis
cystolithic
cystolithotomy
cystometer
    Lewis' c.
cystometric
cystometrogram
cystometrography
cystometry
    flow c.
cystonephrosis
cystoneuralgia
cystoparalysis
cystopexy
cystophotography
cystophthisis
cystoplasty
    cecal c.
cystoplegia
cystoproctostomy
cystoprostatectomy
cystoptosis
cystopyelitis
cystopyelogram
cystopyelography
cystopyelonephritis
cystoradiography
cystorectostomy
cystorrhagia
cystorrhaphy
cystorrhea
cystosarcoma
    c. phyllodes
cystoschisis
cystoscirrhus
cystoscope
    Braasch's c.
    Brown-Buerger c.
    Butterfield's c.
    fiberoptic c.
    Kelly's c.
    Lowsley-Peterson c.

cystoscope (continued)
McCarthy-Campbell c.
McCarthy-Peterson c.
McCarthy's c.
National c.
Nesbit's c.
Ravich's c.
Storz's c.
Wappler's c.
cystoscopic
cystoscopy
cystospasm
cystospermitis
cystostaxis
cystostomy
cystotome
cystotomy
suprapubic c.
cystotrachelotomy
cystoureteritis
cystoureterogram
cystoureteropyelitis
cystoureteropyelonephritis
cystourethrectomy
cystourethritis
cystourethrocele
cystourethrogram
cystourethrography
isotope voiding c.
cystourethropexy
cystourethroscope
cystous
cytology
cytometry
flow c.
cytophilic
cytophotometry
cytoplasm
cytotoxic
Danubian endemic familial
nephropathy
dartoic
dartoid
dartos
dartrous
Daseler's zone
Davat's operation

Davis'
sound
stone dislodger
Deaver's retractor
decapsulation
decortication
renal d.
decubitus
Dees' needle
Defer's method
dehydration
Del Castillo's syndrome
demasculinization
Deming's operation
Demme's method
Dennis-Brown technique
Denonvilliers'
aponeurosis
fascia
operation
denudation
de Pezzer catheter
dermoid
descending
descensus
d. testis
Desjardin's forceps
detrusor
d. urinae
devascularization
diabetes
d. insipidus
d. mellitus
dialysance
dialysate
dialysis
peritoneal d.
renal d.
dialyzer
diaphragm
urogenital d.
Dietl's crisis
diffusion
digitalization
dilatation
dilator
French's d. Nos. 8 to 36

dilator (continued)
    Guyon's d.
    Kollmann's d.
    Leader-Kollmann d.
    Van Buren's d.
    Walther's d.
disease
    Addison's d.
    Bowen's d.
    Bright's d.
    Corbus' d.
    Ducrey's d.
    Durand-Nicholas-Favre d.
    Ebstein's d.
    end-stage renal d.
    Fournier's d.
    Hodgkin's d.
    Klebs' d.
    Lindau's d.
    medullary cystic d.
    Paget's d.
    Peyronie's d.
    polycystic d.
    Reiter's d.
    Stühmer's d.
Dittel's
    operation
    sound
diuresis (diureses)
    tubular d.
diuretic
    hydragogue d.
    refrigerant d.
diuria
diversion
    ileal conduit d.
    ileocecal cutaneous d.
    jejunal cutaneous urinary
        d.
    Leadbetter's ileal
        loop d.
diverticula
    d. ampullae ductus
        deferentis
diverticulectomy
diverticuleve
diverticulitis

diverticulum
    calyceal d.
    vesical d.
Doppler's operation
Dorian's rib stripper
Dormia's
    basket
    stone dislodger
Douglas' pouch
Doyen's operation
drain
    Malecot's d.
    Penrose d.
    Pezzer's d.
    sump d.
dressing. See *General Surgical
    Terms* section.
dribbling
drugs. See *Drugs and Chemistry*
    section.
Ducrey's disease
duct
    Bellini's d's
    ejaculatory d.
    Leydig's d.
    mesonephric d.
    d. of Wolff
    wolffian d.
ductal
ductuli
    d. aberrantes
    d. prostatica
ductulus
    d. aberrans superior
ductus
    d. aberrans
    d. deferens
    d. ejaculatorius
    d. epididymidis
    d. excretorius glandulae
        bulbourethrales
    d. excretorius vesiculae
        seminalis
    d. glandulae
        bulbourethralis
    d. mesonephricus
    d. Muelleri

ductus (continued)
  d. paraurethrales
  d. prostatica
  d. spermaticus
  d. wolffi
Duplay's operation
Dupuytren's hydrocele
Durand-Nicholas-Favre disease
dynamoscope
dynamoscopy
dysgenesis
  gonadal d.
dysgenitalism
dysgerminoma
dysgonesis
dysphagia
dysplasia
dyspnea
dysuresia
dysuria
  psychic d.
  spastic d.
dysuriac
dysuric
dyszoospermia
Ebstein's disease
echinococcosis
ectasia
ectopia
  e. testis
  e. vesicae
Edebohls' operation
edema
efferent
efflux
Eissner's prostatic cooler
ejaculate
ejaculatio
  e. deficiens
  e. praecox
  e. retardata
ejaculation
ejaculatory
ejaculum
electrocystography
electrode
  ball tip e.

electrode (continued)
  bayonet tip e.
  Bugbee's e.
  Collings' e.
  conical tip e.
  Hamm's e.
  McCarthy's e.
  Neil-Moore e.
  ureteral meatotomy e.
electrolyte
electromyography
  ureteral e.
electrotome
  Stern-McCarthy e.
elephantiasis
  e. scroti
Ellik's evacuator
embolism
embolization
embryonal
emission
Emmett-Foley catheter
endocrine
endogenous
endometrioid
endometriosis
  e. vesicae
endopelvic
endoscope
  Kelly's e.
endoscopic
endoscopy
endourethral
end-stage renal disease
enorchia
enteral
enteropathy
enucleation
enucleator
  Young's e.
enuresis
  diurnal e.
  nocturnal e.
enuretic
enzyme
  degradative e's
epicystitis

epicystotomy
epidermal
epidermoid
epididymal
epididymectomy
epididymis
epididymitis
 spermatogenic e.
epididymodeferentectomy
epididymodeferential
epididymo-orchitis
epididymotomy
epididymovasectomy
epididymovasostomy
epinephrectomy
epinephritis
epinephroma
epinephros
epispadia
epispadiac
epispadial
epispadias
 balanitic e.
 penile e.
 penopubic e.
epistaxis
 Gull's renal e.
epithelial
epithelioid
epithelium
Epstein's
 nephrosis
 syndrome
erectile
erection
erythrocytosis
erythroplasia
 e. of Queyrat
 Zoon's e.
Esbach's method
EU—excretory urography
evacuator
 Creevy's e.
 Ellik's e.
 McCarthy's e.
 Toomey's e.
Everett-TeLinde operation

excretion
excretory
 e. cystogram
 e. urogram
exenteration
exogenous
exophytic
exsanguinate
exstrophy
 e. of the bladder
extracellular
extragonadal
extravasation
exudate
exudative
fal-. See words beginning *phal-*.
Fanconi's syndrome
Farr's retractor
fascia
 Buck's f.
 Camper's f.
 Colles' f.
 cremasteric f.
 f. cremasterica
 dartos f. of scrotum
 Denonvilliers' f.
 Gerota's f.
 inferior f.
 f. lata
 f. of prostate
 f. of urogenital trigone
 f. penis profunda
 f. penis superficialis
 f. propria cooperi
 rectovesical f.
 renal f.
 f. renalis
 Scarpa's f.
 spermatic f., external
 spermatic f., internal
 f. spermatica externa
 f. spermatica interna
 subserous f.
 transversalis f.
Feleki's instrument
feminization
 testicular f.

femoral
    f. triangle
feo-. See words beginning *pheo-*.
Ferguson's basket
α-fetoprotein
fi-. See words beginning *phi-*.
fibrinolysis
fibrosarcoma
fibrosis
    retroperitoneal f.
filariasis
filiform
filtration
Fishberg's method
fistula
flagellum
flebo-. See words beginning
    phlebo-.
fluid
    straw-colored f.
fluoresceinuria
Foley
    catheter
    forceps
    Y-type ureteropelvioplasty
Foley-Alcock catheter
Folin and Bell's method
Folin and Berglund's method
Folin and Denis' method
Folin and Farmer's method
Folin and Flander's method
Folin and Hart's method
Folin and Macallum's method
Folin and Wright's method
Folin and Youngburg's method
Folin, Benedict and Myers'
    method
Folin, McEllroy and Peck's
    method
Folin's
    gravimetric method
    method
Follmann's balanitis
follower
forceps
    Allis' f.
    Blake's f.

forceps (continued)
    Bozeman's f.
    Braasch's f.
    Buerger-McCarthy f.
    Bumpus' f.
    Bunim's f.
    Campbell's f.
    Coppridge's f.
    Crenshaw's f.
    Desjardin's f.
    Foley f.
    Harris' f.
    Kelly's f.
    Lewis' f.
    Lewkowitz's f.
    Lowsley's f.
    Mathieu's f.
    McCarthy-Alcock f.
    McCarthy's f.
    McNealy-Glassman-
      Babcock f.
    Millin's f.
    Pitha's f.
    Poutasse's f.
    Randall's f.
    Ratliff-Blake f.
    Ray's f.
    Rochester-Pean f.
    Skillern's f.
    White-Oslay f.
    Young's f.
foreskin
    redundant f.
Formad's kidney
foroblique
fossa
    f. of Morgagni
    navicular f. of male
      urethra
    f. navicularis urethrae
    f. ovalis
    paravesical f.
Fournier's disease
Fowler's sound
Franco's operation
Franklin-Silverman needle
French-McCarthy panendoscope

French-Robinson catheter
French's dilator
frenulum
    f. of prepuce of penis
    f. preputii penis
frenum
frequency
Freyer's operation
friable
frond
FTA-ABS—fluorescent
    treponemal antibody-
    absorption test
fulguration
Fuller's operation
fundic
fundiform
fundus
    f. of bladder
    f. of urinary bladder
    f. vesicae urinariae
fungal
fungating
    f. growth
funiculitis
funiculopexy
funiculus
    f. spermaticus
Furniss' catheter
galactosuria
galacturia
gallium
ganglioneuroblastoma
ganglioneuroma
GC—gonococcus
Gelpi's retractor
genital
genitalia
genitocrural
genitofemoral
genitoinfectious
genitoplasty
genitourinary
germinoma
germinomatous
Gerota's
    capsule

Gerot's (continued)
    fascia
GFR—glomerular filtration rate
Gibbon's hydrocele
Gibbons' stent
Gilbert-Dreyfus syndrome
Gilbert's
    sign
    syndrome
Giraldes' organ
gland
    adrenal g.
    Albarran's g.
    bulbourethral g.
    Cowper's g.
    Littre's g's
    paraurethral g.
    preputial g.
    prostate g.
    Skene's g.
    suprarenal g.
glandular
    g. cystitis
    g. metaplasia
glans
    g. penis
Gleason's grading score
gleet
Glenn's technique
glischruria
globulinuria
globus
    g. major epididymidis
    g. minor epididymidis
glomerular
glomeruli
    g. renis
    Ruysch's g.
glomerulitis
glomerulonephritis
glomerulopathy
glomerulosclerosis
glomerulose
glomerulus
glucose
glycoprotein
glycosuria

Goldblatt's
  clamp
  hypertension
  kidney
Gomco's clamp
gonad
gonadal
gonadectomize
gonadectomy
gonadial
gonadoblastic
gonadoblastoma
gonadopathy
gonadotherapy
gonadotropin
    chorionic g.
gonadotropism
gonaduct
gonangiectomy
gonecyst
gonecystis
gonecystitis
gonecystolith
gonecystopyosis
gonocele
gonococcal
gonococci
gonococcus
gonophore
gonorrhea
gonorrheal
Goodpasture's syndrome
gorget
    Teale's g.
graft
    Thiersch's g.
granular
granuloma
    g. inguinale
granulomatous
    g. prostatitis
gravity
    specific g.
Grawitz's tumor
groin
GU – genitourinary

gubernaculum
    chorda g.
    Hunter's g.
    g. testis
Gull's renal epistaxis
gumma
Guyon-Pean clamp
Guyon's
    clamp
    dilator
    sound
gynandroblastoma
gynecomastia
gynoblastoma
Hacker's operation
Hagner's operation
Halsted's clamp
hamartoma
Hamm's electrode
Harrington's retractor
Harris'
    forceps
    segregator
HCO_3 – bicarbonate
Heintz's method
Heitz-Boyer procedure
Heller-Nelson syndrome
hemangioendothelioma
hemangioma
hemangiopericytoma
hemangiosarcoma
hematocele
    scrotal h.
hematoma
hematoscheocele
hematospermatocele
hematospermia
hematuria
    angioneurotic h.
    endemic h.
    essential h.
    microscopic h.
    renal h.
    urethral h.
    vesical h.
hemaurochrome
hemihypertrophy

heminephrectomy
heminephroureterectomy
hemiscrotectomy
hemodialysis
hemodynamic
hemorrhage
hemospermia
hemostatic bag
    Pilcher's h.b.
Hendrickson's lithotrite
Henle's
    ampulla
    internal cremaster
    loop
    sphincter
    tubules
hermaphrodism
hermaphrodite
hermaphroditism
hernia
    parastomal h.
herpes
    genital h.
    h. praeputialis
    h. progenitalis
    h. simplex
    h. zoster
Herrick's clamp
Hesselbach's triangle
Hess' operation
Heyd's syndrome
Highmore
    corpus of H.
    H.'s body
hilar
hilum (hila)
hilus (hili)
    h. glandulae suprarenalis
    h. of kidney
    h. of suprarenal gland
    h. renalis
hind-kidney
Hinman's reflux
Hippel-Lindau syndrome
hirsutism
histogenesis
Hodgkin's disease

homotransplant
hook
    Kimball's h.
Howard's basket
Huggins' operation
humoral
Hunner's stricture
Hunter's gubernaculum
Hurwitz's trocar
Hutchins' needle
hyaline
Hyams' clamp
hydatid
    h. of Morgagni
    sessile h.
hydatidocele
hydatiduria
hydration
hydrocele
    chylous h.
    h. colli
    communicating h.
    Dupuytren's h.
    encysted h.
    funicular h.
    Gibbon's h.
    Maunoir's h.
    noncommunicating h.
    scrotal h.
hydrocelectomy
Hydroflex penile prosthesis
hydronephrosis
hydronephrotic
hydroperinephrosis
hydropyonephrosis
hydrosarcocele
hydroscheocele
hydrostatic
hydroureter
hydroureterosis
hydrouria
hyperaldosteronism
hyperalimentation
hyperbilirubinemia
hypercalcemia
hypercortisolism
hyperemia

hyperkeratotic
hypermetabolism
hypernephritis
hypernephroid
hypernephroma
hyperorchidism
hyperoxaluria
hyperparathyroidism
hyperplasia
hyperreninemia
hypertension
    adrenal h.
    essential h.
    Goldblatt's h.
    renal h.
    secondary h.
hypertonic
hypertrophy
    prostatic h.
hypocalcemia
hypogastric
hypogonadism
hypokalemia
hypomagnesemia
hypophosphatemia
hypoplasia
hypoproteinemia
hypospadiac
hypospadias
hypothalamic
    h. suppression
hypothermia
hypotonia
hypotonic
Hyrtl's sphincter
Iglesias' resectoscope
ileal
    i. conduit diversion
ileocecal
    i. cutaneous diversion
ileocystoplasty
ileocystostomy
iliac
iliocostal
iliohypogastric
ilioinguinal
Immergut's tube

immune
immunity
immunohistochemistry
immunology
immunoperoxidase
immunosuppression
immunosuppressive
immunosurveillance
immunotherapy
implant
    Silastic i.
implantation
    radioactive isotope i.
impotence
impotentia
    i. coeundi
    i. erigendi
incision. See *General Surgical Terms* section.
incontinence
    i. of urine
    paradoxical i.
    paralytic i.
    stress i.
    urinary i.
incontinent
incontinentia
    i. urinae
indoluria
indoxyl
indoxyluria
induration
    penile i.
indwelling
infarct
    bilirubin i's
    Brewer's i's
    uric acid i.
infarction
    renal i.
inferior vena cava
infiltrating
inflammatory
infundibula
    i. of kidney
infundibular
infundibuliform

infundibulopelvic
infundibulum
    i. of urinary bladder
inguinal
inguinocrural
inguinoscrotal
innervation
insertion
    cystoradium i.
insipidus
instrument
    Feleki's i.
insufficiency
    renal i.
integument
intercostal
intercourse
interlobar
interlobular
interstitial
interureteral
interureteric
intestinal
intrarenal
intratesticular
intrathoracic
intratubular
intraureteral
intraurethral
intravenous
intravesical
intussusception
involution
ipsilateral
irradiation
Isaacs-Ludwig arteriole
ischemia
ischiopubic
ischiorectal
isotope
Israel's operation
isthmus
    i. prostatae
    i. urethrae
isuria
IVCU – isotope voiding
    cystourethrography

IVP – intravenous pyelogram
Jacobson's retractor
jejunal
    j. cutaneous urinary
      diversion
jejunostomy
    needle catheter j.
Jewett's sound
Jewett-Strong system
Johnson's
    basket
    needle holder
    stone dislodger
Judd-Masson retractor
Judd's retractor
junction
    ureteropelvic j.
    ureterovesical j.
juxtaglomerular
K – potassium
Kantor's clamp
Kaposi's sarcoma
Keitzer's urethrotome
Kelly-Deming operation
Kelly's
    cystoscope
    endoscope
    forceps
    operation
Kelly-Stoeckel operation
ketone body
ketonuria
ketosis
Keyes' lithotrite
kidney
    amyloid k.
    arteriosclerotic k.
    artificial k.
    atrophic k.
    cake k.
    cicatricial k.
    cirrhotic k.
    clump k.
    congested k.
    contracted k.
    crush k.
    cyanotic k.

kidney (continued)
  cystic k.
  disk k.
  doughnut k.
  ectopic k.
  fatty k.
  flea-bitten k.
  floating k.
  Formad's k.
  fused k.
  Goldblatt's k.
  granular k.
  hind k.
  horseshoe k.
  hypermobile k.
  hypoplastic k.
  lardaceous k.
  large red k.
  lump k.
  medullary sponge k.
  mortar k.
  mural k.
  myelin k.
  pelvic k.
  polycystic k.
  primordial k.
  putty k.
  Rokitansky's k.
  Rose-Bradford k.
  sacciform k.
  sclerotic k.
  sigmoid k.
  soapy k.
  sponge k.
  k. stone
  supernumerary k.
  wandering k.
  waxy k.
kilo-. See words beginning *chylo-*.
Kimball's hook
Kimmelstiel-Wilson syndrome
Klebs' disease
Klinefelter's syndrome
Kocher's
  maneuver
  retractor
Koch's pouch

Kock's reservoir
Kollmann's dilator
kor-. See words beginning *chor-*.
Korean hemorrhagic
  nephrosonephritis
kraurosis
  penile k.
KUB – kidney, ureter and bladder
Labbé's syndrome
lactosuria
lacuna
  great l. of urethra
  l. magna
lacunae
  l. Morgagnii urethrae
    muliebris
  l. of Morgagni
  l. of urethra
  l. urethrales
lamella
lamina
  l. visceralis tunicae
    vaginalis propriae testis
  l. visceralis tunicae
    vaginalis testis
Lancereaux's nephritis
laparonephrectomy
Lapides' needle holder
laser
Lashmet and Newburgh method
law
  Bell's l.
Leadbetter's ideal loop diversion
Leader-Kollmann dilator
LeFort's
  bougie
  catheter
  sound
Legueu's retractor
leiomyoma
leiomyosarcoma
Leriche's syndrome
leukemia
  testicular l.
leukoplakia
  l. of penis
Levant's stone dislodger

Lewis'
    cystometer
    forceps
Lewkowitz's forceps
leydigarche
Leydig's
    cells
    duct
libidogen
lichen
    l. planus
lienorenal
ligament
    lateral false l.
    lateral puboprostatic l.
    medial puboprostatic l.
    middle umbilical l.
    pubovesical l.
    round l.
Lightwood's syndrome
Lindau's disease
line
    Brödel's l.
linea
    l. alba
lipoma
liposarcoma
liquor
    l. prostaticus
    l. seminis
lithangiuria
lithectasy
lithiasis
lithocenosis
lithoclysmia
lithocystotomy
lithodialysis
lithokonion
litholabe
litholapaxy
litholysis
litholyte
lithometer
lithomyl
lithonephria
lithonephritis
lithonephrotomy

lithophone
lithoscope
lithotripsy
lithotriptic
lithotriptor
lithotriptoscope
lithotriptoscopy
lithotrite
    Alcock's l.
    Alcock-Hendrickson's l.
    Bigelow's l.
    Hendrickson's l.
    Keyes' l.
    Lowenstein's l.
    Lowsley's l.
    Reliquet's l.
    Thompson's l.
lithotrity
lithous
lithoxiduria
lithuresis
lithureteria
lithuria
Littre's glands
liver
    l. dysfunction
    l. scan
Lloyd's sign
lobulation
lobule
    cortical l's of kidney
    l's of testis
lobuli
    l. corticales renis
    l. epididymidis
    l. testis
lobulus
Löhlein's nephritis
Longuet's operation
loop
    Henle's l.
Lowenstein's lithotrite
Lowsley-Peterson cystoscope
Lowsley's
    forceps
    lithotrite
    operation

Lowsley's (continued)
    tractor
Luder-Sheldon syndrome
lumbosacral
lumen
luteinizing
luxation
Luy's segregator
lymphadenectomy
lymphangiogram
lymphangiography
lymphangioma
lymphangiosarcoma
lymphatic
lymphedema
lymphogranuloma
    l. inguinale
    venereal l.
    l. venereum
lymphoma
    Burkitt's l.
    testicular l.
lymphomatous
lymphopathia
    l. venereum
lymphosarcoma
lysosomal
macrophage
magnetic resonance imaging
Maisonneuve's urethrotome
Makka's operation
malacoplakia
    m. vesicae
Malecot's
    catheter
    drain
malignant
malrotation
maneuver
    Kocher's m.
Marañon's syndrome
Marchand's adrenals
Marian's operation
Marshall-Jewett-Strong
    classification
Marshall-Marchetti-Birch
    operation

Marshall-Marchetti-Krantz
    operation
Marshall-Marchetti operation
Marshall's
    surgical sucker
    test
Martin's operation
Martius-Harris operation
Martius' operation
Masson-Judd retractor
Mathieu's forceps
Maunoir's hydrocele
Mayo's clamp
Mays' operation
McCarthy-Alcock forceps
McCarthy-Campbell
    cystoscope
McCarthy-Peterson cystoscope
McCarthy's
    cystoscope
    electrode
    evacuator
    forceps
    foroblique panendoscope
    resectoscope
    telescope
McCrea's sound
McGill's operation
McIver's catheter
McNealy-Glassman-Babcock
    forceps
meatal
meatome
meatometer
meatorrhaphy
meatoscope
meatoscopy
meatotome
meatotomy
meatus
    m. urinarius
median-bar
mediastinum
    m. testis
medications. See *Drugs and*
    Chemistry section.
medorrhea

medulla
    adrenal m.
    m. glandulae suprarenalis
    m. nephrica
    m. of kidney
    m. of suprarenal gland
    m. renis
    suprarenal m.
medullae
medullary
medullectomy
medulliadrenal
medulloadrenal
medulloid
medullosuprarenoma
megabladder
megalopenis
megaloureter
melanoma
melanosis
melasma
    m. addisonii
    m. suprarenale
mellitus
Mercier's
    bar
    operation
mesangium
mesenchymal
mesenchymoma
mesoblastic
mesonephric
mesonephroma
mesonephron
mesonephros
mesothelioma
metanephrine
metanephroi
metanephros
metaplasia
metastasis
method
    acid hematin m.
    Addis' m.
    Arnold and Gunning's m.
    Bence Jones protein m.
    Benedict and Franke's m.

method (continued)
    Benedict and Osterberg's
      m.
    Bertrand's m.
    Defer's m.
    Demme's m.
    Esbach's m.
    Fishberg's m.
    Folin and Bell's m.
    Folin and Berglund's m.
    Folin and Denis' m.
    Folin and Farmer's m.
    Folin and Flander's m.
    Folin and Hart's m.
    Folin and Macallum's m.
    Folin and Wright's m.
    Folin and Youngburg's m.
    Folin, Benedict, and
      Myers' m.
    Folin, McEllroy, and
      Peck's m.
    Folin's gravimetric m.
    Folin's m.
    Heintz's m.
    Lashmet and Newburgh
      m.
    Naunyn-Minkowski m.
    Osborne and Folin's m.
    permutit m.
    Power and Wilder's m.
    Shohl and Pedley's m.
    Sjöqvist's m.
    Sumner's m.
    Volhard and Fahr m.
Metzenbaum's scissors
micrography
    transition electron m.
microrchidia
miction
micturate
micturition
Miller's syndrome
Millin-Bacon
    retractor
    spreader
Millin's
    forceps

Millin's (continued)
    tube
Mitchell's basket
monoclonal
mononephrous
morcellement
Morgagni
    fossa of M.
    hydatid of M.
    lacunae of M.
mosaicism
Mosher's speculum
Moynihan's
    probe
    scoop
MRI – magnetic resonance
  imaging
mucinous
mucosa
Muelleri
    ductus M.
multicentric
muscle
    Bell's m.
    bulbocavernous m.
    cremaster m.
    detrusor urinae m.
    external oblique m.
    internal oblique m.
    ischiocavernous m.
    latissimus dorsi m.
    levator ani m.
    psoas m.
    pubovesicalis m.
    rectourethralis m.
    rectovesicalis m.
    transversalis m.
    transverse perinei m.
musculus
    m. levator prostate
    m. obturatorius externus
    m. obturatorius internus
    m. pubovaginalis
    m. pubovesicalis
    m. quadratus lumborum
    m. rectourethralis
    m. rectovesicalis

musculus (continued)
    m. sphincter urethrae
    m. sphincter vesicae
      urinariae
    m. transversus abdominis
    m. transversus perinei
      superficialis
myelolipoma
myoblastoma
myoma
myosarcoma
myxocystitis
myxoid
myxoma
myxosarcoma
Na – sodium
Narath's operation
National cystoscope
National Prostatic Cancer
    Treatment Group
Naunyn-Minkowski method
necrosis
    renal papillary n.
needle
    Dees' n.
    Franklin-Silverman n.
    Hutchins' n.
    Travenol n.
    Turkel's n.
    Veenema-Gusberg n.
    Vim-Silverman n.
needle holder
    Johnson's n.h.
    Lapides' n.h.
    Stratte's n.h.
    Young-Millin n.h.
    Young's n.h.
Neil-Moore electrode
Nélaton's
    catheter
    sphincter
neoadjuvant
neoplasia
neoplasm
    vascular n.
neoplastic
nephradenoma

nephralgia
  idiopathic n.
nephralgic
nephrapostasis
nephrasthenia
nephratonia
nephratony
nephrauxe
nephrectasia
nephrectasis
nephrectasy
nephrectomize
nephrectomy
  abdominal n.
  lumbar n.
  paraperitoneal n.
  posterior n.
nephredema
nephrelcosis
nephremia
nephremphraxis
nephria
nephric
nephridium
nephrism
nephritic
nephritides
nephritis
  albuminous n.
  arteriosclerotic n.
  azotemic n.
  bacterial n.
  Balkan n.
  capsular n.
  n. caseosa
  catarrhal n.
  cheesy n.
  chloroazotemic n.
  clostridial n.
  congenital n.
  croupous n.
  degenerative n.
  desquamative n.
  diffuse n.
  n. dolorosa
  dropsical n.
  exudative n.

nephritis (continued)
  fibrolipomatous n.
  fibrous n.
  focal n.
  glomerular n.
  glomerulocapsular n.
  n. gravidarum
  hemorrhagic n.
  hydremic n.
  hydropigenous n.
  hypogenetic n.
  idiopathic n.
  indurative n.
  interstitial n.
  Lancereaux's n.
  lipomatous n.
  Löhlein's n.
  n. mitis
  n. of pregnancy
  parenchymatous n.
  phenacetin n.
  pneumococcus n.
  potassium-losing n.
  productive n.
  radiation n.
  n. repens
  salt-losing n.
  saturnine n.
  scarlatinal n.
  subacute n.
  suppurative n.
  syphilitic n.
  tartrate n.
  transfusion n.
  trench n.
  tubal n.
  tuberculous n.
  vascular n.
  Volhard's n.
  war n.
nephritogenic
nephroabdominal
nephroangiosclerosis
nephroblastoma
nephroblastomatosis
nephrocalcinosis
nephrocapsectomy

nephrocardiac
nephrocele
nephrocirrhosis
nephrocolic
nephrocolopexy
nephrocoloptosis
nephrocystanastomosis
nephrocystitis
nephrocystosis
nephroerysipelas
nephrogastric
nephrogenic
nephrogenous
nephrogram
nephrography
nephrohemia
nephrohydrosis
nephrohypertrophy
nephroid
nephrolith
nephrolithiasis
nephrolithotomy
nephrologist
nephrology
nephrolysis
nephroma
    embryonal n.
    mesoblastic n.
nephromalacia
nephromegaly
nephron
nephroncus
nephro-omentopexy
nephroparalysis
nephropathic
nephropathy
    analgesic n.
    Balkan n.
    Danubian endemic
      familial n.
    dropsical n.
    gouty n.
    hypazoturic n.
    hypercalcemic n.
    hypochloruric n.
    toxic n.
nephropexy

nephrophagiasis
nephropoietic
nephropoietin
nephroptosia
nephroptosis
nephropyelitis
nephropyelolithotomy
nephropyeloplasty
nephropyosis
nephrorosein
nephrorrhagia
nephrorrhapy
nephroscleria
nephrosclerosis
    arteriolar n.
    benign n.
    hyaline arteriolar n.
    hyperplastic arteriolar n.
    intercapillary n.
    malignant n.
    senile n.
nephroses
nephrosis
    amyloid n.
    cholemic n.
    Epstein's n.
    glycogen n.
    hydropic n.
    hypokalemic n.
    larval n.
    lipid n.
    lipoid n.
    lower nephron n.
    necrotizing n.
    osmotic n.
    toxic n.
    vacuolar n.
nephrosonephritis
    hemorrhagic n.
    Korean hemorrhagic n.
nephrosonography
nephrospasis
nephrosplenopexy
nephrostomy
nephrotic
nephrotome
nephrotomogram

nephrotomography
nephrotomy
       abdominal n.
       lumbar
nephrotoxic
nephrotoxicity
nephrotoxin
nephrotresis
nephrotropic
nephrotuberculosis
nephrotyphoid
nephrotyphus
nephroureterectomy
nephroureterocystectomy
nephrozymase
nephrozymosis
Nesbit's
       cystoscope
       resectoscope
nest
       Brunn's n's
       von Brunn's n's
neuroblastoma
neuroendocrine
neurofibroma
neurofibromatosis
neurogenic
neuroma
neutropenia
Nisbet's chancre
nitrosamine
nocturia
nodular
Nonnenbruch's syndrome
nonopaque
nonseminomatous
Nourse's syringe
NPCTG–National Prostatic
    Cancer Treatment Group
NSU–nonspecific urethritis
nucleotide
obstruction
obstructive
       o. uropathy
obturator
       Alcock-Timberlake o.
       Timberlake's o.

Ochsner's
       probe
       trocar
Ockerblad's clamp
O'Conor's operation
oligohydruria
oligonecrospermia
oligophosphaturia
oligospermatism
oligospermia
oliguria
Ombrédanne's operation
oncocytoma
oncogene
opacity
opaque
operation
       Andrews' o.
       Bates' o.
       Belfield's o.
       Bennett's o.
       Bergenhem's o.
       Bevan-Rochet o.
       Bevan's o.
       Bigelow's o.
       Boari's o.
       Bottini's o.
       Bricker's o.
       Cecil's o.
       Civiale's o.
       Clark's o.
       Cock's o.
       Davat's o.
       Deming's o.
       Denonvilliers' o.
       Dittel's o.
       Doppler's o.
       Doyen's o.
       Duplay's o.
       Edebohls' o.
       Everett-TeLinde o.
       Franco's o.
       Freyer's o.
       Fuller's o.
       Hacker's o.
       Hagner's o.
       Hess' o.

operation (continued)
    Huggins' o.
    interposition o.
    Israel's o.
    Kelly-Deming o.
    Kelly's o.
    Kelly-Stoeckel o.
    Longuet's o.
    Lowsley's o.
    Makka's o.
    Marian's o.
    Marshall-Marchetti o.
    Marshall-Marchetti-
      Birch o.
    Marshall-Marchetti-
      Krantz o.
    Martin's o.
    Martius-Harris o.
    Martius' o.
    Mays' o.
    McGill's o.
    Mercier's o.
    mika o.
    morcellement o.
    Narath's o.
    O'Conor's o.
    Ombrédanne's o.
    Petersen's o.
    Poncet's o.
    Rigaud's o.
    sling o.
    Spivack's o.
    Stanischeff's o.
    Steinach's o.
    Torek's o.
    Tuffier's o.
    van Hook's o.
    Vidal's o.
    Vogel's o.
    Volkmann's o.
    von Bergmann's o.
    von Hacker's o.
    Voronoff's o.
    Wheelhouse's o.
    White's o.
    Wood's o.
    Young's o.

orchialgia
orchichorea
orchidalgia
orchidectomy
orchidic
orchiditis
orchidocelioplasty
orchidoepididymectomy
orchidoncus
orchidopathy
orchidopexy
orchidoplasty
orchidoptosis
orchidorrhaphy
orchidotherapy
orchidotomy
orchiectomy
orchiencephaloma
orchiepididymitis
orchilytic
orchiocatabasis
orchiocele
orchiococcus
orchiodynia
orchiomyeloma
orchioncus
orchioneuralgia
orchiopathy
orchiopexy
orchioplasty
orchiorrhaphy
orchioscheocele
orchioscirrhus
orchiotomy
orchis
orchitic
orchitis
    metastatic o.
    o. parotidea
    o. variolosa
orchitolytic
orchotomy
organ
    o. of Giraldes
orgasm
orifice
    o. of male urethra

orifice (continued)
  o. of ureter
  o. of urethra
  ureteral o.
  vesicourethral o.
os
  o. penis
  o. pubis
Osborne and Folin's method
osteitis
  o. pubis
osteoma
osteosarcoma
Otis'
  bougie
  sound
  urethrotome
ovary (ovaries)
Owens' catheter
Paget's disease
pampiniform
panendoscope
  French-McCarthy p.
  McCarthy's foroblique p.
panendoscopy
panniculitis
papilla
papillary
papilloma
  squamous cell p.
papulosis
  bowenoid p.
paradidymal
paradidymis
paragenitalis
paraglobulinuria
paralysis
paranephric
paranephritis
  lipomatous p.
paranephroma
paranephros
paraphimosis
pararenal
paratesticular
paraurethra
paraurethral

paraurethritis
paravesical
parenchyma
  p. of kidney
  p. of testis
  p. testis
parenchymal
parietal
pars
  p. abdominalis ureteris
  p. cavernosa urethrae
    virilis
  p. convoluta lobuli
    corticalis renis
  p. membranacea urethrae
    masculinae
  p. membranacea urethrae
    virilis
  p. pelvina ureteris
  p. prostatica urethrae
    masculinae
  p. prostatica urethrae
    virilis
  p. radiata lobuli corticalis
    renis
  p. spongiosa urethrae
    masculinae
partes
  p. genitales externae
    viriles
  p. genitales masculinae
    externae
pedicle
pelves
pelvilithotomy
pelvioileoneocystostomy
pelviolithotomy
pelvioneostomy
pelvioperitonitis
pelvioplasty
pelvioradiography
pelvioscopy
pelviostomy
pelviotomy
pelviradiography
pelvirectal
pelviroentgenography

pelvis
    renal p.
penectomy
penial
penile
penis
    clubbed p.
    ligamentum fundiforme p.
    p. plastica
penischisis
penitis
penoscrotal
Penrose drain
percutaneous
periarteritis
    p. gummosa
    p. nodosa
pericystitis
perineal
perineoscrotal
perineostomy
perinephric
perinephritic
perinephritis
perinephrium
perineum
perineural
periorchitis
    p. adhaesiva
    p. purulenta
periorchium
peripenial
peripheral
periprostatic
periprostatis
perirenal
perispermatitis
    p. serosa
peritoneal
peritoneum
peritonitis
periureteric
periureteritis
periurethral
periurethritis
perivesical
perivesicular

perivesiculitis
permutit method
Petersen's operation
Peyronie's disease
Pezzer's
    catheter
    drain
pH–hydrogen ion
    concentration
phallalgia
phallanastrophe
phallaneurysm
phallectomy
phallic
phallitis
phallocampsis
phallocrypsis
phallodynia
phalloncus
phalloplasty
phallorrhagia
phallorrhea
phallotomy
phallus
Pheifer-Young retractor
phenolsulfonphthalein
phenotype
phenotypic
phenylketonuria
pheochromocyte
pheochromocytoma
Philips'
    bougie
    catheter
phimosiectomy
phimosis
phimotic
phlebolith
photoradiation
photoscan
pielo. See words beginning *pyelo-.*
Pilcher's hemostatic bag
pio. See words beginning *pyo-.*
Pitha's forceps
Pitres' sign
pituitary
PKU—phenylketonuria

plaque
    Randall's p's
plasminogen
plexus
    p. cavernosus penis
    cavernous p. of penis
    hypogastric p.
    pampiniform p.
    p. pampiniformis
    pelvic p.
    prostatic p.
    prostaticovesical p.
    p. prostaticus
    renal p.
    p. renalis
    sacral p.
    Santorini's p.
    spermatic p.
    p. spermaticus
    suprarenal p.
    p. suprarenalis
    testicular p.
    p. testicularis
    ureteric p.
    p. uretericus
    p. venosus prostaticus
    vesical p.
    p. vesicale
    p. vesicalis
    vesicoprostatic p.
plica
    p. pubovesicalis
    p. vesicalis transversa
ploidy
pneumaturia
polycystic
polydipsia
polyorchidism
polyorchis
polyspermia
polyspermism
polyspermy
polyuria
Poncet's operation
porphyria
porphyrinuria
porphyruria

position. See *General Surgical Terms* section.
posthetomy
posthioplasty
posthitis
postholith
postirradiation
Potain's trocar
pouch
    p. of Douglas
    Koch's p.
Poutasse's forceps
Power and Wilder's method
Pratt's sound
Prehn's sign
preperitoneal
prepubertal
prepuce
    p. of penis
preputial
preputiotomy
preputium
    p. penis
preurethritis
prevesical
priapism
priapitis
priapus
probe
    Moynihan's p.
    Ochsner's p.
procedure
    Campbell's p.
    Heitz-Boyer p.
progenital
proliferative
pronephros
properitoneal
prostata
prostatalgia
prostatauxe
prostate
prostatectomy
    perineal p.
    radical p.
    retropubic previscal p.
    suprapubic tranvesical p.

prostatectomy (continued)
    transurethral p.
prostatelcosis
prostateria
prostatic
prostaticovesical
prostaticovesiculectomy
prostatism
    vesical p.
prostatisme
    p. sans prostate
prostatitic
prostatitis
    granulomatous p.
    tuberculous p.
prostatocystitis
prostatocystotomy
prostatodynia
prostatography
prostatolith
prostatolithotomy
prostatomegaly
prostatometer
prostatomy
prostatomyomectomy
prostatorrhea
prostatotomy
prostatotoxin
prostatovesiculectomy
prostatovesiculitis
prosthesis
    Hydroflex penile p.
    semirigid p.
    Silastic testicular p.
proteinuria
    adventitious p.
    Bence Jones p.
    cardiac p.
    colliquative p.
    cyclic p.
    emulsion p.
    enterogenic p.
    febrile p.
    globular p.
    gouty p.
    hematogenous p.
    intrinsic p.

proteinuria (continued)
    nephrogenous p.
    palpatory p.
    postrenal p.
    residual p.
proteinuric
pruritus
pseudocyst
pseudohermaphrodism
pseudohermaphrodite
pseudohermaphroditism
pseudosarcoid
psoas muscle
PSP – phenolsulfonphthalein
ptosis
    p. of kidney
    renal p.
pubes
pubetrotomy
pubic
pubioplasty
pubiotomy
pubis
    symphysis p.
puboprostatic
pubovesical
pudendal
punch
    Turkel's p.
purulent
pustule
PVC – postvoiding cystogram
pyelectasia
pyelectasis
pyelic
pyelitic
pyelitis
    calculous p.
    p. cystica
    defloration p.
    encrusted p.
    p. glandularis
    p. granulosa
    p. gravidarum
    hematogenous p.
    hemorrhagic p.
    suppurative p.

pyelitis (continued)
    urogenous p.
pyelocaliectasis
pyelocystanastomosis
pyelocystitis
pyelocystostomosis
pyelofluoroscopy
pyelogram
        dragon p.
        infusion p.
        intravenous p.
pyelograph
pyelography
        air p.
        ascending p.
        drip p.
        excretion p.
        infusion p.
        intravenous p.
        respiration p.
        retrograde p.
        washout p.
pyeloileocutaneous
pyelointerstitial
pyelolithotomy
pyelometer
pyelometry
pyelonephritis
        acute p.
        chronic p.
        xanthogranulomatous p.
pyelonephrosis
pyelopathy
pyelophlebitis
pyeloplasty
pyeloplication
pyeloscopy
pyelostomy
pyelotomy
pyelotubular
pyeloureterectasis
pyeloureteritis cystica
pyeloureterogram
pyeloureterography
pyeloureterolysis
pyeloureteroplasty
pyelovenous

pyocalix
pyocele
pyogenic
pyonephritis
pyonephrolithiasis
pyonephrosis
pyonephrotic
pyospermia
pyoureter
pyovesiculosis
pyramid
        p's of kidney
        renal p's
pyuria
quadriplegia
Queyrat's erythroplasia
rabdo. See words beginning
        rhabdo-.
radicular
radioactive
radioenzymatic
radiography
radioimmunoassay
radiolucent
radionuclide
radiopaque
radiotherapy
rafe. See *raphe*.
Ralks' adapter
Randall's
        forceps
        plaque
Rankin's retractor
raphe
        r. of perineum
        r. of scrotum
        r. penis
        r. scroti
Ratliff-Blake forceps
Ravich's cystoscope
Ray's forceps
reabsorption
reaction
        Bittorf's r.
recessus
        r. hepatorenalis
rectourethral

rectovesical
rectovestibular
rectum
red Robinson catheter
reflux
      Hinman's r.
      urethrovesiculodifferential
      r.
Reifenstein's syndrome
Reiter's disease
rejection
Reliquet's lithotrite
ren
      r. mobilis
      r. unguliformis
renal
      r. artery
      r. blastema
      r. cell carcinoma
      r. cortex
      r. cortical necrosis
      r. cyst
      r. ectopia
      r. failure
      r. fascia
      r. hyperplasia
      r. insufficiency
      r. lithiasis
      r. osteodystrophy
      r. papillae
      r. pedicle
      r. pelvis
      r. plexus
      r. pouch
      r. rickets
      r. sinus
      r. tubular acidosis
      r. tubule
      r. vein
      r. venogram
renculi
renes
renicapsule
renicardiac
reniculi
reniculus
renin

reninoma
renipelvic
reniportal
renipuncture
renocortical
renocutaneous
renogastric
renogram
renography
renointestinal
renoprival
renopulmonary
renotrophic
renotropic
repair
      Bengt-Johanson r.
      Cecil's r.
resection
resectoscope
      Baumrucker's r.
      Bumpus' r.
      cold punch r.
      Iglesias' r.
      McCarthy's r.
      Nesbit's r.
      Stern-McCarthy r.
      Thompson's r.
reservoir
      Kock's r.
residual
rete
      r. testis
retention
retractor
      Campbell's r.
      Deaver's r.
      Farr's r.
      Gelpi's r.
      Harrington's r.
      Jacobson's r.
      Judd-Masson r.
      Judd's r.
      Kocher's r.
      Legueu's r.
      Masson-Judd r.
      Millin-Bacon r.
      Pheifer-Young r.

retractor (continued)
    Rankin's r.
    self-retaining r.
    Tuffier-Raney r.
    Tuffier's r.
    Veenema's r.
    Young's r.
retrograde
    r. ejaculation
    r. pyelography
    r. urography
retroperitoneal
retropubic
Retzius' space
rhabdoid
rhabdomyoma
rhabdomyomatous
rhabdomyosarcoma
rhabdosarcoma
    renal r.
rib cutter
    Bethune's r.c.
rib stripper
    Dorian's r.s.
ridge
    interureteric r.
Rigaud's operation
RNA – ribonucleic acid
Robinson's stone dislodger
Roche's sign
Rochester-Pean forceps
Rokitansky's kidney
Rose-Bradford kidney
Rosenthal's speculum
RP – retrograde pyelogram
ruga (rugae)
Ruschelit's bougie
Ruysch's glomeruli
sacculation
sacculus
sacral
Santorini's plexus
saphenous
sarcocele
sarcoidosis
sarcoma
    clear cell s.

sarcoma (continued)
    Kaposi's s.
    soft tissue s.
scan/scanning
    gallium s.
    nucleotide s.
    radionuclide s.
scapus
    s. penis
Scardino's ureteropelvioplasty
Scarpa's fascia
schistosomiasis
    urinary s.
    vesical s.
Schmidt's syndrome
schwannoma
scissors
    Metzenbaum's s.
sclerosis
    renal arteriolar s.
scoop
    Moynihan's s.
score
    Gleason's grading s.
scrotal
    s. fat necrosis
    s. hemangioma
    s. lymphangioma
    s. panniculitis
scrotectomy
scrotitis
scrotocele
scrotoplasty
scrotum
    s. lapillosum
    lymph s.
    watering-can s.
secretion
segregator
    Cathclin's
    Harris' s.
    Luy's s.
semen
semenuria
seminal
semination
seminiferous

seminologist
seminology
seminoma
seminomatous
seminuria
sepsis
septa of testis
septum
    s. bulbi urethrae
    s. glandis penis
    s. of glans penis
    s. of scrotum
    s. pectiniforme
    s. penis
    rectovesical s.
    s. rectovesicale
    s. renis
    s. scroti
serosa
Sertoli's
    cell
    column
serum
    s. acid phosphatase
    s. alkaline phosphatase
    s. blocking factor
shangker. See *chancre.*
Shiley's tube
Shohl and Pedley's method
sickle cell trait
sigmoid
    s. conduit
sign
    Bergman's s.
    Gilbert's s.
    Lloyd's s.
    Pitres' s.
    Prehn's s.
    Roche's s.
    Thornton's s.
Silastic
    S. implant
    S. mushroom catheter
    S. testicular prosthesis
sinus
    s. epididymidis
    s. of epididymis

sinus (continued)
    prostatic s.
    s. prostaticus
    renal s.
    s. renalis
Sipple's syndrome
Sjöqvist's method
Skene's gland
Skillern's forceps
skis. See words beginning *schis-.*
smegma
    s. praeputii
sois. See *psoas.*
sound
    Campbell's s.
    Davis' s.
    Dittel's s.
    Fowler's s.
    Guyon's s.
    Jewett's s.
    LeFort's s.
    McCrea's s.
    Otis' s.
    Pratt's s.
    Van Buren's s.
    Walther's s.
space
    intravesical s.
    preperitoneal s.
    prevesical s.
    Retzius' s.
specific gravity
speculum
    Mosher's s.
    Rosenthal's s.
sperm
    muzzled s.
spermacrasia
spermagglutination
spermalist
spermatemphraxis
spermatic
spermaticide
spermatid
spermatin
spermatism
spermatitis

spermatoblast
spermatocele
spermatocelectomy
spermatocidal
spermatocyst
spermatocystectomy
spermatocystitis
spermatocystotomy
spermatocytal
spermatocyte
spermatocytic
spermatocytogenesis
spermatogenesis
spermatogenic
spermatogenous
spermatogeny
spermatogone
spermatogonium
spermatoid
spermatology
spermatolysin
spermatolysis
spermatolytic
spermatomere
spermatomerite
spermatopathia
spermatopoietic
spermatorrhea
spermatoschesis
spermatovum
spermatozoa
spermatozoal
spermatozoon
spermaturia
spermectomy
spermia
spermiation
spermicidal
spermicide
spermiduct
spermiocyte
spermiogenesis
spermioteleosis
spermioteleotic
spermium
spermoblast
spermoculture

spermolith
spermoloropexy
spermolytic
spermoneuralgia
spermophlebectasia
spermoplasm
spermosphere
spermotoxic
spermotoxin
sphincter
    Henle's s.
    Hyrtl's s.
    inguinal s.
    Nélaton's s.
    s. urethrae
    s. vesicae
Spivack's operation
spleen
spreader
    Millin-Bacon s.
squamous
    s. metaplasia
stain
    Ziehl-Neelsen s.
Stanischeff's operation
stasis
    urinary s.
Steinach's operation
stellate
stenosis
    meatal s.
stenotic
stent
    double-J silicone s.
    Gibbons' ureteral s.
    pigtail s.
sterile
sterility
sterilization
Stern-McCarthy
    electrotome
    resectoscope
steroid
Stille's clamp
Stockman's clamp
stoma
    Turnbull's loop s.

stone
  bladder s.
  cystine s.
  kidney s.
  s. searcher
stone dislodger
  Councill's s.d.
  Davis' s.d.
  Dormia's s.d.
  Johnson's s.d.
  Levant's s.d.
  Robinson's s.d.
  woven loop s.d.
Storz's cystoscope
strangulation
  s. of bladder
stranguria
strangury
Stratte's needle holder
stricture
  Hunner's s.
stroma
stromal
Stühmer's disease
stuttering
  urinary s.
stylet
sucker
  Marshall's surgical s.
sulcus
Sulkowitch's test
summit
  s. of bladder
Sumner's method
supraclavicular
suprahilar
suprapubic
suprarenal
suprarenalectomy
suprarenalism
suprarenalopathy
suprarene
suprarenoma
surgical procedures. See
  operation.
suspensory

suture. See *General Surgical
  Terms* section.
symphysis
  s. pubica
  s. pubis
syndrome
  acquired
    immunodeficiency s.
  adrenogenital s.
  Allemann's s.
  Bartter's s.
  Bywaters' s.
  Cacchi-Ricci s.
  Conn's s.
  Cooke-Apert-Gallais s.
  Cushing's s.
  Del Castillo's s.
  Epstein's s.
  Fanconi's s.
  Gilbert-Dreyfus s.
  Gilbert's s.
  Goodpasture's s.
  Heller-Nelson s.
  Heyd's s.
  Hippel-Lindau s.
  Kimmelstiel-Wilson s.
  Klinefelter's s.
  Labbé's s.
  Leriche's s.
  Lightwood's s.
  Luder-Sheldon s.
  Marañon's s.
  Miller's s.
  nephrotic s.
  Nonnenbruch's s.
  Reifenstein's s.
  Schmidt's s.
  Sipple's s.
  suprarenogenic s.
  Thorn's s.
  Turner's s.
  Waterhouse-
    Friderichsen s.
synorchidism
synorchism
synoscheos
syphilis

syphilitic
syringe
> Nourse's s.
> Toomey's s.

system
> Jewett-Strong s.

Tatum's clamp
Teale's gorget
technique
> Dennis-Brown t.
> Glenn's t.

Teilum's tumor
telescope
> McCarthy's t.
> Vest's t.

tenesmus
> vesical t.

teratocarcinoma
teratoma
test
> Albarran's t.
> aldosterone suppression t.
> blood urea nitrogen (BUN) t.
> clonidine suppression t.
> Coombs' t.
> creatinine clearance t.
> FTA-ABS t.
> glucose t.
> immunodiffusion t.
> ketone body t.
> leukocyte adherence inhibition t.
> Marshall's t.
> nitrogen retention t.
> pH t.
> proteinuria t.
> radioisotope renogram t.
> renin stimulation t.
> saline suppression t.
> semen analysis t.
> serum creatinine t.
> specific gravity t.
> specific red cell adherence t.
> Sulkowitch's t.
> urine chloride t.
> urine concentration t.

test (continued)
> VDRL t.
> Watson-Schwartz t.

testes
testicle
testicular
testiculoma
testiculus
testis
> Cooper's irritable t.
> ectopic t.
> inverted t.
> obstructed t.
> pulpy t.
> t. redux
> retained t.
> undescended t.

testitis
testitoxicosis
testoid
testopathy
testosterone
theca granulosa
Thiersch's graft
Thompson's
> lithotrite
> resectoscope

Thomsen-Friedenreich antigen
thoracoabdominal
Thorn's syndrome
Thornton's sign
thrombocytopenia
thrombophlebitis
thrombosis
> renal vein t.

thrombus
Tiemann's catheter
Timberlake's obturator
tomography
> computed t.

Toomey's
> evacuator
> syringe

Torek's operation
torsion
torus
> t. uretericus

tosis. See *ptosis.*
tour
    t. de maitre
trabecula (trabeculae)
    t. corporum
      cavernosorum penis
    t. of corpus spongiosum
      of penis
trabecular
trabeculation
tractor
    Lowsley's t.
    Young's t.
transabdominal
transcutaneous
transillumination
transitional
transperineal
transplant
transplantation
    renal t.
transrectal
transureteroureterostomy
transurethral
transversalis
transverse
transversourethralis
transversus
transvesical
transvestism
transvestite
Travenol needle
triangle
    Hesselbach's t.
trichiasis
Trichomonas
    T. urethritis
trichomoniasis
trigone
    urogenital t.
trigonectomy
trigonitis
trigonotome
trigonum
    t. urogenitale
    t. vesicae
triplication

trocar
    Campbell's t.
    Hurwitz's t.
    Ochsner's t.
    Potain's t.
tube
    Acmi-Valentine t.
    Immergut's t.
    Millin's t.
    rectal t.
    Shiley's t.
    U-t.
    Valentine's t.
tuberculosis
    adrenal t.
    t. of kidney and
      bladder
tuberous
tubular
tubule
    Albarran's t's
    Bellini's t's
    Henle's t's
    mesonephric t's
    metanephric t's
    renal t's
    seminiferous t's
    testicular t's
    urine-collecting t.
    uriniferous t's
    uriniparous t's
Tuffier-Raney retractor
Tuffier's
    operation
    retractor
tuft
    malpighian t.
    renal t.
tumor
    Brenner's t.
    Buschke-Loewenstein t.
    germ cell t.
    Grawitz's t.
    juxtaglomerular t.
    rhabdoid t.
    Teilum's t.
    theca granulosa t.
    thrombus t.

tumor (continued)
  Wilms' t.
  yolk sac t.
tunica
  s. adnata testis
  t. adventitia
  t. adventitia ductus
    deferentis
  t. adventitia ureteris
  t. adventitia vesiculae
    seminalis
  t. albuginea
  t. albuginea corporis
    spongiosi
  t. albuginea corporum
    cavernosorum
  t. albuginea testis
  t. dartos
  t. mucosa ductus
    deferentis
  t. mucosa ureteris
  t. mucosa vesicae urinariae
  t. mucosa vesiculae
    seminalis
  t. muscularis ductus
    deferentis
  t. muscularis renis
  t. muscularis ureteris
  t. muscularis vesicae
    urinariae
  t. muscularis vesiculae
    seminalis
  t. propria tubuli testis
  t. serosa testis
  t. serosa vesicae urinariae
  t. vaginalis communis
    testis et funiculi
    spermatica
  t. vaginalis propria testis
  t. vaginalis testis
  t. vasculosa
tunicae
  t. funiculi spermatici
  t. funiculi spermatici et
    testis
TUR – transurethral resection
turbid

Turkel's
  needle
  punch
Turnbull's loop stoma
Turner's syndrome
TURP – transurethral resection
  of prostate
U/A – urine analysis
ulcer
  decubitus u.
ulceration
ulcus
  u. syphiliticum
ultrasonogram
  renal u.
ultrasonography
undescended testis
undifferentiated
UPJ – ureteropelvic junction
urachal
urachovesical
urachus
uracrasia
uracratia
uragogue
uraturia
urea
uremia
  azotemic u.
  extrarenal u.
  prerenal u.
  retention u.
uremic
ureter
  ectopic u.
  postcaval u.
  retrocaval u.
  retroiliac u.
ureteral
  u. reflux
  u. stent
ureteralgia
ureterectasia
ureterectasis
ureterectomy
ureteric
  u. ridge

ureteritis
  u. cystica
  u. glandularis
ureterocele
ureterocelectomy
ureterocervical
ureterocolostomy
ureterocutaneostomy
ureterocutaneous
ureterocystanastomosis
ureterocystoneostomy
ureterocystoscope
ureterocystostomy
ureterodialysis
ureteroduodenal
ureteroenteric
ureteroenteroanastomosis
ureteroenterostomy
ureterogram
ureterography
ureteroheminephrectomy
ureteroileostomy
ureterointestinal
ureterolith
ureterolithiasis
ureterolithotomy
ureterolysis
ureteromeatotomy
ureteroneocystostomy
ureteroneopyelostomy
ureteronephrectomy
ureteropathy
ureteropelvic
ureteropelvioneostomy
ureteropelvioplasty
  Culp's u.
  Foley Y-type u.
  Scardino's u.
ureterophlegma
ureteroplasty
ureteroproctostomy
ureteropyelitis
ureteropyelography
ureteropyeloneostomy
ureteropyelonephritis
ureteropyelonephrostomy
ureteropyeloplasty

ureteropyelostomy
ureteropyosis
ureterorectal
ureterorectoneostomy
ureterorectostomy
ureterorrhagia
ureterorrhaphy
ureteroscopy
ureterosigmoid
ureterosigmoidostomy
ureterostegnosis
ureterostenoma
ureterostenosis
ureterostoma
ureterostomosis
ureterostomy
  cutaneous u.
ureterotomy
ureterotrigonoenterostomy
ureterotrigonosigmoidostomy
ureteroureteral
ureteroureterostomy
ureterouterine
ureterovaginal
ureterovesical
ureterovesicoplasty
ureterovesicostomy
urethra
  female u.
  u. feminina
  male u.
  u. masculina
  u. muliebris
  u. virilis
urethral
urethralgia
urethratresia
urethrectomy
urethremphraxis
urethreurynter
urethrism
urethritis
  u. cystica
  u. glandularis
  gonorrheal u.
  gouty u.
  u. granulosa

urethritis (continued)
    nonspecific u.
    u. orificii externi
    u. petrificans
    polypoid u.
    prophylactic u.
    specific u.
    u. venerea
urethroblennorrhea
urethrobulbar
urethrocele
urethrocystitis
urethrocystogram
urethrocystography
urethocystopexy
urethrodynia
urethrogram
urethrograph
urethrography
urethrometer
urethrometry
urethropenile
urethroperineal
urethroperineoscrotal
urethropexy
urethrophraxis
urethrophyma
urethroplasty
urethroprostatic
urethrorectal
urethrorrhagia
urethrorrhaphy
urethrorrhea
urethroscope
urethroscopic
urethroscopy
urethroscrotal
urethrospasm
urethrostaxis
urethrostenosis
urethrostomy
urethrotome
    Keitzer's u.
    Maisonneuve's u.
    Otis' u.
urethrotomy
urethrovaginal

urethrovesical
uretic
urhidrosis
uric acid
uricaciduria
uricometer
uricosuria
urina
    u. chyli
    u. cibi
    u. cruenta
    u. galactodes
    u. jumentosa
    u. potus
    u. sanguinus
    u. spastica
urinable
urinacidometer
urinal
urinalysis
urinary
    u. bladder
    u. diversion
    u. fistula
    u. frequency
    u. incontinence
    u. meatus
    u. retention
    u. sphincter
    u. tract
urinate
urination
    precipitant u.
    stuttering u.
urine
    anemic u.
    Bence Jones u.
    black u.
    chylous u.
    clean catch u.
    crude u.
    u. cytology
    diabetic u.
    dyspeptic u.
    febile u.
    gouty u.
    milky u.

urine (continued)
    nebulous u.
    nervous u.
    residual u.
    straw-colored u.
    voided u.
urinemia
urine-mucoid
uriniferous
uriniparous
urinocryoscopy
urinogenital
urinogenous
urinoglucosometer
urinologist
urinology
urinoma
urinometer
urinometry
urinosexual
urinous
urobilinogenuria
urobilinuria
urocele
urochezia
urochrome
urochromogen
uroclepsia
urocrisia
urocrisis
urocriterion
urocyanogen
urocyst
urocystic
urocystis
urocystitis
urodeum
urodialysis
urodochium
urodynia
uroedema
uroerythrin
uroflavin
uroflometer
urofuscin
urofuscohematin

urogenital
    u. trigone
urogenous
uroglaucin
urogram
    excretory u.
    intravenous u.
urography
    ascending u.
    cystoscopic u.
    descending u.
    excretion u.
    excretory u.
    intravenous u.
    oral u.
    retrograde u.
urohematin
urohematonephrosis
urohematoporphyrin
urohypertensin
urokinase
urokinetic
urokymography
urolith
urolithiasis
urolithic
urolithology
urologic
urological
urologist
urology
urolutein
uromancy
uromantia
uromelanin
urometer
uromucoid
uroncus
uronephrosis
uronology
urononcometry
uronophile
uronoscopy
uropathogen
uropathy
    obstructive u.
uropenia

uropepsin
uropepsinogen
urophanic
urophein
urophobia
urophosphometer
uroplania
uropoiesis
uropoietic
uroporphyrin
uropsammus
uropterin
uropyonephrosis
uropyoureter
uroreaction
urorhythmography
urorrhagia
urorrhea
urorrhodin
urorrhodinogen
urorubin
urorubinogen
urorubrohematin
urosaccharometry
uroscheocele
uroschesis
uroscopic
uroscopy
urosemiology
urosepsin
urosepsis
uroseptic
urosis
urospectrin
urostalagmometry
urostealith
urothelial
urothelium
urotherapy
urotoxia
urotoxic
urotoxicity
urotoxin
uroureter
uroxanthin
uterine
uterus

UTI – urinary tract infection
utricle
      prostatic u.
      urethral u.
utricular
utriculi
utriculitis
utriculosaccular
utriculus
      u. masculinus
      u. prostaticus
      u. vestibuli
U-tube
UVJ – ureterovesical junction
uvula
      u. of bladder
      u. vesicae
vaccine
      bacille Calmette-Guérin v.
vagina
Valentine's tube
Van Buren's
      dilator
      sound
van Hook's operation
varicocele
varicocelectomy
varix
vas
      v. aberrans
      v. afferens glomeruli
      v. deferens
      v. efferens glomeruli
      v. epididymidis
vasculature
vasectomized
vasectomy
vasitis
vasodilator
vasoepididymostomy
vasoligation
vaso-orthidostomy
vasopuncture
vasoresection
vasorrhaphy
vasosection
vasostomy

vasotomy
vasovasotomy
vasovesiculectomy
vasovesiculitis
VCU – voiding cystourethrogram
VDRL – Venereal Disease
    Research Laboratory
Veenema-Gusberg needle
Veenema's retractor
vein
        arcuate v.
        interlobar v.
vena cava
venacavography
venacavotomy
venae cavernosae penis
venereal
venogram
        renal v.
ventral
venulae
        v. rectae renis
        v. stellatae renis
venule
        stellate v's of kidney
        straight v's of kidney
verruca (verrucae)
        v. acuminata
verrucous
vertex
        v. of urinary bladder
        v. vesicae urinariae
verumontanitis
verumontanum
Ves. (vesica) – bladder
vesica
        v. prostatica
        v. urinaria
vesicae
vesical
vesicle
        prostatic v.
        seminal v.
        spermatic v.
vesicoabdominal
vesicocele
vesicocervical

vesicoclysis
vesicocolonic
vesicoenteric
vesicofixation
vesicointestinal
vesicoperineal
vesicoprostatic
vesicopubic
vesicopustule
vesicorectal
vesicorenal
vesicosigmoid
vesicosigmoidostomy
vesicospinal
vesicotomy
vesicoumbilical
vesicourachal
vesicoureteral
vesicourethral
vesicouterine
vesicouterovaginal
vesicovaginal
vesicovaginorectal
vesicula
        v. prostatica
        v. seminalis
vesiculase
vesiculectomy
vesiculitis
vesiculogram
vesiculography
vesiculotomy
vessel
        internal spermatic v.
Vest's telescope
Vidal's operation
Vim-Silverman needle
virilizing
visceral
viscus
Vogel's operation
void
voiding
Volhard and Fahr method
Volhard's nephritis
Volkmann's operation
von Bergmann's operation

von Brunn's nest
von Hacker's operation
Voronoff's operation
Walther-Crenshaw
   clamp
Walther's
   clamp
   dilator
   sound
Wappler's cystoscope
waste
   nitrogenous w.
Waterhouse-Friderichsen
   syndrome
Watson-Schwartz test
Wertheim-Cullen clamp
Wertheim-Reverdin
   clamp
Wertheim's clamp
Wheelhouse's operation
White-Oslay forceps
White's operation
Wilms' tumor
Winer's catheter
Wishard's catheter
Wolff
   corpus of W.
   duct of W.

wolffian
   w. body
   w. cyst
   w. duct
Wood's operation
xanthogranuloma
   juvenile x.
xanthogranulomatous
XC–excretory cystogram
XU–excretory urogram
YAG laster therapy
yolk sac tumor
Young-Millin needle holder
Young's
   clamp
   enucleator
   forceps
   needle holder
   operation
   retractor
   tractor
Ziehl-Neelsen stain
Zipser's clamp
zone
   Daseler's z.
Zoon's erythroplasia
zoospermia
Zylytol

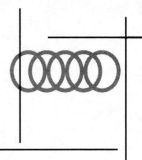

Part Three
Guides to Terminology

Abbreviations and Symbols*

ABBREVIATIONS

A absolute temperature
   absorbance
   accommodation
   acetum
   age
   allergy
   ampere
   Angström unit
   anode
   anterior
   artery
   atropine
   axial
   before (*ante*)
   mass number
   start of anesthesia
   total acidity
   water (*aqua*)
A. *Actinomyces*
   Anopheles
a or A ampere
   anode
A_2 aortic second sound
AA acetic acid
   achievement age
   alveolar-arterial
   aminoacetone
   amplitude of accommodation
   arachidonic acid
   ascending aorta
   of each (*ana*)
aa arteries
A & A aid and attendance
AAA abdominal aortic aneurysm
   amalgam
   androgenic anabolic agent

AACG acute angle closure
   glaucoma
AAL anterior axillary line
AAOS American Academy of
   Orthopaedic Surgeons
AAR antigen-antiglobulin reaction
AAS aortic arch syndrome
AAT alpha-antitrypsin
AAV adeno-associated virus
AB abnormal
   abortion
   alcian blue
   asbestos body
   asthmatic bronchitis
   axiobuccal
A/B acid-base ratio
ABA antibacterial activity
ABC absolute basophil count
   antigen binding capacity
   axiobuccocervical
ABD,
Abd or
abd abdomen
   abdominal
ABDOM,
Abdom or
abdom abdomen
   abdominal
ABE acute bacterial endocarditis
ABG axiobuccogingival
ABL abetalipoproteinemia
   axiobuccolingual
ABLB alternate binaural loudness
   balance
ABMA anti-basement membrane
   antibody
ABN,
Abn or
abn abnormal

---

*Symbols start on page 1069.

997

ABO   blood groups (named for
           agglutinogens)
ABP   arterial blood pressure
ABPA allergic bronchopulmonary
           aspergillosis
ABR   American Board of Radiology
           auditory brain stem evoked
           response
abs feb while the fever is absent
           (*absente febre*)
ABV   Adriamycin, bleomycin and
           vinblastine
AC   acromioclavicular
         adenylate cyclase
         adrenal cortex
         air conduction
         alternating current
         anodal closure
         anterior chamber
         anticoagulant
         anticomplementary
         anti-inflammatory corticoid
         aortic closure
         atriocarotid
         auriculocarotid
         axiocervical
         before meals (*ante cibum*)
ac   acute
         before meals (*ante cibum*)
AC/A ratio accommodative
           convergence/
           accommodation ratio
ACA   adenocarcinoma
ACAD academy
ACC   adenoid cystic carcinoma
           anodal closure contraction
Acc   accommodation
ACCL anodal closure clonus
accom accommodation
ACD   absolute cardiac dullness
           acid, citrate, dextrose
           anterior chest diameter
ACE   adrenocortical extract
ACG   angle closure glaucoma
           acute angle closure glaucoma
           apexcardiogram
AcG   accelerator globulin
ACH   adrenal cortical hormone
ACh   acetylcholine
ACHE acetylcholinesterase
ACl   aspiryl chloride
ACM   albumin-calcium-magnesium
ACO   anodal-closing odor

ACP   acid phosphatase
           acyl-carrier protein
           anodal-closing picture
           aspirin, caffeine, phenacetin
ACR   American College of
           Radiology
ACS   anodal-closing sound
           antireticular cytotoxic serum
ACSM American College of Sports
           Medicine
ACSV aortocoronary saphenous
           vein
ACT   activated coagulation time
           anticoagulant therapy
ACTe anodal-closure tetanus
ACTH adrenocorticotropic
           hormone
ACTP adrenocorticotropic
           polypeptide
ACVD acute cardiovascular disease
AD   admitting diagnosis
         Aleutian disease
         anodal duration
         average deviation
         axiodistal
         axis deviation
         right ear (*auris dextra*)
A & D ascending and descending
ad   add (*adde*)
         let there be added (*addetur*)
ad lib as desired (*ad libitum*)
ADA   adenosine deaminase
           anterior descending artery
ADA# American Diabetes
           Association diet number
ADC   analog-to-digital conversion
           anodal-duration contraction
           average daily census
           axiodistocervical
ADCC antibody-dependent
           cell-mediated cytotoxicity
ADE   acute disseminated
           encephalomyelitis
ADEM acute disseminated
           encephalomyelitis
ADG   atrial diastolic gallop
           axiodistogingival
ADH   alcohol dehydrogenase
           antidiuretic hormone
adhib to be administered
           (*adhibendus*)
ADI   axiodistoincisal
ADL   activities of daily living

ADM administrative medicine
administrator
adm or
admit admission
admov let there be added (*admove*)
ADO axiodisto-occlusal
ADP adenosine diphosphate
automatic data processing
ADPL average daily patient load
ADS antibody deficiency syndrome
antidiuretic substance
ADT adenosine triphosphate
anything desired (*placebo*)
ADV adenovirus
adv against (*adversum*)
ad 2 vic for two doses (*ad duas vices*)
AE above elbow
antitoxineinheit (antitoxin unit)
AEC Atomic Energy Commission
AEF allogeneic effect factor
AEG air encephalogram
aeg the patient (*aeger*)
AEP average evoked potential
AEq age equivalent
AER aldosterone excretion rate
auditory evoked response
average evoked response
AET absorption-equivalent
thickness
aet age (*aetas*)
aetat aged, of age (*aetatis*)
AF acid-fast
aldehyde fuchsin
amniotic fluid
antibody-forming
aortic flow
atrial fibrillation
atrial flutter
AFB acid-fast bacilli
AFC antibody-forming cells
AFI amaurotic familial idiocy
AFIB atrial fibrillation
AFL atrial flutter
AFP anterior faucial pillar
AG antiglobulin
atrial gallop
axiogingival
A/G albumin-globulin ratio
AGA appropriate for gestational
age
AGG agammaglobulinemia
agg aggravated

agit shake (*agita*)
AGL acute granulocytic leukemia
aminoglutethimide
AGMK African green monkey
kidney
AGN acute glomerulonephritis
AGS adrenogenital syndrome
AGT antiglobulin test
AGTT abnormal glucose tolerance
test
AGV aniline gentian violet
AH abdominal hysterectomy
acetohexamide
amenorrhea and hirsutism
aminohippurate
antihyaluronidase
arterial hypertension
hypermetropic astigmatism
AHA acquired hemolytic anemia
autoimmune hemolytic
anemia
AHD arteriosclerotic heart disease
atherosclerotic heart disease
AHF antihemophilic factor
AHG antihemophilic globulin
antihuman globulin
AHH alpha-hydrazine analogue of
histidine
arylhydrocarbon hydroxylase
AHLE acute hemorrhagic
leukoencephalitis
AHLS antihuman lymphocyte
serum
AHM anterior hyaloid membrane
AHP air at high pressure
AHRA American Hospital
Radiology Administrators
AHT augmented histamine test
AI accidentally incurred
aortic incompetence
aortic insufficiency
apical impulse
axioincisal
AIBA aminoisobutyric acid
AIC aminoimidazole carboxamide
AICD automatic implanted
cardioverter defibrillator
AID acute infectious disease
artificial insemination donor
AIDS acquired immunodeficiency
syndrome
AIEP amount of insulin extractable
from the pancreas

AIH artificial insemination,
    homologous
AIHA autoimmune hemolytic
    anemia
AIP acute intermittent porphyria
    average intravascular pressure
AITT arginine insulin tolerance test
AIU absolute iodine uptake
AIUM American Institute of
    Ultrasound in Medicine
AJ   ankle jerk
AK   above knee
AKA above-knee amputation
AL   albumin
    axiolingual
ALA aminolevulinic acid
    axiolabial
ALAD abnormal left axis deviation
    aminolevulinic acid
    dehydrase
ALAG axiolabiogingival
ALAL axiolabiolingual
alb albumin
    white
ALC approximate lethal
    concentration
    axiolinguocervical
ALD aldolase
ALG antilymphocyte globulin
    axiolinguogingival
ALH anterior lobe hormone
    anterior lobe of the
    hypophysis
alk alkaline
alk phos alkaline phosphatase
ALL acute lymphoblastic leukemia
    acute lymphocytic leukemia
all allergies
ALME acetyl-lysine methyl ester
ALMI anterior lateral myocardial
    infarct
ALN anterior lymph node
ALO axiolinguo-occlusal
ALP alkaline phosphatase
    antilymphocyte plasma
ALS amyotrophic lateral sclerosis
    antilymphatic serum
    antilymphocyte serum
ALT alanine aminotransferase
ALTEE acetyl-L-tyrosine ethyl ester
ALW arch-loop-whorl
AM   alveolar macrophage

AM (continued)
    ametropia
    amperemeter
    anovular menstruation
    arithmetic mean
    aviation medicine
    axiomesial
    morning
    myopic astigmatism
am   meter-angle
AMA against medical advice
    American Medical
    Association
AMB ambulatory
AMC axiomesiocervical
AMD alpha-methyldopa
    axiomesiodistal
Ameslan American Sign Language
AmFAR American Foundation for
    AIDS Research
AMG antimacrophage globulin
    axiomesiogingival
AMH automated medical history
Amh mixed astigmatism with
    myopia predominating
AMI acute myocardial infarction
    amitriptyline
    axiomesioincisal
AML acute monocytic leukemia
    acute myelocytic leukemia
AMLS antimouse lymphocyte
    serum
AMM agnogenic myeloid
    metaplasia
    ammonia
AMML acute myelomonocytic
    leukemia
AMO axiomesio-occlusal
A-mode amplitude modulation
AMOL acute monocytic
    leukemia
AMP acid mucopolysaccharide
    adenosine monophosphate
    ampicillin
    amputation
    average mean pressure
amp ampere
AMPPE acute multifocal placoid
    pigment epitheliopathy
AMPS abnormal mucopoly-
    sacchariduria
    acid mucopolysaccharides

AMS aggravated in military service
     antimacrophage serum
     automated multiphasic
        screening
AMT alpha-methyltyrosine
     amethopterin
amt amount
amu atomic mass unit
AMY amylase
An   anisometropia
     anodal
     anode
ANA acetylneuraminic acid
     antinuclear antibodies
     aspartyl naphthylamide
anal analysis
     analyst
anat anatomical
     anatomy
AnCC anodal-closure contraction
AnDTe anodal-duration tetanus
anes anesthesia
     anesthesiology
ANF alpha-naphthoflavone
     antinuclear factor
ang angiogram
ank ankle
ANLL acute nonlymphocytic
        leukemia
AnOC anodal-opening contraction
ANOV analysis of variance
ANS antineutrophilic serum
     arteriolonephrosclerosis
     autonomic nervous system
ant anterior
ante before
ANTR apparent net transfer rate
ANTU alpha-naphthylthiourea
AO   anodal opening
     anterior oblique
     aorta
     aortic opening
     axio-occlusal
     opening of the atrioventricular
        valves
AOB alcohol on breath
AOC anodal-opening contraction
AOCl anodal-opening clonus
AOD arterial occlusive disease
AOO anodal-opening odor
AOP anodal-opening picture
AOS anodal-opening sound

AOTe anodal-opening tetanus
AP   acid phosphatase
     action potential
     acute proliferative
     alkaline phosphatase
     aminopeptidase
     angina pectoris
     antepartum
     anterior pituitary
     anteroposterior
     appendix
     arterial pressure
     association period
     axiopulpal
A & P anterior and posterior
     auscultation and percussion
APA aldosterone-producing
        adenoma
     aminopenicillanic acid
     antipernicious anemia factor
APACHE acute physiology and
        chronic health
        evaluation
APB atrial premature beat
     auricular premature beat
APC acetylsalicylic acid,
        phenacetin, caffeine
     adenoidal-pharyngeal-
        conjunctival
     antigen presenting cell
     aspirin, phenacetin, caffeine
     atrial premature contraction
APC-C aspirin, phenacetin,
        caffeine; with codeine
APD action-potential duration
APE aminophylline, phenobarbital,
        ephedrine
     anterior pituitary extract
APF animal protein factor
APGL alkaline phosphatase activity
        of the granular leukocytes
APH antepartum hemorrhage
APHP anti-*Pseudomonas* human
        plasma
APL accelerated painless labor
     acute promyelocytic leukemia
     anterior pituitary-like
APN average peak noise
ApoE apolipoprotein E
APP alum-precipitated pyridine
app appendix
appy appendectomy

APR   amebic prevalence rate
APT   alum-precipitated toxoid
APTA   American Physical Therapy
          Association
APTT   activated partial
          thromboplastin time
AQ   achievement quotient
aq   water (*aqua*)
AQS   additional qualifying
          symptoms
AR   alarm reaction
          aortic regurgitation
          Argyll Robertson (pupil)
          artificial respiration
          at risk
ARA   American Rheumatism
          Association
ara-C   cytosine arabinoside
ARAS   ascending reticular
          activation system
ARC   AIDS related complex
          anomalous retinal
          correspondence
ARD   acute respiratory disease
          anorectal dressing
ARDMS   American Registry of
          Diagnostic Medical
          Sonographers
ARDS   adult respiratory distress
          syndrome
ARF   acute respiratory failure
          acute rheumatic fever
arg   silver (*argentum*)
ARL   average remaining lifetime
ARM   artificial rupture of the
          membranes
ARP   at risk period
ARRS   American Roentgen Ray
          Society
ARRT   American Registry of
          Radiologic Technologists
ARS   AIDS related syndrome
          antirabies serum
ART   algebraic reconstruction
          technique
art   artery
ARV   AIDS related virus
AS   acetylstrophanthidin
          Adams-Stokes (disease)
          androsterone sulfate
          antistreptolysin
          aortic stenosis

AS (continued)
          arteriosclerosis
          astigmatism
          left ear (*auris sinistra*)
ASA   acetylsalicylic acid
          Adams-Stokes attack
          argininosuccinic acid
          arylsulfatase-A
ASCVD   arteriosclerotic
          cardiovascular disease
          atherosclerotic
          cardiovascular disease
ASD   aldosterone secretion defect
          atrial septal defect
ASF   aniline, sulfur, formaldehyde
ASH   asymmetrical septal
          hypertrophy
AsH   hypermetropic astigmatism
ASHD   arteriosclerotic heart disease
ASIS   anterior superior iliac spine
ASK   antistreptokinase
ASL   antistreptolysin
ASLO   antistreptolysin-O
AsM   myopic astigmatism
ASMI   anteroseptal myocardial
          infarct
ASN   alkali-soluble nitrogen
ASO   antistreptolysin-O
          arteriosclerosis obliterans
ASP   area systolic pressure
ASR   aldosterone secretion rate
          aldosterone secretory rate
ASRT   American Society of
          Radiologic Technologists
ASS   anterior superior spine
asst   assistant
AST   above a selected threshold
          aspartate aminotransferase
Ast   astigmatism
Asth   asthenopia
ASTO   antistreptolysin-O
ASTZ   antistreptozyme
ASV   antisnake venom
AT   antitrypsin
          ataxia telangiectasia
          old tuberculin (alt tuberculin)
AT_{10} dihydrotachysterol
ATA   anti-*Toxoplasma* antibodies
          atmosphere absolute
          aurintricarboxylic acid
ATB   at the time of the bomb
          (A-bomb in Japan)

ATCC   American Type Culture
         Collection
ATD   asphyxiating thoracic
         dystrophy
ATE   adipose tissue extract
ATEE   acetyltyrosine ethyl ester
ATG   antithyroglobulin
ATL   antitension line
ATLL   adult T cell leukemia-
         lymphoma
ATN   acute tubular necrosis
ATP   adenosine triphosphate
ATPS   ambient temperature and
         pressure, saturated
ATR   Achilles tendon reflex
atr fib   atrial fibrillation
ATS   antitetanic serum
         antithymocyte serum
         anxiety tension state
         arteriosclerosis
ATT   aspirin tolerance time
att   attending
at wt   atomic weight
AU   Angström unit
         antitoxin unit
         arbitrary units
         azauridine
Au   Australia (antigen)
au   both ears (*aures unitas*)
         each ear (*auris uterque*)
AUL   acute undifferentiated
         leukemia
aur fib   auricular fibrillation
ausc   auscultation
AV   arteriovenous
         atrioventricular
av   average
AV/AF   anteverted, anteflexed
AVCS   atrioventricular conduction
         system
avdp   avoirdupois
AVF   arteriovenous fistula
AVH   acute viral hepatitis
AVI   air velocity index
AVM   arteriovenous malformation
AVN   atrioventricular node
AVR   aortic valve replacement
AVRP   atrioventricular refractory
         period
AVT   Allen vision test
AW   anterior wall
A & W   alive and well

AWI   anterior wall infarction
AWMI   anterior wall myocardial
         infarction
ax   axis
Az   azote (French for nitrogen)
azg   azaguanine
AZO   (indicates presence of the
         group) –N:N–
AZT   Aschheim-Zondek test
         azidothymidine
         zidovudine
AZ test   Aschheim-Zondek test
AZUR   azauridine
B   bacillus
     base
     bath (*balneum*)
     Baume's scale
     behavior
     Benoist's scale
     bicuspid
     boron
     buccal
     Bucky (film in cassette in
         Potter-Bucky diaphragm)
     symbol for gauss
     tomogram with oscillating Bucky
B4   before
B.   *Brucella*
b   born
BA   bacterial agglutination
     betamethasone acetate
     blocking antibody
     bone age
     bovine albumin
     branchial artery
     bronchial asthma
     buccoaxial
     sand bath (*balneum arenae*)
Ba   barium
BAC   blood alcohol concentration
     bronchioloalveolar
         adenocarcinoma
     buccoaxiocervical
bact   bacterium
BaE   barium enema
BAEE   benzoyl arginine ethyl ester
     benzylarginine ethyl ester
BAEP   brain-stem auditory evoked
         potential
BAER   brain-stem auditory evoked
         response
BAG   buccoaxiogingival

BAIB   beta-aminoisobutyric acid
BAL   British anti-lewisite
bal   bath (*balneum*)
bals   balsam
BAME   benzoylarginine methyl
        ester
BAO   basal acid output
BAP   blood agar plate
        brightness area product
BASH   body acceleration given
        synchronously with the
        heartbeat
baso   basophile
BB   blood bank
        blood buffer base
        blue bloaters (emphysema)
        both bones
        breakthrough bleeding
        breast biopsy
        buffer base
BBA   born before arrival
BBB   blood-brain barrier
        bundle branch block
BBT   basal body temperature
BC   bactericidal concentration
        battle casualty
        bone conduction
        buccocervical
BCB   brilliant cresyl blue
BCD   binary coded decimal
BCE   basal cell epithelioma
BCG   bacille Calmette-Guérin
        (vaccine)
        ballistocardiogram
        bicolor guaiac (test)
BCGF-I   B cell growth Factor I, II
BCNU   bischloroethylnitrosourea
        bischloronitrosourea
BCP   basic calcium phosphate
BCW   biological and chemical
        warfare
BD   base deficit
        base of prism down
        bile duct
        buccodistal
        twice a day (*bis die*)
BDE   bile duct exploration
BDM   border detection method
BE   bacillen emulsion (tuberculin)
        bacterial endocarditis
        barium enema
        base excess

BE (continued)
        bovine enteritis
BEAM   brain electrical activity map
BEI   butanol-extractable iodine
BEV   billion electron volts
BF   blood flow
bf   bouillon filtrate (tuberculin)
B/F   bound-free ratio
BFC   benign febrile convulsion
BFP   biologic false-positive
BFR   biologic false-postitive reactor
        blood flow rate
        bone formation rate
BFT   bentonite flocculation test
BG   blood glucose
        bone graft
        buccogingival
BGH   bovine growth hormone
BGP   beta-glycerophosphatase
BGSA   blood granulocyte-specific
        activity
BGTT   borderline glucose tolerance
        test
BH   benzalkonium and heparin
BHA   butylated hydroxyanisole
BHC   benzene hexachloride
BHI   brain-heart infusion
BHS   beta-hemolytic streptococcus
BHT   butylated hydroxytoluene
BH/VH   body hematocrit-venous
        hematocrit ratio
BI   bacteriological index
        base of prism in
        burn index
bib   drink (*bibe*)
BID or
bid   twice a day (*bis in die*)
BIDLB   block in the posteroinferior
        division of the left branch
BIH   benign intracranial
        hypertension
BIL   bilirubin
bil   bilateral
bilat   bilateral
BIN or
bin   twice a night (*bis in nocte*)
BIP   bismuth iodoform paraffin
bis   twice
BJ   Bence Jones
BJP   Bence Jones protein
BK   below knee
BKA   below-knee amputation

bkfst   breakfast
BL   baseline
   Bessey-Lowry (units)
   bleeding
   blood loss
   buccolingual
   Burkitt's lymphoma
BLB   Boothby, Lovelace, Bulbulian
   (mask)
bl cult   blood culture
BLG   beta-lactoglobulin
BLN   bronchial lymph nodes
bl pr   blood pressure
BLT   blood-clot lysis time
BLU   Bessey-Lowry units
BM   basement membrane
   body mass
   bone marrow
   bowel movement
   buccomesial
bm   sea-water bath (*balneum maris*)
bmk   birthmark
B-mode   brightness modulation
BMR   basal metabolic rate
BMT   bone marrow transplantation
BN   branchial neuritis
BNO   bladder neck obstruction
BNPA   binasal pharyngeal airway
BO   base (of prism) out
   bowel obstruction
   bucco-occlusal
B & O   belladonna and opium
BOBA   beta-oxybutyric acids
BOEA   ethyl biscoumacetate
bol   pill (*bolus*)
BOM   bilateral otitis media
BOOP   bronchiolitis obliterans
   organizing pneumonia
BP   back pressure
   bathroom privileges
   behavior pattern
   benzpyrene
   birthplace
   blood pressure
   boiling point
   bronchopleural
   buccopulpal
   bypass
BPD   biparietal diameter
BPH   benign prostatic hypertrophy
BPL   beta-propiolactone
BPO   benzylpenicilloyl

BPRS   brief psychiatric rating scale
   brief psychiatric reacting
   scale
BPV   benign positional vertigo
BR   bathroom
   bed rest
   bilirubin
Br.   *Brucella*
BRAO   branch retinal artery
   occlusion
BRBC   bovine red blood cells
BRH   Bureau of Radiological Health
brkf or
brkt   breakfast
BRM   biuret reactive material
BRP   bathroom privileges
   bilirubin production
brth   breath
BS   blood sugar
   bowel sounds
   breaking strength
   breath sounds
BSA   bismuth-sulfite agar
   body surface area
   bovine serum albumin
BSAP   brief short-action potential
BSB   body surface burned
BSDLB   block in the anterosuperior
   division of the left branch
BSE   bilateral, symmetrical and
   equal
BSF   back scatter factor
BSF-1,2   B cell stimulating factor 1,2
BSI   bound serum iron
BSO   bilateral salpingo-
   oophorectomy
BSP   Bromsulphalein
BSR   basal skin resistance
BSS   balanced salt solution
   black silk suture
   buffered saline solution
BSV   binocular single vision
BT   bladder tumor
   brain tumor
BTB   breakthrough bleeding
BTE   behind the ear
BTPS   body temperature, ambient
   pressure, saturated
BTR   Bezold-type reflex
BTU   British thermal unit
BU   base (of prism) up
   Bodansky units

BU (continued)
    burn unit
BUDR   bromodeoxyuracil
        bromodeoxyuridine
bull   let it boil (*bulliat*)
BUN   blood urea nitrogen
BUS   Bartholin's, urethral, Skene's
        (glands)
BUT   breakup time
but   butter (*butyrum*)
BV   biologic value
        blood vessel
        blood volume
        bronchovesicular
bv   vapor bath (*balneum vaporis*)
BVA   best corrected visual acuity
BVH   biventricular hypertrophy
BVI   blood vessel invasion
BVV   bovine vaginitis virus
BW   biological warfare
        birth weight
        body water
        body weight
BX   biopsy
C   calculus
    calorie (large)
    canine
    carbohydrate
    cathode
    Caucasian
    Celsius
    centigrade
    certified
    cervical
    chest
    clearance rate
    clonus
    closure
    color sense
    complement
    compound
    contracture
    correct
    curic
    cylinder
    gallon (*congius*)
    hundred
    velocity of light
C.   *Clostridium*
    Cryptococcus
C'   complement
c   calorie (small)

c (continued)
    cup
    curie
    with (*cum*)
C_{alb} albumin clearance
C_{am} amylase clearance
C_{cr} creatinine clearance
C_{in} insulin clearance
C_{pah} para-aminohippurate clearance
C_{u} urea clearance
CA   cancer
    carcinoma
    cardiac arrest
    cathode
    cervicoaxial
    cholic acid
    chronological age
    cold agglutinin
    common antigen
    coronary artery
    corpora amylacea
    croup-associated (virus)
Ca   calcium
ca   about (*circa*)
CAB   cellulose acetate butyrate
        coronary artery bypass
CABG   coronary artery bypass graft
CACC   cathodal closure contraction
CAD   computerized assisted design
        coronary artery disease
CADTe   cathodal-duration tetanus
CAG   chronic atrophic gastritis
CAH   chronic active hepatitis
        congenital adrenal hyperplasia
CAHD   coronary atherosclerotic
            heart disease
CAI   computer-assisted instruction
CAL   computer-assisted learning
Cal   large calorie
cal   small calorie
calef   warmed (*calefactus*)
CALLA   common acute
            lymphocytic leukemia
            antigen
CAM   chorioallantoic membrane
        contralateral axillary
            metastasis
CAMP   computer-assisted menu
            planning
        cyclic adenosine
            monophosphate
CAO   chronic airway obstruction

CAP capsule
cellulose acetate phthalate
chloramphenicol
cystine aminopeptidase
cap let him take (*capiat*)
CAPD continued ambulatory
peritoneal dialysis
CAR cancer-associated retinopathy
card cardiology
CAST cardiac arrhythmia
suppression trial
CAT children's apperception test
chlormerodrin accumulation
test
computed axial tomography
computer of average transients
computerized axial
tomography
cath cathartic
catheter
catheterize
CAV congenital absence of vagina
congenital adrenal virilism
CB chronic bronchitis
cb cardboard or plastic film holder
without intensifying screens
CBA chronic bronchitis with
asthma
CBC complete blood count
CBD common bile duct
CBF cerebral blood flow
coronary blood flow
CBG corticosteroid-binding
globulin
cortisol-binding globulin
CBOC completion bed occupancy
care
CBS chronic brain syndrome
CBV central blood volume
circulating blood volume
corrected blood volume
CBW chemical and biological
warfare
CC cardiac cycle
chief complaint
clinical course
closing capacity
commission certified
compound cathartic
cord compression
costochondral
creatinine clearance

cc cubic centimeter
CCA chick-cell agglutination
chimpanzee coryza agent
common carotid artery
CCAT conglutinating complement
absorption test
CCC cathodal-closing contraction
chronic calculous cholecystitis
consecutive case conference
CCCl cathodal-closure clonus
CCF carotid cavernous fistula
cephalin-cholesterol
flocculation
compound comminuted
fracture
congestive cardiac failure
CCK cholecystokinin
CCK-PZ cholecystokinin-
pancreozymin
CCN coronary care nursing
CCP ciliocytophthoria
CCS casualty clearing station
CCT composite cyclic therapy
cranial computed
tomography
CCTe cathodal-closure tetanus
CCU cardiac care unit
Cherry-Crandall units
community care unit
coronary care unit
CCW counterclockwise
CD cadaver donor
cardiac disease
cardiac dullness
cardiovascular disease
caudal
cluster of differentiation
common duct
conjugata diagonalis
consanguineous donor
curative dose
cystic duct
C/D cigarettes per day
C & D cystoscopy and dilatation
CD_{50} median curative dose
CDC calculated date of
confinement
Centers for Disease Control
chenodeoxycholate
Communicable Disease
Center
CDCA chenodeoxycholic acid

CDD certificate of disability for discharge
CDE canine distemper encephalitis
chlordiazepoxide
common duct exploration
CDH ceramide dihexoside
congenital dislocation of the hip
CDL chlorodeoxylincomycin
CDP coronary drug project
CDR complementarity-determining region
CDSS clinical decision support system
CE California encephalitis
cardiac enlargement
chick embryo
cholesterol esters
contractile element
CEA carcinoembryonic antigen
crystalline egg albumin
CEEV Central European encephalitis virus
CEF chick embryo fibroblast
Cel Celsius
Cent Centigrade
cent centimeter
Cert certified
CES central excitatory state
CF carbolfuchsin
cardiac failure
carrier-free
chemotactic factor
chest and left leg (ECG leads)
Chiari-Frommel syndrome
Christmas factor
citrovorum factor
complement fixation
complement-fixing
contractile force
count fingers
counting finger
cystic fibrosis
cf compare (confer)
CFA complement-fixing antibody
complete Freund adjuvant
CFF critical flicker fusion test
critical fusion frequency
CFP chronic false-positive
cystic fibrosis of the pancreas
CFT clinical full-time
complement-fixation test

CFU colony-forming units
color-forming units
CFU-S colony-forming unit–spleen
CFWM cancer-free white mouse
CG cardiogreen
chorionic gonadotropin
chronic glomerulonephritis
colloidal gold
phosgene (choking gas)
Cg or
cg centigram
CGD chronic granulomatous disease
CGI clinical global impression
CGL chronic granulocytic leukemia
c gl correction with glasses
cgm centigram
CGN chronic glomerulonephritis
CG/OQ cerebral glucose oxygen quotient
CGP choline glycerophosphatide
chorionic growth hormone prolactin
circulating granulocyte pool
CGRP calcitonin gene-related peptide
CGS or
cgs centimeter-gram-second
CGT chorionic gonadotropin
CGTT cortisone glucose tolerance test
CH cholesterol
crown-heel (length of fetus)
wheelchair
CHA congenital hypoplastic anemia
cyclohexylamine
Chart paper (charta)
CHB complete heart block
CHD congestive heart disease
CHE cholinesterase
Chem chemotherapy
CHF congestive heart failure
CHH cartilage-hair hypoplasia
CHI creatinine-height index
CHL chloramphenicol
CHO carbohydrate
Chol cholesterol
Chol est cholesterol esters
CHP child psychiatry
comprehensive health planning
Chr. Chromobacterium

chr   chronic
CHS   Chediak-Higashi syndrome
      cholinesterase
CI   cardiac index
      cardiac insufficiency
      cerebral infarction
      chemotherapeutic index
      clinical investigator
      colloidal iron
      color index
      coronary insufficiency
      crystalline insulin
Ci   curie
cib   food (*cibus*)
CICU   cardiology intensive care unit
      coronary intensive care unit
CID   cytomegalic inclusion disease
CIDS   cellular immunity deficiency
         syndrome
CIE   countercurrent
         immunoelectrophoresis
Ci-INH   Ci inhibitor
CIN   cervical intra-epithelial
         neoplasia
circ   circulation
CIS   carcinoma in situ
      central inhibitory state
CIXU   constant infusion excretory
         urogram
CJD   Creutzfeldt-Jakob disease
CK   creatine kinase
ck   check
CL   chest and left arm
Cl.   *Clostridium*
Cl   chlorine
cl   centiliter
CLAS   congenital localized absence
         of skin
CLBBB   complete left bundle
         branch block
CLD   chronic liver disease
      chronic lung disease
cldy   cloudy
clin   clinic
      clinical
CLL   chronic lymphatic leukemia
      chronic lymphocytic leukemia
CLO   cod liver oil
CLSL   chronic lymphosarcoma
         (cell) leukemia
CLT   clot-lysis time
CM   capreomycin

CM (continued)
      chloroquine-mepacrine
      cochlear microphonic
      complications
      costal margin
      cow's milk
cm   centimeter
      tomorrow morning (*cras mane*)
cM   centiMorgan
cm³   cubic centimeter
CMB   carbolic methylene blue
CMC   carboxymethyl cellulose
      critical micellar concentration
CME   cystoid macular edema
CMF   chondromyxoid fibroma
      Cytoxan, methotrexate, 5-
         fluorouracil
CMGN   chronic membranous
         glomerulonephritis
CMI   carbohydrate metabolism
         index
      cell-mediated immunity
      cellular-mediated immune
         (response)
      cytomegalic inclusion
CMID   cytomegalic inclusion
         disease
c/min   cycles per minute
CML   chronic myelocytic leukemia
      chronic myelogenous
         leukemia
CMM   cutaneous malignant
         melanoma
cmm   cubic millimeter
CMN   cystic medial necrosis
CMN-AA   cystic medial necrosis of
         the ascending aorta
CMO   cardiac minute output
      card made out
CMP   cytidine monophosphate
CMR   carpometacarpal ratio
      cerebral metabolic rate
      crude mortality ratio
CMRG   cerebral metabolic rate of
         glucose
CMRO   cerebral metabolic rate of
         oxygen
CMS   Clyde Mood Scale
cms   to be taken tomorrow
         morning (*cras mane
         sumendus*)
CMU   chlorophenyldimethylurea

CMV cytomegalovirus
CN clinical nursing
  cyanogen
cn tomorrow night (*cras nocte*)
CNE chronic nervous exhaustion
CNH community nursing home
CNHD congenital nonspherocytic
  hemolytic disease
CNL cardiolipin natural lecithin
CNS central nervous system
cns to be taken tomorrow night
  (*cras nocte sumendus*)
CNV conative negative variation
  contingent negative variation
CO carbon monoxide
  cardiac output
  castor oil
  cervicoaxial
  coenzyme
  corneal opacity
  compound
C/O complains of
CO₂ carbon dioxide
CoA coenzyme A
COAG chronic open angle
  glaucoma
coag coagulation
COC cathodal-opening clonus
  coccygeal
  combination-type oral
  contraceptive
cochl spoonful (*cochleare*)
COCL cathodal-opening clonus
coct boiling (*coctio*)
COD cause of death
COGTT cortisone-primed oral
  glucose tolerance test
COHb carboxyhemoglobin
col strain (*cola*)
colat strained (*colatus*)
COLD chronic obstructive lung
  disease
coll eyewash (*collyrium*)
collut mouthwash (*collutorium*)
collyr eyewash (*collyrium*)
COMP complaint
  complication
  compound
COMT catechol-O-methyl
  transferase
ConA concanavalin A
conc concentration

concis cut (*concisus*)
cong gallon (*congius*)
cont continue
  continuously
conv convalescent
COP colloid osmotic pressure
  Cytoxan, Oncovin, prednisone
COPD chronic obstructive
  pulmonary disease
coq boil (*coque*)
coq sa boil properly (*coque
  secundum artem*)
CORA conditioned orientation
  reflex audiometry
cort bark (*cortex*)
  cortex
COT critical off-time
CP candle power
  cerebral palsy
  chemically pure
  chloropurine
  chloroquine and primaquine
  chronic pyelonephritis
  closing pressure
  cochlear potential
  combination product
  combining power
  coproporphyrin
  creatine phosphate
C/P cholesterol-phospholipid ratio
C & P compensation and pension
CPA cerebellar pontine angle
  chlorophenylalanine
CPAP continuous positive airway
  pressure
CPB cardiopulmonary bypass
CPC central posterior curve
  cetylpyridinium chloride
  chronic passive congestion
  clinicopathologic conference
CPD cephalopelvic disproportion
  citrate-phosphate-dextrose
cpd compound
CPE chronic pulmonary
  emphysema
  compensation, pension, and
  education
  cytopathic effect
CPEO chronic progressive external
  ophthalmoplegia
CPI constitutional psychopathic
  inferiority

CPI (continued)
    coronary prognostic index
CPIB   chlorophenoxyisobutyrate
CPK   creatine phosphokinase
CPM   central pontine myelinolysis
cpm   counts per minute
CPN   chronic pyelonephritis
CPP   cyclopentenophenanthrene
CPPB   continuous positive-pressure
    breathing
CPPD   calcium pyrophosphate
    dihydrate
CPR   cardiopulmonary resuscitation
    cerebral-cortex perfusion rate
    cortisol production rate
CPS   clinical performance score
    cumulative probability of
    success
cps   cycles per second
CPT   chest physiotherapy
CPZ   chlorpromazine
CQ   chloroquine-quinine
    circadian quotient
CR   calculus removed
    chest and right arm
    clinical research
    colon resection
    complete remission
    conditioned reflex
    crown-rump (length of fetus)
CR 1,2,3,4   complement receptor
    1,2,3,4
Cr   chromium
CRA   central retinal artery
cran   cranial
CRAO   central retinal artery
    occlusion
CRBBB   complete right bundle
    branch block
CRBP   cellular retinol binding
    protein
CRD   chronic renal disease
    complete reaction of
    degeneration
creat   creatinine
CREST   calcinosis, Raynaud's
    disease, esophageal
    involvement,
    sclerodactyly,
    telangiectasias
CRF   chronic renal failure
    corticotropin-releasing factor

CRI   concentrated rust-inhibitor
    cross-reacting idiotype
CRM   cross-reacting material
CROS   contralateral routing of
    signals
CRP   C-reactive protein
CRS   Chinese restaurant syndrome
    colon-rectal surgery
CRST   calcinosis cutis, Raynaud's
    phenomenon,
    sclerodactyly, and
    telangiectasia
CRT   cathode ray tube
CRU   clinical research unit
CRV   central retinal vein
CRVO   central retinal vein
    occlusion
crys   crystal
CS   Central Service
    Central Supply
    cesarean section
    chondroitin sulfate
    conditioned stimulus
    conscious
    coronary sinus
    corticosteroid
    current strength
    cycloserine
C & S   conjunctiva and sclera
    culture and sensitivity
CSA   canavaninosuccinic acid
    chondroitin sulfate A
CSF   cerebrospinal fluid
    colony-stimulating factor
CSH   chronic subdural hematoma
    cortical stromal hyperplasia
CSL   cardiolipin synthetic lecithin
CSM   cerebrospinal meningitis
    corn-soy milk
CSN   carotid sinus nerve
CSR   Cheyne-Stokes respiration
    corrected sedimentation rate
    cortisol secretion rate
CSS   carotid sinus stimulation
CST   convulsive shock therapy
CT   cardiothoracic (ratio)
    carotid tracing
    carpal tunnel
    cerebral thrombosis
    chlorothiazide
    circulation time
    classic technique

CT (continued)
    clotting time
    coagulation time
    collecting tubule
    computed tomography
    computerized tomography
    connective tissue
    contraction time
    Coombs' test
    coronary thrombosis
    corrected transposition
    corrective therapy
    cover test
    crest time
    cytotechnologist
CTAB cetyltrimethylammonium bromide
CTC chlortetracycline
CTD carpal tunnel decompression
    congenital thymic dysplasia
CTFE chlorotrifluoroethylene
CTH ceramide trihexoside
CTL cytotoxic T lymphocyte
CTR cardiothoracic ratio
CTZ chemoreceptor trigger zone
    chlorothiazide
CU color unit
    convalescent unit
CUC chronic ulcerative colitis
cu cm cubic centimeter
CUG cystourethrogram
cuj of which (*cujus*)
cuj lib of any you desire (*cujus libet*)
cu mm cubic millimeter
CV cardiovascular
    cell volume
    central venous
    cerebrovascular
    closing volume
    coefficient of variation
    color vision
    conjugata vera
    conversational voice
    corpuscular volume
    cresyl violet
cv tomorrow evening (*cras vespere*)
CVA cardiovascular accident
    cerebrovascular accident
    costovertebral angle
CVD cardiovascular disease
    color vision deviant
    color vision deviate

cvd curved
CVF cobra venom factor
CVH combined ventricular hypertrophy
    common variable hypogammaglobulinemia
CVI common variable immunodeficiency
CVO conjugata vera obstetrica
CVOD cerebrovascular obstructive disease
CVP cell volume profile
    central venous pressure
    Cytoxan, vincristine, prednisone
CVR cardiovascular-renal
    cerebrovascular resistance
CVRD cardiovascular renal disease
CVS cardiovascular surgery
    cardiovascular system
    clean-voided specimen
CW cardiac work
    casework
    chemical warfare
    chest wall
    children's ward
    continuous wave
cw clockwise
CWDF cell wall–deficient bacterial forms
CWI cardiac work index
CWP childbirth without pain
cwt hundredweight
CX cervix
Cx or
cx convex
CXR chest x-ray film
Cy cyanogen
cy copy
Cyclo cyclophosphamide
    cyclopropane
cyl cylinder
    cylindrical lens
cysto cystoscopic examination
D daughter
    day
    dead
    deciduous
    density
    dermatology
    deuterium
    deuteron

D (continued)
  dextro
  died
  diopter
  diplomate
  distal
  divorced
  dorsal
  duration
  mean dose
  vitamin D unit
d dose (*dosis*)
  give (*da*)
  right (*dexter*)
D_{CO} diffusing capacity for carbon monoxide
D_L diffusing capacity of lung
DA degenerative arthritis
  dental assistant
  direct agglutination
  disaggregated
  dopamine
  ductus arteriosus
DAB dimethylaminoazobenzene
DAF decay antibody-accelerating factor
DAG diacylglycerol
DAH disordered action of the heart
DALA delta-aminolevulinic acid
DAM degraded amyloid
  diacetyl monoxime
DAN diabetic autonomic neuropathy
D and N distance and near
DAO diamine oxidase
DAP dihydroxyacetone phosphate
  direct agglutination pregnancy (test)
DAPT direct agglutination pregnancy test
Dapt Daptazole
DAT differential agglutination titer
  diphtheria antitoxin
DB date of birth
  dextran blue
  disability
  distobuccal
db decibel
DBA dibenzanthracene
DBC dye-binding capacity
DBCL dilute blood clot lysis (method)

DBI development-at-birth index
DBM dibromomannitol
DBO distobucco-occlusal
DBP diastolic blood pressure
  distobuccopulpal
DC daily census
  deoxycholate
  diagnostic code
  diphenylarsine cyanide
  direct current
  discontinue
  distocervical
D & C dilatation and curettage
  dilation and curettage
DCA deoxycholate-citrate agar
  deoxycholic acid
  desoxycorticosterone acetate
DCC double concave
DCCT Diabetes Control and Complications Trial
DCF direct centrifugal flotation
DCG disodium cromoglycate
DCHFB dichlorohexafluorobutane
DCI dichloroisoproterenol
DCT direct Coombs' test
DCTMA desoxycorticosterone trimethylacetate
DCTPA desoxycorticosterone triphenylacetate
DCx double convex
DD died of the disease
  differential diagnosis
  disk diameter
dd let it be given to (*detur ad*)
DDAVP deamino D-arginine vasopressin
DDC diethyldithiocarbamic acid
  direct display console
DDCT dideoxycytidine
DDD dichlorodiphenyldichloroethane
DDH dissociated double hypertropia
DDS diaminodiphenylsulfone
  dystrophy-dystocia syndrome
DDT dichlorodiphenyltrichloroethane
DE dream elements
  duration of ejection
D & E dilation and evacuation
DEA dehydroepiandrosterone
DEAE diethylaminoethanol

DEAE (continued)
    diethylaminoethyl
DEAE-D diethylaminoethyl
    dextran
DEBA diethylbarbituric acid
DEC dendritic epidermal cell
dec deceased
    deciduous
    decrease
    pour off (*decanta*)
decoct decoction
decr decrease
decub lying down (*decubitus*)
def deficiency
deg degeneration
    degree
deglut let it be swallowed
    (*deglutiatur*)
del delivery
Dem Demerol (meperidine)
dep dependents
DeR reaction of degeneration
derm dermatology
DES diethylstilbestrol
    diffuse esophageal spasm
dest distilled (*destilla*)
DET diethyltryptamine
det give (*detur*)
DEV duck embryo vaccine
DF decapacitation factor
    deficiency factor
    degree of freedom
    desferrioxamine
    diabetic father
    discriminant function
    disseminated foci
DFDT difluorodiphenyl-
    trichloroethane
DFO deferoxamine
DFP diisopropylfluorophosphate
DFU dead fetus in utero
    dideoxyfluorouridine
DG deoxyglucose
    diagnosis
    diastolic gallop
    diglyceride
    distogingival
dg decigram
DGI disseminated gonococcal
    infection
dgm decigram
DH delayed hypersensitivity

DHA dehydroepiandrosterone
    dihydroxyacetone
DHAP dihydroxyacetone
    phosphate
DHAS dehydroepiandrosterone
    sulfate
DHE dihydroergotamine
DHEA dehydroepiandrosterone
DHEAS dehydroepiandrosterone
    sulfate
DHFR dihydrofolate reductase
DHIA dehydroisoandrosterone
DHL diffuse histiocytic lymphoma
DHT dihydrotachysterol
    dihydrotestosterone
DI diabetes insipidus
    diagnostic imaging
diag diagnosis
DIC diffuse intravascular
    coagulation
    disseminated intravascular
    coagulopathy
DID dead of intercurrent disease
DIE died in Emergency Room
diff differential
dig let it be digested (*digeratur*)
dil dilute (*dilue*)
DILD diffuse infiltrative lung
    disease
diluc at daybreak (*diluculo*)
dilut dilute (*dilutus*)
DIM divalent ion metabolism
dim one half (*dimidius*)
DIP desquamative interstitial
    pneumonia
    diisopropyl phosphate
    distal interphalangeal
DIPJ distal interphalangeal joint
dis disease
disc discontinue
disch discharge
DISH diffuse idiopathic skeletal
    hyperostosis
DISI dorsiflexion intercalated
    segment instability
disp dispensatory
    dispense
dist distill
DIT diet-induced thermogenesis
    diiodotyrosine
div divide
DJD degenerative joint disease

DK   decay
        diseased kidney
        dog kidney
DKA   diabetic ketoacidosis
DL   danger list
        difference limen
        diffusing capacity of lung
        distolingual
        Donath-Landsteiner (test)
dl   deciliter
DLA   distolabial
DLAI   distolabioincisal
DLCO   diffusing capacity of lung
           for carbon monoxide
DLE   discoid lupus erythematosus
          disseminated lupus
          erythematosus
DLI   distolinguoincisal
DLO   distolinguo-occlusal
DLP   distolinguopulpal
DM   diabetes mellitus
        diabetic mother
        diastolic murmur
        dopamine
DMA   dimethyladenosine
DMAB   dimethylamino-
             benzaldehyde
DMARD   disease-modifying
               anti-rheumatic drug
DMBA   dimethylbenzanthracene
DMCT   demethylchlortetracycline
DMD   Duchenne's muscular
           dystrophy
DME   dimethyl ether (of D-
           tubocurarine)
DMF   decayed, missing or filled
           (teeth)
DMM   dimethylmyleran
DMN   dimethylnitrosamine
DMO   dimethyloxazolidinedione
DMPA   depomedroxyprogesterone
             acetate
DMPE or
DMPEA   dimethoxyphenylethyla-
               mine
DMPP   dimethylphenyl-
              piperazinium
DMS   dimethylsulfoxide
DMSO   dimethylsulfoxide
DMT   dimethyltryptamine
DN   dextrose-nitrogen (ratio)
DNA   deoxyribonucleic acid

DNase   deoxyribonuclease
DNB   dinitrobenzene
DNC   dinitrocarbanilide
DNCB   dinitrochlorobenzene
DND   died a natural death
DNFB   dinitrofluorobenzene
DNP   deoxyribonucleoprotein
          dinitrophenol
DNPH   dinitrophenylhydrazine
DNPM   dinitrophenylmorphine
DNT   did not test
DO   diamine oxidase
        disto-occlusal
DOA   dead on arrival
DOB   date of birth
DOC   deoxycholate
          deoxycorticosterone
          died of other causes
DOCA   deoxycorticosterone acetate
DOCS   deoxycorticoids
DOD   date of death
          dead of disease
DOE   dyspnea on exercise
          dyspnea on exertion
DOM   deaminated-O-methyl
            metabolite
          dimethoxymethyl
            amphetamine
DOMA   dihydroxymandelic acid
DON   diazo-oxonorleucine
DOPA   dihydroxyphenylalanine
DOPAC   dihydroxyphenylacetic
               acid
DP   dementia praecox
       diastolic pressure
       directional preponderance
       disability pension
       distopulpal
dp   with proper direction (*directione
       propria*)
DPA   dipropylacetate
DPC   delayed primary closure
DPD   diffuse pulmonary disease
DPDL   diffuse poorly differentiated
            lymphoma
DPG   diphosphoglycerate
          displacement placentogram
DPGM   diphosphoglyceromutase
DPGP   diphosphoglycerate
             phosphatase
DPH   diphenylhydantoin
DPI   disposable personal income

DPL distopulpolingual
dpm disintegrations per minute
DPN diphosphopyridine nucleotide
DPO dimethoxyphenyl penicillin
DPS dimethylpolysiloxane
DPT diphtheria, pertussis, and
       tetanus
       dipropyltryptamine
DPTA diethylenetriamine
        penta-acetic acid
DPTI diastolic pressure-time index
DPVNS diffuse pigmented
          villonodular synovitis
DQ developmental quotient
DR diabetic retinopathy
      doctor
      reaction of degeneration
Dr doctor
dr drachm
     dram
DRF dose-reduction factor
DRGs diagnosis-related groups
DRI Discharge Readiness Inventory
DS dead space
      dehydroepiandrosterone sulfate
      dextrose-saline
      Down's syndrome
      dry swallow
D & S dermatology and syphilology
DSA digital subtraction
       angiography
DSAP disseminated superficial
         actinic porokeratosis
DSC or
DSCG disodium cromoglycate
DSM dextrose solution mixture
DST dexamethasone suppression
       test
DT delirium tremens
      distance test
      duration tetany
      dye test
DTBC D-tubocurarine
DTBN di-t-butyl nitroxide
DTC D-tubocurarine
dtd let such a dose be given (*datur
       talis dosis*)
DTH delayed-type hypersensitivity
D time dream time
DTM dermatophyte test medium
DTMP deoxythymidine
          monophosphate

DTN diphtheria toxin normal
DTNB dithiobisnitrobenzoic acid
DTP diphtheria, tetanus, and
       pertussis
       distal tingling on percussion
DTPA diethylenetriaminepenta-
         acetic acid
DTR deep tendon reflex
DTZ diatrizoate
DU deoxyuridine
      diagnosis undetermined
      dog unit
      duodenal ulcer
DUB dysfunctional uterine bleeding
DUMP deoxyuridine
          monophosphate
duod duodenum
DUSN diffuse unilateral subacute
          neuroretinitis
DV double vibration
DVA distance visual acuity
DVD dissociated vertical deviation
DW distilled water
      dry weight
D/W dextrose in water
D5W,
D5 & W or
D₅W 5 per cent dextrose in water
DX dextran
Dx diagnosis
DXD discontinued
DXM dexamethasone
DXT deep x-ray therapy
DZ dizygous
E cortisone (compound E)
     electric charge
     electromotive force
     electron
     emmetropia
     energy
     epinephrine
     erythrocyte
     esotropia
     experimenter
     eye
E. *Entamoeba*
     Escherichia
EA ethacrynic acid
ea each
EAC Ehrlich ascites carcinoma
       external auditory canal
EACA epsilon aminocaproic acid

ead   the same (*eadem*)
EAE   experimental allergic
    encephalomyelitis
EAHF   eczema, asthma, hay
    fever
EAHLG   equine antihuman
    lymphoblast globulin
EAHLS   equine antihuman
    lymphoblast serum
EAM   external auditory meatus
EAP   epiallopregnanolone
EB   elementary body
    epidermolysis bullosa
    Epstein-Barr (virus)
    estradiol benzoate
EBD   epidermolysis bullosa
EBI   emetine bismuth iodide
EBL   estimated blood loss
EBV   Epstein-Barr virus
EC   electron capture
    enteric-coated
    entrance complaint
    enzyme classification
    Escherichia coli
    excitation-contraction
    experimental control
    extracellular
    eyes closed
ECA   ethacrynic acid
ECBO   enteric cytopathogenic
    bovine orphan (virus)
ECBV   effective circulating blood
    volume
ECC   extracorporeal circulation
ECCE   extracapsular cataract
    extraction
ECDO   enteric cytopathogenic dog
    orphan (virus)
ECF   effective capillary flow
    eosinophil chemotactic factor
    extended care facility
    extracellular fluid
ECFA   eosinophil chemotactic
    factor of anaphylaxis
ECFV   extracellular fluid volume
ECG   electrocardiogram
    electrocardiography
ECHO   enteric cytopathogenic
    human orphan (virus)
ECI or
ECIB   extracorporeal irradiation of
    blood

ECIL   extracorporeal irradiation of
    lymph
eclec   eclectic
ECLT   euglobulin clot lysis time
ECM   erythema chronicum migrans
    extracellular material
ECMO   enteric cytopathogenic
    monkey orphan (virus)
E. coli   *Escherichia coli*
ECS   electroconvulsive shock
ECSO   enteric cytopathogenic swine
    orphan (virus)
ECT   electroconvulsive therapy
    emission computed
    tomography
ECV   extracellular volume
ECW   extracellular water
ED   effective dose
    Ehlers-Danlos syndrome
    epileptiform discharge
    erythema dose
ED_{50} median effective dose
EDC   estimated date of confinement
    expected date of confinement
EDD   effective drug duration
    expected date of delivery
EDP   electronic data processing
    end-diastolic pressure
EDR   effective direct radiation
    electrodermal response
EDS   Ehlers-Danlos syndrome
EDTA   edetic acid
    ethylenediaminetetra-
    acetate
EDV   end-diastolic volume
EE   end-to-end
    eye and ear
EEA   electroencephalic audiometry
EEC   enteropathogenic *Escherichia
    coli*
EEE   eastern equine encephalitis
EEG   electroencephalogram
    electroencephalography
EEME   ethinylestradiol methyl ether
EENT   eyes, ears, nose and throat
EER   electroencepahlic response
EF   ectopic focus
    ejection fraction
    encephalitogenic factor
EFA   essential fatty acids
    extrafamily adoptees
EFC   endogenous fecal calcium

EFE   endocardial fibroelastosis
EFV   extracellular fluid volume
EFVC   expiratory flow-volume
       curve
EG   esophagogastrectomy
EGA   estimated gestational age
EGF   epidermal growth factor
EGG   electrogastrogram
EGL   eosinophilic granuloma of the
       lung
EGM   electrogram
EGOT   erythrocyte glutamic oxalo-
       acetic transaminase
EH   essential hypertension
EHBF   estimated hepatic blood flow
       exercise hyperemia blood
       flow
EHC   enterohepatic circulation
       essential hypercholesterolemia
EHDP   ethane hydroxydiphosphate
EHF   exophthalmos-hyperthyroid
       factor
EHL   endogenous hyperlipidemia
EHO   extrahepatic obstruction
EHP   excessive heat production
EI   enzyme inhibitor
E/I   expiration-inspiration ratio
EIA   enzyme immunoassay
EIAL   exercise induced airflow
       limitation
EID   egg-infective dose
       electroimmunodiffusion
EIP   extensor indicis proprius
EIT   erythrocyte iron turnover
EK   erythrokinase
EKC   epidemic keratoconjunctivitis
EKG   electrocardiogram
EKY   electrokymogram
el   elixir
E-LAM endothelial-leukocyte
       adhesion molecule
elb   elbow
ELISA enzyme-linked
       immunosorbent assay
elix   elixir
ELT   euglobulin lysis time
EM   ejection murmur
       electron microscopy
       erythrocyte mass
Em   emmetropia
EMB   embryology
       eosin methylene blue

EMB (continued)
       ethambutol
       ethambutol-myambutol
EMC   electron microscopy
       encephalomyocarditis
EMD   electromechanical
       dissociation
EMF   electromagnetic flowmeter
       electromotive force
       endomyocardial fibrosis
       erythrocyte maturation factor
EMG   electromyogram
       electromyography
       exophthalmos, macroglossia,
       gigantism
EMI   Electric and Musical Industries
emp   a plaster (*emplastrum*)
       as directed (*ex modo
       prescripto*)
emul   emulsion
EN   enema
       erythema nodosum
ENA   extractable nuclear antigen
enem   enema
ENG   electronystagmograph
       electronystagmography
ENL   erythema nodosum leprosum
ENT   ear, nose, and throat
EO   eosinophils
       ethylene oxide
       eyes open
EOD   entry on duty
eod   every other day
EOG   electro-oculogram
EOM   extraocular movement
eos   eosinophils
EOT   effective oxygen transport
EP   ectopic pregnancy
       erythrocyte protoporphyrin
EPA   eicosapentaenoic acid
EPC   epilepsia partialis continua
EPEC   enteropathogenic
       Escherichia coli
EPF   exophthalmos-producing
       factor
Epi   epinephrine
EPI   Expanded Programme on
       Immunization
epith   epithelium
EPL   extracorporeal piezoelectric
       lithotriptor
EPP   end-plate potential

EPP (continued)
  erythropoietic protoporphyria
EPR   electron paramagnetic
        resonance
      electrophrenic respiration
      estradiol production rate
EPS   exophthalmos-producing
        substance
      expressed prostatic secretions
EPSP excitatory postsynaptic
        potential
EPTE existed prior to enlistment
EPTS existed prior to service
eq   equivalent
ER   ejection rate
      emergency room
      endoplasmic reticulum
      estrogen receptors
      external resistance
      evoked response
ERA   evoked response audiometry
ERBF effective renal blood flow
ERC   endoscopic retrograde
        cholangiography
ERCP endoscopic retrograde
        cholangiopancreatography
ERG   electroretinogram
ERP   effective refractory period
      equine rhinopneumonitis
      estrogen receptor proteins
ERPF effective renal plasma flow
ERV   expiratory reserve volume
ES   end-to-side
      Expectation Score
ESB   electrical stimulation to brain
ESC   electromechanical slope
        computer
Esch. Escherichia
ESD   electronic summation device
ESF   erythropoietic-stimulating
        factor
ESL   end-systolic length
ESM   ejection systolic murmur
eso   esophagoscopy
      esophagus
ESP   end-systolic pressure
      extrasensory perception
ESR   erythrocyte sedimentation rate
ESS   erythrocyte-sensitizing
        substance
ess   essential
ess neg essentially negative

EST   electroshock therapy
est   estimated
ESU   electrostatic unit
ESV   end-systolic volume
ET   effective temperature
      ejection time
      endotracheal
      esotropia
      etiology
      eustachian tube
Et   ethyl
ETA   ethionamide
ETAF epithelial thymic-activating
        factor
et al   and others (et alii)
ETF   eustachian tube function
ETH   elixir terpin hydrate
ETH/C elixir terpin hydrate with
        codeine
etiol   etiology
ETKM every test known to man
ETM   erythromycin
ETOH ethyl alcohol
ETOX ethylene oxide
ETP   entire treatment period
      eustachian tube pressure
ETT   extrathyroidal thyroxine
ETV   educational television
EU   Ehrlich units
      enzyme units
      excretory urography
EUA   examination under anesthesia
EV   extravascular
ev   electron volt
eval evaluation
EVLW extravascular lung water
EW   Emergency Ward
ew   elsewhere
EWB   estrogen withdrawal bleeding
EWL   egg-white lysozyme
ex   excision
      exophthalmos
exam examination
EXBF exercise hyperemia blood
        flow
exc   excision
exhib let it be given (exhibeatur)
exp or
expir expired
      expiration
      expiratory
ext   exterior

ext (continued)
    external
    extract
    spread (*extende*)
F Fahrenheit
    fat
    father
    fellow
    female
    field of vision
    foramen
    formula
    French (catheter size)
    gilbert (unit of magnetomotive
      force)
    hydrocortisone (compound F)
F. *Filaria*
    Fusiformis
f make (*fiat*)
F_1 first filial generation
F_2 second filial generation
FA far advanced
    fatty acid
    femoral artery
    field ambulance
    first aid
    fluorescent antibody
    forearm
    free acid
FACS fluorescence-activated cell
      sorting
FAD flavin adenine dinucleotide
FADF fluorescent antibody
      dark-field
FAE follicle-associated epithelium
Fahr Fahrenheit
FAIDS feline AIDS
fam doc family doctor
FAN fuchsin, amido black, and
      naphthol yellow
FANA fluorescent antinuclear
      antibody
FAP familial adenomatous
      polyposis
FAT fluorescent antibody test
FAV feline ataxia virus
FB fingerbreadth
    foreign body
FBE full blood examination
FBP femoral blood pressure
    fibrinogen breakdown
      products

FBS fasting blood sugar
    fetal bovine serum
FC finger clubbing
    finger counting
fc foot candles
FCA ferritin-conjugated antibodies
FD fatal dose
    focal distance
    foot drape
    forceps delivery
    freeze-dried
FD_{50} median fatal dose
FDA frontodextra anterior
FDE final drug evaluation
FDG 2-fluoro-2-deoxyglucose
FDP fibrin degradation product
    flexor digitorum profundus
    frontodextra posterior
    fructose 1,6-diphosphate
FDS flexor digitorum superficialis
FDT frontodextra transversa
feb dur while the fever lasts (*febre
      durante*)
FEC free erythrocyte
      coproporphyrin
FECG fetal electrocardiogram
FECP free erythrocyte
      coproporphyria
FECV functional extracellular fluid
      volume
FEF forced expiratory flow
FEKG fetal electrocardiogram
FeLV feline leukemia virus
fem female
FEP or
FEPP free erythrocyte
      protoporphyrin
FES forced expiratory spirogram
FET forced expiratory time
FETS forced expiratory time, in
      seconds
FEV familial exudative
      vitreoretinopathy
    forced expiratory volume
FF fat free
    father factor
    fecal frequency
    filtration fraction
    finger-to-finger
    flat feet
    force fluids
    forearm flow

FF (continued)
    foster father
FFA   free fatty acids
FFDW   fat-free dry weight
fff fields   flicker, fusion, frequency
    fields
FFM   fat-free mass
FFP   fresh frozen plasma
FFT   flicker fusion threshold
FFWW   fat-free wet weight
FG   fibrinogen
FGD   fatal granulomatous
    disease
FGF   father's grandfather
    fresh gas flow
FGM   father's grandmother
FH   family history
    fetal head
    fetal heart
fh   let a draft be made (*fiat haustus*)
FHR   fetal heart rate
FHS   fetal heart sound
FHT   fetal heart
    fetal heart tones
FI   fever caused by infection
    fibrinogen
    forced inspiration
FIA   fluoroimmunoassay
fib   fibrillation
    fibrinogen
FID   free induction decay
    flame ionization detector
FIF   forced inspiratory flow
fig   figure
FIGE   field inversion gel
    electrophoresis
FIGLU   formiminoglutamic acid
FIGO   International Federation of
    Gynecology and Obstetrics
filt   filter
fist   fistula
FJN   familial juvenile
    nephrophthisis
fl   fluid
FLA   left frontoanterior
    (*frontolaevo anterior*)
fla   according to rule (*fiat lege artis*)
FLASH   fast low-angle shot
fld   fluid
fl dr   fluid dram
flor   flowers
fl oz   fluid ounce

FLP   left frontoposterior
    (*frontolaevo posterior*)
FLSA   follicular lymphosarcoma
FLT   left frontotransverse
    (*frontolaeva transversa*)
Fl up   flare-up
FM   flowmeter
fm   make a mixture (*fiat mistura*)
FMD   foot and mouth disease
FME   full-mouth extraction
FMF   familial Mediterranean fever
FMG   foreign medical graduate
FMN   flavin mononucleotide
FMR   fetal-to-maternal ratio
FMS   fat-mobilizing substance
    full-mouth series
FN   false-negative
    finger-to-nose
FO   foramen ovale
    fronto-occipital
FOAVF   failure of all vital forces
FOD   free of disease
fol   leaves (*folia*)
FONAR   focused nuclear magnetic
    resonance
FP   false-positive
    family practice
    freezing point
    frontoparietal
    frozen plasma
fp   let a potion be made (*fiat potio*)
FPA   fluorophenylalanine
fpa   far point of accommodation
FPC   familial polyposis coli
    fish protein concentrate
F pil   let pills be made (*fiant pilulae*)
FPM   filter paper microscopic (test)
FPP   familial paroxysmal
    polyserositis
fps   frames per second
FR   Fisher-Race (notation)
    flocculation reaction
    flow rate
Fr   French (catheter gauge)
F & R   force and rhythm
fract   fracture
frag   fragility
Fr BB   fracture of both bones
FRC   frozen red cells
    functional reserve capacity
    functional residual capacity
frict   friction

FROM   full range of motion
FRP   functional refractory period
FRS   furosemide
FS   full scale (IQ)
 function study
FSA   fetal sulfoglycoprotein antigen
fsa   let it be made skillfully (*fiat secundum artem*)
FSD   focal skin distance
FSF   fibrin-stabilizing factor
FSH   follicle-stimulating hormone
FSP   fibrinogen split products
 fibrinolytic split products
FSR   fusiform skin revision
FSW   field service worker
FT   false transmitter
 family therapy
 fibrous tissue
 free thyroxine
 full term
ft   foot
 make (*fiat*)
FTA   fluorescent treponemal antibody
FTA-AB or
FTA-ABS   fluorescent treponemal antibody absorption test
FTI   free thyroxine index
FTLB   full term living birth
FTND   full term normal delivery
ft pulv   make a powder (*fiat pulvis*)
FTT   failure to thrive
FU   fecal urobilinogen
 fluorouracil
 follow-up
FUDR   fluorodeoxyuridine
FUO   fever of undetermined origin
 fever of unknown origin
FUR   fluorouracil riboside
FV   fluid volume
FVC   forced vital capacity
FVL   femoral vein ligation
f vs   let the patient be bled (*fiat venaesectio*)
FW   Felix-Weil (reaction)
 Folin and Wu's (method)
 fragment wound
FWHM   full width at half-maximum
FWR   Felix-Weil reaction
fx   fracture

FY   fiscal year
FYI   for your information
FZ   focal zone
G   an immunoglobulin
 gauge
 gingival
 glucose
 gonidial (colony)
 good
 gravida
 Greek
g   force (the pull of gravity)
 gram
GA   Gamblers Anonymous
 gastric analysis
 general anesthesia
 gestational age
 gingivoaxial
 glucuronic acid
 gut-associated
Ga   gallium
GABA   gamma-aminobutyric acid
GAG   glycosaminoglycan
gal   gallon
GALT   gastrointestinal-associated lymphoid tissue
 gut-associated lymphoid tissue
galv   galvanic
GAPD or
GAPDH   glyceraldehyde phosphate dehydrogenase
garg   gargle
GB   gallbladder
 Guillain-Barré syndrome
GBA   ganglionic-blocking agent
 gingivobuccoaxial
GBH   graphite-benzalkonium-heparin
GBM   glomerular basement membrane
GBS   gallbladder series
GC   ganglion cells
 gas chromatography
 glucocorticoid
 gonococcus
 gonorrhea
 granular casts
 guanine cytosine
g-cal   gram-calorie
g-cm   gram-centimeter
GCS   general clinical service

GCSF   granulocyte colony-
      stimulating factor
GDA   germine diacetate
GDH   glycerophosphate
      dehydrogenase
GDS   Gradual Dosage Schedule
GE   gastroemotional
      gastroenterology
      gastroenterostomy
G/E   granulocyte-erythroid ratio
GEMS   good emergency mother
      substitute
gen   general
GER   gastroesophageal reflux
ger   geriatrics
GERD   gastroesophageal reflux
      disease
GERL   Golgi-endoplasmic
      reticulum-lysosomes
GET   gastric emptying time
GET½   gastric emptying half-time
GF   germ-free
      gluten-free
      grandfather
GFD   gluten-free diet
GFR   glomerular filtration rate
GG   gamma globulin
GGA   general gonadotropic activity
GGG   gamboge
GG or S   glands, goiter, or stiffness
      (the neck)
GGT   gamma glutamyl transferase
GGTP   gamma-glutamyl
      transpeptidase
GH   growth hormone
GHD   growth hormone deficiency
GHRF   growth hormone-releasing
      factor
GI   gastrointestinal
      globin insulin
GIK   glucose, insulin, and
      potassium
GIM   gonadotropin-inhibitory
      material
GIP   gastric inhibitory peptides
GIS   gas in stomach
      gastrointestinal system
GIT   gastrointestinal tract
GITT   glucose-insulin tolerance test
GK   glycerol kinase
GL   greatest length
Gl   gill

Gl (continued)
    gland
GLA   gingivolinguoaxial
GLC   gas-liquid chromatography
GLNS   gay lymph node syndrome
glob   globulin
GLP   group-living program
glu or
gluc   glucose
GM   gastric mucosa
      general medical
      geometric mean
      grandmother
      grand multiparity
gm   gram
g-m   gram-meter
GMA   glyceryl methacrylate
GMC   general medical council
GM-CSF   granulocyte-macrophage
      colony-stimulating
      factor
GMK   green monkey kidney
GM & S   general medical and
      surgical
GMT   geometric mean titer
GMW   gram-molecular weight
GN   glomerulonephritis
      glucose nitrogen (ratio)
      gram-negative
GNB   gram-negative bacilli
GNID   gram-negative intracellular
      diplococci
GnRH   gonadotropin-releasing
      hormone
GOE   gas, oxygen and ether
GOK   God only knows
GOT   glutamic oxaloacetic
      transaminase
GP   general paresis
      general practice
      general practitioner
      glycoprotein
      guinea pig
      gutta-percha
gp   group (muscle)
GPA   grade-point averages
GPAIS   guinea pig anti-insulin
      serum
GPC   giant papillary conjunctivitis
GPD or
GPDH   glucose phosphate
      dehydrogenase

G6PD or
G6PDH   glucose-6-phosphate
        dehydrogenase
GPI   general paralysis of the insane
      glucose phosphate isomerase
GPIPID   guinea pig intraperitoneal
       infectious dose
GPK   guinea pig kidney (antigen)
GPKA   guinea pig kidney
       absorption (test)
GPS   guinea pig serum
GPT   glutamic pyruvic transaminase
GPUT   galactose phosphate uridyl
       transferase
GR   gastric resection
      glutathione reductase
gr   grain
GRA   gonadotropin-releasing agent
grad   gradually, by degrees
GRAS   generally recognized as
       safe
GRASS   gradient recalled acquisi-
       tion in a steady state
grav I   pregnancy one
       primigravida
GRF   gonadotropin-releasing factor
GRID   gay-related
       immunodeficiency disease
GRP   gastrin-releasing peptide
GS   general surgery
G/S   glucose and saline
GSA   Gross virus antigen
       guanidinosuccinic acid
GSC   gas-solid chromatography
       gravity-settling culture
GSD   genetically significant dose
       glycogen storage disease
GSE   gluten-sensitive enteropathy
GSH   glomerular-stimulating
       hormone
      (reduced) glutathione
GSR   galvanic skin response
      generalized Shwartzman
       reaction
GSSG   (oxidized) glutathione
GSSR   generalized Sanarelli-
       Shwartzman reaction
GSW   gunshot wound
GT   gingiva, treatment of
      glucose tolerance
      glutamyl transpeptidase
G & T   gowns and towels

gt   drop
GTH   gonadotropic hormone
GTN   gestational trophoblastic
       neoplasia
      glyceryl trinitrate
GTP   glutamyl transpeptidase
      guanosine triphosphate
GTT   glucose tolerance test
gtt   drops
GU   gastric ulcer
      genitourinary
      gonococcal urethritis
GUS   genitourinary system
GV   gentian violet
GVH   graft versus host
GVHD   graft-versus-host disease
GVHR   graft-versus-host reaction
GW   group work
GXT   graded exercise test
gyn   gynecology
GZ   Guilford-Zimmerman
       personality test
H   a draft (*haustus*)
      height
      henry
      high
      Holzknecht unit
      horizontal
      hormone
      hour
      hypermetropia
      hyperphoria
      hypo
H   Hauch (motile microorganism)
H.   *Hemophilus*
H^+ hydrogen ion
HA   headache
      height age
      hemagglutinating antibody
      hemagglutination
      hemolytic anemia
      high anxiety
      hospital admission
      Hounsfield unit
      hyaluronic acid
      hydroxyapatite
HAA   hepatitis-associated antigen
HABA   hydroxybenzeneazobenzoic
       acid
HAD   hemadsorption
HAE   hereditary angioneurotic
       edema

HAHTG   horse antihuman thymus
          globulin
HAI   hemagglutination inhibition
          hemagglutinin inhibition
hal   halothane
HAP   heredopathia atactica
          polyneuritiformis
          histamine phosphate acid
HAPA   hemagglutinating
          antipenicillin antibody
HASHD   hypertensive
          arteriosclerotic heart
          disease
haust   a draft (*haustus*)
HB   heart block
          housebound
Hb   hemoglobin
HBABA   hydroxybenzene-
          azobenzoic acid
HBB   hydroxybenzyl benzimidazole
HBD or
HBDH   hydroxybutyrate
          dehydrogenase
HBF   heaptic blood flow
HBI   high-serum-bound iron
HBLV   human B lymphotropic
          virus
HBO   hyperbaric oxygen
HBP   high blood pressure
HBV   hepatitis B virus
HBW   high birth weight
HC   hair cell
          head compression
          hepatic catalase
          house call
          Huntington's chorea
          hyaline casts
          hydroxycorticoid
HCA   hypothalamic chronic
          anovulation
HCC   hepatocellular carcinoma
          hydroxycholecalciferol
hCG   human chorionic
          gonadotropin
HCH   hexachlorocyclohexane
HCL   hard contact lenses
HCO₃   the bicarbonate radical
HCP   hepatocatalase peroxidase
          hereditary coproporphyria
hCS or
hCSM   human chorionic
          somatomammotropin

HCT   hematocrit
          homocytotrophic
          hydrochlorothiazide
HCU   homocystinuria
HCVD   hypertensive cardiovascular
          disease
HD   hearing distance
          heart disease
          high dosage
          Hodgkin's disease
          hydatid disease
hd   at bedtime (*hora decubitus*)
HDBH   hydroxybutyric
          dehydrogenase
HDC   histidine decarboxylase
HDH   heart disease history
HDI   hexamethylene diisocyanate
HDL or
HDLP   high-density lipoprotein
HDLW   distance at which a watch
          is heard by the left ear
HDN   hemolytic disease of the
          newborn
HDP   hydroxydimethylpyrimidine
HDRW   distance at which a watch
          is heard by the right ear
HDS   herniated disk syndrome
HE   hereditary elliptocytosis
          human enteric
H & E   hematoxylin and eosin
HEAT   human erythrocyte
          agglutination test
hebdom   a week (*hebdomada*)
HEC   hydroxyergo-
          calciferol
HED   unit of roentgen-ray dosage
          (*Haut-Einheits-Dosis*)
HEENT   head, eyes, ears, nose and
          throat
HEK   human embryo kidney
          human embryonic kidney
HEMA   hydroxy-ethyl methacrylate
hematol   hematology
HEPA   high-efficiency particulate
          air (filter)
HES   hydroxyethyl starch
HET   helium equilibration time
HETE   hydroxy-eicosatetraenoic
          acid
HETP   hexaethyltetraphosphate
HF   Hageman factor
          hay fever

HF (continued)
  heart failure
  hemorrhagic fever
  high flow
  high frequency
HFI hereditary fructose intolerance
HFP hexafluoropropylene
Hg or
Hgb hemoglobin
HGF hyperglycemic-glycogenolytic
    factor
hGG human gamma globulin
hGH human growth hormone
HGPRT hypoxanthine-guanine
    phosphoribosyl
    transferase
HH hydroxyhexamide
HHA hereditary hemolytic anemia
HHb un-ionized hemoglobin
HHD hypertensive heart disease
H & Hm compound hypermetropic
    astigmatism
HHT hereditary hemorrhagic
    telangiectasia
HI hemagglutination inhibition
  high impulsiveness
  hydroxyindole
HIA hemagglutination-inhibition
    antibody
HIAA hydroxyindoleacetic acid
HIHA high impulsiveness, high
    anxiety
HILA high impulsiveness, low
    anxiety
HIOMT hydroxyindole-*O*-methyl
    transferase
HIT hemagglutination-inhibition
    test
  hypertrophic infiltrative
    tendinitis
HIV human immunodeficiency
    virus
HJ Howell-Jolly (bodies)
HK heat-killed
  heel-to-knee
  hexokinase
HKLM heat-killed *Listeria*
    monocytogenes
HL hearing level
  hearing loss
  histocompatibility locus
  hypermetropia, latent

H & L heart and lungs
HLA histocompatibility complex
  human leukocyte antigen
HLDH heat-stable lactic
    dehydrogenase
hLH human luteinizing hormone
H-L-K heart, liver, kidney
HLR heart-lung resuscitator
HLT human lymphocyte
    transformation
hlth health
HLV herpes-like virus
HM hand motion
  hand movement
  human milk
  hydatidiform mole
Hm manifest hyperopia
HMD hyaline membrane disease
HME heat and moisture
    exchanger
HMF hydroxymethylfurfural
HMG human menopausal
    gonadotropin
  hydroxymethylglutaryl
HMK high molecular weight
    kininogen
HML human milk lysozyme
HMM hexamethylolmelamine
HMP hexose monophosphate
  hexose monophosphate
    pathway
  hot moist packs
HMPG hydroxymethoxy-
    phenylglycol
HMPS hexose monophosphate
    shunt
HMSAS hypertrophic muscular
    subaortic stenosis
HMSN hereditary motor and
    sensory neuropathy
HN hereditary nephritis
  hilar node
hn tonight (*hac nocte*)
HN$_2$ nitrogen mustard,
    mechlorethamine
HNP herniated nucleus pulposus
HNSHA hereditary nonspherocytic
    hemolytic anemia
HO high oxygen
  hyperbaric oxygen
H/O history of
H$_2$O water

HOA hypertrophic
    osteoarthroscopy
HOC hydroxycorticoid
HOCM hypertrophic obstructive
    cardiomyopathy
HOOD hereditary osteo-
    onychodysplasia
HOP high oxygen pressure
hosp hospital
HP high protein
    human pituitary
H & P history and physical
hp haptoglobin
HPA hypothalamic-pituitary-
    adrenal
HPAA hydroxyphenylacetic acid
HPE history and physical
    examination
HPF heparin-precipitable fraction
    high-power field
hPFSH human pituitary follicle-
    stimulating hormone
hPG human pituitary gonadotropin
HPI history of present illness
hPL human placental lactogen
HPLA hydroxyphenyllactic acid
HPLC high-performance liquid
    chromatography
HPO high pressure oxygen
HPP hereditary pyropoikilocytosis
    hydroxypyrazolopyrimidine
HPPA hydroxyphenylpyruvic acid
HPPH hydroxyphenyl-
    phenylhydantoin
HPS hematoxylin-phloxine-saffron
    hypertrophic pyloric stenosis
HPT hyperparathyroidism
HPV *Haemophilus pertussis*
    vaccine
    human papillomavirus
HPVD hypertensive pulmonary
    vascular disease
HPVG hepatic portal venous gas
HR heart rate
    hospital record
    hospital report
Hr blood type factor
hr hour
H & R hysterectomy and radiation
HRBC horse red blood cells
HRIG human rabies immune
    globulin

HRR Hardy-Rand-Ritter plates
HRS Hamilton Rating Scale
HRT heart rate
HS heat stable
    heme synthetase
    hereditary spherocytosis
    herpes simplex
    horse serum
    Hurler's syndrome
hs on retiring (*hora somni*)
HSA human serum albumin
HSE herpes simplex encephalitis
HSG hysterosalpingogram
HSV herpes simplex virus
HT hemagglutination titer
    histologic technician
    hydroxytryptamine
    hypermetropia, total
    hypertension
    hypodermic tablet
    hypothalamus
Ht total hyperopia
ht heart
    height
HTA hydroxytryptamine
HTC homozygous typing cell
HTHD hypertensive heart disease
HTLA human thymus lymphocyte
    antigen
HTLV human T cell leukemia virus
    human T cell lymphotropic
    virus
HTOH hydroxytryptophol
HTP hydroxytryptophan
HTV herpes-type virus
HU hemagglutinating unit
    Hounsfield unit
    hydroxyurea
    hyperemia unit
HUS hemolytic-uremic syndrome
    hyaluronidase unit for semen
HUTHAS human thymus
    antiserum
HV hepatic vein
    herpes virus
    hospital visit
H & V hemigastrectomy and
    vagotomy
HVA homovanillic acid
HVD hypertensive vascular disease
HVE high-voltage electrophoresis
HVH herpes virus hominis

HVL   half-value layer
HVM   high-velocity missile
HVSD   hydrogen-detected
          ventricular septal defect
Hx   history
Hy   hypermetropia
hy   hysteria
hypo   injection
          under
hys   hysteria
HZ   herpes zoster
Hz   hertz
HZV   herpes zoster virus
I   intensity of magnetism
     permanent incisor
^{131}I   radioactive iodine
i   deciduous incisor
    optically inactive
IA   impedance angle
     internal auditory
     intra-aortic
     intra-arterial
IABP   intra-aortic balloon pump
IAC   internal auditory canal
IADH   inappropriate antidiuretic
          hormone
IADHS   inappropriate antidiuretic
          hormone syndrome
IAM   internal auditory meatus
IAS   interatrial septum
     intra-amniotic saline infusion
IASD   interatrial septal defect
IASP   International Association for
          the Study of Pain
IAT   invasive activity test
     iodine-azide test
IB   inclusion body
IBB   intestinal brush border
IBC   iron-binding capacity
IBD   inflammatory bowel disease
IBR   infectious bovine
          rhinotracheitis
IBS   irritable bowel syndrome
IBU   international benzoate unit
IC   immune complex
     inspiratory capacity
     intensive care
     intercostal
     intermediate care
     intermittent claudication
     intracavitary
     intracellular

IC (continued)
     intracerebral
     intracranial
     intracutaneous
     irritable colon
     isovolumic contraction
ICA   internal carotid artery
     intracranial aneurysm
ICAM-1   intercellular adhesion
          molecule-1
ICAO   internal carotid artery
          occlusion
ICC   immunocompetent cells
     Indian childhood cirrhosis
     intensive coronary care
ICCE   intracapsular cataract
          extraction
ICCU   intensive coronary care unit
ICD or
ICDH   isocitric dehydrogenase
ICF   intensive care facility
     intracellular fluid
ICG   indocyanine green
ICM   intercostal margin
ICP   intracranial pressure
ICRP   International Commission
          on Radiological Protection
ICRU   International Commission
          on Radiation Units and
          Measures
ICS   immotile cilia syndrome
     intercostal space
ICSH   interstitial cell-stimulating
          hormone
ICT   indirect Coombs' test
     inflammation of connective
          tissue
     insulin coma therapy
     isovolumic contraction time
ict ind   icterus index
ICU   intensive care unit
ICW   intracellular water
ID   identification
     immunodeficiency
     infant deaths
     infective dose
     inside diameter
     internal diameter
     intradermal
id   the same (*idem*)
I & D   incision and drainage
ID$_{50}$ median infective dose

IDA image display and analysis
iron deficiency anemia
IDDM insulin-dependent diabetes
mellitus
IDI induction-delivery interval
IDL intermediate-density
lipoproteins
IDM infant of diabetic mother
IDP initial dose period
IDR intradermal reaction
IDS immunity deficiency state
IDU idoxuridine
iododeoxyuridine
IDVC indwelling venous catheter
IE immunizing unit (*immunitäts
Einheit*)
I/E inspiratory-expiratory ratio
IEF isoelectric focusing
IEL intraepithelial lymphocytes
IEMG integrated electromyogram
IEOP immunoelectro-osmophoresis
IEP immunoelectrophoresis
IF immunofluorescence
interstitial fluid
intrinsic factor
IFA immunofluorescent assay
indirect fluorescent antibody
IFC intrinsic factor concentrate
IFN interferon
IFR inspiratory flow rate
IFRA indirect fluorescent rabies
antibody (test)
IFV intracellular fluid volume
IG immune globulin
intragastric
Ig immunoglobulin
IgA gamma A immunoglobulin
IgD gamma D immunoglobulin
IgE gamma E immunoglobulin
IgG gamma G immunoglobulin
IgM gamma M immunoglobulin
IgY gamma Y immunoglobulin
IGDM infant of gestational
diabetic mother
IGF-1 insulin-like growth factor-1
IGV intrathoracic gas volume
IH idiopathic hyperprolactinemia
infectious hepatitis
inner half
IHA indirect hemagglutination
IHBTD incompatible hemolytic
blood transfusion disease

IHC idiopathic hypercalciuria
immunohistochemistry
inner hair cell
IHD ischemic heart disease
IHO idiopathic hypertrophic
osteoarthropathy
IHR intrinsic heart rate
IHSA iodinated human serum
albumin
IHSS idiopathic hypertrophic
subaortic stenosis
IIF indirect immunofluorescent
IJP internal jugular pressure
IL-1,2,3 interleukin-1,2,3
ILA insulin-like activity
ILB or
ILBW infant, low birth weight
ILD ischemic leg disease
ischemic limb disease
IL-2R interleukin-2 receptor
IM infectious mononucleosis
internal medicine
intramedullary
intramuscular
im- (indicates presence of) NH
group
IMA internal mammary artery
IMAA iodinated macroaggregated
albumin
IMB intermenstrual bleeding
IMBC indirect maximum breathing
capacity
IMH idiopathic myocardial
hypertrophy
IMHP 1-iodomercuri-2-
hydroxypropane
IMI intramuscular injection
imp impression
improved
IMR infant mortality rate
IMRAD introduction, methods,
results, and discussion
IMS incurred in military service
IN intranasal
in inch
INAD infantile neuroaxonal
dystrophy
INAH isonicotinic acid hydrazide
inc increase
incurred
incr increase
ind independents

in d   daily (*in die*)
INDM   infant of nondiabetic
          mother
INE   infantile necrotizing
          encephalomyelopathy
inf   inferior
          infusion
          pour in (*infunde*)
info   information
INH   isoniazid
          isonicotinic acid hydrazide
inj   inject
inl   inlay
INO   internuclear ophthalmoplegia
inoc   inoculate
INPV   intermittent negative-
          pressure assisted
          ventilation
INS   idiopathic nephrotic syndrome
inspir   inspiration
int   intermediates
          intermittent
          internal
int med   internal medicine
IO   internal os
          intestinal obstruction
          intraocular
I & O   in and out
          intake and output
IOFB   intraocular foreign body
IOP   intraocular pressure
IOU   intensive therapy observation
          unit
IP   incisioproximal
          incubation period
          instantaneous pressure
          interphalangeal
          intraperitoneal
          isoelectric point
I-para   primipara
IPC   isopropyl chlorophenyl
IPD   inflammatory pelvic disease
IPG   impedance plethysmography
IPH   idiopathic pulmonary
          hemosiderosis
IPL   intrapleural
IPP   intermittent positive pressure
IPPB   intermittent positive-pressure
          breathing
IPPI   interruption of pregnancy for
          psychiatric indication

IPPO   intermittent positive-pressure
          inflation with oxygen
IPPR   intermittent positive-pressure
          respiration
IPPV   intermittent positive-pressure
          ventilation
IPRT   interpersonal reaction test
IPS   initial prognostic score
IPSP   inhibitory postsynaptic
          potential
IPU   inpatient unit
IPV   inactivated poliovaccine
IQ   intelligence quotient
IR   immunoreactive
          index of response
          internal resistance
IRBBB   incomplete right bundle
          branch block
IRDS   idiopathic respiratory distress
          syndrome
IRG   immunoreactive glucagon
IRHCS   immunoradioassayable
          human chorionic
          somatomammotropin
IRhGH   immunoreactive human
          growth hormone
IRI   immunoreactive insulin
IRMA   intraretinal microvascular
          abnormalities
irr   irradiation
IRS   infrared spectrophotometry
IRV   inspiratory reserve volume
IS   intercostal space
          interspace
is   in place (*in situ*)
ISA   intrinsic sympathomimetic
          activity
ISC   irreversible sickled cells
ISD or
ISDN   isosorbide dinitrate
ISF   interstitial fluid
ISG   immune serum globulin
ISH   icteric serum hepatitis
iso   isoproterenol
ISP   interspace
IST   insulin sensitivity test
          insulin shock therapy
ISW   interstitial water
IT   implantation test
          inhalation test
          inhalation therapy

IT (continued)
 intradermal test
 intrathecal
 intratracheal
 intratracheal tube
 intratumoral
 isomeric transition
ITC imidazolyl-thioguanine
     chemotherapy
ITE in the ear
ITLC instant thin-layer
     chromatography
ITP idiopathic thrombocytopenic
     purpura
ITPA Illinois Test of
     Psycholinguistic Abilities
ITT insulin tolerance test
ITU intensive therapy unit
IU immunizing unit
    international unit
    intrauterine
IUCD intrauterine contraceptive
     device
IUD intrauterine death
     intrauterine device
IUDR iododeoxyuridine
IUFB intrauterine foreign body
IUGR intrauterine growth rate
     intrauterine growth
     retardation
IUM intrauterine fetally
     malnourished
IUT intrauterine transfusion
IV interventricular
    intervertebral
    intravascular
    intravenous
    intraventricular
    invasive
IVAP in vivo adhesive platelet
IVC inferior vena cava
     intravenous cholangiogram
IVCC intravascular consumption
     coagulopathy
IVCD intraventricular conduction
     defect
IVCP inferior vena cava pressure
IVCU isotope voiding
     cystourethrography
IVCV inferior venacavography
IVD intervertebral disk

IVF intravascular fluid
IVGTT intravenous glucose
     tolerance test
IVH intraventricular hemorrhage
IVM intravascular mass
IVP intravenous pyelogram
IVS interventricular septum
IVSD interventricular septal defect
IVT intravenous transfusion
IVTTT intravenous tolbutamide
     tolerance test
IVU intravenous urography
IWL insensible water loss
IWMI inferior wall myocardial
     infarction
J Joule's equivalent
   journal
JA juvenile arthritis
JBE Japanese B encephalitis
JCA juvenile chronic arthritis
JCAH Joint Commission on
     Accreditation of Hospitals
jej jejunum
JG juxtaglomerular
JGC juxtaglomerular cell
JGI juxtaglomerular granulation
     index
JND just noticeable difference
JPS joint position sense
JRA juvenile rheumatoid arthritis
jt joint
JV jugular vein
    jugular venous
JVP jugular venous pulse
JXG juvenile xanthogranuloma
K absolute zero
   electrostatic capacity
   kathode (cathode)
   Kell blood system
   Kelvin
   killer cell
   potassium
KA kathode
    ketoacidosis
    King-Armstrong (units)
KAP knowledge, attitudes, and
     practice
KAU King-Armstrong units
KB ketone bodies
kb kilobase
KC kathodal closing

kc   kilocycle
kcal   kilocalorie
KCC   kathodal-closing contraction
KCG   kinetocardiogram
KCl   potassium chloride
kcps   kilocycles per second
KCT   kathodal-closing tetanus
KD   kathodal duration
KDT   kathodal-duration tetanus
KE   kinetic energy
kev   kilo electron volts
KeV   electron volts
KFAB   kidney-fixing antibody
KFS   Klippel-Feil syndrome
kg   kilogram
kg-cal   kilogram-calorie
KGS   ketogenic steroid
kHz   kilohertz
KIA   Kliger iron agar
KIU   kallikrein-inhibiting unit
KJ   knee jerk
KK   knee kick
KLH   keyhole limpet hemocyanin
KLS   kidney, liver, spleen
KM   kanamycin
km   kilometer
KMnO   potassium permanganate
KMV   killed measles virus vaccine
kn   knee
KOC   kathodal-opening contraction
KOH   potassium hydroxide
KP   keratitic precipitates
KPTT   kaolin partial
        thromboplastin time
KRB   Krebs-Ringer bicarbonate
        buffer
KRP   Kolmer's test with Reiter
        protein
        Krebs-Ringer phosphate
KS   Kaposi's sarcoma
        ketosteroid
        Klinefelter's syndrome
        Kveim-Siltzbach (test)
KU   Karmen units
KUB   kidney, ureter, and bladder
KV   killed vaccine
kv   kilovolt
kvp   kilovolt peak
KW   Keith-Wagener
kw   kilowatt
KWB   Keith, Wagener, Barker
        (classification)
kw-hr   kilowatt-hour

L   coefficient of induction
      Latin
      left
      length
      levo-
      ligament
      light sense
      liter
      low
      lower
      lumbar
L.   Lactobacillus
      Leishmania
l   lethal (letha)
      liter
      pound (libra)
LA   lactic acid
      latex agglutination (test)
      left arm
      left atrial
      left atrium
      leucine aminopeptidase
      linguoaxial
      local anesthesia
      low anxiety
L & A   light and accommodation
LAA   leukocyte ascorbic acid
lab   laboratory
LAD   left anterior descending
      left axis deviation
      leukocyte adhesion deficiency
LAE   left atrial enlargement
LAF   laminar air flow
LAG   labiogingival
      lymphangiogram
LAH   lactalbumin hydrolysate
      left atrial hypertrophy
LAI   labioincisal
LAIT   latex agglutination-inhibition
        test
LAL   limulus amebocyte lysate
LAO   left anterior oblique
LAP   left atrial pressure
      leucine aminopeptidase
      leukocyte alkaline phosphatase
      lyophilized anterior pituitary
LAR   left arm recumbent
LAS   linear alkylate sulfonate
      lymphadenopathy syndrome
LASER   light amplification by
        stimulated emission of
        radiation
lat   lateral

LATS   long-acting thyroid
    stimulator
LAV   lymphadenopathy-associated
    virus
LB   laboratory data
    lipid body
    live births
    loose body
lb   pound (*libra*)
LBB   left bundle branch
LBBB   left bundle branch block
LBCD   left border of cardiac
    dullness
LBF   *Lactobacillus bulgaricus*
    factor
LBI   low serum-bound iron
LBM   lean body mass
LBNP   lower-body negative
    pressure
LBW   low birth weight
LBWI   low birth weight infant
LBWR   lung-body weight ratio
LC   Langerhans' cells
    late clamped
    lethal concentration
    lipid cytosomes
    living children
LCA   left coronary artery
    lithocholic acid
L-CA   leukocyte common antigen
LCAT   lecithin-cholesterol-acyl-
    transferase
LCD   liquor carbonis detergens
LCFA   long-chain fatty acid
LCL   Levinthal-Coles-Lillie
    (bodies)
    lymphocytic lymphosarcoma
LCM   left costal margin
    lymphatic choriomeningitis
    lymphocytic choriomeningitis
LCT   long-chain triglyceride
LD   labyrinthine defect
    lactic dehydrogenase
    left deltoid
    lethal dose
    light difference
    linguodistal
    living donor
    low dosage
    lymphocyte-defined
L-D   Leishman-Donovan (bodies)
L/D   light-dark ratio
LD_{50} median lethal dose

LDA   left dorsoanterior
    linear displacement analysis
LDD   light-dark discrimination
LDDS   local dentist
LDH   lactic dehydrogenase
LDL   loudness discomfort level
    low-density lipoprotein
LDLP   low-density lipoprotein
LDP   left dorsoposterior
LDV   lactic dehydrogenase virus
LE   left eye
    leukoerythrogenetic
    lower extremity
    lupus erythematosus
LED   lupus erythematosus
    disseminatus
LES   local excitatory state
LET   linear energy transfer
LF   laryngofissure
    limit flocculation
    low forceps
LFA   left femoral artery
    left frontoanterior
LFA-1,2,3   lymphocyte function-
    associated
    antigen-1,2,3
LFD   lactose-free diet
    least fatal dose
    low forceps delivery
LFN   lactoferrin
LFP   left frontoposterior
LFT   latex flocculation test
    left frontotransverse
    liver function test
LG   laryngectomy
    left gluteal
    linguogingival
lg   large
LGB   Landry-Guillain-Barré
    (syndrome)
    lateral geniculate body
LGN   lateral geniculate nucleus
LGV   lymphogranuloma
    venereum
LH   lower half
    luteinizing hormone
LHL   left hepatic lobe
LHRF   luteinizing hormone-
    releasing factor
LHRH   luteinizing hormone-
    releasing hormone
LI   linguoincisal
    low impulsiveness

LIAFI   late infantile amaurotic familial idiocy
lib   pound (*libra*)
LIBC   latent iron-binding capacity
LIF   left iliac fossa
    leukocyte inhibiting factor
lig   ligament
LIHA   low impulsiveness, high anxiety
LILA   low impulsiveness, low anxiety
LIP   lymphocytic interstitial pneumonitis
LIQ   lower inner quadrant
liq   liquid
    liquor
LIS   lobular in situ
LK   left kidney
LKP   lamellar keratoplasty
LL   left leg
    left lower
    left lung
    lower lobe
    lysolecithin
LLC   lymphocytic leukemia
LLF   Laki-Lorand factor
LLL   left lower lobe
LLM   localized leukocyte mobilization
LLQ   left lower quadrant
LM   light microscopy
    linguomesial
LMA   left mentoanterior
LMD   local medical doctor
    low molecular weight dextran
LMDX   low molecular weight dextran
LMK   low molecular weight kininogen
LMP   last menstrual period
    left mentoposterior
LMR   localized magnetic resonance
LMT   left mentotransverse
LMW   low molecular weight
LMWD   low molecular weight dextran
LN   lipoid nephrosis
    lupus nephritis
    lymph node
L/N   letter-numerical (system)
LNMP   last normal menstrual period

LNPF   lymph node permeability factor
LO   linguo-occlusal
    low
LOA   leave of absence
    left occipitoanterior
loc dol   to the painful spot (*loco dolenti*)
LOD   line of duty
LOM   limitation of motion
    loss of motion
LOP   left occipitoposterior
LOQ   lower outer quadrant
LOT   left occipitotransverse
LOWBI   low birth weight infant
LP   latency period
    leukocyte-poor
    light perception
    linguopulpal
    lipoprotein
    low protein
    lumbar puncture
    lymphoid plasma
L/P   lactate-pyruvate ratio
LPA   left pulmonary artery
LPC   late positive component
LPE   lipoprotein electrophoresis
LPF   leukocytosis-promoting factor
    localized plaque formation
    low-power field
    lymphocytosis-promoting factor
LPL   lipoprotein lipase
lpm   liters per minute
LPO   left posterior oblique
    light perception only
LPS   lipopolysaccharide
LPV   left pulmonary veins
LR   laboratory references
    lactated Ringer's solution
    light reaction
L/R   left to right ratio
L & R   left and right
L→R   left to right
LRF   luteinizing hormone-releasing factor
LRH   luteinizing hormone-releasing hormone
LRQ   lower right quadrant
LRS   lactated Ringer's solution
LRT   lower respiratory tract
LS   left side

LS (continued)
   legally separated
   liver and spleen
   lumbosacral
   lymphosarcoma
LSA left sacroanterior
   lymphosarcoma
LSA/RCS lymphosarcoma-
       reticulum cell sarcoma
LSB left sternal border
LScA left scapuloanterior
LScP left scapuloposterior
LSCS lower segment cesarean
     section
LSD lysergic acid diethylamide
LSM late systolic murmur
LSP left sacroposterior
LST left sacrotransverse
LSV left subclavian vein
LT left thigh
   leukotriene
   levothyroxine
   long-term
   lymphotoxin
lt left
LTB laryngotyracheobronchitis
LTB$_4$ leukotriene B$_4$
LTH lactogenic hormone
   luteotropic hormone
lt lat left lateral
LTPP lipothiamide pyrophosphate
LU left upper
L & U lower and upper
LUF luteinized unruptured follicle
    (syndrome)
LUL left upper lobe
LUQ left upper quadrant
LV left ventricle
   leukemia virus
   live virus
LVAD left ventricular assist device
LVDP left ventricular diastolic
     pressure
LVE left ventricular enlargement
LVEDP left ventricular end-
     diastolic pressure
LVEDV left ventricular end-
     diastolic volume
LVET left ventricular ejection time
LVF left ventricular failure
   low-voltage fast
   low-voltage foci

LVH left ventricular hypertrophy
LVP left ventricular pressure
   lysine-vasopressin
LVS left ventricular strain
LVSP left ventricular systolic
     pressure
LVSV left ventricular stroke
     volume
LVSW left ventricular stroke work
LVW left ventricular work
LVWI left ventricular work index
LW lacerating wound
   Lee-White (method)
L & W or
L/W living and well
LX local irradiation
lymphs lymphocytes
lzm lysozyme
M macerate (*macerare*)
   male
   married
   minim
   minute
   mix
   molar
   month
   mother
   multipara
   murmur
   muscle
   myopia
   permanent molar
   strength of pole
   thousand (*mil, milli*)
M. *Micrococcus*
   Microsporum
   Mycobacterium
   Mycoplasma
M$_1$ mitral first sound
m deciduous molar
   handful (*manipulus*)
   meter
   minim
μ micron
MA mandelic acid
   mean arterial (blood pressure)
   medical audit
   mental age
   Miller-Abbott (tube)
   moderately advanced
ma meter-angle
   milliampere

MAA   macroaggregated albumin
MABP   mean arterial blood pressure
MAC   maximum allowable
         concentration
       membrane attack complex
       minimum alveolar
         concentration
mac   macerate
MAF   macrophage-activating factor
MAFH   macroaggregated ferrous
         hydroxide
magn   large (*magnus*)
MAI   *Mycobacterium avium-
         intracellulare*
MAM   methylazomethanol
M + Am   myopic astigmatism
mam   milliampere-minute
man   handful (*manipulus*)
       manipulate
manip   manipulation
MANOVA   multivariate analysis of
         variance
man pr   early in the morning
         (*mane primo*)
MAO   maximal acid output
       monoamine oxidase
MAOI   monoamine oxidase
         inhibitor
MAP   mean aortic pressure
       mean arterial pressure
       megaloblastic anemia of
         pregnancy
       methylacetoxyprogesterone
       methylaminopurine
       muscle-action potential
MAPF   microatomized protein
         food
mas   milliampere-second
MASER   microwave amplification
         by stimulated emission
         of radiation
       molecular application by
         stimulated emission of
         radiation
matut   in the morning (*matutinus*)
max   maximum
MB   mesiobuccal
       methylene blue
mb   mix well (*misce bene*)
MBA   methylbovine albumin
MBAS   methylene blue active
         substance

MBC   maximal breathing capacity
       minimal bactericidal
         concentration
MBD   methylene blue dye
       minimal brain damage
       minimal brain dysfunction
       Morquio-Brailsford
         disease
MBF   myocardial blood flow
MBFLB   monaural bifrequency
         loudness balance
MBL   minimal bactericidal level
MBO   mesiobucco-occlusal
MBP   antigen prepared from
         melitensis
       mean blood pressure
       mesiobuccopulpal
       myelin basic protein
MBSA   methylated bovine serum
         albumin
MC   mast cell
       maximum concentration
       metacarpal
       mineralocorticoid
       myocarditis
       mytomycin-C
Mc   megacurie
       megacycle
mc or mCi   millicurie
MCA   methylcholanthrene
       middle cerebral artery
MCB   membranous cytoplasmic
         body
MCBR   minimum concentration of
         bilirubin
MCC   mean corpuscular hemo-
         globin concentration
       minimum complete-killing
         concentration
MCCU   mobile coronary care unit
MCD   mean cell diameter
       mean corpuscular diameter
       medullary cystic disease
MCF   mononuclear cell factor
MCFA   medium-chain fatty acid
mcg or
μg   microgram
MCH   mean corpuscular
         hemoglobin
mch   millicurie-hour
MCHC   mean corpuscular hemo-
         globin concentration

MCI   mean cardiac index
mCi   millicurie
MCL   midclavicular line
      midcostal line
      most comfortable loudness
        level
MCP   metacarpophalangeal
      mitotic-control protein
mc p s   megacycles per second
MCQ   multiple choice question
MCR   message competition ratio
      metabolic clearance rate
M-CSF   macrophage colony-
        stimulating factor
MCT   mean circulation time
      mean corpuscular thickness
      medium-chain triglyceride
      medullary carcinoma of
        thyroid
MCTD   mixed connective tissue
        disease
MCV   mean clinical value
      mean corpuscular volume
MD   malic dehydrogenase
      manic depressive
      Mantoux diameter
      Marek's disease
      maternal deprivation
      medium dosage
      movement disorder
      muscular dystrophy
      myocardial damage
      myocardial disease
MDA   mentodextra anterior
      methylenedioxy-
        amphetamine
      motor discriminative acuity
MDC   minimum detectable
        concentration
MDD   mean daily dose
MDF   mean dominant frequency
      myocardial depressant factor
MDH   malic dehydrogenase
MDHV   Marek's disease herpesvirus
m dict   as directed (moro dicto)
MDM   minor determinant mixture
MDP   mentodextra posterior
      muramyl dipeptide
MDT   median detection threshold
      mentodextra transversa
MDTR   mean diameter-thickness
        ratio

MDUO   myocardial disease of
         unknown origin
MDY   month, date, year
ME   medical education
      mercaptoethanol
      middle ear
M/E   myeloid-erythroid ratio
Me   methyl
MEA   mercaptoethylamine
      multiple endocrine
        adenomatosis
MED   minimal effective dose
      minimal erythema dose
med   median
      medical
      medicine
MEDAC   multiple endocrine
         deficiency-autoimmune
         candidiasis
meds   medications
       medicines
MEF   maximal expiratory flow
MEFR   maximum expiratory flow
        rate
MEFV   maximum expiratory flow
        volume
MEG   mercaptoethylguanidine
meg   megakaryocytes
MEM   minimum essential medium
MEN   multiple endocrine neoplasia
mep   meperidine
MEPP   miniature end-plate
        potential
mEq or
meq   milliequivalent
MER   mean ejection rate
      methanol-extruded residue
MER-29   triparanol
Mets   metastases
m et sig   mix and label (misce et
            signa)
mev   million electron volts
MF   medium frequency
      mycosis fungoides
      myelin figures
M/F   male-female ratio
M & F   mother and father
mf   microfilaria
μf   microfarad
MFB   metallic foreign body
MFD   midforceps delivery
      minimum fatal dose

μfd   microfarad
MFP   monofluorophosphate
MFR   mucus flow rate
m ft   make a mixture (*mistura fiat*)
MFW   multiple fragment wounds
MG   mesiogingival
    methyl glucoside
    muscle group
    myasthenia gravis
Mg   magnesium
mg   milligram
mg%   milligrams per 100 milliliters;
    milligrams per deciliter
MGF   mother's grandfather
MGGH   methylglyoxal
    guanylhydrazone
MGH or
mgh   milligram-hour
MGM   mother's grandmother
mgm   milligram
MGN   membranous
    glomerulonephritis
MGP   marginal granulocyte pool
MGR   modified gain ratio
mgtis   meningitis
MGUS   monoclonal
    grammopathies of
    undetermined
    significance
MH   mammotropic hormone
    marital history
    medical history
    mental health
MHA   methemalbumin
    microangiopathic hemolytic
    anemia
    mixed hemadsorption
MHB   maximum hospital benefit
MHb   methemoglobin
MHC   major histocompatibility
    complex
MHD   mean hemolytic dose
    minimum hemolytic dose
MHN   massive hepatic necrosis
MHP   1-mercuri-2-hydroxypropane
MHPG   methoxyhydroxy-
    phenylglycol
MHR   maximal heart rate
MI   mercaptoimidazole
    mitral incompetence
    mitral insufficiency
    myocardial infarction

MIC   Maternity and Infant Care
    minimum inhibitory
    concentration
mic pan   bread crumb (*mica panis*)
MICU   mobile intensive care unit
MID   maximum inhibiting dilution
    mesioincisodistal
    minimum infective dose
midnoc   midnight
MIF   macrophage-inhibiting factor
    migration inhibitory factor
    mixed immunofluorescence
    müllerian inhibitory factor
MIFR   maximal inspiratory flow
    rate
mIg   membrane immunoglobulin
MIH   migratory inhibitory hormone
MILIS   Multicenter Investigation
    for the Limitation of
    Infarct Size
min   minim
    minimal
    minute
MIO   minimum identifiable odor
MIP   maximum inspiratory
    pressure
MIRD   medical internal radiation
    dose
MIRU   myocardial infarction
    research unit
mist   mixture (*mistura*)
MIT   monoiodotyrosine
mit   send (*mitte*)
mixt   mixture
MK   monkey kidney
MKS   meter-kilogram-second
MKV   killed-measles vaccine
ML   mesiolingual
    middle lobe
    midline
M:L   monocyte-lymphocyte ratio
ml   milliliter
MLA   mentolaeva anterior
    mesiolabial
    monocytic leukemia, acute
MLAI   mesiolabioincisal
MLAP   mean left atrial pressure
MLC   minimum lethal
    concentration
    mixed leukocyte culture
    mixed lymphocyte culture
    multilamellar cytosome

MLC (continued)
    myelomonocytic leukemia,
      chronic
MLD metachromatic
    leukodystrophy
    minimum lethal dose
MLF medial longitudinal fasciculus
MLI mesiolinguoincisal
MLN mesenteric lymph node
MLO mesiolinguo-occlusal
MLP left mentoposterior
    (*mentolaeva posterior*)
    mesiolinguopulpal
MLR mixed lymphocyte reaction
MLS mean lifespan
    myelomonocytic leukemia,
      subacute
MLSI multiple line scan imaging
MLT left mentotransverse
    (*mentolaeva transversa*)
MLV Moloney's leukemogenic
    virus
    mouse leukemia virus
MM malignant melanoma
    Marshall-Marchetti
    medial malleolus
    mucous membrane
    multiple myeloma
    muscularis mucosa
    myeloid metaplasia
M & M milk and molasses
mM millimolar
    millimole
mm millimeter
    muscles
MMA methylmalonic acid
MMC migrating motor complex
    minimum medullary
      concentration
MMD minimum morbidostatic
      dose
MMEF maximal midexpiratory
      flow
MMEFR maximal midexpiratory
      flow rate
MMF maximal midexpiratory flow
MMFR maximal midexpiratory
      flow rate
    maximal midlfow rate
mmHg millimeters of mercury
mM/L or
mM/l millimoles per liter

MMM myeloid metaplasia with
    myelofibrosis
    myelosclerosis with myeloid
      metaplasia
MMPI Minnesota Multiphasic
    Personality Inventory
mmpp millimeters partial pressure
MMPR methylmercaptopurine
    riboside
MMR mass miniature radiography
    mobile mass x-ray
    myocardial metabolic rate
mμ millimicron
mμc millimicrocurie (nanocurie)
mμg millimicrogram (nanogram)
MN midnight
    multinodular
    myoneural
M/N or
M & N morning and night
Mn manganese
mN millinormal
mn midnight
MNA maximum noise area
MNCV motor nerve conduction
    velocity
MNU methylnitrosourea
MO mesio-occlusal
    mineral oil
mo month
MOD mesio-occlusodistal
mod moderate
mol wt molecular weight
moll soft (*mollis*)
MOM milk of magnesia
MOMA methoxyhydroxymandelic
    acid
Monos monocytes
MOPP nitrogen mustard, Oncovin,
    prednisone, procarbazine
MOPV monovalent oral poliovirus
    vaccine
mor dict in the manner directed
    (*more dicto*)
mor sol in the usual way (*more
    solito*)
mOs milliosmolal
mOsm milliosmol, milliosmole
MP mean pressure
    melting point
    menstrual period
    mercaptopurine

MP (continued)
   mesiopulpal
   metacarpophalangeal
   monophosphate
   mucopolysaccharide
   multiparous
6-MP 6-mercaptopurine
mp as directed (*modo prescripto*)
MPA main pulmonary artery
   medroxyprogesterone acetate
   methylprednisolone acetate
MPAP mean pulmonary arterial
    pressure
MPC marine protein concentrate
   maximum permissible
    concentration
   meperidine, promethazine,
    chlorpromazine
   minimum mycoplasmacidal
    concentration
MPD maximum permissible dose
MPEH methylphenyl-
    ethylhydantoin
MPGN membranoproliferative
    glomerulonephritis
MPJ metacarpophalangeal joint
MPL mesiopulpolingual
MPLA mesiopulpolabial
MPMV Mason Pfizer monkey virus
MPN most probable number
MPO myeloperoxidase
MPP mercaptopyrazidopyrimidine
MPS mucopolysaccharide
MPSS methylprednisolone sodium
    succinate
MR mental retardation
   metabolic rate
   methyl red
   mitral reflux
   mitral regurgitation
   mortality rate
   mortality ratio
   muscle relaxant
mr milliroentgen
MRAP mean right atrial pressure
MRD minimum reacting dose
MRF mesencephalic reticular
    formation
   mitral regurgitant flow
MRFIT Multiple-Risk Factor
    Intervention Trial
MRI magnetic resonance imaging

mRNA messenger RNA
MRT median recognition threshold
   milk-ring test
MRVP mean right ventricular
    pressure
MS mental status
   mitral stenosis
   morphine sulfate
   mucosubstance
   multiple sclerosis
   musculoskeletal
ms manuscript
msec millisecond
MSER mean systolic ejection rate
MSG monosodium glutamate
MSH medical self-help
   melanocyte-stimulating
    hormone
   melanophore-stimulating
    hormone
MSK medullary sponge kidney
MSL midsternal line
MSLA mouse-specific lymphocyte
    antigen
MSN mildly subnormal
MSRPP multidimensional scale for
    rating psychiatric
    patients
MSS mental status schedule
MSU monosodium urate
MSUD maple syrup urine disease
MSV Moloney sarcoma virus
   murine sarcoma virus
MSVC maximal sustained
    ventilatory capacity
MT empty
   malignant teratoma
   maximal therapy
   medical technologist
   membranea tympani
   metatarsal
   methyltyrosine
   more than
   music therapy
MTD maximum tolerated dose
MTDT modified tone decay test
MTF maximum terminal flow
   modulation transfer function
MTHF methyltetrahydrofolic acid
MTI malignant teratoma
    intermediate
   minimum time interval

MTP   metatarsophalangeal
MTR   Meinicke turbidity reaction
MTT   malignant teratoma
          trophoblastic
          marrow transit time
          mean transit time
          monotetrazolium
MTU   methylthiouracil
MTV   mammary tumor virus
MTX   methotrexate
MU   Mache unit
          Montevideo unit
mU   milliunit
mu   micron
          mouse unit
muc   mucilage
multip   pregnant woman who has
          borne two or more
          children
μl microliter
μmg micromilligram
μmm micromillimeter
$\mu\mu$ micromicron
$\mu\mu c$ micromicrocurie (picocurie)
$\mu\mu g$ micromicrogram (picogram)
MUST   medical unit,
          self-contained,
          transportable
MUU   mouse uterine units
MV   minute volume
          mitral valve
          mixed venous
mV   millivolt
MVM   microvillose membrane
MVP   mitral valve prolapse
MVR   massive vitreous retraction
MVV   maximum voluntary
          ventilation
MW   molecular weight
mw   microwave
My   myopia
my   mayer (unit of heat capacity)
MyG   myasthenia gravis
MZ   monozygotic
N   nasal
          neurology
          normal
          size of sample
          unit of neutron dosage
N.   Neisseria
          Nocardia
n   index of refraction

n (continued)
          nerve
NA   neutralizing antibody
          Nomina Anatomica
          noradrenaline
          not admitted
          not applicable
          not available
          numerical aperture
Na   sodium
NAA   no apparent abnormalities
NAD   nicotinamide adenine
          dinucleotide
          no appreciable disease
          normal axis deviation
NADH   nicotinamide adenine
          dinucleotide (reduced
          form)
NADP   nicotinamide adenine
          dinucleotide phosphate
NADPH   nicotinamide adenine
          dinucleotide phosphate
          (reduced form)
NANA   N-acetylneuraminic acid
NAPA   N-acetyl-p-aminophenol
NB   newborn
          nitrous oxide-barbiturate
nb   note well (nota bene)
NBM   nothing by mouth
NBO   nonbed occupancy
NBS   normal blood serum
NBT   nitroblue tetrazolium
NBTE   nonbacterial thrombotic
          endocarditis
NBW   normal birth weight
NC   no casualty
          no change
          noise criterion
          noncontributory
          not cultured
N/C   no complaints
nc   nanocurie
NCA   neurocirculatory asthenia
NCD   not considered disabling
NCF   neutrophil chemotactic factor
nCi   nanocurie
NCRPM   National Council on
          Radiation Protection
          and Measurements
NCV   nerve conduction velocity
ND   neonatal death
          neurotic depression

ND (continued)
    Newcastle disease
    New Drugs
    no data
    no disease
    nondisabling
    normal delivery
    not detectable
    not detected
    not determined
    not done
n_D refractive index
NDA   no data available
    no demonstrable antibodies
NDF   new dosage form
NDGA   nordihydroguaiaretic acid
NDI   nephrogenic diabetes insipidus
NDMA   nitrosodimethylaniline
NDP   net dietary protein
NDV   Newcastle disease virus
NE   nerve ending
    neurologic examination
    no effect
    nonelastic
    norepinephrine
    not evaluated
    not examined
NEC   not elsewhere classifiable
    not elsewhere classified
NED   no evidence of disease
NEFA   nonesterified fatty acid
NEG   negative
NEM   *N*-ethylmaleimide
NER   no evidence of recurrence
NERD   no evidence of recurrent
      disease
neur   neurology
neuro   neurologic
neurol   neurologic
NF   none found
    normal flow
    not found
NFTD   normal full-term delivery
NG   nasogastric
ng   nanogram
NGF   nerve growth factor
NGU   nongonococcal urethritis
NH   nonhuman
    nursing home
NHA   nonspecific hepatocellular
      abnormality
NHL   non-Hodgkin's lymphoma

NHS   normal horse serum
    normal human serum
NI   no information
    not identified
    not isolated
NIA   no information available
NIAID   National Institute of
      Allergy and Infectious
      Disease
NIH   National Institutes of Health
NK   natural killer
    not known
NKH   nonketotic hyperosmotic
NI   normal
NLA   neuroleptanalgesia
NLP   no light perception
NLT   normal lymphocyte transfer
      test
NM   neuromuscular
    not measurable
    not measured
    not mentioned
    nuclear medicine
nm   nanometer
    nutmeg (*nux moschata*)
NMA   neurogenic muscular atrophy
NMP   normal menstrual period
NMR   nuclear magnetic resonance
N:N   (indicates presence of) the
      azo group
nn   nerves
NND   neonatal death
    New and Nonofficial Drugs
NNI   noise and number index
NNM   Nicolle-Novy-MacNeal
      (medium)
NO   none obtained
No   number
noc   night
noct   at night (*nocte*)
non-REM   nonrapid eye movement
non rep   do not repeat (*non
      repetatur*)
NOS   not otherwise specified
NP   nasopharyngeal
    nasopharynx
    neuropathology
    neuropsychiatric
    normal plasma
    not performed
    nucleoplasmic index
    nucleoprotein

NP (continued)
    nursing procedure
NPA   near point of accommodation
NPB   nodal premature beat
NPC   near point of convergence
NPD   Niemann-Pick disease
NPDL   nodular, poorly
          differentiated lymphocytes
NPH   neutral protamine Hagedorn
          (insulin)
NPN   nonprotein nitrogen
NPO, npo   nothing by mouth
          (*nulla per os*)
NPO/HS   nothing by mouth at
          bedtime (*nulla per os*
          hora somni)
NPT   neoprecipitin test
    nocturnal penile tumescence
NPU   net protein utilization
NR   do not repeat (*non repetatur*)
    no radiation
    no response
    nonreactive
    normal
    not readable
    not recorded
    not resolved
nr   do not repeat (*non repetatur*)
NRBC   nucleated red blood cell
NRC   National Radiological
        Commission
    National Research Council
    normal retinal
        correspondence
NRD   nonrenal death
NREM   nonrapid eye movement
NRPB   National Radiological
        Protection Board
NRS   normal rabbit serum
    normal reference serum
NS   nephrotic syndrome
    nervous system
    neurologic survey
    neurosurgery
    nonspecific
    nonsymptomatic
    normal saline
    no sample
    no specimen
    not significant
    not sufficient
N/S   normal saline

NSA   no serious abnormality
    no significant abnormality
NSAID   non-steroidal anti-
        inflammatory drug
NSC   no significant change
    not service-connected
NSCD   nonservice-connected
        disability
NSCLC   non-small cell lung
        carcinoma
NSD   nominal single dose
    normal spontaneous delivery
    no significant defect
    no significant deviation
    no significant difference
    no significant disease
NSE   neuron-specific enolase
nsg   nursing
NSM   neurosecretory material
NSND   nonsymptomatic,
        nondisabling
NSQ   not sufficient quantity
NSR   normal sinus rhythm
NSS   normal saline solution
    not statistically significant
NSU   nonspecific urethritis
NT   nasotracheal
    neutralization test
    neutralizing
    nontypable
    not tested
NTAB   nephrotoxic antibody
NTG   nontoxic goiter
NTN   nephrotoxic nephritis
NTP   normal temperature and
        pressure
NUD   non-ulcer dyspepsia
NUG   necrotizing ulcerative
        gingivitis
NV   negative variation
N & V   nausea and vomiting
Nv   naked vision
NVA   near visual acuity
NVD   nausea, vomiting, and
        diarrhea
    Newcastle virus disease
NWB   no weight bearing
NYD   not yet diagnosed
NZB   New Zealand black mouse
NZW   New Zealand white mouse
O   eye (*oculus*)
    none

O (continued)
    obstetrics
    opening
    oral
    orderly
    oxygen
    respirations (anesthesia chart)
    suture size (zero)
O nonmotile organism
O_2 both eyes
    oxygen
o pint (*octarius*)
o- ortho-
OA occipital artery
    osteoarthritis
    oxalic acid
OAAD ovarian ascorbic acid
       depletion
OAD obstructive airway disease
OAF osteoclast-activating factor
OAP osteoarthropathy
OAR other administrative reasons
OAV oculoauriculovertebral
       dysplasia
OB objective benefit
    obstetrics
O & B opium and belladonna
OBG or
OB-GYN obstetrics and gynecology
obl oblique
OBS obstetrical service
    organic brain syndrome
obs or
obst obstetrics
OC occlusocervical
    office call
    on call
    oral contraceptive
    original claim
O_2cap oxygen capacity
occ occasional
OCG oral cholecystogram
OCR optical character recognition
OCT ornithine carbamyl transferase
OCV ordinary conversational voice
OD once a day
    optical density
    outside diameter
    overdose
    right eye (*oculus dexter*)
ODA occipitodextra anterior
ODD oculodentodigital dysplasia

ODN ophthalmodynamometry
ODP occipitodextra posterior
ODT occipitodextra transversa
O & E observation and examination
OER oxygen enhancement ratio
OF Ovenstone factor
Off official
OFC occipitofrontal circumference
OFD oral-facial digital
OG or
O & G obstetrics and gynecology
OGS oxogenic steroid
OGTT oral glucose tolerance test
OH hydroxycorticosteroids
    occupational history
OHC outer hair cell
OHCS hydroxycorticosteroid
OHP oxygen under high pressure
OI osteogenesis imperfecta
OIF oil immersion field
OIH orthoiodohippurate
OJ orange juice
OKN optokinetic nystagmus
OL left eye (*oculus laevus*)
ol oil
ol res oleoresin
OLA occipitolaeva anterior
OLH ovine lactogenic hormone
OLP occipitolaeva posterior
OL & T owners, landlords, and
       tenants
OM otitis media
om every morning (*omni mane*)
OMD ocular muscular dystrophy
OMI old myocardial infarction
omn bih every two hours (*omni
       bihora*)
omn hor every hour (*omni hora*)
OMPA octamethyl-
       pyrophosphoramide
    otitis media, purulent, acute
ON,
On or
on every night (*omni nocte*)
OOB out of bed
OP opening pressure
    operation
    osmotic pressure
    outpatient
O & P ova and parasites
OPC outpatient clinic
OPD outpatient department

OPG   oxypolygelatin
oph or
ophth   ophthalmology
OPK   optokinetic
OPS   outpatient service
OPT   outpatient
         outpatient treatment
OPV   oral poliovaccine
         oral poliovirus vaccine
OR   operating room
ORF   open reading frame
ORS   orthopedic surgery
orth or
ortho   orthopedics
OS   left eye (*oculus sinister*)
       opening snap
       oral surgery
os   mouth (*os*)
OSA   obstructive sleep apnea
OSM   oxygen saturation meter
OST   object sorting test
OT   occlusion time
       occupational therapy
       old term
       old terminology
       old tuberculin
       orotracheal
       otolaryngology
OTC   ornithine transcarbamylase
         over-the-counter
         oxytetracycline
OTD   organ tolerance dose
oto   otolaryngology
       otology
otol   otology
otolar   otolaryngology
OTR   Ovarian Tumor Registry
OU   both eyes (*oculi unitas*)
       each eye (*oculus uterque*)
OURQ   outer upper right quadrant
OV   office visit
ov   egg (*ovum*)
OW   out of wedlock
O/W   oil in water
         oil-water ratio
OWS   overwear syndrome
ox   oxymel
oz   ounce
P   by weight (*pondere*)
     near (*proxium*)
     partial pressure
     pharmacopeia

P (continued)
     phosphorus
     position
     postpartum
     premolar
     presbyopia
     pressure
     primipara
     properdin
     protein
     psychiatry
     pulse
     pupil
P.   *Pasteurella*
         Plasmodium
         Proteus
P_1 parental generation
P_2 pulmonic second sound
^{32}P radioactive phosphorus
p   after (*post*)
     handful (*pugillus*)
     probability
p-   para-
PA   paralysis agitans
       pathology
       pernicious anemia
       phakic-aphakic
       posteroanterior
       primary amenorrhea
       primary anemia
       pulmonary artery
       pulpoaxial
P & A   percussion & auscultation
pa   yearly (*per annum*)
PAB or
PABA   para-aminobenzoic acid
PAC   premature auricular
         contraction
p ae   in equal parts (*partes aequales*)
PAF   platelet-activating factor
         pulmonary arteriovenous
         fistula
PAFIB   paroxysmal atrial fibrillation
PAGMK   primary African green
         monkey kidney
PAH   para-aminohippurate
         polycyclic aromatic
         hydrocarbon
         pulmonary artery
         hypertension
PAHA   para-aminohippuric acid
PAIDS   pediatric AIDS

PAL   posterior axillary line
PAM   crystalline penicillin G in 2
         per cent aluminum
         monostearate
       phenylalanine mustard
       pralidoxime
       pulmonary alveolar
         macrophage(s)
       pulmonary alveolar
         microlithiasis
       pyridine aldoxime methiodide
PAN   periarteritis nodosa
       periodic alternating
         nystagmus
       peroxyacetyl nitrate
       polyarteritis nodosa
PANS   puromycin aminonucleoside
PAO   peak acid output
PAOD   peripheral arterial occlusive
         disease
       peripheral arteriosclerotic
         occlusive disease
PAP   Papanicolaou (stain, smear,
         test)
       positive airway pressure
       primary atypical pneumonia
       prostatic acid phosphatase
       pulmonary alveolar
         proteinosis
       pulmonary artery pressure
PAPP   para-aminopropiophenone
PAPS   phosphoadenosyl-
         phosphosulfate
PAPVC partial anomalous
         pulmonary venous
         connection
PAR   postanesthesia room
       pulmonary arteriolar
         resistance
para   number of pregnancies
par aff   the part affected (*pars
         affecta*)
PAS   para-aminosalicylic acid
       periodic acid–Schiff (method,
         stain, technique, test)
       peripheral anterior synechia
       pulmonary artery stenosis
PASA   para-aminosalicylic acid
PAS-C para-aminosalicylic acid
         crystallized with ascorbic
         acid
PASD   after diastase digestion

PASM   periodic acid-silver
         methenamine
PAST   periodic acid-Schiff
         technique
Past.   *Pasteurella*
PAT   paroxysmal atrial tachycardia
       prism adaptation test
path   pathology
PB   phenobarbital
       phonetically balanced
PBA   pulpobuccoaxial
PBC   prebed care
       primary biliary cirrhosis
PBF   pulmonary blood flow
PBG   porphobilinogen
PBI   protein-bound iodine
PBL   peripheral blood lymphocytes
PBN   paralytic brachial neuritis
PBO   penicillin in beeswax
       placebo
PBS   phosphate-buffered saline
PBSP   prognostically bad signs
         during pregnancy
PBT_4 protein-bound thyroxine
PBV   predicted blood volume
       pulmonary blood volume
PBZ   pyribenzamine
PC   pentose cycle
       phosphate cycle
       phosphocreatine
       platelet concentrate
       platelet count
       portacaval
       pubococcygeus
       pulmonic closure
pc   after meals (*post cibum*)
       avoirdupois weight (*pondus
         civile*)
       picocurie
PCA   passive cutaneous
         anaphylaxis
PCB   paracervical block
PcB   near point of convergence
PCc   periscopic concave
PCD   phosphate-citrate-dextrose
       polycystic disease
       posterior corneal deposits
PCE   pseudocholinesterase
PCF   posterior cranial fossa
PCG   phonocardiogram
PCH   paroxysmal cold
         hemoglobinuria

PCI   pneumatosis cystoides
          intestinalis
pCi   picocurie
PCM   protein-calorie malnutrition
PCN   penicillin
PCNA   proliferating cell nuclear
          antigen
PCO_2 or
pCO_2 carbon dioxide pressure
PCP   parachlorophenate
          phencyclidine
          Pneumocystis carinii
          pneumonia
PCPA   parachlorophenylalanine
pcpt   perception
PCR   polymerase chain reaction
PCS   portacaval shunt
pcs   preconscious
PCT   plasmacrit
          porphyria cutanea tarda
          portacaval transposition
PCV   packed cell volume
          polycythemia vera
PCV-M   myeloid metaplasia with
          polycythemia vera
PCx   periscopic convex
PD   papilla diameter
          Parkinson's disease
          patent ductus
          pediatrics
          phosphate dehydrogenase
          plasma defect
          poorly differentiated
          potential difference
          pressor dose
          prism diopter
          progression of disease
          psychotic depression
          pulmonary disease
          pulpodistal
          pupillary distance
PDA   patent ductus arteriosus
          pediatric allergy
PDAB   para-dimethyl-
          aminobenzaldehyde
PDC   pediatric cardiology
PDD   pyridoxine-deficient diet
PDGF   platelet-derived growth
          factor
PDH   packaged disaster hospital
          phosphate dehydrogenase
pdl   pudendal

PDP   piperidino-pyrimidine
PDR   Physician's Desk Reference
          proliferative diabetic
          retinopathy
PE   pharyngoesophageal
          phenylephrine
          physical evaluation
          physical examination
          pleural effusion
          polyethylene
          probable error
          pulmonary edema
          pulmonary embolism
PEBG   phenethylbiguanide
ped or
peds   pediatrics
PEEP   positive end-expiratory
          pressure
PEF   peak expiratory flow
PEFR   peak expiratory flow rate
PEG   pneumoencephalography
          polyethylene glycol
PEI   phosphate excretion index
          physical efficiency index
pen   penicillin
pent   pentothal
PEO   progressive external
          ophthalmoplegia
PEP   pre-ejection period
PEPP   positive expiratory pressure
          plateau
PER   protein efficiency ratio
PERLA   pupils equal, react to light
          and accommodation
perpad   perineal pad
PERRLA   pupils equal, round,
          regular, react to light
          and accommodation
PET   positron emission tomography
          pre-eclamptic toxemia
PETN   pentaerythritol tetranitrate
PETT   positron emission transverse
          tomography
PF   personality factor
          picture-frustration (study)
          platelet factor
P/F   pass-fail system
PFC   plaque-forming cell
PFGE   pulsed field gradient gel
          electrophoresis
PFIB   perfluoroisobutylene
PFK   phosphofructokinase

PFO   patent foramen ovale
PFQ   personality factor
        questionnaire
PFR   peak flow rate
PFS   primary fibromyalgia
        syndrome
PFT   posterior fossa tumor
        pulmonary function test
PFU   plaque-forming units
PG   plasma triglyceride
        postgraduate
        pregnant
        prostaglandin
        pyoderma gangrenosum
pg   picogram
PGA   pteroylglutamic acid
PGC   pontine gaze center
PGD   phosphogluconate
        dehydrogenase
        phosphoglyceraldehyde
        dehydrogenase
PGDH phosphogluconate
        dehydrogenase
PGDR plasma-glucose
        disappearance rate
PGH   pituitary growth hormone
PGI   phosphoglucoisomerase
        potassium, glucose, and insulin
PGK   phosphoglycerate kinase
PGL   persistent generalized
        lymphadenopathy
PGM   phosphoglucomutase
        phosphoglycerate mutase
PGP   postgamma proteinuria
PGTR plasma glucose tolerance
        rate
PH   past history
        personal history
        pharmacopeia
        prostatic hypertrophy
        public health
        pulmonary hypertension
Ph   phenyl
pH   hydrogen ion concentration
PHA   phytohemagglutinin
phar or
pharm   pharmacy
PHBB propylhydroxybenzyl
        benzimidazole
PHC   posthospital care
PHI   phosphohexoisomerase
PHK   platelet phosphohexokinase

PHLA postheparin lipolytic activity
PHM   posterior hyaloid membrane
PHP   primary hyperparathyroidism
        pseudohypoparathyroidism
phys physiology
PI   pacing impulse
        performance intensity
        peripheral iridectomy
        pre-induction (examination)
        present illness
        protamine insulin
        pulmonary incompetence
        pulmonary infarction
PIA   plasma insulin activity
PICA posterior inferior cerebellar
        artery
PICU pulmonary intensive care
        unit
PID   pelvic-inflammatory disease
        plasma-iron disappearance
PIDT plasma-iron disappearance
        time
PIE   pulmonary infiltration and
        eosinophilia
        pulmonary interstitial
        emphysema
PIF   peak inspiratory flow
        prolactin-inhibiting factor
PIFR peak inspiratory flow rate
PII   plasma inorganic iodine
pil   pill
PIP   proximal interphalangeal
PIPJ proximal interphalangeal joint
PIT   plasma iron transport rate
        plasma iron turnover
PITR plasma iron turnover rate
pixel picture element
PK   Prausnitz-Küstner (reaction)
        psychokinesis
        pyruvate kinase
PKP   penetrating keratoplasty
PKU   phenylketonuria
PKV   killed poliomyelitis vaccine
PL   light perception
        phospholipid
        placebo
        placental lactogen
        pulpolingual
PLA   pulpolinguoaxial
        pulpolabial
PLD   platelet defect
PLS   prostaglandin-like substance

pls please
PLT primed, lymphocyte typing
PLV live poliomyelitis vaccine
　　panleukopenia virus
　　phenylalanine-lysine-
　　　vasopressin
PM after noon
　　night
　　physical medicine
　　polymorphs
　　postmortem
　　pulpomesial
PMA phorbol myristate acetate
　　prevalence of gingivitis
　　　(papillary, marginal,
　　　attached)
　　progressive muscular atrophy
PMB para-hydroxymercuribenzoate
　　polymorphonuclear basophil
PMC pseudomembranous
　　　enterocolitis
PMD primary myocardial disease
　　progressive muscular
　　　dystrophy
PME polymorphonuclear
　　　eosinophil
PMH past medical history
PMI point of maximal impulse
　　point of maximal intensity
PML polymorphous light eruption
　　progressive multifocal
　　　leukoencephalopathy
PMN polymorphonuclear
　　　neutrophil
PMP past menstrual period
　　previous menstrual period
PMR perinatal mortality rate
　　physical medicine and
　　　rehabilitation
　　polymyalgia rheumatica
　　proportionate morbidity ratio
PMS phenazine methosulfate
　　postmitochondrial
　　　supernatant
　　pregnant mare serum
　　premenstrual syndrome
PMSG pregnant mare serum
　　　gonadotropin
PMT Porteus maze test
PMV prolapse of mitral valve
PN perceived noise
　　percussion note

PN (continued)
　　periarteritis nodosa
　　peripheral neuropathy
　　pneumonia
　　positional nystagmus
　　pyelonephritis
P_{NA} plasma sodium
PND paroxysmal nocturnal
　　　dyspnea
　　postnasal drainage
　　postnasal drip
pnd pound
PNH paroxysmal nocturnal
　　　hemoglobinuria
PNI Prognostic Nutritional Index
　　psychoneuroimmunology
PNP para-nitrophenol
　　purine nucleoside
　　　phosphorylase
PNPP para-nitrophenylphosphate
PNS partial nonprogressing stroke
　　peripheral nervous system
PNU protein nitrogen unit
PO by mouth (*per os*)
　　parieto-occipital
　　period of onset
　　phone order
　　posterior
　　postoperative
po by mouth (*per os*)
PO_2 or
pO_2 oxygen partial pressure
　　　(tension)
POA point of application
POB phenoxybenzamine
　　place of birth
POC postoperative care
pocul cup (*poculum*)
POD place of death
　　postoperative day
PODx preoperative diagnosis
pOH hydroxyl concentration
poik poikilocyte
polio poliomyelitis
poly polymorphonuclear leukocyte
POMC pro-opiomelanocortin
POMP prednisone, Oncovin,
　　　methotrexate, 6-
　　　mercaptopurine
POP plasma oncotic pressure
POPOP 1,4-bis-(5-phenox-
　　　azole)-benzene

pos   positive
pos pr   positive pressure
poss   possible
post   posterior
        postmortem
postop   postoperative
pot   potassa
        portion
PP   near point (*punctum
        proximum*) of
        accommodation
        partial pressure
        pellagra preventive
        permanent partial
        pink puffers (emphysema)
        pinpoint
        postpartum
        postprandial
        private practice
        prothrombin-proconvertin
        protoporphyrin
        proximal phalanx
        pulse pressure
        pyrophosphate
PPA   phenylpyruvic acid
PPA,
Ppa or
ppa   first shake well (*phiala prius
        agitata*)
PPB   platelet-poor blood
        positive-pressure breathing
ppb   parts per billion
PPBS   postprandial blood sugar
PPC   progressive patient care
PPD   paraphenylenediamine
        phenyldiphenyloxadiazole
        purified protein derivative
PPD-S   purified protein derivative-
        standard
ppg   picopicogram
PPH   primary pulmonary
        hypertension
        protocollagen proline
        hydroxylase
        postpartum hemorrhage
PPHP   pseudopseudo-
        hypoparathyroidism
PPLO   pleuropneumonia-like
        organism
ppm   parts per million
PPNG   penicillinase-producing
        Neisseria gonorrhoeae

PPP   pentose phosphate pathway
PPPI   primary private practice
        income
PPR   Price precipitation reaction
PPS   postpump syndrome
PPT   plant protease test
Ppt or
ppt   precipitate
PPTT   prepubertal testicular tumor
PPV   positive-pressure ventilation
PQ   permeability quotient
        pyrimethamine-quinine
PR   far point (*punctum remotum*)
        partial remission
        peer review
        peripheral resistance
        pregnancy rate
        production rate
        professional relations
        protein
        public relations
        pulse rate
Pr   presbyopia
        prism
pr or
Pr   far point (*punctum remotum*)
pr   through the rectum (*per rectum*)
PRA   plasma renin activity
PRBV   placental residual blood
        volume
PRC   packed red cells
PRCA   pure red cell agenesis
PRD   partial reaction of
        degeneration
        postradiation dysplasia
pre   preliminary
preg   pregnant
preop   preoperative
prep   prepare
PRFM   prolonged rupture of fetal
        membranes
PRI   phosphoribose isomerase
primip   woman bearing first child
PRIST   paperradioimmunosorbent
PRL   prolactin
PRM   phosphoribomutase
        preventive medicine
prn   as the occasion arises (*pro
        renata*)
pro   prothrombin
proct   proctology
prog   prognosis

PROM   premature rupture of
        membranes
        prolonged rupture of
        membranes
prot   protein
prox   proximal
PRP   panretinal photocoagulation
        pityriasis rubra pilaris
        platelet-rich plasma
        progesterone receptor proteins
        Psychotic Reaction Profile
PRPP   phosphoribosyl-
        pyrophosphate
PRRE   pupils round, regular, and
        equal
PRT   phosphoribosyltransferase
PRU   peripheral resistance unit
PS   performing scale (IQ)
      periodic syndrome
      physical status
      plastic surgery
      population sample
      Porter-Silber (chromogen)
      prescription
      psychiatric
      pulmonary stenosis
      pyloric stenosis
Ps.   *Pseudomonas*
P/S   polyunsaturated to saturated
      fatty acids ratio
ps   per second
PSA   apply to the affected region
      polyethylene sulfonic acid
PSC   Porter-Silber chromogen
      posterior subcapsular cataract
      primary sclerosing cholangitis
PSD   peptone-starch-dextrose
PSE   portal-systemic
      encephalopathy
PSG   peak systolic gradient
      presystolic gallop
PSGN   poststreptococcal
      glomerulonephritis
psi   pounds per square inch
PSP   periodic short pulse
      phenolsulfonphthalein
      positive spike pattern
      progressive supranuclear palsy
PSS   physiological saline solution
      progressive systemic sclerosis
PST   penicillin, streptomycin, and
      tetracycline

psy or
psych   psychiatry
      psychology
PT   parathyroid
      paroxysmal tachycardia
      permanent and total
      pharmacy and therapeutics
      physical therapy
      physical training
      pneumothorax
      prothrombin time
pt   patient
    pint
PTA   persistent truncus arteriosus
      phosphotungstic acid
      plasma thromboplastin
      antecedent
      post-traumatic amnesia
      prior to admission
      prior to arrival
PTAH   phosphotungstic acid
      hematoxylin
PTAV   percutaneous transluminal
      atrial valvuloplasty
PTB   patellar tendon bearing
      prior to birth
PTBD   percutaneous biliary
      drainage
PTC   percutaneous transhepatic
      cholangiography
      phenylthiocarbamide
      plasma thromboplastin
      component
PTCA   percutaneous transluminal
      coronary angioplasty
PTD   permanent and total disability
PTE   parathyroid extract
      pulmonary thromboembolism
PTED   pulmonary thromboembolic
      disease
PTH   parathormone
      parathyroid hormone
      post-transfusion hepatitis
PTHS   parathyroid hormone
      secretion (rate)
PTI   persistent tolerant infection
PTM   post-transfusion
      mononucleosis
PTMA   phenyltrimethylammonium
PTMV   percutaneous transluminal
      mitral valvuloplasty
PTP   post-tetanic potentiation

PTP (continued)
    prior to program
PTR   peripheral total resistance
PTRA percutaneous transluminal
    renal angioplasty
PTS   para-toluenesulfonic acid
PTT   partial thromboplastin time
    particle transport time
PTU   propylthiouracil
PTX   parathyroidectomy
PU   peptic ulcer
    pregnancy urine
PUD   pulmonary disease
PUE   pyrexia of unknown etiology
PUFA polyunsaturated fatty acid
pul   pulmonary
pulm gruel (*pulmentum*)
    pulmonary
pulv   powder (*pulvis*)
PUO   pyrexia of unknown origin
PV   peripheral vascular
    peripheral vein
    peripheral vessels
    plasma volume
    polycythemia vera
    portal vein
    postvoiding
    through the vagina (*per
    vaginam*)
P & V pyloroplasty and vagotomy
PVA   polyvinyl alcohol
PVC   polyvinyl chloride
    postvoiding cystogram
    premature ventricular
    contraction
    pulmonary venous congestion
PVD   peripheral vascular disease
PVE   prosthetic valve endocarditis
PVF   portal venous flow
PVM   pneumonia virus of mice
PVP   penicillin V potassium
    peripheral vein plasma
    polyvinylpyrrolidone
    portal venous pressure
PVR   peripheral vascular resistance
    pulmonary vascular resistance
PVS   premature ventricular systole
PVT   paroxysmal ventricular
    tachycardia
    portal vein thrombosis
pvt   private
PW   posterior wall

PWA   person with AIDS
PWB   partial weight-bearing
PWC   physical work capacity
PWI   posterior wall infarct
Px   physical examination
    pneumothorax
    prognosis
PXE   pseudoxanthoma elasticum
PZ   pancreozymin
PZA   pyrazinamide
PZ-CCK pancreozymin-
    cholecystokinin
PZI   protamine zinc insulin
Q   coulomb (electric quantity)
q   every (*quaque*)
    quart
qAM   every morning
QC   quinine-colchicine
qd   every day (*quaque die*)
qh   every hour (*quaque hora*)
q2h   every two hours
q3h   every three hours
q4h   every four hours
qhs   every hour of sleep
qid   four times a day (*quater in die*)
ql   as much as desired (*quantum
    libet*)
qm   every morning (*quaque mane*)
qn   every night (*quaque nocte*)
QNS   quantity not sufficient
qod   every other day
QO_2 or
qO_2 oxygen quotient
QP   quanti-Pirquet reaction
qp,
Qp or
QP   at will (*quantum placeat*)
qPM   every night
qq   each (*quaque*)
qqh   every four hours (*quaque
    quarta hora*)
qqhor   every hour (*quaque hora*)
QRZ   wheal reaction time
qs,
Qs or
QS   enough (*quantum satis*)
qsad   to a sufficient quantity
qsuff   as much as suffices (*quantum
    sufficit*)
qt   quiet
    quart
quant   quantity

quat four (*quattuor*)
QUICHA quantitative inhalation challenge apparatus
quint fifth (*quintus*)
quotid daily (*quotidie*)
qv as much as you like (*quantum vis*)
    which see (*quod vide*)
R Behnken's unit
    far point (*remotum*)
    organic radical
    radiology
    Rankine (scale)
    Réaumur (scale)
    rectal
    regression coefficient
    remote
    resistance
    respiration
    right
    Rinne test
    roentgen
    rough (colony)
    take (*recipe*)
R. *Rickettsia*
RA renal artery
    rheumatoid arthritis
    right arm
    right atrial
    right atrium
R_A airway resistance
RAD radiation absorbed dose
    right axis deviation
rad radial
    root (*radix*)
RADTS rabbit antidog thymus serum
RAE right atrial enlargement
RAF rheumatoid arthritis factor
RAH right atrial hypertrophy
RAI radioactive iodine
RAIU radioactive iodine uptake
RAMT rabbit antimouse thymocyte
RAO right anterior oblique
RAP rheumatoid arthritis precipitin
    right atrial pressure
RAR right arm recumbent
RARLS rabbit antirat lymphocyte serum
RAS renal artery stenosis
ras scrapings (*rasurae*)
RAST radioallergosorbent test

RATHAS rat thymus antiserum
RATx radiation therapy
RB rating board
RBA rose bengal antigen
RBB right bundle branch
RBBB right bundle branch block
RBC red blood cell
    red blood count
RBCM red blood cell mass
RBCV red blood cell volume
RBE relative biological effectiveness
RBF renal blood flow
RBL Reid's base line
RC red cell
    red cell casts
    retrograde cystogram
RCA right coronary artery
RCBV regional cerebral blood volume
RCC red cell count
RCD relative cardiac dullness
RCF red cell folate
    relative centrifugal force
RCM red cell mass
    right costal margin
RCR respiratory control ratio
RCS reticulum cell sarcoma
RCU respiratory care unit
RCV red cell volume
RD Raynaud's disease
    reaction of (to) degeneration
    resistance determinant
    respiratory disease
    retinal detachment
    right deltoid
rd rutherford
RDA recommended daily allowance
    recommended dietary allowance
    right dorsoanterior
RDDA recommended daily dietary allowance
RDE receptor-destroying enzyme
RDI rupture-delivery interval
RDP right dorsoposterior
RDS respiratory distress syndrome
RE radium emanation
    regional enteritis
    resting energy
    reticuloendothelial
    right eye

R & E   research and education
rec   fresh (*recens*)
rect   rectified
REE   resting energy expenditure
REF   renal erythropoietic factor
REG   radioencephalogram
rehab   rehabilitation
REM   rapid eye movement
        roentgen-equivalent–man
rem   removal
REMP   roentgen-equivalent–man
        period
REP   roentgen equivalent–physical
rep or
rept   let it be repeated (*repetatur*)
RER   rough endoplasmic reticulum
res   research
RES   reticuloendothelial system
resp   respectively
        respiratory
retic   reticulocyte
RF   radio frequency
        Reitland-Franklin (unit)
        relative fluorescence
        releasing factor
        rheumatic fever
        rheumatoid factor
        root canal, filling of
RFA   right femoral artery
        right frontoanterior
RFB   retained foreign body
RFLA   rheumatoid factor-like
        activity
RFLP   restriction fragment length
        polymorphism
RFP   right frontoposterior
RFS   renal function study
RFT   right frontotransverse
        rod-and-frame test
RFW   rapid filling wave
RG   right gluteal
RH   reactive hyperemia
        relative humidity
Rh   Rhesus (factor)
rh   rheumatic
RHBF   reactive hyperemia blood
        flow
RHD   relative hepatic dullness
        rheumatic heart disease
rheum   rheumatic
RHL   right hepatic lobe
RHLN   right hilar lymph node

rhm   roentgen (per) hour (at one)
        meter
Rh neg   Rhesus factor negative
Rh pos   Rhesus factor positive
RI   refractive index
        regional ileitis
        respiratory illness
RIA   radioimmunoassay
RIF   right iliac fossa
RIFA   radioiodinated fatty acid
RIHSA   radioactive iodinated
        human serum albumin
RIND   reversible ischemic
        neurologic disability
RIP   radioimmunoprecipitation
RISA   radioactive iodinated serum
        albumin
RIST   radioimmunosorbent test
RITC   rhodamine isothiocyanate
RIU   radioactive iodine uptake
RK   rabbit kidney
        radial keratotomy
        right kidney
RKY   roentgen kymography
RL   right leg
        right lung
R-L, R→L   right-to-left
RLC   residual lung capacity
RLD   related living donor
RLF   retrolental fibroplasia
RLL   right lower lobe
RLN   recurrent laryngeal nerve
RLP   radiation-leukemia-protection
RLQ   right lower quadrant
RLS   Ringer's lactate solution
RM   radical mastectomy
        respiratory movement
RMA   right mentoanterior
RMK   rhesus monkey kidney
RML   right middle lobe
RMP   rapidly miscible pool
        right mentoposterior
RMS   root-mean-square
RMSF   Rocky Mountain spotted
        fever
RMT   retromolar trigone
        right mentotransverse
RMV   respiratory minute volume
RNA   ribonucleic acid
RNase   ribonuclease
RND   radical neck dissection
RNP   ribonucleoprotein

RO   Ritter-Oleson (technique)
      rule out
ROA   right occipitoanterior
roent roentgenology
ROH   rat ovarian hyperemia (test)
ROM   range of motion
      rupture of membranes
ROP   right occipitoposterior
ROS   review of systems
ROT   right occipitotransverse
rot   rotating
RP   reactive protein
      refractory period
      rest pain
      resting pressure
      retinitis pigmentosa
      retrograde pyelogram
Rp   pulmonary resistance
RPA   right pulmonary artery
RPCF Reiter protein complement-
      fixation
RPCFT Reiter protein
      complement-fixation test
RPE   retinal pigment epithelium
RPF   renal plasma flow
RPG   retrograde pyelogram
RPGN rapidly progressive
      glomerulonephritis
RPM   rapid processing mode
rpm   revolutions per minute
RPO   right posterior oblique
RPR   rapid plasma reagin
RPR-CT rapid plasma reagin circle
      card test
RPS   renal pressor substance
RPV   right pulmonary veins
RQ   respiratory quotient
RR   radiation response
      recovery room
      renin release
      respiratory rate
      response rate
R & R rest and recuperation
RRA   radioreceptor assay
RR & E round, regular, and equal
RR-HPO rapid recompression – high
      pressure oxygen
RRP   relative refractory period
RRR   renin-release rate
RS   rating schedule
      respiratory syncytial
      right side

RSA   relative specific activity
      right sacroanterior
RSB   right sternal border
RSC   rested-state contraction
RScA right scapuloanterior
RScP right scapuloposterior
RSP   right sacroposterior
RSR   regular sinus rhythm
RST   radiosensitivity test
      right sacrotransverse
RSTL relaxed skin tension lines
RSV   respiratory syncytial virus
      right subclavian vein
      Rous sarcoma virus
RT   radiation therapy
      radiotherapy
      radium therapy
      reaction time
      reading test
      recreational therapy
      right thigh
      room temperature
rt   right
RTA   renal tubular acidosis
RTD   routine test dilution
rtd   retarded
RTF   replication and transfer
      resistance transfer factor
      respiratory tract fluid
rt lat right lateral
rtn   return
RU   rat unit
      resistance unit
      retrograde urogram
      right upper
      roentgen unit
rub   red (*ruber*)
RUL   right upper lobe
RUQ   right upper quadrant
RUR   resin-uptake ratio
RURTI recurrent upper respiratory
      tract infection
RV   rat virus
      residual volume
      respiratory volume
      right ventricle
      rubella virus
RVB   red venous blood
RVD   relative vertebral density
RVE   right ventricular enlargement
RVEDP right ventricular end-
      diastolic pressure

RVH   right ventricular hypertrophy
RVI   relative value index
RVP   red veterinary petrolatum
RVR   renal vascular resistance
          resistance to venous return
RVRA   renal vein renin activity
            renal venous renin assay
RVRC   renal vein renin
              concentration
RVS   Relative Value Schedule
          Relative Value Study
RVT   renal vein thrombosis
RW   ragweed
R_x prescription
          take (*recipe*)
          therapy
          treatment
S   half (*semis*)
    label (*signa*)
    left (*sinister*)
    sacral
    screen-containing cassette
    second
    single
    smooth (colony)
    soluble
    spherical lens
    subject
    supravergence
    surgery
    Svedberg unit of sedimentation
        coefficient
    write (*sigma*)
S.   *Salmonella*
        Schistosoma
        Spirillum
        Staphylococcus
        Streptococcus
s̄   without (*sine*)
SA   salicylic acid
        sarcoma
        secondary amenorrhea
        secondary anemia
        serum albumin
        sinoatrial
        slightly active
        specific activity
        Stokes-Adams
        surface area
        sustained action
        sympathetic activity

sa   according to art (*secundum
        artem*)
SAA   serum amyloid A component
SAB   significant asymptomatic
            bacteriuria
SACD   subacute combined
              degeneration
SAD   source to axis distance
SAG   Swiss agammaglobulinemia
SAH   subarachnoid hemorrhage
SAIDS   simian AIDS
sal   according to the rule of art
        (*secundum artis leges*)
        saline
SAM   sulfated acid
            mucopolysaccharide
SAP   serum alkaline phosphatase
          serum amyloid P component
          systemic arterial pressure
SAS   supravalvular aortic stenosis
SAT   Scholastic Aptitude Test
sat   saturated
SB   serum bilirubin
        single breath
        Stanford-Binet (test)
        sternal border
        stillbirth
SBE   subacute bacterial endocarditis
SBF   splanchnic blood flow
SBFT   small bowel follow-through
SBP   systemic blood pressure
          systolic blood pressure
SBS   social-breakdown syndrome
SBT   serum bacterial titer
          single-breath test
SBTI   soybean trypsin inhibitor
SC   closure of the semilunar valves
        sacrococcygeal
        self-care
        semicircular
        semiclosed
        service-connected
        sick call
        sickle cell
        single chemical
        special care
        sternoclavicular
        subcutaneous
        succinylcholine
        sugar-coated
SCAT   sheep cell agglutination test

scat   a box (*scatula*)
SCC   squamous cell carcinoma
SCD   service-connected disability
ScDA   scapulodextra anterior
ScDP   scapulodextra posterior
SCG   serum chemistry graft
SCH   succinylcholine
sched   schedule
schiz   schizophrenia
SCI   structured clinical interview
SCID   severe combined
           immunodeficiency
SCK   serum creatine kinase
ScLA   scapulolaeva anterior
SCLC   small cell lung cancer
           squamous cell, large cell
           (carcinoma)
ScLP   scapulolaeva posterior
scop   scopolamine
SCP   single-celled protein
SCPK   serum creatine
           phosphokinase
scr   scruple
SCT   sex chromatin test
           staphylococcal clumping test
SCUBA   self-contained underwater
           breathing apparatus
SD   septal defect
       serum defect
       skin dose
       spontaneous delivery
       standard deviation
       streptodornase
       sudden death
S/D   systolic to diastolic
SDA   sacrodextra anterior
           specific dynamic action
SDCL   symptom distress check list
SDH   serine dehydrase
           sorbitol dehydrogenase
           succinate dehydrogenase
SDM   standard deviation of the
           mean
SDO   sudden-dosage onset
SDP   sacrodextra posterior
SDS   Self-Rating Depression Scale
           sensory deprivation
               syndrome
           sodium dodecyl sulfate
           sudden death syndrome
SDT   sacrodextra transversa

SE   standard error
       Starr-Edwards (prosthesis)
se   himself, itself (*se*)
sec   second
SED   skin erythema dose
           spondyloepiphyseal dysplasia
sed   stool (*sedes*)
sed rate   sedimentation rate
SEE   Seeing Essential English
           standard error of the estimate
SEG   sonoencephalogram
seg   segmented (leukocyte)
SEGS   segmented neutrophils
SEM   scanning electron microscopy
           standard error of the mean
semi   half
semid   half a drachm (dram)
semih   half an hour
SEP   sensory evoked potential
           systolic ejection period
seq   sequela
           sequestrum
SER   smooth endoplasmic reticulum
           systolic ejection rate
serv   keep, preserve (*serva*)
SES   socioeconomic status
SET   systolic ejection time
sev   severe
           severed
SF   scarlet fever
       shell fragment
       shrapnel fragment
       spinal fluid
Sf   Svedberg flotation units
SFP   screen filtration pressure
           spinal fluid pressure
SFS   split function study
SFT   skinfold thickness
SFW   shell fragment wound
           shrapnel fragment wound
SG   serum globulin
       signs
       skin graft
       specific gravity
       surgeon general
S-G   Sachs-Georgi (test)
SGA   small for gestational age
s gl   without correction
SGOT   serum glutamic-oxaloacetic
               transaminase
SGP   serine glycerophosphatide

SGPT   serum glutamic-pyruvic
          transaminase
SGV   salivary gland virus
SH   serum hepatitis
       sex hormone
       sinus histiocytosis
       social history
       sulfhydryl
       surgical history
sh   shoulder
SHB   sulfhemoglobin
SHBD   serum hydroxybutyrate
            dehydrogenase
SHBG   sex hormone–binding
             globulin
SHG   synthetic human gastrin
SHO   secondary hypertrophic
            osteoarthropathy
SI   sacroiliac
      saturation index
      self-inflicted
      seriously ill
      serum iron
      soluble insulin
      stroke index
SIADH   syndrome of inappropriate
             antidiuretic hormone
SICD   serum isocitric dehydrogenase
SID   sudden infant death
SIDS   sudden infant death syndrome
sIg   secreted immunoglobulin
sig   let it be labeled (*signetur*)
      significant
SIJ   sacroiliac joint
simul   at the same time
sing   of each (*singuli*)
SISI   short-increment sensitivity
           index
SIW   self-inflicted wound
SJR   Shinawora-Jones-Reinhart
          (units)
SK   streptokinase
SKSD   streptokinase-streptodornase
SL   sensation level
      streptolysin
sl   according to law (*secundum
       legem*)
      slight
SLA   sacrolaeva anterior
SLD or
SLDH   serum lactic dehydrogenase
SLE   St. Louis encephalitis

SLE (continued)
        systemic lupus erythematosus
SLEV   St. Louis encephalitis virus
SLI   splenic localization index
SLKC   superior limbic
             keratoconjunctivitis
SLN   superior laryngeal nerve
SLO   streptolysin-O
SLP   sacrolaeva posterior
        sex-limited protein
SLR   straight leg raising
        Streptococcus lactis R
SLT   sacrolaeva transversa
SM   simple mastectomy
       skim milk
       streptomycin
       submucous
       suction method
       symptoms
       systolic mean
       systolic murmur
sm   small
SMA   superior mesenteric artery
          supplementary motor area
SMC   special monthly
            compensation
SMD   senile macular
            degeneration
SMO   slip made out
SMON   subacute myelo-optical
             neuropathy
SMP   slow-moving protease
        special monthly pension
SMR   somnolent metabolic rate
        standard mortality ratio
        submucous resection
SMRR   submucous resection and
             rhinoplasty
SN   serum-neutralizing
      suprasternal notch
sn   according to nature (*secundum
       naturam*)
SNB   scalene node biopsy
SNR   signal-to-noise ratio
SO   salpingo-oophorectomy
SOA-MCA   superficial occipital
                artery to middle
                cerebral artery
SOB   short(ness) of breath
SOC   sequential-type oral
            contraceptive
SOD   superoxide dismutase

SOL or Sol   solution
    space-occupying lesion
sol or
soln   solution
solv   dissolve (*solve*)
SOM   secretory otitis media
    serous otitis media
SOP   standard operating procedure
s op s   if necessary (*si opus sit*)
sos   if it is necessary (*si opus sit*)
SOTT   synthetic medium old
      tuberculin trichoracetic
      acid precipitated
SP   shunt procedure
    skin potential
    status post
    steady potential
    summating potential
    suprapubic
    symphysis pubis
    systolic pressure
sp   species
    spirit (*spiritus*)
SPA   suprapubic aspiration
SPAI   steroid protein activity index
SPBI   serum protein-bound iodine
SPCA   serum prothrombin
      conversion accelerator
SPE   serum protein electrophoresis
SPECT   single photon emission
      computed tomography
SPEP   serum protein electrophoresis
SPF   specific pathogen-free
    split products of fibrin
sp gr   specific gravity
SPH   secondary pulmonary
      hemosiderosis
sph   spherical
    spherical lens
SPI   serum precipitable iodine
spir   spirit (*spiritus*)
SPL   sound pressure level
    spontaneous lesion
spont   spontaneous (delivery)
SPP   suprapubic prostatectomy
spt   spirit
SPTI   systolic pressure-time index
SQ   social quotient
    subcutaneous
sq   square
SR   sarcoplasmic reticulum
    secretion rate

SR (continued)
    sedimentation rate
    sensitization response
    service record
    sigma reaction
    sinus rhythm
    skin resistance
    superior rectus
    systemic resistance
    system review
    systems research
SRBC   sheep red blood cells
SRC   sedimented red cells
    sheep red cells
SRF   somatotropin-releasing factor
    split renal function
    subretinal fluid
SRFS   split renal function study
SRIF   somatotropin release-
      inhibiting factor
SRNA   soluble ribonucleic acid
SRP   short rib polydactyly
SRR   slow rotation room
SRS   slow-reacting substance
SRS-A   slow-reacting substance of
      anaphylaxis
SRT   speech reception test
    speech reception threshold
SS   saturated solution
    side-to-side
    signs and symptoms
    Sjögren's syndrome
    soapsuds
    statistically significant
    subaortic stenosis
    sum of squares
    supersaturated
ss   one-half (*semis*)
SSA   salicylsalicylic acid
    skin-sensitizing antibody
    sulfosalicylic acid (test)
SSc   systemic sclerosis
SSD   source to skin distance
    sum of square deviations
SSE   soapsuds enema
SSKI   saturated solution of
      potassium iodide
SSN   severely subnormal
SSP   Sanarelli-Shwartzman
      phenomenon
    subacute sclerosing
      panencephalitis

SSPE subacute sclerosing panencephalitis
SSS specific soluble substance
sss layer upon layer (*stratum super stratum*)
SSSS staphylococcal scalded skin syndrome
SSU sterile supply unit
SSV under a poison label (*sub signo veneni*)
ST esotropia
sternothyroid
subtalar
subtotal
surface tension
st let it stand (*stet*)
stage (of disease)
straight
STA serum thrombotic accelerator
standard tube agglutination
STA-MCA superficial temporal artery to middle cerebral artery
stab stab nuclear neutrophil
staph staphylococcus
stat German unit of radium emanation
immediately (*statim*)
STC soft tissue calcification
STD sexually transmitted disease
skin test dose
skin to tumor distance
std saturated
standard
STH somatotropic hormone
STK streptokinase
STM streptomycin
STP scientifically treated petroleum
standard temperature and pressure
STPD standard temperature and pressure, dry (0°C, 760 mm Hg)
str or
strep streptococcus
STS serologic test for syphilis
standard test for syphilis
STSG split thickness skin graft
STT serial thrombin time
STU skin test unit
STVA subtotal villose atrophy
SU sensation unit

su let the person take (*sumat*)
SUA serum uric acid
single umbilical artery
subcu,
subcut or
subq subcutaneous
SUD sudden unexpected death
sudden unexplained death
SUID sudden unexplained infant death
sum let the person take (*sumat*)
SUN serum urea nitrogen
sup superficial
superior
surg surgery
SUS stained urinary sediment
SUUD sudden unexpected, unexplained death
SV severe
simian virus
snake venom
stroke volume
subclavian vein
supravital
sv alcoholic spirit (*spiritus vini*)
SVAS supravalvular aortic stenosis
SVC slow vital capacity
superior vena cava
SVCG spatial vectorcardiogram
SVD spontaneous vaginal delivery
spontaneous vertex delivery
SVI stroke volume index
SVM syncytiovascular membrane
SVR systemic vascular resistance
svr rectified spirit of wine (*spiritus vini rectificatus*)
svt proof spirit (*spiritus vini tenuis*)
SW spiral wound
stroke work
SWI stroke work index
Sx signs
symptoms
sym symmetrical
symptoms
symp symptoms
syr syrup
Sz schizophrenia
T temperature
tension (intraocular)
thoracic
thorax

T (continued)
  time
  tumor
T. *Taenia*
   Treponema
   Trichophyton
   Trypanosoma
t temporal
  three times (*ter*)
  tertiary
  test of significance
T+ increased tension
T− decreased tension
T½ half-life
T_3 triiodothyronine
T_4 thyroxine
TA alkaline tuberculin
  therapeutic abortion
  titratable acid
  toxin-antitoxin
T & A tonsillectomy &
    adenoidectomy
TA-AB teichoic acid antibody
TA-AIDS transfusion associated
    AIDS
TAB typhoid, paratyphoid A, and
    paratyphoid B
tab tablet
TACE chlorotrianisene
TAD thoracic asphyxiant dystrophy
TADAC therapeutic abortion,
    dilation, aspiration,
    curettage
TAF albumose-free tuberculin
  toxoid-antitoxin floccules
  trypsin-aldehyde-fuchsin
TAH total abdominal hysterectomy
TAL tendo Achillis lengthening
  thymic alymphoplasia
tal of such (*talis*)
TAM toxoid-antitoxin mixture
TAME toluene-sulfo-trypsin
    arginine methyl ester
TAMI thrombolysis and
    angioplasty in myocardial
    infarction (trial)
TAO thromboangiitis obliterans
  triacetyloleandomycin
TAP tension by applanation
TAPVD total anomalous
    pulmonary venous
    drainage

TAR thrombocytopenia with
    absence of the radius
TAT tetanus antitoxin
  thematic apperception test
  thromboplastin activation test
  total antitryptic activity
  toxin-antitoxin
  turn-around time
  tyrosine aminotransferase
TB toluidine blue
  total base
  total body
  tracheobronchitis
  tubercle bacillus
  tuberculosis
TBA tertiary butylacetate
  testosterone-binding affinity
  thiobarbituric acid
TBC tuberculosis
TBD total body density
TBF total body fat
TBG thyroxine-binding globulin
TBGP total blood granulocyte pool
TBI thyroxine-binding index
  total body irradiation
TBK total body potassium
TBM tuberculous meningitis
TBN bacillus emulsions
TBP thyroxine-binding protein
TBPA thyroxine-binding
    prealbumin
TB-RD tuberculosis-respiratory
    disease
TBS total body solute
  tribromosalicylanilide
  triethanolamine-buffered
    saline
Tbsp tablespoonful
TBT tolbutamide test
  tracheobronchial toilet
TBV total blood volume
TBW total body water
  total body weight
TBX whole body irradiation
TC taurocholate
  temperature compensation
  tetracycline
  tissue culture
  to contain
  total capacity
  total cholesterol
  transhepatic cholangiography

TC (continued)
    tubocurarine
TC2   transcobalamin 2
Tc   technetium
TCA   tricarboxylic acid
    trichloroacetate
    trichloroacetic acid
TCAP   trimethylcetylammonium
      pentachlorophenate
TCC   trichlorocarbanilide
TCD   tissue culture dose
TCD_{50} median tissue culture dose
TCE   trichloroethylene
TCF   total coronary flow
TCGF   T-cell growth factor
TCH   total circulating hemoglobin
TCI   to come in
    transient cerebral ischemia
TCID   tissue culture infective dose
$TCID_{50}$ median tissue culture
      infective dose
TCIE   transient cerebral ischemic
      episode
TCM   tissue culture medium
TCP   therapeutic continuous
      penicillin
TCPA   tetrachlorophthalic
      anhydride
TcR   T-cell receptor
TCSA   tetrachlorosalicylanilide
TCT   thrombin-clotting time
    thyrocalcitonin
TD   tetanus-diphtheria
    therapy discontinued
    thoracic duct
    three times a day
    threshold of discomfort
    thymus-dependent
    time disintegration
    to deliver
    tone decay
    torsion dystonia
    total disability
    transverse diameter
    treatment discontinued
TDF   thoracic duct fistula
    thoracic duct flow
TDI   toluene-diisocyanate
    total-dose infusion
TDL   thoracic duct lymph
TDP   thoracic duct pressure
    thymidine diphosphate

TDS or
tds   three times a day (*ter die
      sumendum*)
TDT   tone decay test
TE   threshold energy
    tissue-equivalent
    tooth extracted
    total estrogen (excretion)
    tracheo-esophageal
Te   tetanus
TEA   tetraethylammonium
TEAC   tetraethylammonium
      chloride
TED   threshold erythema dose
    thromboembolic disease
TEE   tyrosine ethyl ester
TEF   tracheoesophageal fistula
TEIB   triethylene-
      iminobenzoquinone
TEL   tetraethyl lead
TEM   transmission electron
      microscopy
    triethylenemelamine
TEN   toxic epidermal necrolysis
tenac   tenaculum
TENS   transcutaneous electrical
      nerve stimulator
TEP   thromboendophlebectomy
TEPP   tetraethyl pyrophosphate
TER   three times
    threefold
TES   trimethylaminoethane-sulfonic
      acid
Tet   tetanus
    tetralogy of Fallot
tet   tetanus
TETD   tetraethylthiuram disulfide
TF   tactile fremitus
    tetralogy of Fallot
    thymol flocculation
    tissue-damaging factor
    to follow
    total flow
    transfer factor
    tuberculin filtrate
    tubular fluid
TFA   total fatty acids
TFE   tetrafluoroethylene
TFS   testicular feminization
      syndrome
TG   thioguanine
    thyroglobulin

TG (continued)
    toxic goiter
    triglyceride
TGA   transient global amnesia
    transposition of the great
      arteries
TgAb's thyroglobulin antibodies
TGAR total graft area rejected
TGF   transforming growth factor
TGFA triglyceride fatty acid
TGL   triglyceride
    triglyceride lipase
TGT   thromboplastin generation
      test
    thromboplastin generation
      time
TGV   thoracic gas volume
    transposition of the great
      vessels
TH   thyrohyoid
th   thoracic
THA   total hydroxyapatite
THAM trihydroxymethyl-
      aminomethane
THBR thyroid hormone–binding
      ratio
THC   tetrahydrocannabinol
THDOC tetrahydrodeoxy-
      corticosterone
THE   tetrahydrocortisone
ther   therapy
THF   humoral thymic factor
    tetrahydrocortisol
    tetrahydrofolic acid
THFA tetrahydrofolic acid
THO   titrated water
THP   total hydroxyproline
TI   thoracic index
    time interval
    transverse inlet
    tricuspid incompetence
    tricuspid insufficiency
TIA   transient ischemic attack
TIBC total iron-binding capacity
TIC   trypsin-inhibitory capacity
TID   titrated initial dose
tid   three times a day (*ter in die*)
TIE   transient ischemic episode
TIG   tetanus immunoglobulin
TIMI II thrombolysis in
      myocardial infarction
      (trial)

tin   three times a night (*ter in nocte*)
tinct   tincture
TIS   tumor in situ
TIT   triiodothyronine
TIVC thoracic inferior vena cava
TKA   transketolase activity
TKD   tokodynamometer
TKG   tokodynagraph
TL   time lapse
    time-limited
    total lipids
    tubal ligation
TLA   translumbar aortogram
TLC   tender loving care
    thin-layer chromatography
    total L-chain concentration
    total lung capacity
    total lung compliance
TLD   thermoluminescent dosimeter
    tumor lethal dose
T/LD_{100} minimum dose causing
      death or malformation
      of 100 per cent of fetuses
TLE   thin-layer electrophoresis
TLQ   total living quotient
TLV   threshold limit value
TM   temporomandibular
    time motion
    trademark
    transmetatarsal
    tympanic membrane
T_m maximal tubular excretory
      capacity of the kidneys
TMAb thyroid microsomal
      antibody
TMAS Taylor Manifest Anxiety
      Scale
Tm_G or
TmG   maximal tubular
      reabsorption of glucose
TMJ   temporomandibular joint
TML   tetramethyl lead
TMP   thymidine monophosphate
    trimethoprim
TMTD tetramethylthiuram
      disulfide
TMV   tobacco mosaic virus
TN   total negatives
    true negative
Tn   normal intraocular tension
TND   term normal delivery
TNF   tumor necrosis factor

TNI   total nodal irradiation

TNM   (primary) tumor, (regional lymph) nodes, (remote) metastases – cancer grading system

TNT   trinitrotoluene

TNTC   too numerous to count

TO   original tuberculin
telephone order
tincture of opium

TOA   tubo-ovarian abscess

TOCP   triorthocresyl phosphate

tonoc   tonight

TOPS   Take Off Pounds Sensibly

TOPV   trivalent oral poliovirus vaccine

TORCH   toxoplasmosis, other (syphilis), rubella, cytomegalovirus, herpes simplex

TORP   total ossicular replacement prosthesis

tot prot   total protein

TP   temperature and pressure
thrombocytopenic purpura
total positives
total protein
true positive
tryptophan
tube precipitin
tuberculin precipitation

TPA   tetradecanoylphorbol-13-acetate
tissue plasminogen activator
Treponema pallidum agglutination

TPBF   total pulmonary blood flow

TPCF   *Treponema pallidum* complement-fixation

TPG   transplacental gradient

TPH   transplacental hemorrhage

TPHA   treponemal hemagglutination (test)

TPI   *Treponema pallidum* immobilization
treponemal immobilization test (cardiolipin)
triose phosphate isomerase

TPIA   *Treponema pallidum* immobilization (immune) adherence

TPM   triphenylmethane

TPN   total parenteral nutrition
triphosphopyridine nucleotide

TPNH   reduced triphosphopyridine nucleotide

TPP   thiamine pyrophosphate

TPR   temperature, pulse, and respiration
testosterone production rate
total peripheral resistance
total pulmonary resistance

TPS   tumor polysaccharide substance

TPT   typhoid-paratyphoid (vaccine)

TPTZ   tripyridyltriazine

TPVR   total pulmonary vascular resistance

TQ   tourniquet

TR   tetrazolium reduction
therapeutic radiology
time release
total resistance
total response
tuberculin R (new tuberculin)

tr   tincture
trace

TRA   transaldolase

TRAIDS   transfusion-related AIDS

TRAM   Treatment Rating Assessment Matrix
Treatment Response Assessment Method

TRBF   total renal blood flow

TRC   tanned red cell
total ridge-count

TRF   thymus-replacing factor
thyrotropin-releasing factor

TRH   thyrotropin-releasing hormone

TRI   tetrazolium reduction inhibition

TRIC   trachoma-inclusion conjunctivitis

trit   triturate

TRK   transketolase

TRMC   tetramethylrhodamino-isothiocyanate

tRNA   transfer RNA

TRNG   tetracycline-resistant *Neisseria gonorrhoea*

troch   troche (*trochiscus*)

TRP   tubular reabsorption of phosphate

TRPT   theoretical renal phosphorus
   threshold
TRU   turbidity-reducing unit
TS   test solution
  thoracic surgery
  total solids
  triple strength
  tropical sprue
TSA   technical surgical assistance
  trypticase soy agar
  tumor-specific antigen
T_4SA thyroxine-specific activity
TSB   trypticase soy broth
TSC   technetium sulfur colloid
  thiosemicarbizide
TSD   target skin distance
  Tay-Sachs disease
  theory of signal detectability
TSE   trisodium edetate
TSF   tissue-coding factor
TSH   thyroid-stimulating hormone
TSI   triple sugar iron (agar)
TSP   total serum protein
tsp   teaspoonful
TSPAP   total serum prostatic acid
   phosphatase
TSR   thyroid-to-serum ratio
TSS   toxic shock syndrome
  tropical splenomegaly
  syndrome
TST   tumor skin test
TSTA   tumor-specific
   transplantation antigen
TSY   trypticase soy yeast
TT   tetrazol
  thrombin time
  thymol turbidity
  tooth, treatment of
  total thyroxine
  total time
  transit time
  transthoracic
TTC   triphenyltetrazolium chloride
TTD   tissue tolerance dose
TTH   thyrotropic hormone
  tritiated thymidine
TTI   time-tension index
  tension-time index
TTP   thrombotic thrombocytopenic
  purpura
  thymidine triphosphate
TTR   transacting transcriptional
  regulation

TTS   temporary threshold shift
TTT   tolbutamide tolerance
  test
TU   thiouracil
  toxic unit
  tuberculin unit
tuberc   tuberculosis
TUG   total urinary gonadotropin
TUR   transurethral resection
TURB   transurethral resection of
  the bladder
TURP   transurethral resection of
  the prostate
tus   cough (*tussis*)
TV   tidal volume
  trial visit
  tuberculin volutin
TVC   timed vital capacity
  total volume capacity
  transvaginal cone
TVH   total vaginal hysterectomy
TW   tap water
TWL   transepidermal water loss
Tx   traction
  treatment
Ty   type
  typhoid
TZ   tuberculin zymoplastiche
U   unit
  unknown
  upper
  urology
UA   umbilical artery
  unaggregated
  uric acid
  urine analysis
  uterine aspiration
UAP   uterine arterial pressure
UB   ultimobranchial body
UBBC   unsaturated vitamin
  B_{12}-binding capacity
UBF   uterine blood flow
UBI   ultraviolet blood
  irradiation
UC   ulcerative colitis
  ultracentrifugal
  unchanged
  unclassifiable
  unit clerk
  urea clearance
  urethral catheterization
  uterine contractions
U & C   usual and customary

UCD usual childhood diseases
UCG urinary chorionic
    gonadotropin
UCHD usual childhood diseases
UCO urethral catheter out
UCP urinary coproporphyrin
UCS unconditioned stimulus
    unconscious
UCTS undifferentiated connective
    tissue syndrome
UD urethral discharge
    uroporphyrinogen
    decarboxylase
UDCA ursodeoxycholic acid
UDP uridine diphosphate
UDPG uridine diphosphoglucose
UDPGA uridine diphospho-
    glucuronic acid
UDPGT uridine diphospho-
    glycyronyl transferase
UE upper extremity
UFA unesterified fatty acid
UG urogenital
UGI upper gastrointestinal
UH upper half
UI uroporphyrin isomerase
UIBC unsaturated iron-binding
    capacity
UIF undegraded insulin factor
UIQ upper inner quadrant
UK unknown
    urokinase
UL upper lobe
U & L upper and lower
ULN upper limits of normal
ULQ upper left quadrant
UM uracil mustard
umb umbilicus
UMP uridine monophosphate
UN urea nitrogen
ung ointment (*unguentum*)
uni- one (prefix)
unk or
unkn unknown
UOQ upper outer quadrant
UP upright posture
    ureteropelvic
    uroporphyrin
U/P urine-plasma ratio
UPG uroporphyrinogen
UPI uteroplacental insufficiency
UPJ ureteropelvic junction
UPOR usual place of residence

UPP uterine perfusion pressure
    uvulopalatopharyngoplasty
UR upper respiratory
    utilization review
ur urine
URD upper respiratory disease
URF unidentified reading frame
URI upper respiratory infection
urol urology
URQ upper right quadrant
URTI upper respiratory tract
    infection
US ultrasonic
USN ultrasonic nebulizer
USO unilateral salpingo-
    oophorectomy
USR unheated serum reagin (test)
UTBG unbound thyroxine-binding
    globulin
ut dict as directed (*ut dictum*)
utend to be used (*utendus*)
UTI urinary tract infection
UTP uridine triphosphate
UU urine urobilinogen
UUN urine urea nitrogen
UV ultraviolet
    umbilical vein
    urinary volume
UVJ ureterovesical junction
UVL ultraviolet light
UVP uterine venous pressure
V vein
    vision
    visual acuity
    voice
    volume
V. *Vibrio*
v see (*vide*)
    very
    volt
VA vacuum aspiration
    ventriculoatrial
    vertebral artery
    visual acuity
Va alveolar ventilation
    visual acuity
vag vagina
    vaginal
VALE visual acuity, left eye
VAMP vincristine, amethopterine,
    6-mercaptopurine, and
    prednisone
var variation

VARE   visual acuity, right eye
VASC   Verbal Auditory Screen for
      Children
vasc   vascular
VB   viable birth
    vinblastine
VBL   vinblastine
VBS   veronal-buffered saline
VBS:FBS   veronal-buffered saline-
      fetal bovine serum
VC   acuity of color vision
    vena cava
    ventilatory capacity
    vincristine
    vital capacity
VCA   viral capsid antigen
VCG   vectorcardiogram
    vectorcardiography
VCR   vincristine
VCU   voiding cystourethrogram
VD   vapor density
    venereal disease
VDA   visual discriminatory acuity
VDBR   volume of distribution of
      bilirubin
VDG   venereal disease–gonorrhea
vdg   voiding
VDH   valvular disease of the heart
VDL   visual detection level
VDM   vasodepressor material
VDP   vincristine, daunorubicin,
      prednisone
VDRL   Venereal Disease Research
      Laboratory
VDRS   Verdun Depression Rating
      Scale
VDS   venereal disease–syphilis
VE   visual efficiency
    volumic ejection
V & E   Vinethene and ether
VEE   Venezuelan equine
      encephalomyelitis (virus)
VEM   vasoexcitor material
vent   ventricular
VEP   visual evoked potential
VER   visual evoked response
ves   bladder (*vesica*)
    vesicular
vesic   blister (*vesicula*)
VF   left leg (electrode)
    ventricular fibrillation
    ventricular fluid
    visual field

VF (continued)
    vocal fremitus
VFP   ventricular fluid pressure
VG   ventricular gallop
VH   vaginal hysterectomy
    venous hematocrit
    viral hepatitis
VHD   viral hematodepressive
      disease
VHF   visual half-field
VI   volume index
VIA   virus-inactivating agent
vib   vibration
VIG   vaccinia-immune globulin
vin   wine (*vinum*)
VIP   vasoactive intestinal
      polypeptide
    very important patient
    voluntary interruption of
      pregnancy
VIS   vaginal irrigation smear
VISC   vitreous infusion suction
      cutter
vit   vitamin
    yolk (*vitellus*)
vit cap   vital capacity
VL   left arm (electrode)
VLA   very late appearing antigen
VLDL or
VLDLP   very low density
      lipoprotein
VM   viomycin
    voltmeter
VMA   vanillylmandelic acid
VMR   vasomotor rhinitis
VN   virus-neutralizing
VNS   villonodular synovitis
VO   verbal order
VOD   vision, right eye (*visio oculus*
      dextra)
vol   volume
vos   dissolved in yolk of egg (*vitello*
      ovi solutus)
    vision, left eye (*visio oculus*
      sinister)
VOU   vision, each eye (*visio oculus*
      uterque)
voxel   volume element
VP   vasopressin
    venipuncture
    venous pressure
    Voges-Proskauer (reaction)
    volume-pressure

VP (continued)
  vulnerable period
V & P vagotomy and pyloroplasty
VPB ventricular premature beat
VPC ventricular premature
      contraction
  volume per cent
VPRC volume of packed red cells
V/Q ventilation-perfusion
VR right arm (electrode)
  valve replacement
  vascular resistance
  venous return
  ventilation ratio
  vocal resonance
  vocational rehabilitation
VRBC red blood cell volume
VR & E vocational rehabilitation
      and education
VRI viral respiratory infection
VRP very reliable product (written
      on prescription)
VS vaccination scar
  venisection
  verbal scale (IQ)
  vital signs
  volumetric solution
  without glasses
vs against (*versus*)
  vibration seconds
  voids
VsB bleeding in the arm
      (*venaesectio brachii*)
VSD ventricular septal defect
VSOK vital signs normal
VSS vital signs stable
VSULA vaccination scar upper left
      arm
VSV vesicular stomatitis virus
VSW ventricular stroke work
VT tidal volume
  vacuum tuberculin
  ventricular tachycardia
V & T volume and tension
V_T tidal volume
VTSRS Verdun Target Symptom
      Rating Scale
VV viper venom
vv veins
v/v volume for volume
V/VI grade 5 on a 6-grade basis
VW vessel wall

VW (continued)
  von Willebrand's disease
VZ varicella-zoster
VZV varicella-zoster virus
W water
  Weber (test)
  week
  wehnelt (unit of roentgen ray
      penetrating ability)
  weight
  widowed
  wife
W+ weakly positive
w watt
  with
WAIS Wechsler's Adult Intelligence
      Scale
WAS Wiskott-Aldrich syndrome
WB weight bearing
  Willowbrook (virus)
  whole blood
  whole body
WBC white blood cell
  white blood count
WBF whole-blood folate
WBH whole-blood hematocrit
WBR whole-body radiation
WC water closet
  white cell
  white cell casts
  whooping cough
  work capacity
WC' whole complement
WCC white cell count
WD wallerian degeneration
  well-developed
  well-differentiated
  with disease
WDWN well-developed, well-
      nourished
WE western encephalitis
  western encephalomyelitis
WEE western equine encephalitis
WF Weil-Felix (reaction)
  white female
WFR Weil-Felix reaction
WG water gauge
WH well-healed
WHO World Health Organization
WIA wounded in action
WISC Wechsler's Intelligence Scale
      for Children

WK   Wernicke-Korsakoff
       (syndrome)
wk   weak
       week
WL   waiting list
       wavelength
       work load
WM   white male
       whole milk
WMF   white middle-aged female
WMM   white middle-aged male
WMR   work metabolic rate
WN   well-nourished
WNF   well-nourished female
WNL   within normal limits
WNM   well-nourished male
wo   without
W/O   water in oil
WP   weakly positive
       working point
WPRS   Wittenborn Psychiatric
       Rating Scale
WPW   Wolff-Parkinson-White
       (syndrome)
WR   Wassermann reaction
       weakly reactive
wr   wrist
WRC   washed red cells
WRE   whole ragweed extract
WS   water swallow
ws   watts-second
wt   weight
       white
WV   whispered voice
w/v   weight per volume
X   homeopathic symbol for the
       decimal scale of potencies
       Kienbock's unit of x-ray dosage

X (continued)
       magnification
       removal of
       respirations (anesthesia chart)
       start of anesthesia
       times
XC   excretory cystogram
XDP   xeroderma pigmentosum
XLA   X-linked
       agammaglobulinemia
XM   crossmatch
XP   xeroderma pigmentosum
XR   x-ray
XS   excess
       xiphisternum
XT   exotropia
XU   excretory urogram
Xu   x-unit
Y   year
yd   yard
YF   yellow fever
YO   year old
YOB   year of birth
yr   year
YS   yellow spot (of the retina)
       yolk sac
YST   yolk sac tumor
Z   atomic number
       zero
       Zuckung (contraction)
Z/D   zero defects
ZE   Zollinger-Ellison (syndrome)
Z/G   or
ZIG   zoster immune globulin
ZSR   zeta sedimentation rate
Zz   ginger (*zingiber*)
Z,Z', Z"   increasing degrees of
       contraction

SYMBOLS

Ⓛ	left	⊙	start of operation
Ⓜ	murmur	⊗	end of operation
®	right trademark	□	male

○	female	#	gauge number weight
♂	male		
♀	female	24°	24 hours
*	birth	Δt	time interval
†	death	3 = D	delayed double diffusion (test)
τ	life (time)		
τ½	half-life (time)	606	arsphenamine
p̄	after	914	neoarsphenamine
ā	before	℞	take
c̄	with	6-MP	6-mercaptopurine
s̄	without	³HT	H₃T, tritiated thymidine
?	possible question of questionable	2d	second
~	approximate	2°	secondary
±	not definite	2ndry	secondary
↓	decreased depression	2×	twice
↑	elevation increased	×2	twice
⇑	up	1×	once
→	causes transfer to	°	degree
←	is due to	′	foot
⊖	normal	″	inch
✓c̄	check with	˙ı̈ı	two
φ	none	/	of per
V	systolic blood pressure	: or /	ratio (is to)
∧	diastolic blood pressure	+	positive present
		−	absent negative

$\overline{X}$	average of all X's	$\mu\mu$g	micromicrogram (picogram)
α	alpha particle is proportional to	μM	micromolar
$\neq$	does not equal	μr	microroentgen
$>$	greater than	μsec	microsecond
$<$	less than	μu	microunit
χ^2	chi square (test)	μv	microvolt
σ	1/100 of a second standard deviation	μw	microwatt
℈	scruple	$\mu\gamma$	milligamma (nanogram)
℥	ounce	mμc	millimicrocurie (nanocurie)
f℥	fluid ounce	mμg	millimicrogram (nanogram)
μ	micron	mμ	millimicron
$\mu\mu$	micromicron	ʒ	drachm dram
μc	microcurie	fʒ	fluidrachm fluidram
μEq	microequivalent		
μf	microfarad	$\triangle$	prism diopter
μg	microgram	∞	infinity
μl	microliter	⌒	combined with
$\mu\mu$c	micromicrocurie (picocurie)		

Combining Forms in Medical Terminology*

The following is a list of combining forms encountered frequently in the vocabulary of medicine. A dash or dashes are appended to indicate whether the form usually precedes (as *ante-*) or follows (as *-agra*) the other elements of the compound or usually appears between the other elements (as *-em-*). Following each combining form, the first item of information is the Greek or Latin word, or both a Greek and a Latin word, from which it is derived. Greek words have been transliterated into Roman characters. Latin words are identified by [L.], Greek words by [Gr.]. Information necessary to an understanding of the form appears next in parentheses. Then the meaning or meanings of the words are given, followed where appropriate by reference to a synonymous combining form. Finally, an example is given to illustrate the use of the combining form in a compound English derivative.

a-	*a-* [L.] (*n* is added before words beginning with a vowel) negative prefix. Cf. in-³. *a*metria		beginning with those consonants) to. *ad*renal
		aden-	*adēn* [Gr.] gland. Cf. gland-. *aden*oma
ab-	*ab* [L.] away from. Cf. apo-, *ab*ducent	adip-	*adeps, adipis* [L.] fat. Cf. lip- and stear-. *adip*ocellular
abdomin-	*abdomen, abdominis* [L.] abdomen. *abdomin*oscopy	aer-	*aēr* [Gr.] air. an*aer*obiosis
		aesthe-	See esthe-. *aesthe*sioneurosis
ac-	See ad-, *ac*cretion		
acet-	*acetum* [L.] vinegar. *acet*ometer	af-	See ad-. *af*ferent
		ag-	See ad-. *ag*glutinant
acid-	*acidus* [L.] sour. *acid*uric	-agogue	*agōgos* [Gr.] leading, inducing. galact*agogue*
acou-	*akouō* [Gr.] hear. *acou*esthesia. (Also spelled acu-)	-agra	*agra* [Gr.] catching, seizure. pod*agra*
acr-	*akron* [Gr.] extremity, peak, *acr*omegaly	alb-	*albus* [L.] white. Cf. leuk-. *alb*ocinereous
act-	*ago, actus* [L.] do, drive, act. re*act*ion	alg-	*algos* [Gr.] pain. neur*alg*ia
actin-	*aktis, aktinos* [Gr.] ray, radius. Cf. radi-. *actin*ogenesis	all-	*allos* [Gr.] other, different. *all*ergy
		alve-	*alveus* [L.] trough, channel, cavity. *alve*olar
acu-	See acou-. osteo*acu*sis	amph-	See amphi-. *amph*eclexis
ad-	*ad* [L.] (*d* changes to *c, f, g, p, s,* or *t* before words	amphi-	*amphi* [Gr.] (*i* is dropped before words beginning

---

*Compiled by Lloyd W. Daly, A.M., Ph.D., Litt. D., Allen Memorial Professor of Greek Emeritus, University of Pennsylvania.

amyl- — *amylon* [Gr.] starch. *amylo*synthesis

an-¹ — See ana-. *ana*gogic

an-² — See a-. *an*omalous

ana- — *ana* [Gr.] (final *a* is dropped before words beginning with a vowel) up, positive. *ana*phoresis

ancyl- — See ankyl-. *ancylo*stomiasis

andr- — *anēr, andros* [Gr.] man. gyn*andr*oid

angi- — *angeion* [Gr.] vessel. Cf. vas-. *angi*emphraxis

ankyl- — *unkylos* [Gr.] crooked, looped. *ankylo*dactylia. (Also spelled ancyl-)

ant- — See anti-. *ant*ophthalmic

ante- — *ante* [L.] before. *ante*flexion

anti- — *anti* [Gr.] (*i* is dropped before words beginning with a vowel) against, counter. Cf. contra-. *anti*pyogenic

antr- — *antron* [Gr.] cavern. *antro*dynia

ap-¹ — See apo-. *ap*heter

ap-² — See ad-. *ap*pend

-aph- — *haptō, haph-* [Gr.] touch. dys*aph*ia. (See also hapt-)

apo- — *apo* [Gr.] (*o* is dropped before words beginning with a vowel) away from, detached. Cf. ab-. *apo*physis

arachn- — *arachnē* [Gr.] spider. *arachno*dactyly

arch- — *archē* [Gr.] beginning, origin. *arch*enteron

arter(i)- — *arteria* [L.] windpipe, artery. *arterio*sclerosis, peri*arter*itis

arthr- — *arthron* [Gr.] joint. Cf. articul-. syn*arthro*sis

articul- — *articulus* [L.] joint. Cf. arthr-. dis*articul*ation

as- — See ad-. *as*similation

at- — See ad-. *at*trition

aur- — *auris* [L.] ear. Cf. ot-. *auri*nasal

aux- — *auxō* [Gr.] increase. enter*auxe*

ax- — *axōn* [Gr.] or *axis* [L.] axis. *axo*fugal

axon- — *axōn* [Gr.] axis. *axon*ometer

ba- — *bainō, ba-* [Gr.] go, walk, stand. hypno*ba*tia

bacill- — *bacillus* [L.] small staff, rod. Cf. bacter-. actino*bacill*osis

bacter- — *bactērion* [Gr.] small staff, rod. Cf. bacill-. *bacter*iophage

ball- — *ballō, bol-* [Gr.] throw. *ball*istics. (See also bol-)

bar- — *baros* [Gr.] weight. pedo*bar*ometer

bi-¹ — *bios* [Gr.] life. Cf. vit-. aero*bi*c

bi-² — *bi-* [L.] two (see also di-¹). *bi*lobate

bil- — *bilis* [L.] bile. Cf. chol-. *bil*iary

blast- — *blastos* [Gr.] bud, child, a growing thing in its early stages. Cf. germ-. *blast*oma, zygoto*blast*

blep- — *blepō* [Gr.] look, see. hemia*blep*sia

blephar- — *blepharon* [Gr.] (from *blepō;* see blep-) eyelid. Cf. cili-. *blephar*oncus

bol- — See ball-. em*bol*ism

brachi- — *brachiōn* [Gr.] arm. *brachio*cephalic

brachy- — *brachys* [Gr.] short, *brachy*cephalic

brady- — *bradys* [Gr.] slow. *brady*cardia

brom- — *brōmos* [Gr.] stench. podo*brom*idrosis

bronch- — *bronchos* [Gr.] windpipe. *bronch*oscopy

bry- — *bryō* [Gr.] be full of life. em*bry*onic

bucc- — *bucca* [L.] cheek. disto*bucc*al

cac- — *kakos* [Gr.] bad, abnormal. Cf. mal*cac*odontia. arthro*cac*e. (See also dys-)

calc-¹ — *calx, calcis* [L.] stone (cf. lith-). limestone, lime. *calc*ipexy

calc-² — *calx, calcis* [L.] heel. *calc*aneotibial

calor- — *calor* [L.] heat. Cf. therm-. *calor*imeter

cancr- — *cancer, cancri* [L.] crab, cancer. Cf. carcin-. *cancr*ology (Also spelled chancr-)

capit- — *caput, capitis* [L.] head. Cf. cephal-. de*capit*ator

caps- — *capsa* [L.] (from *capio;* see cept-) container. en*caps*ulation

carbo(n)- — *carbo, carbonis* [L.] coal,

charcoal. *carbo*hydrate,
*carbon*uria

carcin- *karkinos* [Gr.] crab,
cancer. Cf. cancr-.
*carcin*oma

cardi- *kardia* [Gr.] heart.
lipo*cardi*ac

cary- See kary-. *cary*okinesis

cat- See cata-. *cat*hode

cata- *kata* [Gr.] (final *a* is
dropped before words
beginning with a vowel)
down, negative. *cata*batic

caud- *cauda* [L.] tail. *caud*ad

cav- *cavus* [L.] hollow. Cf.
coel-. con*cav*e

cec- *caecus* [L.] blind. Cf.
typhl-. *ceco*pexy

cel-¹ See coel-. amphi*cel*ous

cel-² See -cele. *cel*ectome

-cele *kēlē* [Gr.] tumor, hernia.
gastro*cele*

cell- *cella* [L.] room, cell. Cf.
cyt-. *cell*iferous

cen- *koinos* [Gr.] common.
*cen*esthesia

cent- *centum* [L.] hundred. Cf.
hect-. Indicates fraction
in metric system. [This
exemplifies the custom
in the metric system of
identifying fractions of
units by stems from the
Latin, as centimeter,
decimeter, and
millimeter, and multiples
of units by the similar
stems from the Greek, as
hectometer, decameter,
and kilometer.]
*cent*imeter, *cent*ipede

cente- *kenteō* [Gr.] to puncture.
Cf. punct-. entero*cente*sis

centr- *kentron* [Gr.] or *centrum*
[L.] point, center.
neuro*centr*al

cephal- *kephalē* [Gr.] head. Cf.
capit-. en*cephal*itis

cept- *capio, -cipientis, -ceptus*
[L.] take, receive. re*cept*or

cer- *kēros* [Gr.] or *cera* [L.]
wax. *cer*oplasty, *cer*omel

cerat- See kerat-. a*cerat*osis

cerebr- *cerebrum* [L.] brain.
*cerebr*ospinal

cervic- *cervix, cervicis* [L.] neck.
Cf. trachel-. *cervic*itis

chancr- See cancr-. *chancr*iform

cheil- *cheilos* [Gr.] lip. Cf. labi-.

*cheilo*schisis

cheir- *cheir* [Gr.] hand. Cf. man-.
macro*cheiria* (Also
spelled chir-)

chir- See cheir-. *chiro*megaly

chlor- *chlōros* [Gr.] green.
a*chlor*opsia

chol- *cholē* [Gr.] bile. Cf. bil-.
hepato*chol*angeitis

chondr- *chondros* [Gr.] cartilage.
*chondr*omalacia

chord- *chordē* [Gr.] string, cord.
peri*chord*al

chori- *chorion* [Gr.] protective
fetal membrane.
endo*chori*on

chro- *chrōs* [Gr.] color.
poly*chro*matic

chron- *chronos* [Gr.] time.
syn*chron*ous

chy- *cheō, chy-* [Gr.] pour.
ec*chy*mosis

-cid(e) *caedo, -cisus* [L.] cut, kill.
infanti*cide*, germi*cid*al

cili- *cilium* [L.] eyelid. Cf.
blephar-. super*cili*ary

cine- See kine-. auto*cine*sis

-cipient See cept-. in*cipient*

circum- *circum* [L.] around. Cf.
peri-. *circum*ferential

-cis- *caedo, -cisus* [L.] cut, kill.
ex*cis*ion

clas- *klaō* [Gr.] break. cranio*clast*

clin- *klinō* [Gr.] bend, incline,
make lie down.
*clin*ometer

clus- *claudo, -clusus* [L.] shut.
malo*clus*ion

co- See con-. *co*hesion

cocc- *kokkos* [Gr.] seed, pill.
gono*cocc*us

coel- *koilos* [Gr.] hollow. Cf.
cav-. *coel*enteron (Also
spelled cel-)

col-¹ See colon-. *col*ic

col-² See con-. *col*lapse

colon- *kolon* [Gr.] lower intestine.
*colon*ic

colp- *kolpos* [Gr.] hollow,
vagina. Cf. sin-.
endo*colp*itis

com- See con-. *com*masculation

con- *con-* [L.] (becomes co-
before vowels or *h;* col-
before *l;* com- before *b,*
m, or *p;* cor- before r)
with, together. Cf. syn-.
*con*traction

contra- *contra* [L.] against,

counter. Cf. anti-. *contra*indication

copr- *kopros* [Gr.] dung. Cf. sterco-. *copr*oma

cor-¹ *korē* [Gr.] doll, little image, pupil. iso*cor*ia

cor-² See con-. *cor*rugator

corpor- *corpus, corporis* [L.] body. Cf. somat-. intra*corpor*al

cortic- *cortex, corticis* [L.] bark, rind. *cortic*osterone

cost- *costa* [L.] rib. Cf. pleur-. inter*cost*al

crani *kranion* [Gr.] or *cranium* [L.] skull. peri*crani*um

creat- *kreas, kreato-* [Gr.] meat, flesh. *creat*orrhea

-crescent *cresco, crescentis, cretus* [L.] grow. ex*crescent*

cret- *cerno, cretus* [L.] distinguish. separate off. Cf. crin-. dis*crete*

cret- See -crescent. ac*cret*ion

crin- *krinō* [Gr.] distinguish, separate off. Cf. cret-¹. endo*crin*ology

crur- *crus, cruris* [L.] shin, leg. brachio*crur*al

cry- *kryos* [Gr.] cold. *cry*esthesia

crypt- *kryptō* [Gr.] hide, conceal. *crypt*orchism

cult- *colo, cultus* [L.] tend, cultivate. *cult*ure

cune- *cuneus* [L.] wedge. Cf. sphen-. *cune*iform

cut- *cutis* [L.] skin. Cf. derm(at)-. sub*cut*aneous

cyan- *kyanos* [Gr.] blue. antho*cyan*in

cycl- *kyklos* [Gr.] circle, cycle. *cycl*ophoria

cyst- *kystis* [Gr.] bladder. Cf. vesic-. nephro*cyst*itis

cyt- *kytos* [Gr.] cell. Cf. cell-. plasmo*cyt*oma

dacry- *dakry* [Gr.] tear. *dacry*ocyst

dactyl- *daktylos* [Gr.] finger, toe. Cf. digit-. hexa*dactyl*ism

de- *de* [L.] down from. *de*composition

dec-¹ *deka* [Gr.] ten. Indicates multiple in metric system. Cf. dec-². *dec*agram

dec-² *decem* [L.] ten. Indicates fraction in metric system. Cf. dec-¹. *deci*para, *deci*meter

dendr- *dendron* [Gr.] tree. neuro*dendr*ite

dent- *dens, dentis* [L.] tooth. Cf. odont-. inter*dent*al

derm(at)- *derma, dermatos* [Gr.] skin. Cf. cut-. endo*derm*, *dermat*itis

desm- *desmos* [Gr.] band, ligament. syn*desm*opexy

dextr- *dexter, dextr-* [L.] right-hand. ambi*dextr*ous

di-¹ *di-* [Gr.] two. *di*morphic. (See also bi-²)

di-² See dia-. *di*uresis

di-³ See dis-. *di*vergent

dia- *dia* [Gr.] (*a* is dropped before words beginning with a vowel) through, apart. Cf. per-. *dia*gnosis

didym- *didymos* [Gr.] twin. Cf. gemin-. epi*didym*al

digit- *digitus* [L.] finger, toe. Cf. dactyl-. *digit*igrade

diplo- *diploos* [Gr.] double. *diplo*myelia

dis- *dis-* [L.] (*s* may be dropped before a word beginning with a consonant) apart, away from. *dis*location

disc- *diskos* [Gr.] or *discus* [L.] disk. *disc*oplacenta

dors- *dorsum* [L.] back. ventro*dors*al

drom- *dromos* [Gr.] course. hemo*drom*ometer

-ducent See duct-. ad*ducent*

-duct *duco, ducentis, ductus* [L.] lead, conduct. ovi*duct*

dur- *durus* [L.] hard. Cf. scler-. in*dur*ation

dynam(i)- *dynamis* [Gr.] power, *dynam*oneure, neuro*dynam*ic

dys- *dys-* [Gr.] bad, improper. Cf. mal-. *dys*trophic. (See also cac-)

e- *e* [L.] out from. Cf. ec- and ex-. *e*mission

ec- *ek* [Gr.] out of. Cf. e-. *ec*centric

-ech- *echō* [Gr.] have, hold, be. syn*ech*otomy

ect- *ektos* [Gr.] outside. Cf. extra-. *ect*oplasm

ede- *oideō* [Gr.] swell. *ede*matous

ef- See ex-. *ef*florescent

-elc-	*helkos* [Gr.] sore, ulcer, enter*elc*osis. (See also *helc*-)	fibr-	*fibra* [L.] fiber. Cf. in-¹. chondro*fibr*oma
electr-	*ēlectron* [Gr.] amber. *electr*otherapy	fil-	*filum* [L.] thread. *fili*form
em-	See en-. *em*bolism, *em*pathy, *em*phlysis	fiss-	*findo, fissus* [L.] split. Cf. schis-. *fiss*ion
-em-	*haima* [Gr.] blood. an*em*ia. (See also hem(at)-)	flagell-	*flagellum* [L.] whip. *flagell*ation
en-	*en* [Gr.] (*n* changes to *m* before *b, p* or *ph*) in, on. Cf. in-². *en*celitis	flav-	*flavus* [L.] yellow. Cf. xanth-. ribo*flav*in
		-flect-	*flecto, flexus* [L.] bend, divert. de*flect*ion
end-	*endon* [Gr.] inside. Cf. intra-. *end*angium	-flex-	See -flect-. re*flex*ometer
enter-	*enteron* [Gr.] intestine. dys*enter*y	flu-	*fluo, fluxus* [L.] flow. Cf. rhe-. *flu*id
ep-	See epi-. *ep*axial	flux-	See flu-. af*flux*ion
epi-	*epi* [Gr.] (*i* is dropped before words beginning with a vowel) upon, after, in addition. *epi*glottis	for-	*foris* [L.] door, opening. per*for*ated
		-form	*forma* [L.] shape. Cf.-oid. ossi*form*
		fract-	*frango, fractus* [L.] break. re*fract*ive
erg-	*ergon* [Gr.] work, deed, en*erg*y	front-	*frons, frontis* [L.] forehead, front. naso*front*al
erythr-	*erythros* [Gr.] red. Cf. rub(r)-. *erythr*ochromia	-fug(e)	*fugio* [L.] flee, avoid. vermi*fuge*, centri*fug*al
eso-	*esō* [Gr.] inside. Cf. intra-. *eso*phylactic	funct-	*fungor, functus* [L.] perform, serve, function. mal*funct*ion
esthe-	*aisthanomai, aisthē-* [Gr.] perceive, feel. Cf. sens-. an*esthe*sia	fund-	*fundo, fusus* [L.] pour. in*fund*ibulum
eu-	*eu* [Gr.] good, normal. *eu*pepsia	fus-	See fund-. dif*fus*ible
		galact-	*gala, galactos* [Gr.] milk. Cf. lact-. dys*galact*ia
ex-	*ex* [Gr.] or *ex* [L.] out of. Cf. e-. *ex*cretion	gam-	*gamos* [Gr.] marriage, reproductive union. aga*gam*ont
exo-	*exō* [Gr.] outside. Cf. extra-. *exo*pathic		
extra-	*extra* [L.] outside of, beyond. Cf. ect- and exo-. *extra*cellular	gangli-	*ganglion* [Gr.] swelling, plexus. neuro*gangli*itis
		gastr-	*gastēr, gastros* [Gr.] stomach. cholangio*gastr*ostomy
faci-	*facies* [L.] face. Cf. prosop-. brachio*faci*olingual	gelat-	*gelo, gelatus* [L.] freeze, congeal. *gelat*in
-facient	*facio, facientis, factus, -fectus* [L.] make. Cf. poie-. cale*facient*	gemin-	*geminus* [L.] twin, double. Cf. didym-. quadri*gemin*al
-fact-	See facient-. arte*fact*	gen-	*gignomai, gen-, gon-* [Gr.] become, be produced, originate, or *gennaō* [Gr.] produce. originate, cyto*gen*ic
fasci-	*fascia* [L.] band. *fasci*orrhaphy		
febr-	*febris* [L.] fever. Cf. pyr-. *febr*icide	germ-	*germen, germinis* [L.] bud, a growing thing in its early stages. Cf. blast-. *germ*inal, ovi*germ*
-fect-	See -facient. de*fect*ive		
-ferent	*fero, ferentis, latus* [L.] bear, carry. Cf. phor-. ef*ferent*	gest-	*gero, gerentis, gestus* [L.] bear, carry. con*gest*ion
ferr-	*ferrum* [L.] iron. *ferr*oprotein	gland-	*glans, glandis* [L.] acorn.

Cf. aden-. intra*gland*ular
-glia   *glia* [Gr.] glue. neuro*glia*
gloss-   *glōssa* [Gr.] tongue. Cf.
      lingu-. tricho*gloss*ia
glott-   *glōtta* [Gr.] tongue,
      language. *glott*ic
gluc-   See glyc(y)-
      *gluc*ophenetidin
glutin-   *gluten, glutinis* [L.] glue.
      ag*glutin*ation
glyc(y)-   *glykys* [Gr.] sweet.
      *glyc*emia, *glyc*yrrhizin.
      (Also spelled gluc-)
gnath-   *gnathos* [Gr.] jaw.
      orthog*nath*ous
gno-   *gignōsiō, gnō* [Gr.] know,
      discern. diag*no*sis
gon-   See gen-. anphi*gon*y
grad-   *gradior* [L.] walk, take
      steps. retro*grad*e
-gram   *gramma* [Gr.] letter,
      drawing. cardio*gram*
gran-   *granum* [L.] grain, particle.
      lipo*gran*uloma
graph-   *graphō* [Gr.] scratch, write,
      record. histo*graph*y
grav-   *gravis* [L.] heavy.
      multi*grav*ida
gyn(ec)-   *gynē, gynaikos* [Gr.]
      woman, wife. andro*gyn*y
      *gyne*cologic
gyr-   *gyros* [Gr.] ring, circle.
      *gyr*ospasm
haem(at)-   See hem(at)-.
      *haem*orrhagia,
      *haemat*oxylon
hapt-   *haptō* [Gr.] touch.
      *hapt*ometer
hect-   *hekt-* [Gr.] hundred. Cf.
      cent-. Indicates multiple
      in metric system. *hecto*-
      meter
helc-   *helkos* [Gr.] sore, ulcer.
      *helc*osis
hem(at)-   *haima, haimatos* [Gr.]
      blood. Cf. sanguin-.
      *hem*angioma,
      *hemat*ocyturia. (See also
      -em-)
hemi-   *hēmi-* [Gr.] half. Cf. semi-.
      *hemi*ageusia
hen-   *heis, henos* [Gr.] one. Cf.
      un-. *hen*ogenesis
hepat-   *hēpar, hēpatos* [Gr.] liver.
      gastro*hepat*ic
hept(a)-   *hepta* [Gr.] seven. Cf.
      sept-[2]. *hept*atomic,
      *hept*avalent

hered-   *heres, heredis* [L.] heir.
      *hered*oimmunity
hex-[1]   *hex* [Gr.] six. Cf. sex-.
      *hex*yl-. An *a* is added in
      some combinations
hex-[2]   *echō, hex-* [Gr.] (added to
      s becomes *hex*-) have,
      hold, be. cac*hex*ia
hexa-   See hex-[1]. *hexa*chromic
hidr-   *hidros* [Gr.] sweat.
      hyper*hidr*osis
hist-   *histos* [Gr.] web, tissue.
      *hist*odialysis
hod-   *hodos* [Gr.] road, path,
      *hod*oneuromere. (See
      also od- and -ode[1])
hom-   *homos* [Gr.] common,
      same. *hom*omorphic
horm-   *ormē* [Gr.] impetus,
      impulse. *horm*one
hydat-   *hydōr, hydatos* [Gr.] water.
      *hydat*ism
hydr-   *hydōr, hydr-* [Gr.] water.
      Cf. lymph-. anclor*hydr*ia
hyp-   See hypo-. *hyp*axial
hyper-   *hyper* [Gr.] above, beyond,
      extreme. Cf. super-.
      *hyper*trophy
hypn-   *hypnos* [Gr.] sleep. *hypn*otic
hypo   *hypo* [Gr.] (*o* is dropped
      before words beginning
      with a vowel) under,
      below. Cf. sub-.
      *hypo*metabolism
hyster-   *hystera* [Gr.] womb.
      colpo*hyster*opexy
iatr-   *iatros* [Gr.] physician.
      ped*iatr*ics
idi-   *idios* [Gr.] peculiar,
      separate, distinct.
      *idi*osyncrasy
il-   See in-[2, 3]. *il*linition (in,
      on), *il*legible (negative
      prefix)
ile-   See ili- [ile- is commonly
      used to refer to the
      portion of the intestines
      known as the ileum].
      *ile*ostomy
ili-   *ilium (ileum)* [L.] lower
      abdomen, intestines [ili-
      is commonly used to
      refer to the flaring part
      of the hip bone known
      as the ilium]. *ili*osacral
im-   See in-[2, 3]. *im*mersion (in,
      on). *im*perforation
      (negative prefix)

in-¹   *is, inos* [Gr.] fiber. Cf. fibr-. *in*osteatoma

in-²   *in* [L.] (*n* changes to *l, m,* or *r* before words beginning with those consonants) in, on. Cf. en-. *in*sertion

in-³   *in-* [L.] (*n* changes to *l, m,* or *r* before words beginning with those consonants) negative prefix. Cf. a-. *in*valid

infra-   *infra* [L.] beneath. *infra*orbital

insul-   *insula* [L.] island. *insul*in

inter-   *inter* [L.] among, between. *inter*carpal

intra-   *intra* [L.] inside. Cf. end- and eso-. *intra*venous

ir-   See in-²,³. *ir*radiation (in, on). *ir*reducible (negative prefix)

irid-   *iris, iridos* [Gr.] rainbow, colored circle. kerato*irid*ocyclitis

is-   *isos* [Gr.] equal. *is*otope

ischi-   *ischion* [Gr.] hip, haunch. *ischi*opubic

jact-   *iacio, iactus* [L.] throw. *jact*itation

-ject   *iacio, -iectus* [L.] throw. in*ject*ion

jejun-   *ieiunus* [L.] hungry, not partaking of food. gastro*jejun*ostomy

jug-   *iugum* [L.] yoke. con*jug*ation

junct-   *iungo, iunctus* [L.] yoke, join. con*junct*iva

kary-   *karyon* [Gr.] nut, kernel, nucleus. Cf. nucle-. mega*kary*ocyte. (Also spelled cary-)

kerat-   *keras, keratos* [Gr.] horn. *kerat*olysis. (Also spelled cerat-)

kil-   *chilioi* [Gr.] one thousand. Cf. mill-. Indicates multiple in metric system. *kil*ogram

kine-   *kineō* [Gr.] move. *kine*matograph. (Also spelled cine-)

labi-   *labium* [L.] lip. Cf. cheil-. gingivo*labi*al

lact-   *lac, lactis* [L.] milk. Cf. galact-. gluco*lact*one

lal-   *laleō* [Gr.] talk, babble.

glosso*lal*ia

lapar-   *lapara* [Gr.] flank. *lapar*otomy

laryng-   *larynx, laryngos* [Gr.] windpipe. *laryng*endoscope

lat-   *fero, latus* [L.] bear, carry. See -ferent, trans*lat*ion

later-   *latus, lateris* [L.] side. ventro*later*al

lent-   *lens, lentis* [L.] lentil. Cf. phac-. *lent*iconus

lep-   *lambanō, lēp-* [Gr.] take, seize. cata*lep*tic

leuc-   See leuk-. *leuc*inuria

leuk-   *leukos* [Gr.] white. Cf. alb-. *leuk*orrhea. (Also spelled leuc-)

lien-   *lien* [L.] spleen. Cf. splen-. *lien*ocele

lig-   *ligo* [L.] tie, bind. *lig*ate

lingu-   *lingua* [L.] tongue. Cf. gloss-. sub*lingu*al

lip-   *lipos* [Gr.] fat. Cf. adip-. glyco*lip*in

lith-   *lithos* [Gr.] stone. Cf. calc-¹. nephro*lith*otomy

loc-   *locus* [L.] place. Cf. top-. *loc*omotion

log-   *legō, log-* [Gr.] speak, give an account. *log*orrhea, embryo*log*y

lumb-   *lumbus* [L.] loin. dorso*lumb*ar

lute-   *luteus* [L.] yellow. Cf. xanth-. *lute*oma

ly-   *lyō* [Gr.] loose, dissolve. Cf. solut-. kerato*ly*sis

lymph-   *lympha* [Gr.] water. Cf. hydr-. *lymph*adenosis

macr-   *makros* [Gr.] long, large. *macr*omyeloblast

mal-   *malus* [L.] bad, abnormal. Cf. cac- and dys-. *mal*function

malac-   *malakos* [Gr.] soft. osteo*malac*ia

mamm-   *mamma* [L.] breast. Cf. mast-. sub*mamm*ary

man-   *manus* [L.] hand. Cf. cheir-. *man*iphalanx

mani-   *mania* [Gr.] mental aberration. *mani*graphy, klepto*mani*a

mast-   *mastos* [Gr.] breast. Cf. mamm-. hyper*mast*ia

medi-   *medius* [L.] middle. Cf. mes-. *medi*frontal

mega- *megas* [Gr.] great, large. Also indicates multiple (1,000,000) in metric system. *mega*colon, *mega*dyne. (See also megal-)

megal- *megas, megalou* [Gr.] great, large. acro*megaly*

mel- *melos* [Gr.] limb, member. sym*melia*

melan- *melas, melanos* [Gr.] black. hippo*melanin*

men- *mēn* [Gr.] month. dys*men*orrhea

mening- *mēninx, mēningos* [Gr.] membrane. encephalo*mening*itis

ment- *mens, mentis* [L.] mind. Cf. phren-, psych- and thym-. de*mentia*

mer- *meros* [Gr.] part. poly*meric*

mes- *mesos* [Gr.] middle. Cf. medi-. *mes*oderm

met- See meta-. *met*allergy

meta- *meta* [Gr.] (*a* is dropped before words beginning with a vowel) after, beyond, accompanying. *meta*carpal

metr-[1] *metron* [Gr.] measure. stereo*metry*

metr-[2] *metra* [Gr.] womb. endo*metr*itis

micr- *mikros* [Gr.] small. photo*micr*ograph

mill- *mille* [L.] one thousand. Cf. kil-. Indicates fraction in metric system. *mill*igram, *milli*pede

miss- See -mittent. intro*mission*

-mittent *mitto, mittentis, missus* [L.] send. inter*mittent*

mne- *mimnērcō, mnē-* [Gr.] remember. pseudo*mnesia*

mon- *monos* [Gr.] only, sole. *mon*oplegia

morph- *morphē* [Gr.] form, shape. poly*morph*onuclear

mot- *moveo, motus* [L.] move. vaso*motor*

my- *mys, myos* [Gr.] muscle. inoleio*myoma*

-myces *mykēs, mykētos* [Gr.] fungus. myelo*myces*

myc(et)- See -myces. asco*mycetes*, strepto*mycin*

myel- *myelos* [Gr.] marrow. polio*myelitis*

myx- *myxa* [Gr.] mucus. *myx*edema

narc- *narkē* [Gr.] numbness. topo*narc*osis

nas- *nasus* [L.] nose. Cf. rhin-. palato*nasal*

ne- *neos* [Gr.] new, young. *ne*ocyte

necr- *nekros* [Gr.] corpse. *necr*ocytosis

nephr- *nephros* [Gr.] kidney. Cf. ren-. para*nephr*ic

neur- *neuron* [Gr.] nerve. esthesio*neure*

nod- *nodus* [L.] knot. *nod*osity

nom- *nomos* [Gr.] (from *nemō* deal out, distribute) law, custom. taxo*nomy*

non- *nona* [L.] nine. *non*acosane

nos- *nosos* [Gr.] disease. *nos*ology

nucle- *nucleus* [L.] (from *nux, nucis* nut) kernel. Cf. kary-. *nucle*ide

nutri- *nutrio* [L.] nourish. mal*nutri*tion

ob- *ob* [L.] (*b* changes to *c* before words beginning with that consonant) against, toward, etc. *ob*tuse

oc- See ob-. *oc*clude

ocul- *oculus* [L.] eye. Cf. ophthalm-. *ocul*omotor

-od- See -ode[1]. peri*od*ic

-ode[1] *hodos* [Gr.] road, path. cath*ode*. (See also hod-)

-ode[2] See -oid. nemat*ode*

odont- *odous, odontos* [Gr.] tooth. Cf. dent-. ortho*dont*ia

-odyn- *odynē* [Gr.] pain, distress. gastro*dyn*ia

-oid *eidos* [Gr.] form. Cf. -form. hy*oid*

-ol See ole-. cholester*ol*

ole- *oleum* [L.] oil. *ole*oresin

olig- *oligos* [Gr.] few, small. *olig*ospermia

omphal- *omphalos* [Gr.] navel. peri*omphal*ic

onc- *onkos* [Gr.] bulk, mass. hemat*onc*ometry

onych- *onyx, onychos* [Gr.] claw, nail. an*onych*ia

oo- *ōon* [Gr.] egg. Cf. ov-. peri*oo*thecitis

op- *horaō, op-* [Gr.] see. erythr*op*sia

ophthalm- *ophthalmos* [Gr.] eye. Cf.

ocul-. ex*ophthalm*ic

*per*nasal

or-   *os, oris* [L.] mouth. Cf. *stom*(at)-. intra*oral*

peri-   *peri* [Gr.] around. Cf. circum-. *peri*phery

orb-   *orbis* [L.] circle. sub*orb*ital

pet-   *peto* [L.] seek, tend toward. centri*pet*al

orchi-   *orchis* [Gr.] testicle. Cf. test-. *orchi*opathy

pex-   *pēgnumi. pēg-* [Gr.] (added to *s* becomes *pēx*) fix, make fast. hepato*pex*y

organ-   *organon* [Gr.] implement, instrument. *organ*oleptic

orth-   *orthos* [Gr.] straight, right, normal. *orth*opedics

pha-   *phēmi, pha-* [Gr.] say, speak. dys*pha*sia

oss-   *os, ossis* [L.] bone. Cf. ost(e)-. *oss*iphone

phac-   *phakos* [Gr.] lentil, lens. Cf. lent-. *phac*osclerosis. (Also spelled phak-)

ost(e)-   *osteon* [Gr.] bone. Cf. oss-. en*ost*osis, *oste*anaphysis

phag-   *phagein* [Gr.] eat. lipo*phag*ic

ot-   *ous, ōtos* [Gr.] ear. Cf. aur-. par*ot*id

phak-   See phac-. *phak*itis

ov-   *ovum* [L.] egg. Cf. oo-. syn*ov*ia

phan-   See phen-. dia*phan*oscopy

pharmac-   *pharmakon* [Gr.] drug. *pharmac*ognosy

oxy-   *oxys* [Gr.] sharp. *oxy*cephalic

pharyng-   *pharynx, pharyng-* [Gr.] throat. glosso*pharyng*eal

pachy(n)-   *pachynō* [Gr.] thicken. *pachy*derma, myo*pachyn*sis

phen-   *phainō, phan-* [Gr.] show, be seen. phos*phen*e

pher-   *pherō, phor-* [Gr.] bear, support. peri*pher*y

pag-   *pēgnymi, pag-* [Gr.] fix, make fast. thoraco*pag*us

phil-   *phileō* [Gr.] like, have affinity for. eosino*phil*ia

par-[1]   *pario* [L.] bear, give birth to. primi*par*ous

phleb-   *phleps, phlebos* [Gr.] vein. peri*phleb*itis

par-[2]   See para-. *par*epigastric

phleg-   *phlogō, phlog-* [Gr.] burn, inflame. adeno*phleg*mon

para-   *para* [Gr.] (final *a* is dropped before words beginning with a vowel) beside, beyond. *para*mastoid

phlog-   See phleg-. anti*phlog*istic

phob-   *phobos* [Gr.] fear, dread. claustro*phob*ia

part-   *pario, partus* [L.] bear, give birth to. *part*urition

phon-   *phōne* [Gr.] sound. echo*phon*y

path-   *pathos* [Gr.] that which one undergoes, sickness. psycho*path*ic

phor-   See pher-. Cf. -ferent. exo*phor*ia

pec-   *pēgnymi, pēg-* [Gr.] (*pēk-* before *t*) fix, make fast. sym*pec*tothiene. (See also pex-)

phos-   See phot-. *phos*phorus

phot-   *phōs, phōtos* [Gr.] light. *phot*erythrous

ped-   *pais, paidos* [Gr.] child. ortho*ped*ic

phrag-   *phrassō, phrag-* [Gr.] fence, wall off, stop up. Cf. sept-[1]. dia*phrag*m

pell-   *pellis* [L.] skin, hide. *pell*agra

phrax-   *phrassō, phrag-* [Gr.] (added to *s* becomes *phrax-*) fence, wall off, stop up. em*phrax*is

-pellent   *pello, pellentis, pulsus* [L.] drive. re*pellent*

pen-   *penomai* [Gr.] need, lack. erythrocyto*pen*ia

phren-   *phrēn* [Gr.] mind, midriff. Cf. ment-. meta*phren*ia, meta*phren*on

pend-   *pendeo* [L.] hang down. ap*pend*ix

phthi-   *phthinō* [Gr.] decay, waste away. *phthi*sis

pent(a)-   *pente* [Gr.] five. Cf. quinque-. *pent*ose, *penta*ploid

phy-   *phyō* [Gr.] beget, bring forth, produce, be by nature. noso*phy*te

peps-   *peptō, peps-* [Gr.] digest. brady*peps*ia

phyl-   *phylon* [Gr.] tribe, kind. *phyl*ogeny

pept-   *peptō* [Gr.] digest. dys*pept*ic

-phyll   *phyllon* [Gr.] leaf.

per-   *per* [L.] through. Cf. dia-.

xantho*phyll*

phylac-   *phylax* [Gr.] guard.
pro*phylac*tic

phys(a)-   *physaō* [Gr.] blow, inflate.
*physo*cele, *physa*lis

physe-   *physaō, physē-* [Gr.] blow, inflate. em*physe*ma

pil-   *pilus* [L.] hair. e*pil*ation

pituit-   *pituita* [L.] phlegm, rheum. *pituit*ous

placent-   *placenta* [L.] (from *plakous* [Gr.]) cake. extra*placent*al

plas-   *plassō* [Gr.] mold, shape. cine*plas*ty

platy-   *platys* [Gr.] broad, flat. *platy*rrhine

pleg-   *plēssō* [Gr.] strike. di*pleg*ia

plet-   *pleo, -pletus* [L.] fill. de*plet*ion

pleur-   *pleura* [Gr.] rib, side. Cf. cost-. peri*pleur*al

plex-   *plēssō, plēg-* (added to *s* becomes *plēx-*) strike. apo*plex*y

plic-   *plico* [L.] fold. com*plic*ation

pne-   *pneuma, pneumatos* [Gr.] breathing. traumato*pne*a

pneum(at)-   *pneuma, pneumatos* [Gr.] breath, air. *pneum*odynamics, *pneumat*othorax

pneumo(n)-   *pneumōn* [Gr.] lung. Cf. pulmo(n)-. *pneumo*centesis, *pneumono*tomy

pod-   *pous, podos* [Gr.] foot. *pod*iatry

poie-   *poieō* [Gr.] make, produce. Cf. -facient. sarco*poie*tic

pol-   *polos* [Gr.] axis of a sphere. peri*pol*ar

poly-   *polys* [Gr.] much, many. *poly*spermia

pont-   *pons, pontis* [L.] bridge. *ponto*cerebellar

por-¹   *poros* [Gr.] passage. myelo*por*e

por-²   *poros* [Gr.] callus. *por*ocele

posit-   *pono, positus* [L.] put, place. re*posit*or

post-   *post* [L.] after, behind in time or place. *post*natal, *post*oral

pre-   *prae* [L.] before in time or place. *pre*natal, *pre*vesical

press-   *premo, pressus* [L.] press. *press*oreceptive

pro-   *pro* [Gr.] or *pro* [L.] before in time or place. *pro*gamous, *pro*cheilon, *pro*lapse

proct-   *prōktos* [Gr.] anus. entero*proct*ia

prosop-   *prosōpon* [Gr.] face. Cf. faci-. di*prosop*us

pseud-   *pseudēs* [Gr.] false. *pseudo*paraplegia

psych-   *psychē* [Gr.] soul, mind. Cf. ment-. *psycho*somatic

pto-   *piptō, ptō-* [Gr.] fall. nephro*pto*sis

pub-   *pubes* and *puber, puberis* [L.] adult. ischio*pub*ic. (See also puber-)

puber-   *puber* [L.] adult. *puber*ty

pulmo(n)-   *pulmo, pulmonis* [L.] lung. Cf. pneumo(n)-. *pulmo*lith, cardio*pulmon*ary

puls-   *pello, pellentis, pulsus* [L.] drive. pro*puls*ion

punct-   *pungo, punctus* [L.] prick, pierce. Cf. cente-. *punct*iform

pur-   *pus, puris* [L.] pus. Cf. py-. sup*pur*ation

py-   *pyon* [Gr.] pus. Cf. pur-. nephro*py*osis

pyel-   *pyelos* [Gr.] trough, basin, pelvis. nephro*pyel*itis

pyl-   *pylē* [Gr.] door, orifice. *pyl*ephlebitis

pyr-   *pyr* [Gr.] fire. Cf. febr-. galacto*pyr*a

quadr-   *quadr-* [L.] four. Cf. tetra-. *quadr*igeminal

quinque-   *quinque* [L.] five. Cf. pent(a)-. *quinque*cuspid

rachi-   *rachis* [Gr.] spine. Cf. spin-. encephalo*rachi*dian

radi-   *radius* [L.] ray. Cf. actin-. ir*radi*ation

re-   *re-* [L.] back, again. *re*traction

ren-   *renes* [L.] kidneys. Cf. nephr-. ad*ren*al

ret-   *rete* [L.] net. *ret*othelium

retro-   *retro* [L.] backward. *retro*deviation

rhag-   *rhēgnymi, rhag-* [Gr.] break, burst. hemor*rhag*ic

rhaph-   *rhaphē* [Gr.] suture. gastror*rhaph*y

rhe-
: *rhaphē* [Gr.] flow. Cf. flu-. diar*rhe*al

rhex-
: *rhēgnymi, rhēg-* [Gr.] (added to *s* becomes *rhēx*) break, burst. metror*rhex*is

rhin-
: *rhis, rhinos* [Gr.] nose. Cf. nas-. basi*rhin*al

rot-
: *rota* [L.] wheel. *rot*ator

rub(r)-
: *ruber, rubri* [L.] red. Cf. erythr-. bili*rub*in, *rub*rospinal

salping-
: *salpinx, salpingos* [Gr.] tube, trumpet. *salping*itis

sanguin-
: *sanguis, sanguinis* [L.] blood. Cf. hem(at)-. *sanguin*eous

sarc-
: *sarx, sarkos* [Gr.] flesh. *sarc*oma

schis-
: *schizō, schid-* [Gr.] (before *t* or added to *s* becomes *schis-*) split. Cf. fiss-. *schis*torachis, rachi*schis*is

scler-
: *sklēros* [Gr.] hard. Cf. dur-. *scler*osis

scop-
: *skopeō* [Gr.] look at, observe. endo*scop*e

sect-
: *seco, sectus* [L.] cut. Cf. tom-. *sect*ile

semi-
: *semi* [L.] half. Cf. hemi-. *semi*flexion

sens-
: *sentio, sensus* [L.] perceive, feel. Cf. esthe-. *sens*ory

sep-
: *sepō* [Gr.] rot, decay. *sep*sis

sept-¹
: *saepio, saeptus* [L.] fence, wall off, stop up. Cf. phrag-. naso*sept*al

sept-²
: *septem* [L.] seven. Cf. hept(a)-. *sept*an

ser-
: *serum* [L.] whey, watery substance. *ser*osynovitis

sex-
: *sex* [L.] six. Cf. hex-¹. *sex*digitate

sial-
: *sialon* [Gr.] saliva. poly*sial*ia

sin-
: *sinus* [L.] hollow, fold. Cf. colp-. *sin*obronchitis

sit-
: *sitos* [Gr.] food. para*sit*ic

solut-
: *solvo, solventis, solutus* [L.] loose, dissolve, set free. Cf. ly-. dis*solut*ion

-solvent
: See solut-. dis*solvent*

somat-
: *sōma, somatōs* [Gr.] body. Cf. corpor-. psycho*somat*ic

-some
: See somat-. dictyo*some*

spas-
: *spaō, spas-* [Gr.] draw, pull. *spas*m, *spas*tic

spectr-
: *spectrum* [L.] appearance, what is seen. micro*spectr*oscope

sperm(at)-
: *sperma, spermatos* [Gr.] seed. *sperma*crasia, *spermat*ozoon

spers-
: *spargo, -spersus* [L.] scatter. di*spers*ion

sphen-
: *sphēn* [Gr.] wedge. Cf. cune-. *sphen*oid

spher-
: *sphaira* [Gr.] ball. hemi*spher*e

sphygm-
: *sphygmos* [Gr.] pulsation. *sphygm*omanometer

spin-
: *spina* [L.] spine. Cf. rachi-. cerebro*spin*al

spirat-
: *spiro, spiratus* [L.] breathe. in*spirat*ory

splanchn-
: *splanchna* [Gr.] entrails, viscera. neuro*splanchn*ic

splen-
: *splēn* [Gr.] spleen. Cf. lien-. *splen*omegaly

spor-
: *sporos* [Gr.] seed. *spor*ophyte, zygo*spor*e

squam-
: *squama* [L.] scale. de*squam*ation

sta-
: *histēmi, sta-* [Gr.] make stand, stop. genesi*sta*sis

stal-
: *stellō, stal-* [Gr.] send. peri*stal*sis. (See also stol-)

staphyl-
: *staphylē* [Gr.] bunch of grapes, uvula. *staphyl*ococcus, *staphyl*ectomy

stear-
: *stear, steatos* [Gr.] fat. Cf. adip-. *stear*odermia

steat-
: See stear-. *steat*opygous

sten-
: *stenos* [Gr.] narrow, compressed. *sten*ocardia

ster-
: *stereos* [Gr.] solid. chole*ster*ol

sterc-
: *stercus* [L.] dung. Cf. copr-. *sterc*oporphyrin

sthen-
: *sthenos* [Gr.] strength. a*sthen*ia

stol-
: *stellō, stol-* [Gr.] send. dia*stol*e

stom(at)-
: *stoma, stomatos* [Gr.] mouth, orifice. Cf. or-. ana*stom*osis, *stomat*ogastric

strep(h)-
: *strephō, strep-* (before t) [Gr.] twist. Cf. tors-. *streph*osymbolia, *strep*tomycin. (See also stroph-)

strict-
: *stringo, stringentis, strictus* [L.] draw tight,

	compress, cause pain.		quadr-. *tetra*genous
	con*stric*tion	the-	*tithēmi, thē-* [Gr.] put,
-stringent	See strict-. a*stringent*		place. syn*the*sis
stroph-	*strephō, stroph-* [Gr.] twist.	thec-	*thēkē* [Gr.] repository,
	ana*stroph*ic. (See also		case. *thec*ostegnosis
	strep(h)-)	thel-	*thēlē* [Gr.] teat, nipple.
struct-	*struo, structus* [L.] pile up		*thel*erethism
	(against). ob*struc*tion	therap-	*therapeia* [Gr.] treatment.
sub-	*sub* [L.] (*b* changes to *f* or		hydro*therap*y
	p before words	therm-	*thermē* [Gr.] heat. Cf.
	beginning with those		calor-. dia*therm*y
	consonants) under,	thi-	*theion* [Gr.] sulfur.
	below. Cf. hypo-.		*thi*ogenic
	*sub*lumbar	thorac-	*thōrax, thōrakos* [Gr.]
suf-	See sub-. *suf*fusion		chest. *thorac*oplasty
sup-	See sub-. *sup*pository	thromb-	*thrombos* [Gr.] lump, clot.
super-	*super* [L.] above, beyond,		*thromb*openia
	extreme. Cf. hyper-.	thym-	*thymos* [Gr.] spirit. Cf.
	*super*motility		ment-. dys*thym*ia
sy-	See syn-. *sy*stole	thyr-	*thyreos* [Gr.] shield
syl-	See syn-. *syl*lepsiology		(shaped like a door
sym-	See syn-. *sym*biosis,		*thyra*). *thyr*oid
	*sym*metry, *sym*pathetic,	tme-	*temnō, tmē-* [Gr.] cut.
	*sym*physis		axono*tme*sis
syn-	*syn* [Gr.] (*n* disappears	toc-	*tokos* [Gr.] childbirth.
	before *s*, changes to *l*		dys*toc*ia
	before *l*, and changes to	tom-	*temnō, tom-* [Gr.] cut. Cf.
	m before *b, m, p,* and		sect-. appendec*tom*y
	ph) with, together. Cf.	ton-	*teino, ton-* [Gr.] stretch,
	con-. myo*syn*izesis		put under tension. Cf.
ta-	See ton-. ec*ta*sis		tens-. peri*ton*eum
tac-	*tassō, tag-* [Gr.] (*tak-*	top-	*topos* [Gr.] place. Cf. loc-.
	before *t*) order, arrange.		*top*esthesia
	a*tac*tic	tors-	*torqueo, torsus* [L.] twist.
tact-	*tango, tactus* [L.] touch.		Cf. strep-. ec*tors*ion
	con*tact*	tox-	*toxicon* [Gr.] (from *toxon*
tax-	*tassō, tag-* [Gr.] (added to		bow) arrow poison,
	s becomes *tax-*) order,		poison. *tox*emia
	arrange. a*tax*ia	trache-	*tracheia* [Gr.] windpipe.
tect-	See teg-. pro*tect*ive		*trache*otomy
teg-	*tego, tectus* [L.] cover.	trachel-	*trachēlos* [Gr.] neck. Cf.
	in*teg*ument		cervic-. *trachel*opexy
tel-	*telos* [Gr.] end. *tel*osynapsis	tract-	*traho, tractus* [L.] draw,
tele-	*tēle* [Gr.] at a distance.		drag. pro*tract*ion
	*tele*ceptor	traumat-	*trauma, traumatos* [Gr.]
tempor-	*tempus, temporis* [L.] time,		wound. *traumat*ic
	timely or fatal spot,	tri-	*treis, tria* [Gr.] or *tri-* [L.]
	temple. *tempor*omalar		three. *tri*gonid
ten(ont)-	*tenon, tenontos* [Gr.] (from	trich-	*thrix, trichos* [Gr.] hair.
	teinō stretch) tight		*trich*oid
	stretched band.	trip-	*tribō* [Gr.] rub. en*trip*sis
	*teno*dynia, *teno*nitis,	trop-	*trepō, trop-* [Gr.] turn,
	*tenont*agra		react. sito*trop*ism
tens-	*tendo, tensus* [L.] stretch.	troph-	*trepō, troph-* [Gr.] nurture.
	Cf. ton-. ex*tens*or		a*troph*y
test-	*testis* [L.] testicle. Cf.	tuber-	*tuber* [L.] swelling, node.
	orchi-. *test*itis		*tuber*cle
tetra-	*tetra-* [Gr.] four. Cf.	typ-	*typos* [Gr.] (from *typto*

strike) type. a*typ*ical

typh-	*typhos* [Gr.] fog, stupor. adeno*typh*us	vit-	cyst-. *vesic*ovaginal *vita* [L.] life. Cf. bi-[1]. devi*tal*ize
typhl-	*typhlos* [Gr.] blind. Cf. cec-. *typhl*ectasis	vuls-	*vello, vulsus* [L.] pull, twitch. convul*sion*
un-	*unus* [L.] one. Cf. hen-. *un*ioval	xanth-	*xanthos* [Gr.] yellow, blond. Cf. flav- and lute-. *xanth*ophyll
ur-	*ouron* [Gr.] urine. poly*ur*ia		
vacc-	*vacca* [L.] cow. *vacc*ine	-yl-	*hylē* [Gr.] substance. cacod*yl*
vagin-	*vagina* [L.] sheath. in*vagin*ated	zo-	*zoē* [Gr.] life, *zōon* [Gr.] animal. micro*zo*aria
vas-	*vas* [L.] vessel. Cf. angi-. *vas*cular	zyg-	*zygon* [Gr.] yoke, union. *zyg*odactyly
vers-	See vert-. in*vers*ion	zym-	*zymē* [Gr.] ferment. en*zym*e
vert-	*verto, versus* [L.] turn. di*vert*iculum		
vesic-	*vesica* [L.] bladder. Cf.		

(Courtesy of Miller, B. F., and Keane, C. B.: Encyclopedia and Dictionary of Medicine, Nursing, and Allied Health, 4th ed. Philadelphia, W. B. Saunders Company, 1987.)

Rules for Forming Plurals

The rules for commonly forming plurals of medical terms are as follows:

1. For words ending in **is**, drop the **is** and add **es**:

   Examples:

Singular	Plural
anastomosis	anastomoses
metastasis	metastases
epiphysis	epiphyses
prosthesis	prostheses

2. For words ending in **um**, drop the **um** and add **a**:

   Examples:

Singular	Plural
bacterium	bacteria
diverticulum	diverticula
ovum	ova

3. For words ending in **us**, drop the **us** and add **i**:

   Examples:

Singular	Plural
calculus	calculi
bronchus	bronchi
nucleus	nuclei

   Some exceptions to this rule include viruses and sinuses.

4. For words ending in **a**, retain the **a** and add **e**:

   Examples:

Singular	Plural
vertebra	vertebrae
bursa	bursae
bulla	bullae

5. For words ending in **ix** and **ex**, drop the **ix** or **ex** and add **ices**:

Examples:

Singular	Plural
ape*x*	ap*ices*
var*ix*	var*ices*

6. For words ending in **on**, drop the **on** and add **a**:

Examples:

Singular	Plural
gangli*on*	gangli*a*
spermatozo*on*	spermatozo*a*

(Courtesy of Chabner, D.-E.: Language of Medicine, 3rd ed. Philadelphia, W. B. Saunders Company, 1985, p. i.)

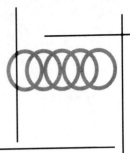

Appendix

Table of Elements

NAME	SYMBOL	AT. NO.	AT. WT.*
Actinium . . . . Ac	89	227.028
Aluminum . . . . Al	13	26.982
Americium. . . . . Am	95	(243)
Antimony . . . . Sb	51	121.75
Argon. . . . . Ar	18	39.948
Arsenic. . . . . As	33	74.922
Astatine . . . . At	85	(210)
Barium . . . . Ba	56	137.33
Berkelium . . . . Bk	97	(247)
Beryllium . . . . Be	4	9.012
Bismuth . . . . Bi	83	208.980
Boron. . . . . B	5	10.811
Bromine . . . . Br	35	79.904
Cadmium. . . . . Cd	48	112.41
Calcium. . . . . Ca	20	40.08
Californium . . . . Cf	98	(251)
Carbon C	6	12.011
Cerium . . . . Ce	58	140.12
Cesium . . . . Cs	55	132.905
Chlorine Cl	17	35.453
Chromium. . . . . Cr	24	51.996
Cobalt. . . . . Co	27	58.933
Copper . . . . Cu	29	63.546
Curium. . . . . Cm	96	(247)
Dysprosium . . . . Dy	66	162.50
Einsteinium . . . . Es	99	(252)
Element 106.	106	(263)
Erbium. . . . . Er	68	167.26
Europium . . . . Eu	63	151.96
Fermium. . . . . Fm	100	(257)
Fluorine . . . . F	9	18.998
Francium. . . . . Fr	87	(223)
Gadolinium . . . . Gd	64	157.25
Gallium. . . . . Ga	31	69.72
Germanium . . . . Ge	32	72.59
Gold. . . . . Au	79	196.967
Hafnium . . . . Hf	72	178.49
Hahnium. . . . . Ha	105	(261)
Helium . . . . He	2	4.003
Holmium. . . . . Ho	67	164.930
Hydrogen . . . . H	1	1.008
Indium . . . . In	49	114.82
Iodine. I	53	126.905
Iridium . . . . Ir	77	192.22
Iron . . . . Fe	26	55.847
Krypton . . . . Kr	36	83.80
Lanthanum . . . . La	57	138.906
Lawrencium. . . . . Lw	103	(260)
Lead. . . . . Pb	82	207.2
Lithium. Li	3	6.941
Lutetium. . . . . Lu	71	174.967
Magnesium . . . . Mg	12	24.312
Manganese. . . . . Mn	25	54.938

*Atomic weights are corrected to conform with the 1979 values of the International Union of Pure and Applied Chemistry, expressed to the fourth decimal point, rounded off to the nearest thousandth. The numbers in parentheses are the mass numbers of the most stable or most common isotope.

NAME	SYMBOL	AT. NO.	AT. WT.*
Mendelevium	Md	101	(258)
Mercury	Hg	80	200.59
Molybdenum	Mo	42	95.94
Neodymium	Nd	60	144.24
Neon	Ne	10	20.179
Neptunium	Np	93	237.0482
Nickel	Ni	28	58.69
Niobium	Nb	41	92.906
Nitrogen	N	7	14.007
Nobelium	No	102	259
Osmium	Os	76	190.2
Oxygen	O	8	15.999
Palladium	Pd	46	106.42
Phosphorus	P	15	30.974
Platinum	Pt	78	195.08
Plutonium	Pu	94	(244)
Polonium	Po	84	(209)
Potassium	K	19	39.098
Praseodymium	Pr	59	140.908
Promethium	Pm	61	(145)
Protactinium	Pa	91	231.036
Radium	Ra	88	226.025
Radon	Rn	86	(222)
Rhenium	Re	75	186.207
Rhodium	Rh	45	102.906
Rubidium	Rb	37	85.468
Ruthenium	Ru	44	101.07
Rutherfordium	Rf	104	(261)
Samarium	Sm	62	150.36
Scandium	Sc	21	44.956
Selenium	Se	34	78.96
Silicon	Si	14	28.086
Silver	Ag	47	107.868
Sodium	Na	11	22.990
Strontium	Sr	38	87.62
Sulfur	S	16	32.064
Tantalum	Ta	73	180.948
Technetium	Tc	43	(98)
Tellurium	Te	52	127.60
Terbium	Tb	65	158.925
Thallium	Tl	81	204.383
Thorium	Th	90	232.038
Thulium	Tm	69	168.934
Tin	Sn	50	118.60
Titanium	Ti	22	47.88
Tungsten	W	74	183.85
Uranium	U	92	238.029
Vanadium	V	23	50.942
Xenon	Xe	54	131.29
Ytterbium	Yb	70	173.04
Yttrium	Y	39	88.906
Zinc	Zn	30	65.38
Zirconium	Zr	40	91.22

TABLES OF WEIGHTS AND MEASURES*

MEASURES OF MASS

AVOIRDUPOIS WEIGHT

Grains	Drams	Ounces	Pounds	Metric Equivalents, Grams
1	0.0366	0.0023	0.00014	0.0647989
27.34	1	0.0625	0.0039	1.772
437.5	16	1	0.0625	28.350
7000	256	16	1	453.5924277

APOTHECARIES' WEIGHT

Grains	Scruples (℈)	Drams (ʒ)	Ounces (℥)	Pounds (lb.)	Metric Equivalents, Grams
1	0.05	0.0167	0.0021	0.00017	0.0647989
20	1	0.333	0.042	0.0035	1.296
60	3	1	0.125	0.0104	3.888
480	24	8	1	0.0833	31.103
5760	288	96	12	1	373.24177

TROY WEIGHT

Grains	Pennyweights	Ounces	Pounds	Metric Equivalents, Grams
1	0.042	0.002	0.00017	0.0647989
24	1	0.05	0.0042	1.555
480	20	1	0.083	31.103
5760	240	12	1	373.24177

METRIC WEIGHT

Micro-gram	Milli-gram	Centi-gram	Deci-gram	Gram	Deka-gram	Hecto-gram	Kilo-gram	Equivalents Avoir-dupois	Apothe-caries'
1	—	—	—	—	—	—	—	0.000015 grains	
10^3	1	—	—	—	—	—	—	0.015432 grains	
10^4	10	1	—	—	—	—	—	0.154323 grains	
10^5	10^2	10	1	—	—	—	—	1.543235 grains	
10^6	10^3	10^2	10	1	—	—	—	15.432356 grains	
10^7	10^4	10^3	10^2	10	1	—	—	5.6438 dr.	7.7162 scr.
10^8	10^5	10^4	10^3	10^2	10	1	—	3.527 oz.	3.215 oz.
10^9	10^6	10^5	10^4	10^3	10^2	10	1	2.2046 lb.	2.6792 lb.
10^{12}	10^9	10^8	10^7	10^6	10^5	10^4	10^3	2204.6223 lb.	2679.2285 lb.

MEASURES OF CAPACITY

APOTHECARIES' (WINE) MEASURE

Minims	Fluid Drams	Fluid Ounces	Gills	Pints	Quarts	Gal-lons	Equivalents Cubic Inches	Milli-liters	Cubic Centi-meters
1	0.0166	0.002	0.0005	0.00013	—	—	0.00376	0.06161	0.06161
60	1	0.125	0.0312	0.0078	0.0039	—	0.22558	3.6967	3.6967
480	8	1	0.25	0.0625	0.0312	0.0078	1.80468	29.5737	29.5737
1920	32	4	1	0.25	0.125	0.0312	7.21875	118.2948	118.2948
7680	128	16	4	1	0.5	0.125	28.875	473.179	473.179
15360	256	32	8	2	1	0.25	57.75	946.358	946.358
61440	1024	128	32	8	4	1	231	3785.434	3785.434

*Courtesy of Miller, B. F. and Keane, C. B.: Encyclopedia and Dictionary of Medicine, Nursing, and Allied Health, 4th ed. Philadelphia, W. B. Saunders Company, 1987.

Metric Measure

Microliter	Milliliter	Centiliter	Deciliter	Liter	Dekaliter	Hectoliter	Kiloliter	Myrialiter	Equivalents (Apothecaries' Fluid)
1	—	—	—	—	—	—	—	—	0.01623108 minim
10^3	1	—	—	—	—	—	—	—	16.23 minims
10^4	10	1	—	—	—	—	—	—	2.7 fluid drams
10^5	10^2	10	1	—	—	—	—	—	3.38 fluid ounces
10^6	10^3	10^2	10	1	—	—	—	—	2.11 pints
10^7	10^4	10^3	10^2	10	1	—	—	—	2.64 gallons
10^8	10^5	10^4	10^3	10^2	10	1	—	—	26.418 gallons
10^9	10^6	10^5	10^4	10^3	10^2	10	1	—	264.18 gallons
10^{10}	10^7	10^6	10^5	10^4	10^3	10^2	10	1	2641.8 gallons

1 liter = 2.113363738 pints (Apothecaries').

Measures of Length

Metric Measure

Micrometer	Millimeter	Centimeter	Decimeter	Meter	Dekameter	Hectometer	Kilometer	Myriameter	Megameter	Equivalents
1	0.001	10^{-4}	—	—	—	—	—	—	—	0.000039 inch
10^3	1	10^{-1}	—	—	—	—	—	—	—	0.03937 inch
10^4	10	1	—	—	—	—	—	—	—	0.3937 inch
10^5	10^2	10	1	—	—	—	—	—	—	3.937 inches
10^6	10^3	10^2	10	1	—	—	—	—	—	39.37 inches
10^7	10^4	10^3	10^2	10	1	—	—	—	—	10.9361 yards
10^8	10^5	10^4	10^3	10^2	10	1	—	—	—	109.3612 yards
10^9	10^6	10^5	10^4	10^3	10^2	10	1	—	—	1093.6121 yards
10^{10}	10^7	10^6	10^5	10^4	10^3	10^2	10	1	—	6.2137 miles
10^{12}	10^9	10^8	10^7	10^6	10^5	10^4	10^3	10^2	1	621.37 miles

CONVERSION TABLES

AVOIRDUPOIS–METRIC WEIGHT

Ounces	Grams	
1/16	1.772	
1/8	3.544	
1/4	7.088	
1/2	14.175	
1	28.350	
2	56.699	
3	85.049	
4	113.398	
5	141.748	
6	170.097	
7	198.447	
8	226.796	
9	255.146	
10	283.495	
11	311.845	
12	340.194	
13	368.544	
14	396.893	
15	425.243	
16 (1 lb.)	453.59	
Pounds		
1 (16 oz.)	453.59	
2	907.18	
3	1360.78	(1.36 kg.)
4	1814.37	(1.81 kg.)
5	2267.96	(2.27 kg.)
6	2721.55	(2.72 kg.)
7	3175.15	(3.18 kg.)
8	3628.74	(3.63 kg.)
9	4082.33	(4.08 kg.)
10	4535.92	(4.54 kg.)

METRIC–AVOIRDUPOIS WEIGHT

Grams	Ounces
0.001 (1 mg.)	0.000035274
1	0.035274
1000 (1 kg.)	35.274 (2.2046 lb.)

APOTHECARIES'–METRIC LIQUID MEASURE

Minims	Milliliters
1	0.06
2	0.12
3	0.19
4	0.25
5	0.31
10	0.62
15	0.92
20	1.23
25	1.54
30	1.85
35	2.16
40	2.46
45	2.77
50	3.08
55	3.39
60 (1 fl. dr.)	3.70
Fluid Drams	
1	3.70
2	7.39
3	11.09
4	14.79
5	18.48
6	22.18
7	25.88
8 (1 fl. oz.)	29.57
Fluid Ounces	
1	29.57
2	59.15
3	88.72
4	118.29
5	147.87
6	177.44
7	207.01
8	236.58
9	266.16
10	295.73
11	325.30
12	354.88
13	384.45
14	414.02
15	443.59
16 (1 pt.)	473.18
32 (1 qt.)	946.36
128 (1 gal.)	3785.43

METRIC–APOTHECARIES' LIQUID MEASURE

Milliliters	Minims	Milliliters	Fluid Drams	Milliliters	Fluid Ounces
1	16.231	5	1.35	30	1.01
2	32.5	10	2.71	40	1.35
3	48.7	15	4.06	50	1.69
4	64.9	20	5.4	500	16.91
5	81.1	25	6.76	1000 (1 L.)	33.815
		30	7.1		

Apothecaries'–Metric Weight		Metric–Apothecaries' Weight	
Grains	Grams	Milli-grams	Grains
1/150	0.0004	1	0.015432
1/120	0.0005	2	0.030864
1/100	0.0006	3	0.046296
1/80	0.0008	4	0.061728
1/64	0.001	5	0.077160
1/50	0.0013	6	0.092592
1/48	0.0014	7	0.108024
1/30	0.0022	8	0.123456
1/25	0.0026	9	0.138888
1/16	0.004	10	0.154320
1/12	0.005	15	0.231480
1/10	0.006	20	0.308640
1/9	0.007	25	0.385800
1/8	0.008	30	0.462960
1/7	0.009	35	0.540120
1/6	0.01	40	0.617280
1/5	0.013	45	0.694440
1/4	0.016	50	0.771600
1/3	0.02	100	1.543240
1/2	0.032		
1	0.065	Grams	
1 1/2	0.097 (0.1)	0.1	1.5432
2	0.125	0.2	3.0864
3	0.20	0.3	4.6296
4	0.25	0.4	6.1728
5	0.30	0.5	7.7160
6	0.40	0.6	9.2592
7	0.45	0.7	10.8024
8	0.50	0.8	12.3456
9	0.60	0.9	13.8888
10	0.65	1.0	15.4320
15	1.00	1.5	23.1480
20 (1ℨ)	1.30	2.0	30.8640
30	2.00	2.5	38.5800
Scruples		3.0	46.2960
1	1.296 (1.3)	3.5	54.0120
2	2.592 (2.6)	4.0	61.728
3 (1ℨ)	3.888 (3.9)	4.5	69.444
Drams		5.0	77.162
1	3.888	10.0	154.324
2	7.776		
3	11.664		Equivalents
4	15.552	10	2.572 drams
5	19.440	15	3.858 drams
6	23.328	20	5.144 drams
7	27.216	25	6.430 drams
8 (1 ℥)	31.103	30	7.716 drams
Ounces		40	1.286 oz.
1	31.103	45	1.447 oz.
2	62.207	50	1.607 oz.
3	93.310	100	3.215 oz.
4	124.414	200	6.430 oz.
5	155.517	300	9.644 oz.
6	186.621	400	12.859
7	217.724	500	1.34 lb.
8	248.828	600	1.61 lb.
9	279.931	700	1.88 lb.
10	311.035	800	2.14 lb.
11	342.138	900	2.41 lb.
12 (1 lb.)	373.242	1000	2.68 lb.

Metric	LIQUID MEASURE *Approx. Apothecary Equivalents*	Metric		LIQUID MEASURE *Approx. Apothecary Equivalents*
1000 ml.	1 quart	3	ml.	45 minims
750 ml.	1 1/2 pints	2	ml.	30 minims
500 ml.	1 pint	1	ml.	15 minims
250 ml.	8 fluid ounces	0.75	ml.	12 minims
200 ml.	7 fluid ounces	0.6	ml.	10 minims
100 ml.	3 1/2 fluid ounces	0.5	ml.	8 minims
50 ml.	1 3/4 fluid ounces	0.3	ml.	5 minims
30 ml.	1 fluid ounce	0.25	ml.	4 minims
15 ml.	4 fluid drams	0.2	ml.	3 minims
10 ml.	2 1/2 fluid drams	0.1	ml.	1 1/2 minims
8 ml.	2 fluid drams	0.06	ml.	1 minim
5 ml.	1 1/4 fluid drams	0.05	ml.	3/4 minim
4 ml.	1 fluid dram	0.03	ml.	1/2 minim

Metric		WEIGHT *Approx. Apothecary Equivalents*	Metric		WEIGHT *Approx. Apothecary Equivalents*
30	gm.	1 ounce	30	mg.	1/2 grain
15	gm.	4 drams	25	mg.	3/8 grain
10	gm.	2 1/2 drams	20	mg.	1/3 grain
7.5	gm.	2 drams	15	mg.	1/4 grain
6	gm.	90 grains	12	mg.	1/5 grain
5	gm.	75 grains	10	mg.	1/6 grain
4	gm.	60 grains (1 dram)	8	mg.	1/8 grain
3	gm.	45 grains	6	mg.	1/10 grain
2	gm.	30 grains (1/2 dram)	5	mg.	1/12 grain
1.5	gm.	22 grains	4	mg.	1/15 grain
1	gm.	15 grains	3	mg.	1/20 grain
0.75	gm.	12 grains	2	mg.	1/30 grain
0.6	gm.	10 grains	1.5	mg.	1/40 grain
0.5	gm.	7 1/2 grains	1.2	mg.	1/50 grain
0.4	gm.	6 grains	1	mg.	1/60 grain
0.3	gm.	5 grains	0.8	mg.	1/80 grain
0.25	gm.	4 grains	0.6	mg.	1/100 grain
0.2	gm.	3 grains	0.5	mg.	1/120 grain
0.15	gm.	2 1/2 grains	0.4	mg.	1/150 grain
0.12	gm.	2 grains	0.3	mg.	1/200 grain
0.1	gm.	1 1/2 grains	0.25	mg.	1/250 grain
75	mg.	1 1/4 grains	0.2	mg.	1/300 grain
60	mg.	1 grains	0.15	mg.	1/400 grain
50	mg.	3/4 grains	0.12	mg.	1/500 grain
40	mg.	2/3 grain	0.1	mg.	1/600 grain

Note: A milliliter (ml.) is the approximate equivalent of a cubic centimeter (cc.).
Adopted by the latest Pharmacopeia, National Formulary, and New and Nonofficial Remedies, and approved by the Federal Food and Drug Administration.